Oral Cancer - Current Concepts and Future Perspectives

Edited by Gokul Sridharan

Published in London, United Kingdom

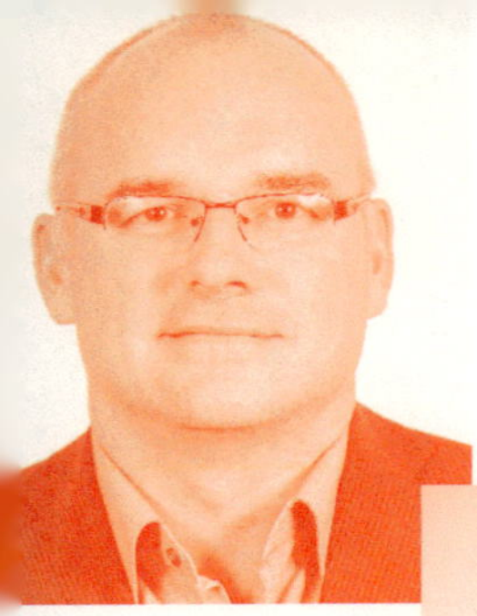
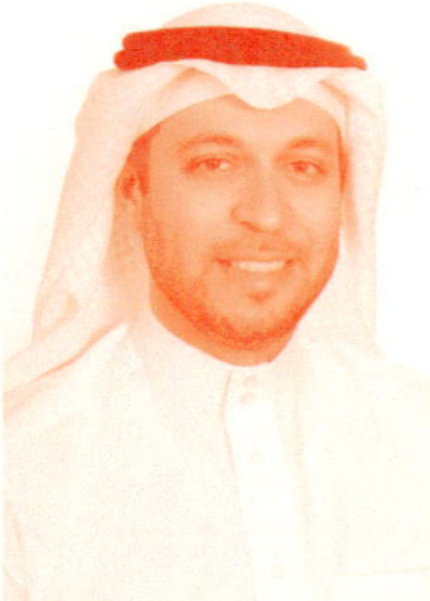
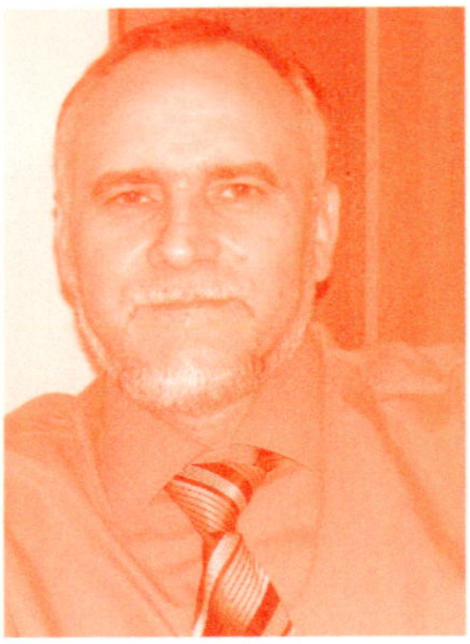
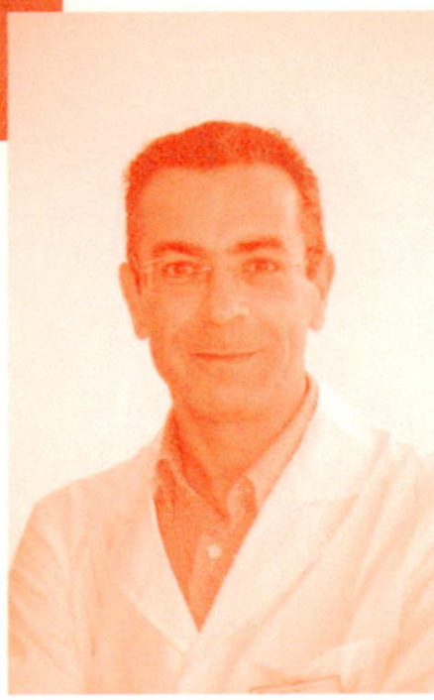
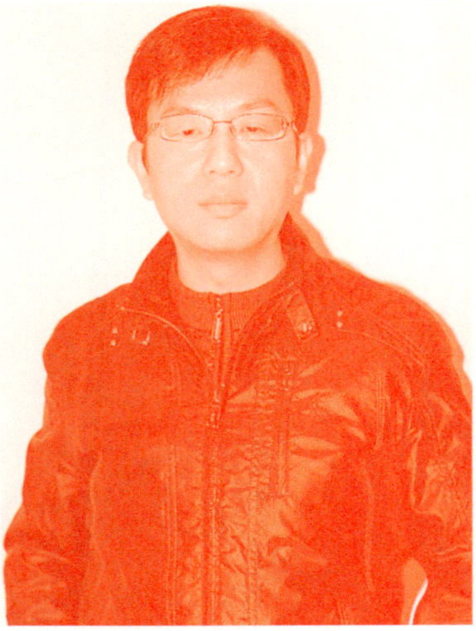
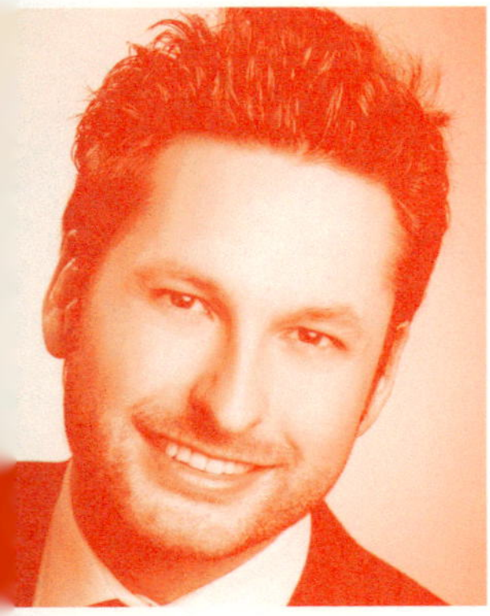
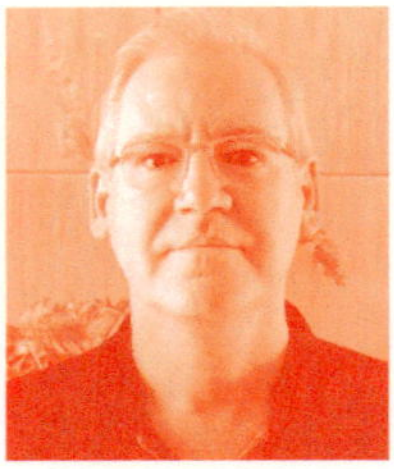

IntechOpen

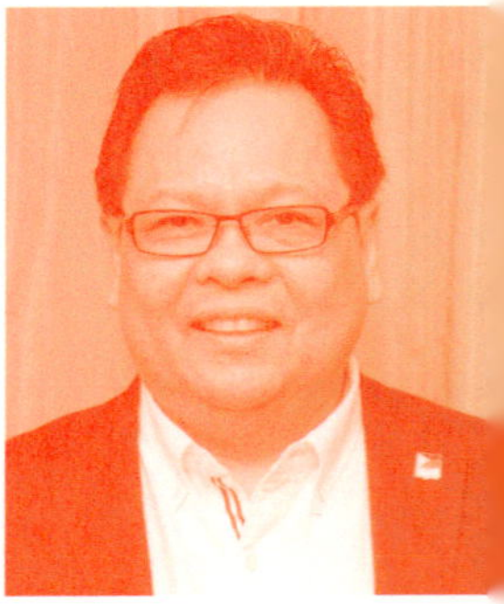
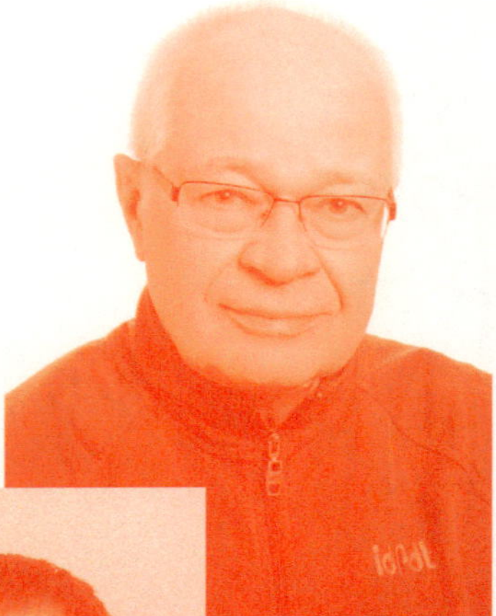
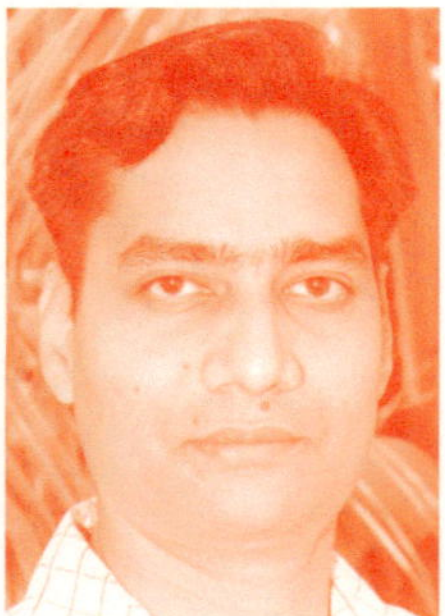
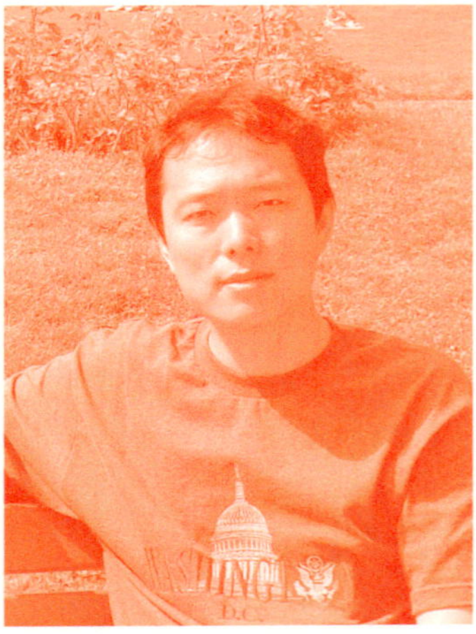
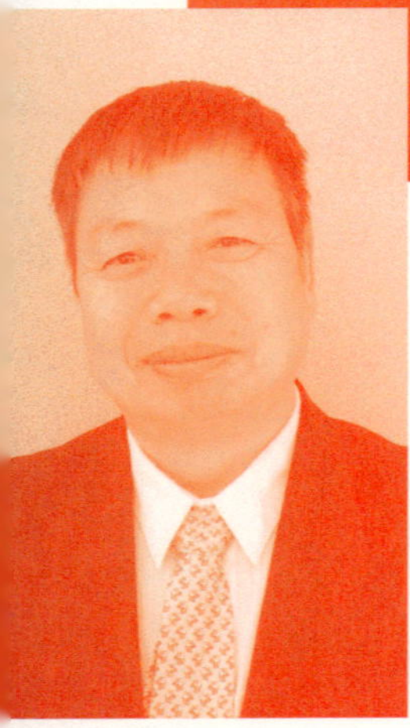
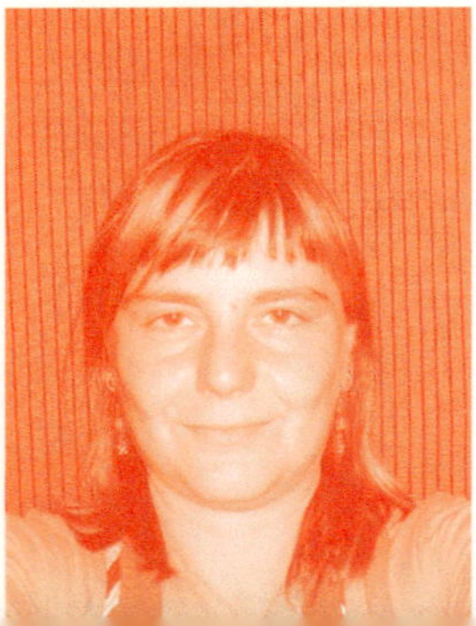

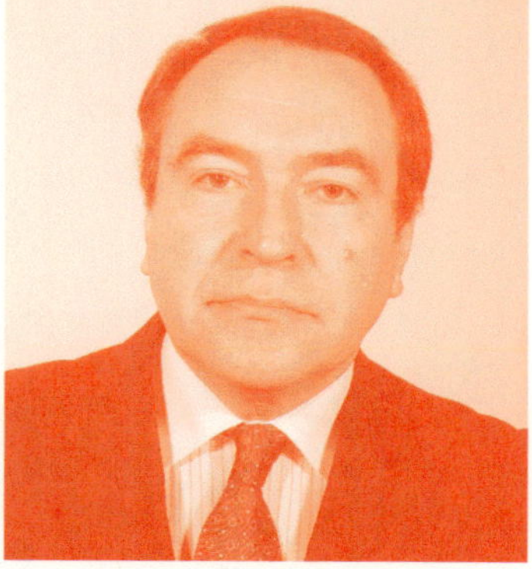
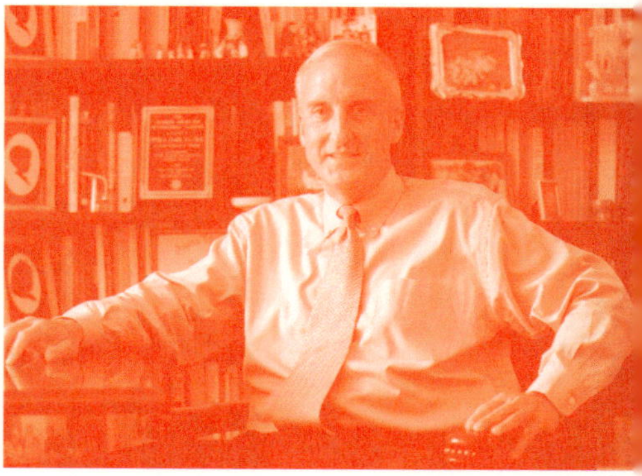
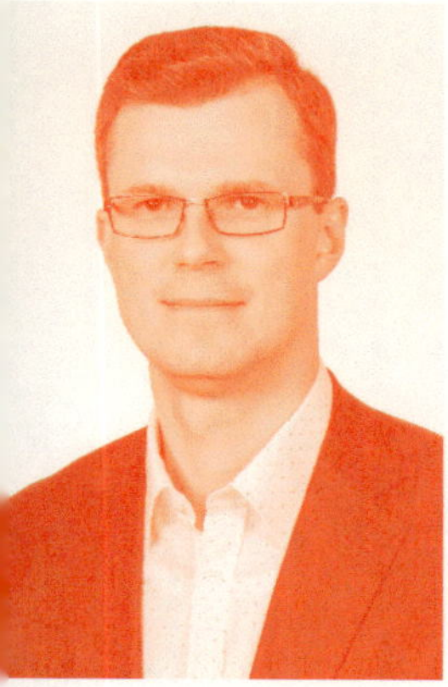
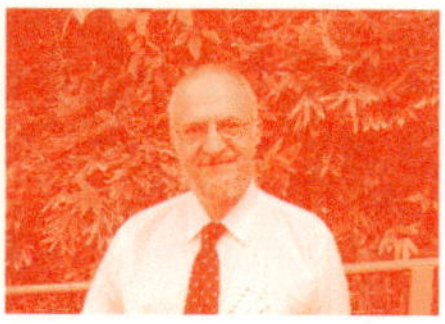
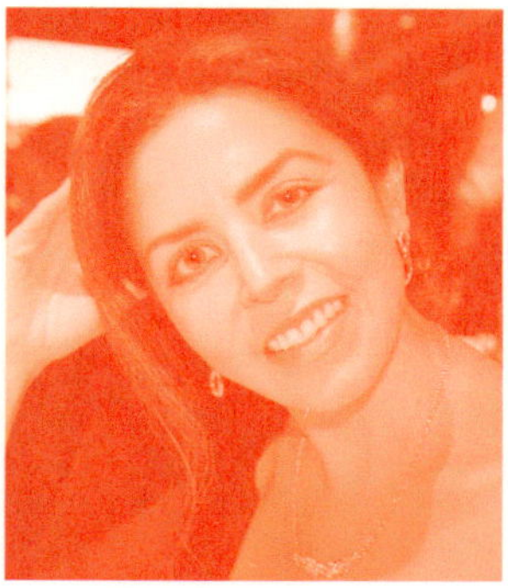

Supporting open minds since 2005

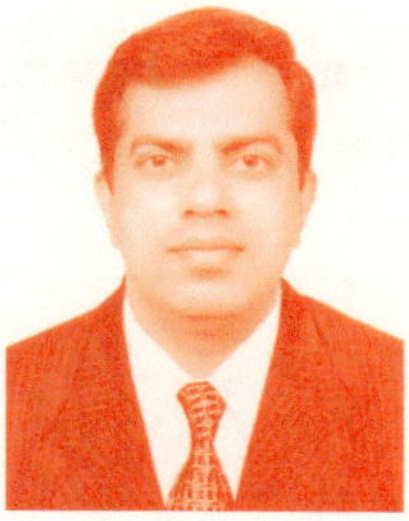
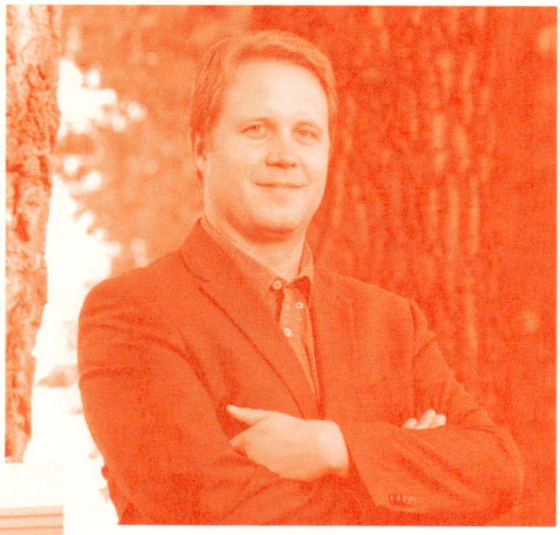
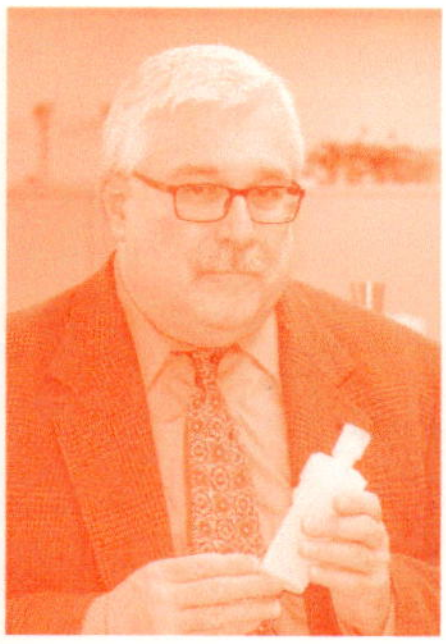
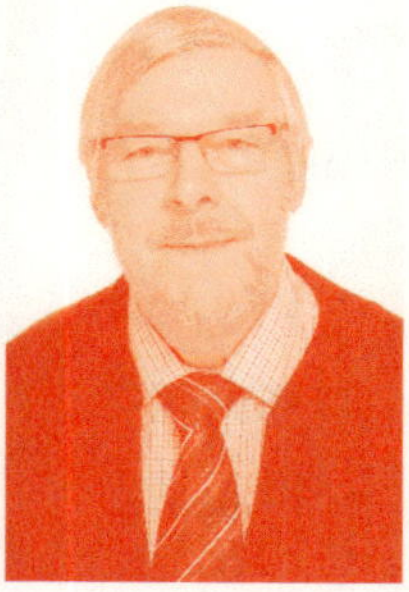
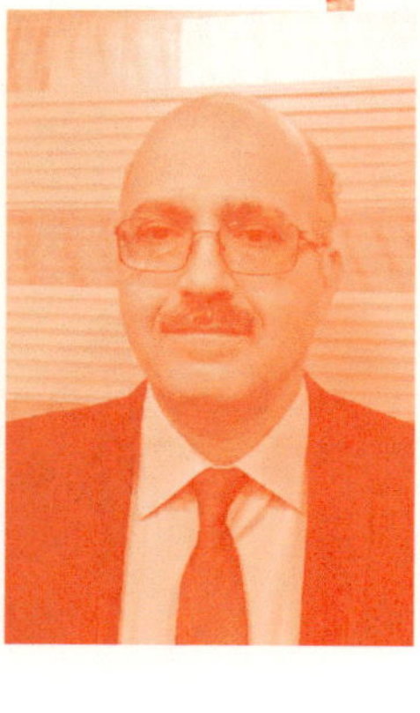
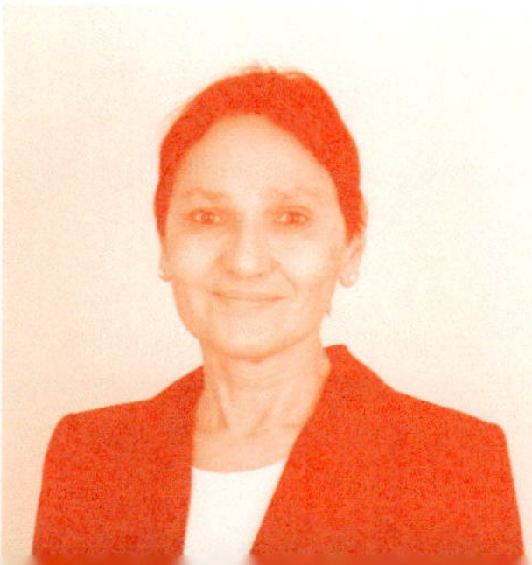
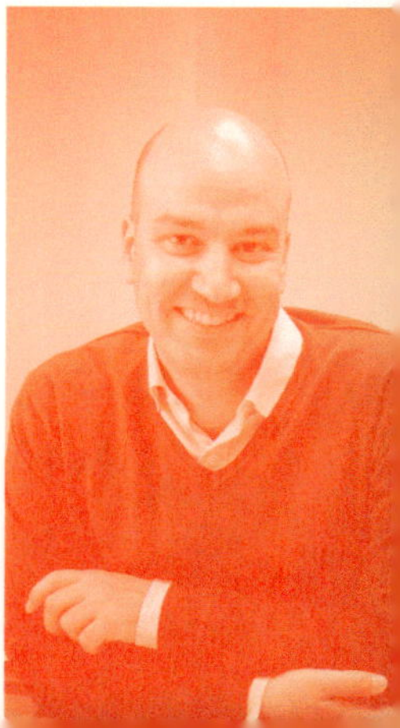

Oral Cancer - Current Concepts and Future Perspectives
http://dx.doi.org/10.5772/intechopen.94817
Edited by Gokul Sridharan

Contributors
Haly Holmes, Henry Ademola Adeola, Dada Oluwaseyi Oluwaseyi Temilola, A.S. Kirthi Koushik, Ram Charith Alva, Jai Kumar Chaurasia, Neelkamal Kapoor, Deepa Patil, Rakesh Nagaraju, Muzib Abdul-Razak, Rajith Mendis, ali khani jeihooni, Fatemeh Jafari, Sankha Bhattacharya

Notice
Statements and opinions expressed in the chapters are these of the individual contributors and not necessarily those of the editors or publisher. No responsibility is accepted for the accuracy of information contained in the published chapters. The publisher assumes no responsibility for any damage or injury to persons or property arising out of the use of any materials, instructions, methods or ideas contained in the book.

First published in London, United Kingdom, 2022 by IntechOpen
IntechOpen is the global imprint of INTECHOPEN LIMITED, registered in England and Wales, registration number: 11086078, 5 Princes Gate Court, London, SW7 2QJ, United Kingdom
Printed in Croatia

British Library Cataloguing-in-Publication Data
A catalogue record for this book is available from the British Library

Additional hard and PDF copies can be obtained from orders@intechopen.com

Oral Cancer - Current Concepts and Future Perspectives
Edited by Gokul Sridharan
p. cm.
Print ISBN 978-1-78984-670-6
Online ISBN 978-1-78984-671-3
eBook (PDF) ISBN 978-1-78985-657-6

For EU product safety concerns:
IN TECH d.o.o., Prolaz Marije Krucifikse Kozulić 3, 51000 Rijeka, Croatia, info@intechopen.com or visit our website at intechopen.com.

Meet the editor

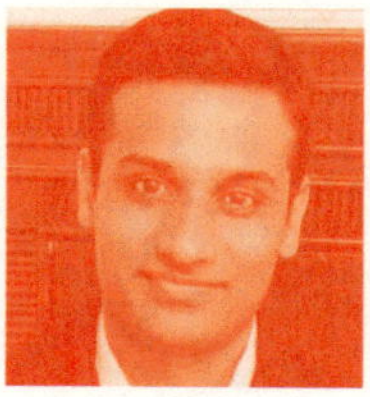

Dr. Gokul Sridharan is currently an associate professor in the Department of Oral Pathology and Microbiology, YMT Dental College and Hospital, Navi Mumbai. He obtained a Ph.D. for his work titled "Salivary and serum metabolomics in oral leukoplakia and oral squamous cell carcinoma." His fields of interest include oral pre-cancer, oral cancer, salivary diagnostics, metabolomics, and oxidative stress. He has several scientific publications to his credit and actively contributes as a peer reviewer to numerous journals. He is an active member of the editorial boards of several journals of repute. Dr. Sridharan has undergone training and is a qualified diploma holder in medical law and ethics and is also certified in tobacco cessation and control.

Contents

Preface

"The eyes do not see what the mind does not know"

Oral cancer is one of the most prevalent diseases worldwide with significant morbidity and mortality. The term oral cancer is a broad term that encompasses malignancies arising from epithelial tissue, mesenchymal tissue, and salivary glands, to name a few. The complex nature of the head and neck anatomy poses a challenge to understanding the various malignancies occurring in this region and thereby challenging the treatment and prognosis of oral cancer. Despite technological advancements in the 21st century, there is little improvement in the five-year survival rate and post-treatment quality of life. The current challenge facing the scientific community and clinicians is to identify means of early diagnosis of oral cancers and improve treatment strategies that could minimize morbidity and improve quality of life. Various technologies for early diagnosis such as identification of tumor biomarkers in saliva and serum, determination of genetic and molecular alterations to predict the behavior and prognosis of oral cancer, implementation of newer methods of treatment such as targeted therapy, immunotherapy, and so on, are being evaluated constantly for clinical application in oral cancer therapy. This book reviews the current concepts concerning oral cancer as well as future perspectives directed towards understanding scientific advancements in managing the disease.

Chapters cover a range of topics such as prevention of oral cancer in hookah smokers, novel methods of cancer detection using salivary exosomes, the role of cytopathology in intra-oral salivary gland tumors, precision personalized medicine, sentinel lymph node biopsy, and applications of various molecular markers and radiotherapy in the treatment of oral cancers.

Dr. Gokul Sridharan MDS, PhD, PGD (Medical Law and Ethics)
Associate Professor,
Department of Oral Pathology and Microbiology,
Dr. G. D. Pol Foundation YMT Dental College and Hospital,
Mumbai, India

Chapter 1

Oral Cancer: Epidemiology, Prevention, Early Detection, and Treatment

Ali Khani Jeihooni and Fatemeh Jafari

Abstract

One of the most common types of cancer is head and neck cancer. Head and neck cancers are the sixth most common cancer worldwide and the most common cancer in developing countries. Oral cancer, which is a subset of head and neck cancers, refers to any cancerous growth in the oral cavity. Risk factors for oral cancer include age, malnutrition, genetic factors, family history, X-rays, papilloma virus, alcohol, smoking, tobacco, which three last are the strongest risk factors. The destructive link between tobacco products and human cancers stems from a powerful combination of two factors - nicotine and carcinogens. The highest incidence of tobacco related oral cancer is seen in low and middle income countries. The chance of curing oral cancers increases if they are diagnosed and treated early. At least three-quarters of all oral cancers can be prevented by quitting smoking and drinking alcohol. Screening programs can be valuable in patients from high-risk groups (smokers and alcoholics) or in patients with a previous diagnosis of cancer outside the head and neck.

Keywords: head and neck cancer, oral cancer, smoking, tobacco, screening

1. Introduction

In the present century, the rapid growth of non-communicable diseases is considered as a serious health challenge that threatens the socio-economic development of communities and people's health [1]. The most common types of non-communicable diseases are cardiovascular disease, diabetes, chronic respiratory disease and cancer [2]. Cancers have been known as life-threatening conditions all over the world [3] and recognized as one of the most significant reasons of death around the world and every year, more than 10 million infections and 6 million deaths caused by cancers are reported [4].

One of the most common types of cancer is head and neck cancer [5]. Head and neck cancers are the sixth most common cancer worldwide and the most common cancer in developing countries. While head and neck cancers are one of the most common cancers in South and Southeast Asia, they account for only 1% -4% of all cancers in the Western world [6].

Oral cancer, which is a subset of head and neck cancers, refers to any cancerous growth in the oral cavity. This cancer includes tumors of the lips, tongue, cheeks, gum, floor of the mouth, soft and hard palate, sinuses, tonsils, salivary glands and throat that can be fatal if left untreated. More than 90% of types of oral cancers originate in the squamous cells that line the inside of the mouth. When the growth of these cells gets out of control, it causes a cancer called squamous cell carcinoma or squamous cell carcinoma. Other types of oral cancers, such as partial malignancies of the salivary glands, sarcomas, odontogenic malignancies, melanoma, and lymphoma, make up less than 10% of oral cancers [7] and approximately 1% of metastatic cancers are lung, breast, prostate and kidney [8]. Squamous cell carcinoma can have various levels of differentiation and often give rise to node metastases. Lymphatic spreading into the neck is directly related to the T stage as well as the depth of invasion and tumor thickness [9].

2. Clinical forms

Tumors may appear in various forms of ulcers, prominent fungal masses, papillary, wart-like, white and red plaques, or a combination of both. Many primary

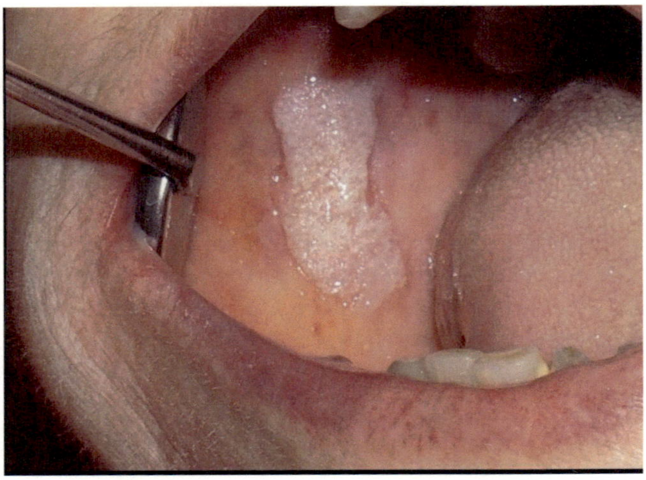

Figure 1.
Verrucous leukoplakia in the right buccal surface of a 72-year-old woman.

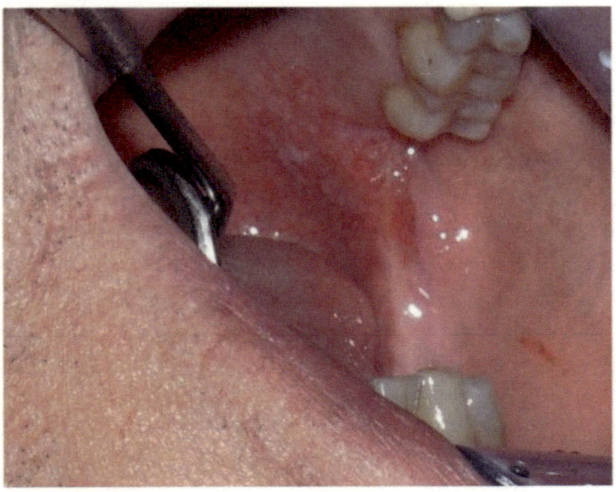

Figure 2.
Erythroplasia of the posterior hard palate, on histopathological examination in a 61-year-old man.

DOI: http://dx.doi.org/10.5772/intechopen.99236

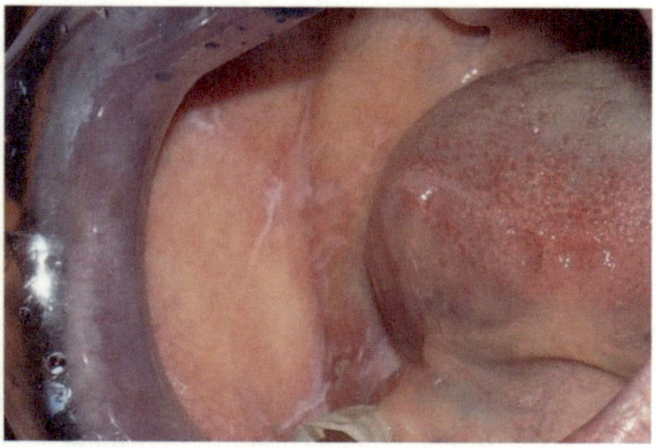

Figure 3.
White reticular striae on the right cheek mucosa of a 52-year-old man with oral lichen planus.

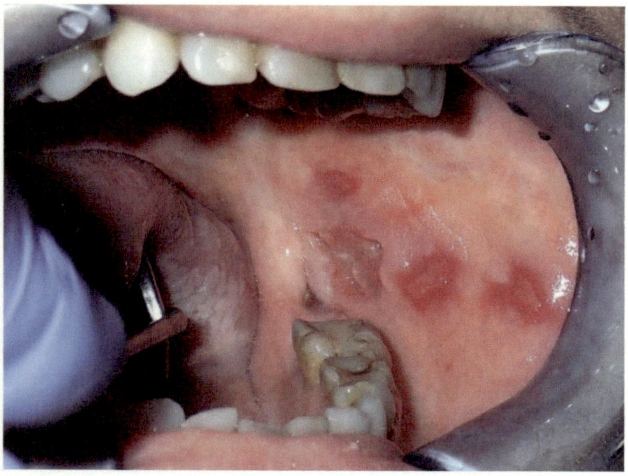

Figure 4.
Multiple areas of erythroplakia with ulceration in the left buccal mucosa because of chronic traumatic ulcer from self-biting in a 53-year-old woman.

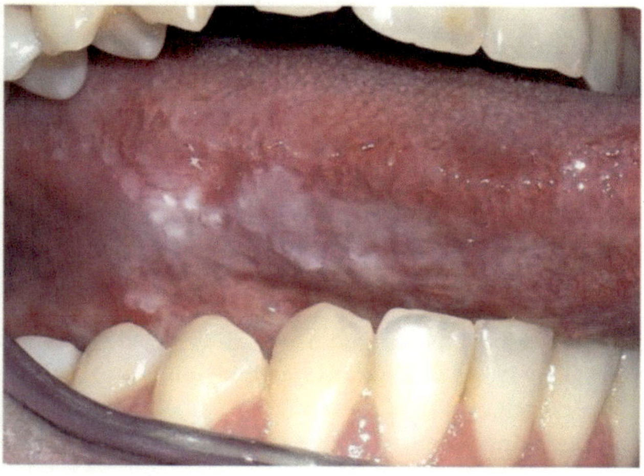

Figure 5.
Leukoplakia in the right border of the tongue with severe dysplasia in a 25-year-old woman.

cancers of the mouth are asymptomatic, while advanced lesions are often ulcerative and have prominent, hard margins. Pain is often absent in the later stages of the disease [8]. Potentially malignant oral epithelial lesions (PMOEL) are a group of oral diseases that may exist before the onset of oral squamous cell carcinoma (OSCC) and include a group of clinically oral mucosal lesions such as leukoplakia, erythroplakia, submucosal fibrosis, and lichen planus. However, most PMOELs do not progress to cancer (**Figures 1–5**) [10].

3. The place of conflict

The most common site of oral cancer is the lip. Lip cancer often occurs in light-skinned older men and most often affects the lower lip. Risk factors for lip cancer include sun exposure, certain occupations such as agriculture, socioeconomic status, smoking and pipe. Inside the mouth, the high-risk sites for cancer are the abdominal surface, the posterior sides of the tongue, the floor of the mouth, and the soft palate. Tongue cancer is the most common malignancy in the mouth. Tongue cancer is more common in men in their sixth and seventh decades of life. Tongue lesions are often aggressive. The second most common intraoral site for cancerous changes is the floor of the mouth. Tumors in this area occur in older men, especially in smokers and alcoholics. Involvement of the cheeks and gums is also common, especially in areas where there are certain habits such as chewing tobacco [8].

4. Risk factors

Oral cancer usually occurs in people over the age of 40 with an average age of 60, and their risk increases with age. It affects most men, but may increase as women smoke. Racially, black Americans are at higher risk for oral and throat cancer than whites. This increase in risk seems to be due to the influence of environmental factors, because the role of genetic factors in its occurrence has not been determined. Patients who smoke or chew a lot of tobacco and people who drink a lot of alcohol are at higher risk for oral cancer. Exposure to UV rays in people who stay in the sun for long periods of time is more likely to develop lip cancer. This is why the incidence of lip cancer is high in Australia. Other factors such as immunosuppression (such as AIDS and organ transplantation), viral papillomavirus infection (especially type 16, which accounts for 63% of new cases of oral cancer), Plummer–Vinson syndrome, and vitamin A deficiency also increase the risk of oral and pharyngeal cancer. The prevalence of HPV-related oral and pharyngeal cancers (mainly HPV type 16) has been increasing in North America and Northern Europe [11]. Other factors, including arsenic compounds used to treat syphilis, nutritional deficiencies, exposure to compounds such as wood and metal particles, and Candida infection, play a lesser role in cancer [8].

4.1 Hookah

In recent years, hookah has spread to Europe and the United States. In most countries, the increasing trend of hookah consumption is due to the increase in fruit and flavored tobacco products [12]. In a study conducted in Iran, the prevalence of hookah use among young people was reported to be 33.9%, which is higher than the number of people who smoke [13]. The side effects of hookah are many because the smoke produced from tobacco is composed of 4000 different chemicals and more than 40 carcinogens [14]. Tobacco smoke and hookah use are the most important risk factors for oral cancers and dysplastic lesions [3]. Cigarettes or other tobacco-related compounds are associated with about 75% of oral cancers. Tobacco contains more than 60 known carcinogens. The use of tobacco, whether in a smoky or chewable form alone, and especially with heavy alcohol consumption, is a very important risk factor for oral cancer. Smokers are 7 times more likely to develop oral cancer than non-smokers. The relative risk of developing cancer in people who consume a lot of alcohol is 6 times higher, and this risk is 38 times higher for patients who use alcohol and tobacco together [8].

The association of tobacco with the risk of cancer may differ among the head and neck cancer subtypes [15]. In some studies, it was demonstrated that smoking had a stronger association with larynx and pharynx than the oral cavity. This may be due to the higher exposure of larynx and pharynx to smoke than the oral cavity [15, 16].

The destructive link between tobacco products and human cancers stems from a powerful combination of two factors - nicotine and carcinogens. Nicotine is addictive and toxic, but there is no scientific evidence that nicotine is carcinogenic, and the IARC does not classify nicotine as a carcinogen. However, this addiction causes people to use tobacco products constantly, and these products contain many carcinogens. Cigarette smoke contains more than 60 carcinogens and unburned tobacco contains at least 16 carcinogens. Among these, tobacco-specific nitrosamines such as 4-(methylnitrosamino)-1-(3-pyridyl)-1-butanone (NNK) and N′-nitrosonornicotine (NNN), polycyclic aromatic hydrocarbons (such as benzoapyrene) and aromatic amines (such as 4-aminobiphenyl) seem to play an important role as causes of oral cancer [17].

Some believe that filtering hookah smoke through water reduces nicotine. However, contrary to popular belief, studies have shown that only 5% of nicotine is removed by water. In addition, hookah users may tend to increase the duration of smoking, thereby increasing the concentration of nicotine in their bloodstream. Therefore, considering the aforementioned harmful effects of hookah use and the results of a recent study, it seems that the use of this smoking device may cause changes in the oral mucosa [3].

Studies have shown that tobacco users, including slaked lime in the betel quid or with areca nut, experience carcinogenic and genotoxic effects on human oral epithelial cells. These products produce reactive oxygen species (ROS) in the chewing mouth [18]. Areca nut is composed of phenolic compounds and tobacco releases various nitrosamines in the mouth that are responsible for proliferative abrasions and damage to DNA and fibroblasts [19, 20]. The N-nitroso compound extracted from Areca nuts, which contains the active ingredient 3- (methyl nitrosamino) proprionityl, has been shown to cause gene poisoning and cytotoxicity responsible for tumors in the buccal cavity of smokeless smokers [21].

The long-lasting and frequent presence of paan and gutkha in the mouth around the gums leads to inflammation of the oral mucosa, which causes the activation of T-cells and macrophages, and ultimately the release of prostaglandins.

Prostaglandin production in buccal keratinocytes occurs due to Arka nut extract, which plays an important role in oral tissue fibrosis and cancer. Cytokines such as interferon-α, tumor necrosis factor (TNF), interleukin-6, and growth factor-like transforming growth factor-beta have been found to be produced at the sites of irritation [22]. The nitrosamine in tobacco is metabolized by cytochrome P450 enzymes, which may lead to the formation of N-nitrosonornicotine, a major carcinogen, which can lead to DNA damage and eventually oral cancer [23].

The consumption of tobacco is closely associated not only with the development of oral cancer, but also with the course of disease evolving a poor prognosis. The most widespread form of tobacco is chewing of betel-quid with tobacco and this has been demonstrated as a major risk factor of cancer of oral cavity [24].

Evidence from many studies shows that smoking in any way doubles the risk of oral cancer in men and women. The risk increases significantly with the duration and frequency of smoking. The risk among former smokers is consistently lower than current smokers, and the risk decreases as the years of quitting increase [25].

The highest incidence of tobacco related oral cancer is seen in low and middle income countries. People in the lower socioeconomic strata are more commonly affected. In India almost 21 people per 100 000 of the population are affected [26]. Data from a pioneering study by Taiwanese researchers show that people with a habit of smoking, drinking and chewing betel nuts at the same time are 123 times more likely to develop oral cancer than the general population [27]. More than 50 percent of oral cancers in India, Sudan and the Republic of South Sudan and about four percent of oral cancers in the United States are due to smokeless tobacco products. Smoking smoke-free tobacco is on the rise among young people in South Asia with the marketing of well-packaged products made from areca nuts and tobacco. As a result, oral precancerous conditions are significantly increased in young adults [28, 29].

4.2 Cigarette

Smoking helps to spread the tumor by suppressing immunity and tumor suppressor genes, most importantly p53 and PTEN [5]. The benefit of quitting smoking may be a time-dependent advantage. It was found that the risk of oral cancer among non-smokers is similar to that of former smokers after 10 years of smoking cessation. In addition, quitting smoking later or in middle age may significantly reduce the risk of oral cancer [30, 31].

A study in China, which included 210 cases, reported a strong association between long-term smoking and OSCC [32]. In the study by Ahmed et al. they have reported an increase in nuclear size, nuclearcytoplasmic (N/C) ratio and multi-lobed nuclei, while a decrease in size of cytoplasm in smokers as compared to non smokers [33]. The study of Woyceichoski et al. has also revealed an increase in cytoplasmic size and N/C ratio, while a decrease in size of cytoplasm in cocaine users as compared to the control group [34].

4.3 Alcohol

Tobacco and alcohol are the most well-known reasons for oral and throat cancers [35]. The synergistic effects of alcohol and tobacco smoke increase the risk of OSCC by increasing the permeability of the oral epithelium, tobacco solution, and increasing its permeability [36]. However, chronic alcohol use alone may lead to OSCC through several mechanisms, including the formation of DNA adducts, the production of ethanol-related reactive oxygen species, and interference with the DNA repair mechanism [37].

4.4 Shammah

Shamma consumption is increasing in many countries [38]. It is a combination of smokeless powder tobacco with ingredients such as lime, pepper, ash and flavorings, and people use it by placing it in the buccal cavity until the taste penetrates [39]. Another study of Yemeni shammah users found that there was a strong link between daily consumption of leukoplakia [40].

4.5 Chewing of khat

Khat is a plant that is mostly used for chewing and is amixture of cathine and norephidrine [41]. In an earlier case report of one patient, a strong affiliation between khat chewing and growth of OSCC was reported [42]. Sawair *et al*. also reported a strong association between khat chewing and OSCC development in their study, which included 649 Yemeni patients [43].

4.6 Shisha (water pipe) smoking

Shisha is commonly available in restaurants, cafes, and other eatery shops in many countries and it contains a high concentration of nicotine, tar, and carbon monoxide [44].

Smoking with water (WPS) is a type of smoking that has traditionally been used for many years in Asia and the eastern Mediterranean. However, in the 1990s, it became global with increasing popularity in other parts of the world, including Western countries [45].

A recent study found a strong link between water pipe smoking and head and neck cancers [45]. In a study from Syria and Lebanon, Zaid et al. Reported that mutations in the p53 gene are smoking in the water tube at OSCC63 [46].

Al-Amad conducted a study in Jordan that found that 36% of those with oral cancer had a habit of smoking in a water pipe [47].

5. Protective factors

Recent studies show that the consumption of coffee, vegetables, fruits, folic acid have a protective effect [8]. A study by Ding et al. In 2013 shows that the use of polyphenols, especially in black and green tea, is effective in preventing oral cancer [48].

6. Disease epidemiology in the world

Oral cancer is a serious and growing problem in many countries. Epidemiological studies show that the incidence of oral cancer and its mortality varies in different parts of the world [49]. In Australia, more than 4,000 new cases of head and neck cancer (including lip cancer) are diagnosed each year. Over 600 of these cancers are oral cavity cancers. In developing countries, oral cancer is the sixth cancer among men and the tenth cancer in women. Worldwide, more than 400,000 new cases of oral cancer are diagnosed each year, two-thirds of which occur in Asian countries such as Sri Lanka, Indonesia, India, Pakistan and Bangladesh [50]. In these high-risk countries, oral cancer is the most common malignancy, accounting for over 25% of all new cases of cancer each year [51]. According to the International Agency for Research on Cancer, some countries in Asia and the Pacific had the top three rates of oral cancer in 2018 [52].

7. Control and prevention measures

Due to recent developments in the diagnosis and treatment of cancers, the survival of patients with cancers of the breast, colon and ovary has increased. However, over the past 50 years, the survival of patients with oral cancer has not changed [53]. In other words, oral cancer has a poor prognosis and the overall 5-year survival rate is 40%, although if diagnosed at an early stage (I and II), the survival rate can exceed 80% [54]. Up to 50% of oral cancers are diagnosed at an advanced stage (stages III and IV) because most patients are asymptomatic in the early stages and do not seek medical help until they see clear symptoms such as pain, bleeding or a mass in the mouth or neck [55]. When the diagnostic delay is more than a month, the risk of having an advanced stage of oral cancer increases significantly [56]. In most cases, the patient is responsible for a large part of the diagnostic delay. However, delays can also be the result of an incorrect medical approach, as there is no suspicion of oral malignancy and it is not diagnosed and treated in a timely and sufficient manner [56, 57]. Clinical and pathological stage in diagnosis is the most important factor in prognosis [11].

Prevention of this devastating disease can be due to fundamental changes in the socio-economic situation, as well as measures to reduce demand, production, marketing and use of tobacco and alcohol products [58]. A healthy diet, oral hygiene and awareness of the signs and symptoms of the disease are important. Success depends on the political will, intersectoral actions, and culturally sensitive public health messages that are disseminated through educational campaigns and mass media initiatives [59].

Primary prevention of oral cancer therefore consists in education of people on the lifestyle changes such as non-smoking and alcohol consumption and protection from sunlight can reduce the risk of oral cancer [8]. Despite the increasing awareness of oral cancer in the general population, in the last 40 years the percentage of patients seeking medical attention with advanced disease has not changed significantly [51]. At least three-quarters of all oral cancers can be prevented by quitting smoking and drinking alcohol. Eliminating these two known factors also reduces cancer recurrence. In India and Sri Lanka, non-smoking tobacco education programs are designed specifically for adolescents to reduce the incidence of oral cancer. HPV vaccination can also be of importance, even though its effectiveness in not as well defined as it is in the prevention of anogenital and cervical cancer [11].

The goal of secondary prevention is early detection of cancer in the oral cavity in one of accessible places. The chance of curing oral cancers increases if they are diagnosed and treated early. Treatment of early-stage oral cancer increases patient survival. Unfortunately, most oral cancers are diagnosed at a more advanced stage and when they become symptomatic, which greatly reduces a person's chances of recovery, so early detection of precancerous lesions or early-stage oral cancer is very valuable. Diagnosis of suspected cases of oral cancer is made by assessing the patient's demographic characteristics and assessing specific habits, especially tobacco and alcohol consumption and other irritating factors that may play a role in causing oral cancer.

Routine biopsy in people with clinically characteristic precancerous lesions may lead to early detection of the underlying cause of oral cancer. In addition to history, physical examination, and biopsy, simultaneous evaluation of the upper aerodigestive tract is essential because patients with oral cancer are at risk for cancer of other parts of the head, neck, and lungs [25].

Oral health status and family history should also be evaluated for any syndromes that may increase the risk of oral cancer. In addition to the history, a complete examination of the head and neck is performed to carefully examine the location and spread of the primary tumor and identify metastases. It is noteworthy that early-stage cancerous lesions may be red or white plaques and non-ulcerative. More advanced cancers are ulcerative, aggressive, fungal, and prominent, or both. Cancer may develop within precancerous lesions such as leukoplakia or erythroplakia. Therefore, increasing the awareness of dentists is very important in getting a complete history and examination of the head and neck. Symptoms to consider include:

- Swelling or lumps on the lips or inside the mouth

- Wounds on the face, neck or mouth that do not heal within 2 weeks.

- Wounds under the denture
- White, red lesions
- Bleeding in the mouth for no reason
- Numbness or tenderness and unexplained pain in any area of the face, mouth and neck
- Difficulty swallowing, chewing, talking or moving the jaw or tongue
- Hoarseness, persistent sore throat or voice change
- Weight Loss [8].

Unlike other frequent cancers (for example, colon or cervical cancer), a standard population-based screening program for oral cancer is not cost-effective and cannot be recommended [51]. Screening programs can be valuable in patients from high-risk groups (smokers and alcoholics) or in patients with a previous diagnosis of cancer outside the head and neck [60]. In countries with regular dental practice attendance, opportunistic screening for oral mucosal lesions (early-stage cancer or precancerous lesions) in general dental practice could also be relevant in reducing diagnostic delay [61].

Visual screening involves regular visual and physical examination of the intraoral mucosa under intense light to observe the symptoms of oral potentially malignant disorders (OPMD) as well as early oral cancer, followed by careful examination and digital palpation of the neck for lymph node enlargement. This is a provider-dependent mental test. Accordingly, its performance in detecting lesions varies among providers. Comprehensive knowledge of oral anatomy, natural history of oral carcinogenesis, and clinical-pathological features of OPMDs and preclinical cancers are important prerequisites for effective oral vision screening providers [59]. A significant 34% reduction in oral cancer mortality among a high-risk group of smokers and alcoholics after three rounds of oral vision screening has been shown in a randomized controlled cluster trial in India [62, 63]. A 15-year follow-up showed a steady decline in oral cancer mortality, with a further decline in those who adhere to frequent screening courses. 38% reduction in oral cancer incidence (95% CI 8–59%) and 81% reduction in oral cancer mortality (95% CI 69–89%) in tobacco and /or alcohol users who They were screened four times [62].

Known risk factors, long natural history, easy diagnosis of precancerous lesions by oral examination make oral cavity cancer very suitable for population screening. Oral cancer usually occurs in accessible places, which can be diagnosed early by visual inspection and touch. Therefore, oral self-examination is possible for everyone because it is a method for early detection of precancerous oral lesions without the need for a simple, non-invasive and inexpensive healthcare professional [64]. It should be strongly supported for ordinary people, especially high-risk people [52]. A quasi-experimental study in Australia found the importance of oral self-examination in reducing the incidence and mortality of oral cancers [65].

Also, prompt treatment is essential for successful secondary prevention. Secondary prevention is also called cancer control [66]. Surgery and radiation therapy are widely used to treat premature oral cancer, either alone or in combination. The choice of method depends on the location of the tumor, cosmetic and functional outcomes, patient age, comorbidities, patient preference, and specialization [59].

The third prevention targets the final stages. More than 70% of advanced cancers have severe pain and other distressing symptoms. Pain control and palliative care are the third most important prevention strategies [67].

8. Conclusion

Since oral cancer is the sixth most common cancer in men and the tenth most common cancer in women and puts a lot of burden on health care providers and the public, and on the other hand many of its risk factors such as smoking and hookah can be controlled, including screening and diagnosis Early in the health care system and educational intervention programs are recommended.

Conflict of interest

The authors declare no conflict of interest.

Abbreviation

PMOEL	Potentially malignant oral epithelial lesions
OSCC	oral squamous cell carcinoma
OPMD	observe the symptoms of potentially malignant oral disorders

Author details

Ali Khani Jeihooni[1*] and Fatemeh Jafari[2]

1 Department of Public Health, School of Health, Shiraz University of Medical Sciences, Shiraz, Iran

2 Student Research Committee, Shiraz University of Medical Sciences, Shiraz, Iran

*Address all correspondence to: khani_1512@yahoo.com

References

[1] Zinat Motlagh SF, Chaman R, Ghafari SR, Parisay Z, Golabi MR, Eslami AA, et al. Knowledge, treatment, control, and risk factors for hypertension among adults in Southern Iran. International journal of hypertension. 2015;2015.

[2] GHAJARIEH SS, Kamangar F, Poustchi H, Malekzadeh R. Reducing the burden of chronic diseases: a neglected agenda in Iranian health care system, requiring a plan for action. 2010.

[3] Taghibakhsh M, Farhadi S, Babaee A, Sheikhi M. The effect of hookah use on buccal mucosa: Evaluation of repair index. Asian Pacific journal of cancer prevention: APJCP. 2019;20(4):1109.

[4] Jeihooni AK, Harsini PA. The Effect of an Educational Intervention Based on PRECEDE Model on Oral Cancer Prevention Behaviors in Hookah Users. Journal of Cancer Education. 2020; 35(6):1250-60.

[5] Bugshan A, Farooq I. Oral squamous cell carcinoma: metastasis, potentially associated malignant disorders, etiology and recent advancements in diagnosis. F1000Research. 2020;9.

[6] Joshi P, Dutta S, Chaturvedi P, Nair S. Head and neck cancers in developing countries. Rambam Maimonides medical journal. 2014;5(2).

[7] Wong T, Wiesenfeld D. Oral cancer. Australian dental journal. 2018;63: S91-S9.

[8] Contributing authors supervised by Dr. Parvin Yavari. Epidemiology textbook of prevalent diseases in Iran (cancers). first edition. volume 3. Tehran. 2014.

[9] Rivera C. Essentials of oral cancer. International journal of clinical and experimental pathology. 2015;8(9): 11884.

[10] Villa A, Villa C, Abati S. Oral cancer and oral erythroplakia: an update and implication for clinicians. Australian dental journal. 2011;56(3):253-6.

[11] Chow LQ. Head and neck cancer. New England Journal of Medicine. 2020;382(1):60-72.

[12] Rastam S, Ward KD, Eissenberg T, Maziak W. Estimating the beginning of the waterpipe epidemic in Syria. BMC public health. 2004;4(1):1-5.

[13] Khalil J, Heath RL, Nakkash RT, Afifi RA. The tobacco health nexus? Health messages in narghile advertisements. BMJ Publishing Group Ltd; 2009.

[14] Kuper H, Adami HO, Boffetta P. Tobacco use, cancer causation and public health impact. Journal of internal medicine. 2002;251(6):455-66.

[15] Dhull AK, Atri R, Dhankhar R, Chauhan AK, Kaushal *V. Major* risk factors in head and neck Cancer: a retrospective analysis of 12-year experiences. World journal of oncology. 2018;9(3):80.

[16] Maasland DH, van den Brandt PA, Kremer B, Goldbohm RAS, Schouten LJ. Alcohol consumption, cigarette smoking and the risk of subtypes of head-neck cancer: results from the Netherlands Cohort Study. BMC cancer. 2014;14(1):1-14.

[17] Hecht SS. Tobacco carcinogens, their biomarkers and tobacco-induced cancer. Nature Reviews Cancer. 2003;3(10):733-44.

[18] Babu S, Sesikeran B, Bhat R. Oral fibrosis among teenagers chewing tobacco, areca nut, and pan masala. The Lancet. 1996;348(9028):692.

[19] Nair J, Ohshima H, Friesen M, Croisy A, Bhide SV, Bartsch H. Tobacco-specific and betel nut-specific N-nitroso compounds: occurrence in saliva and urine of betel quid chewers and formation in vitro by nitrosation of betel quid. Carcinogenesis. 1985;6(2): 295-303.

[20] Bhide S, Gothoskar S, Shivapurkar N. Arecoline tumorigenicity in Swiss strain mice on normal and vitamin B deficient diet. Journal of cancer research and clinical oncology. 1984;107(3):169-71.

[21] Chiu C-J, Chang M-L, Chiang C-P, Hahn L-J, Hsieh L-L, Chen C-J. Interaction of collagen-related genes and susceptibility to betel quid-induced oral submucous fibrosis. Cancer Epidemiology and Prevention Biomarkers. 2002;11(7):646-53.

[22] Kandasamy M, Anisa N, Rahman A, Rajan MA, Prakash A, Lal J. Etiopathogenesis of oral submucous fibrosis-review of literature. Journal of Advanced Medical and Dental Sciences Research. 2015;3(3):53.

[23] Nair U, Bartsch H, Nair J. Alert for an epidemic of oral cancer due to use of the betel quid substitutes gutkha and pan masala: a review of agents and causative mechanisms. Mutagenesis. 2004;19(4):251-62.

[24] Mathur A, Jain M, Shiva M, Navlakha M, Kulkarni S. Tobacco habits and risk of oral cancer: A retrospective study in India. Iranian Journal of Blood and Cancer. 2009;1(3):111-6.

[25] Sankaranarayanan R, Ramadas K, Amarasinghe H, Subramanian S, Johnson N. Oral cancer: prevention, early detection, and treatment. 2015.

[26] Chaturvedi P, Singh A, Chien C-Y, Warnakulasuriya S. Tobacco related oral cancer. BMJ. 2019;365.

[27] Guo S-E, Huang T-J, Huang J-C, Lin M-S, Hong R-M, Chang C-H, et al. Alcohol, betel-nut and cigarette consumption are negatively associated with health promoting behaviors in Taiwan: a cross-sectional study. BMC public health. 2013;13(1):1-8.

[28] Sinha D, Palipudi K, Rolle I, Asma S, Rinchen S. Tobacco use among youth and adults in member countries of South-East Asia region: review of findings from surveys under the Global Tobacco Surveillance System. Indian journal of public health. 2011;55(3): 169-76.

[29] Gupta B, Ariyawardana A, Johnson NW. Oral cancer in India continues in epidemic proportions: evidence base and policy initiatives. International dental journal. 2013;63(1): 12-25.

[30] Porter S, Gueiros LA, Leão JC, Fedele S. Risk factors and etiopathogenesis of potentially premalignant oral epithelial lesions. Oral surgery, oral medicine, oral pathology and oral radiology. 2018;125(6):603-11.

[31] Warnakulasuriya S, Dietrich T, Bornstein MM, Peidró EC, Preshaw PM, Walter C, et al. Oral health risks of tobacco use and effects of cessation. International dental journal. 2010;60(1):7-30.

[32] Wang X, Xu J, Wang L, Liu C, Wang H. The role of cigarette smoking and alcohol consumption in the differentiation of oral squamous cell carcinoma for the males in China. Journal of cancer research and therapeutics. 2015;11(1):141.

[33] Ahmad H, Ebnoof S. Oral epithelial atypical changes in apparently healthy oral mucosa exposed oral mucosa to smoking, alcohl, peppers and hot meals, using the AgNOR and papanicolaou staining techniques. 2009.

[34] Woyceichoski IEC, de Arruda EP, Resende LG, Machado MAN, Grégio AMT, Azevedo LR, et al. Cytomorphometric analysis of crack cocaine effects on the oral mucosa. Oral Surgery, Oral Medicine, Oral Pathology, Oral Radiology, and Endodontology. 2008;105(6):745-9.

[35] Fu YS, Wenig BM, Abemayor E. Head and neck pathology with clinical correlations: Churchill Livingstone; 2001.

[36] Feller L, Chandran R, Khammissa R, Meyerov R, Lemmer J. Alcohol and oral squamous cell carcinoma: clinical review. South African Dental Journal. 2013;68(4): 176-80.

[37] Liu Y, Chen H, Sun Z, Chen X. Molecular mechanisms of ethanol-associated oro-esophageal squamous cell carcinoma. Cancer letters. 2015;361(2):164-73.

[38] Alharbi F. Incidence of head and neck cancers in Jazan province, Saudi Arabia. Saudi Journal of Otorhinolaryngology Head and Neck Surgery. 2017;19(2):47.

[39] Quadri MFA, Alharbi F, Bajonaid AMS, Moafa IHY, Sharwani AA, Alamir AHA. Oral squamous cell carcinoma and associated risk factors in Jazan, Saudi Arabia: a hospital based case control study. Asian Pacific Journal of Cancer Prevention. 2015;16(10):4335-8.

[40] Scheifele C, Nassar A, Reichart P. Prevalence of oral cancer and potentially malignant lesions among shammah users in Yemen. Oral oncology. 2007;43(1):42-50.

[41] Al-Hebshi N, Skaug N. Khat (*Catha edulis*)—an updated review. Addiction biology. 2005;10(4):299-307.

[42] Fasanmade A, Kwok E, Newman L. Oral squamous cell carcinoma associated with khat chewing. Oral Surgery, Oral Medicine, Oral Pathology, Oral Radiology, and Endodontology. 2007;104(1):e53-e5.

[43] Sawair FA, Al-Mutwakel A, Al-Eryani K, Al-Surhy A, Maruyama S, Cheng J, et al. High relative frequency of oral squamous cell carcinoma in Yemen: qat and tobacco chewing as its aetiological background. International journal of environmental health research. 2007;17(3):185-95.

[44] Shafagoj YA, Mohammed FI. Levels of maximum end-expiratory carbon monoxide and certain cardiovascular parameters following hubble-bubble smoking. Saudi medical journal. 2002;23(8):953-8.

[45] Patil S, Awan KH, Arakeri G, Aljabab A, Ferrari M, Gomes CC, et al. The relationship of "shisha"(water pipe) smoking to the risk of head and neck cancer. Journal of Oral Pathology & Medicine. 2019;48(4):278-83.

[46] Zaid K, Azar-Maalouf E, Barakat C, Chantiri M. p53 overexpression in oral mucosa in relation to Shisha smoking in Syria and Lebanon. Asian Pacific journal of cancer prevention: APJCP. 2018;19(7):1879.

[47] Al-Amad SH, Awad MA, Nimri O. Oral cancer in young Jordanians: potential association with frequency of narghile smoking. Oral surgery, oral medicine, oral pathology and oral radiology. 2014;118(5):560-5.

[48] Ding Y, Yao H, Yao Y, Fai LY, Zhang Z. Protection of dietary polyphenols against oral cancer. Nutrients. 2013;5(6):2173-91.

[49] Jeihooni AK, Dindarloo SF, Harsini PA. Effectiveness of health belief model on oral cancer prevention in smoker men. Journal of Cancer Education. 2019;34(5):920-7.

[50] Montero PH, Patel SG. Cancer of the oral cavity. Surgical Oncology Clinics. 2015;24(3):491-508.

[51] Abati S, Bramati C, Bondi S, Lissoni A, Trimarchi M. Oral Cancer and Precancer: A Narrative Review on the Relevance of Early Diagnosis. International Journal of Environmental Research and Public Health. 2020;17(24):9160.

[52] Hung L-C, Kung P-T, Lung C-H, Tsai M-H, Liu S-A, Chiu L-T, et al. Assessment of the risk of oral cancer incidence in a high-risk population and establishment of a predictive model for oral cancer incidence using a population-based cohort in Taiwan. International journal of environmental research and public health. 2020;17(2):665.

[53] Wong DT. Towards a simple, saliva-based test for the detection of oral cancer. 'Oral fluid (saliva), which is the mirror of the body, is a perfect medium to be explored for health and disease surveillance.'. Expert review of molecular diagnostics. 2006;6(3):267-72.

[54] Silverman S, Kerr AR, Epstein JB. Oral and pharyngeal cancer control and early detection. Journal of Cancer Education. 2010;25(3):279-81.

[55] McCullough M, Prasad G, Farah C. Oral mucosal malignancy and potentially malignant lesions: an update on the epidemiology, risk factors, diagnosis and management. Australian dental journal. 2010;55:61-5.

[56] Gómez I, Seoane J, Varela-Centelles P, Diz P, Takkouche B. Is diagnostic delay related to advanced-stage oral cancer? A meta-analysis. European journal of oral sciences. 2009;117(5):541-6.

[57] Groome PA, Rohland SL, Hall SF, Irish J, Mackillop WJ, O'Sullivan B. A population-based study of factors associated with early versus late stage oral cavity cancer diagnoses. Oral oncology. 2011;47(7):642-7.

[58] Johnson NW, Warnakulasuriya S, Gupta P, Dimba E, Chindia M, Otoh E, et al. Global oral health inequalities in incidence and outcomes for oral cancer: causes and solutions. Advances in dental research. 2011;23(2):237-46.

[59] Sankaranarayanan R, Ramadas K, Amarasinghe H, Subramanian S, Johnson N. Oral cancer: prevention, early detection, and treatment. Cancer: disease control priorities, third edition (volume 3). 2015.

[60] Van der Waal I, de Bree R, Brakenhoff R, Coebegh J. Early diagnosis in primary oral cancer: is it possible? Medicina oral, patologia oral y cirugia bucal. 2011;16(3):e300-e5.

[61] Lim K, Moles D, Downer M, Speight P. Opportunistic screening for oral cancer and precancer in general dental practice: results of a demonstration study. British dental journal. 2003;194(9):497-502.

[62] Sankaranarayanan R, Ramadas K, Thara S, Muwonge R, Thomas G, Anju G, et al. Long term effect of visual screening on oral cancer incidence and mortality in a randomized trial in Kerala, India. Oral oncology. 2013;49(4):314-21.

[63] Sankaranarayanan R, Ramadas K, Thomas G, Muwonge R, Thara S, Mathew B, et al. Effect of screening on oral cancer mortality in Kerala, India: a cluster-randomised controlled trial. The Lancet. 2005;365(9475):1927-33.

[64] Shrestha G, Maharjan L. Mouth Self-Examination for Prevention and Control of Oral Cavity Cancer. JNMA; journal of the Nepal Medical Association. 2020;58(225):360-2.

[65] Jornet PL, Garcia FG, Berdugo ML, Perez FP, Lopez APF. Mouth self-examination in a population at risk of oral cancer. Australian dental journal. 2015;60(1):59-64.

[66] Alonge O, Narendran S. Opinions about oral cancer prevention and early detection among dentists practising along the Texas–Mexico border. Oral diseases. 2003;9(1):41-5.

[67] Mangalath U, Aslam SA, Khadar AHKA, Francis PG, Mikacha MSK, Kalathingal JH. Recent trends in prevention of oral cancer. Journal of International Society of Preventive & Community Dentistry. 2014;4(Suppl 3):S131.

Chapter 2

Diagnostic Potential of Salivary Exosomes in Oral Cancer

Henry Ademola Adeola, Haly Holmes and Dada Oluwaseyi Temilola

Abstract

"Omics" based concepts and techniques are gaining momentum in the field of oral medicine, spurred on by rapid advancements within the field of precision diagnostics and therapeutics. Oral cancer, specifically oral squamous cell carcinoma is the most common head and neck cancer, posing both diagnostic and prognostic challenges globally. Saliva offers several advantages as a diagnostic tool and has gained recognition as a biological medium for liquid biopsy. Salivary biomarkers, such as exosomes not only contain the full spectrum of genomic, lipidomic and proteomic material from its cell of origin, but are also more stable and consistently measurable in saliva due to their phospholipid structural protection of their merchandise/contents. Salivary exosomes are mediators in communication and transfer of contents between cancer and normal cells and thus key role players in mediating the tumor environment. Even though exosomes have been widely employed to investigate systemic diseases including head and neck cancers, unraveling the biologic mechanisms, scope of application of salivary tumor-derived exosomes and overcoming restrictions in this emergent field of saliva-exosomics warrants further investigation.

Keywords: Saliva, exosomes, oral cancer, exosomics, omics-based approaches

1. Introduction

Despite the fact, that there is a relatively wider coverage and application of several emerging molecular and omics-based techniques, in the field of medicine; many of these concepts (and techniques) are only beginning to gain recognition in the field of dentistry [1]. The completion of the human genome project [2–4], has expanded the trajectory for precision diagnostic and therapeutic potential thereof across many biomedical fields [5, 6]. The clinical lexicon in the post-genomic era is now burgeoning with various personalized application of genomics (and phenomics) to improving the cancer management pipelines [1, 6–9].

Orthogonal (but complementary) multimodal approaches to conventional histopathology [10, 11], such as liquid biopsies technologies have emerged as useful tools for clinical oncology [11–13], early tumor diagnosis and biomonitoring [14–17], as well as therapeutic decision making and delivery [18]. Nano-scaled multivesicular exosomes have emerged as important components of the tumor circulome that has significantly improved the cancer diagnostic field [11, 14]. Furthermore, salivary exosomes have been applied to improve the diagnosis of various cancers [19–26],

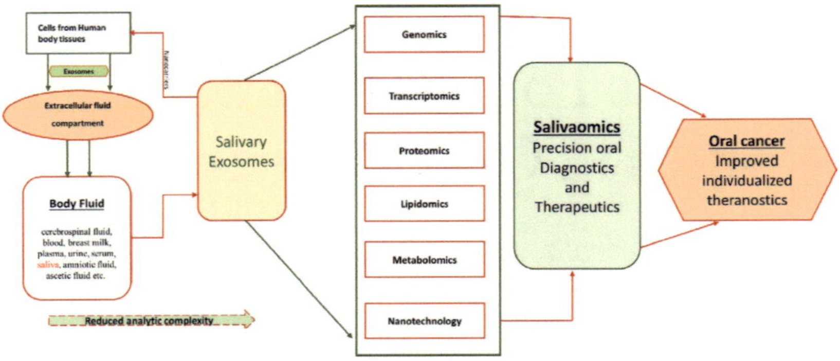

Figure 1.
Overview of origin and theranostic value of exosomes in oral cancer.

including oral cancers [25, 26]. The focus of this chapter is to review the applications and prospects of salivary exosomes in oral cancer detection (**Figure 1**).

2. Salivary diagnostics

Human saliva is a multifunctional biological fluid, which facilitates digestion, swallowing, tasting, tissue lubrication and protection against infectious organisms. It is comprised largely of water (99%) and other biochemical substances such as proteins, nucleic acids, mucins, immunoglobulins, a variety of electrolytes and lipids [27, 28]. Whole saliva production is derived from all the salivary glands including the gingival crevicular fluid [29]. Saliva, which has been used for diagnostic purposes for over 2000 years, plays a key role in the maintenance of general and particularly oral health homeostasis [30]. The health of individuals has been determined by salivary changes such as amount produced, smell, ropiness and gustatory sensation [31, 32].

Components of the salivary glands are responsible for production, modification, transportation and secretion of saliva into the oral cavity (via acinar cells, various ductal system cells, and myoepithelial cells) [33]. The close proximity of a network of highly permeable blood capillaries to the saliva producing acinar cells facilitates the free exchange of blood-derived molecules into the acinar cells [34], which enter the salivary tissues either via transcellular (passive and active transport) or paracellular (extracellular ultrafiltration) routes [35, 36]. This transfer potentially influences the molecular constituency of oral fluids. Diffusion is the most common transport mechanism of molecules from blood into the saliva and this process is driven/influenced by the size and the electric charge of the molecules [37]. Active transport involves the transcellular transportation of blood into saliva via secretory acinar cells of the salivary glands. Ultra-filtration is the major mode by which molecules are transported into saliva via the paracellular route, whereby small sized blood molecules filter into saliva through the spaces between ductal and acinar cells [37]. Salivary acini secrete saliva into collecting ducts, where sodium reabsorption, and bicarbonate and potassium are secretion takes place, thus altering the composition of the saliva [38, 39]. Even though blood molecules transported through ultra-filtration into saliva are usually in low concentration in comparison to their levels in blood, this mode of transport enables blood molecules such as DNA, RNA, proteins, metabolites and exosomes into saliva through the salivary gland. This confers the possibility for oral fluids to harbor molecular information indicative of an individual's current state of health. This information may be reflected by changes in the concentrations of these molecules or mutation in the genetic constitution of the molecules which are also present in saliva - serving as potential salivary biomarkers for diagnosis, prognosis and monitoring of therapeutic responses [40].

Many body fluids have been explored as alternative sources for biomarkers in molecular diagnosis of cancers, genetic, immunological and other systemic diseases [41–45]. However, blood, urine and saliva are the most used media for discovery of biomarkers [46]. Saliva is a rich source of proteins and its DNA, RNA, and protein content is analogous to that of blood with significant commonality in hormones, antibodies and other molecules. Most of the resident salivary protein constituents are synthesized within the salivary glands, with the rest transported from blood or lymph into saliva and used as biomarkers for disease diagnosis and screening purposes [47].

Saliva has the advantages over blood in that it is a readily available specimen which can be collected by non-invasive techniques and is recommended as the diagnostic medium in vulnerable populations such as children. The retrieval of multiple salivary samples from the same individual is possible with minimal discomfort and saliva is safer to work with when compared with blood samples. For example, there are some factors in saliva which help to inhibit HIV infectivity thereby limiting the rate of HIV transmission through the oral cavity [48]. Saliva sample processing is more economical and does not clot making it easier to store and ship with less manipulation. However, the low level of protein detection in saliva is sensitive to the method of saliva collection and specimen contamination. Normal high-abundance salivary constituents such as amylase and proline rich proteins (during stimulated salivary collection methods especially), may dilute the presence of low-level proteins, which may be more important biomarkers.

Salivary biomarkers are miniscule and measured in (picograms), detection of which can only be achieved by techniques which are both sensitive and specific enough to discriminate between them [49]. Technological advances in diagnostic detection methods (next generation sequencing, mass spectrometry, genome wide association studies and other screening techniques) have paralleled the demand for improved diagnostic test accuracy of salivary genomic and proteomic biomarkers, thereby conferring distinct advantages for saliva in the diagnosis and monitoring of diseases such as oral cancer and precancer.

Salivary exosomes, which are nano-sized salivary biomarkers equipped with all the molecular cargo from the parent cells, have become increasingly detectable due to their stability in the circulation and bodily fluids. They have been extensively explored as diagnostic tools for local and systemic diseases [50].

2.1 Salivary exosome physiology

Fusion of nano-sized (30–100 nm in diameter) multivesicular bodies (MVB) [51] derived from the endocytic pathway with plasma membrane was discovered over 30 years ago [52]. Johnstone et al., detected the release of small vesicles into extracellular spaces by reticulocyte MVB's and observed that their enzymatic activity mirrored that of the cell culture from which they were shed [52]. These bodies (exosomes), originally believed to be involved in waste disposal, due to their resistance to degradation by lysozymes, is now more understood to subserve vital biological functions when released as extracellular vesicles [53]. These functions are influenced/determined by their target cell with which they interact and include cellular communication and homeostasis, immune control (they contain IgA), RNA processing and transport of drugs [53–55].

Exosomal release (after formation of intraluminal vesicles), can be compared to the reversal of the endocytosis process, permits their evaluation in the extracellular body fluid environments [56]. The exocytotic release of exosomes into the extracellular domain, reveals that they naturally contain key molecular components derived from the parent cell relating to membrane transport, lipid metabolism and extracellular matrix formation [21, 57]. In addition, cytoplasmic nucleic acid contents such as mRNA and microRNA have been found in exosomes [21, 58, 59]. Considering the important contents as highlighted here, exosomes have been identified to play crucial roles in cell-to-cell communication [21]. All exosomes regardless of their origin possess both shared conserved and cell-specific proteins. Emerging knowledge has associated exosomes with the development of physiological and pathological perturbations [60, 61]. For instance, cancer exosomes have been found to be capable of a range of tumor-promoting activities, such as immunomodulation, development of pre-metastatic niches, as well as dysregulation of angiogenesis [62–64]. Furthermore, cancer exosomes are vital indicators of potentially malignant events in the tumor microenvironment and may exhibit pheno-genomic perturbation biomarkers of cancer [65, 66].

2.2 Diagnostic benefits of exosomes in body fluids

Due to exosomal release into the extracellular compartment, they are abundantly found in most body fluids such as cerebrospinal fluids, blood, breast milk, plasma, urine, serum, saliva, amniotic fluid, semen and ascetic fluid [21, 52–55]. Exosomes are highly suitable substrates for biomarker signature discovery. Because of the content-protective packaging of their rich cargo (by lipid membranes) from extracellular lytic enzymes, and significantly lower complexity of its contents in comparison to whole tissue analysis [53].

Analyzing exosomal shuttle RNA (esRNA) in maternal blood, has been proposed as a potential surrogate prenatal diagnostic tool, to avoid risky invasive procedures such as chorionic villus sampling and amniocentesis [54]. This could potentially lower the risk of surgical injuries and miscarriages. Even though, cell free fetal DNA (cffDNA) has been previously used for the prenatal diagnostic purposes, the low content of fetal cffDNA has reduced the accuracy of this method [54, 56]. Information about cancer risk and genetic disease predisposition can be potentially gleaned from exosomal esRNA content analysis.

The use of novel liquid biopsy-based cancer diagnostic tools has significantly improved the precision and efficacy of individualized medicine, particularly in resource-limited settings [11]. Exosomes are capable of providing robust molecular tumor information about cells of origin, are retrievable from easily accessible body fluids; and hence are highly useful for early detection and follow-up of cancer [55].

2.3 Salivary exosomes and oral cancer

Exosomes have been successfully isolated from saliva [19–25]; and the presence of lipids, proteins and nucleic acids in exosomes, makes salivary exosomes attractive substrates for omics analysis (a.k.a Salivaomics) [57–60]. It has become emergent, that salivary constituents (e.g. mRNAs, proteins, miRNAs, microbes and metabolites such as lipids) may be detected in exosomes and be used as biomarkers for diseases (both local and distal) [54]. Structural, proteomics and transcriptomics analysis of salivary exosomes has been successfully carried out [61–65]; and salivary exosomes are fast becoming key tools in cancer biomarker theranostics. Exosomes have been revealed as valuable indicators of the micro-environments and perpetrators of cancer intercellular communication [25].

The mean diameter and protein content are used as the basis upon which exosomes isolated from saliva are structurally subdivided into two types (I and II which are ca. 85 nm and 40 nm in diameter, respectively) [20]. Since epithelial barriers between blood vessels and salivary gland structures can be crossed by exosomes [66, 67], they have become important tools for essential transport of key signatures between blood and saliva (which is believed to be an ultrafiltrate of blood) [67–69]. Important molecular information may be exchanged via transudation, ultrafiltration or selective transport based on their size or presence of transporter molecules [67].

Of all the head and neck cancers, oral squamous cell carcinoma is the most prevalent, often diagnosed in advanced stage and is associated with a low survival and poor prognosis. Early detection of oral cancer is a key goal in epidemiological cancer control and successful management thereof. Using salivary exosomes for identification of oral cancer biomarkers is potentially a highly sensitive, cost-effective and non-invasive point-of-care technique for detecting oral cancer that may be subclinical or missed by routine histological diagnostic approaches [70]. Evaluation of these vesicles shed by cancer cells via multivesicular bodies (MVB's) into saliva is a viable approach for biomarker detection in oral cancer (**Figure 2**). Salivary exosomes have played key roles in diagnosis of systemic diseases [51] and have been key player in the molecular characterization of cancer [24]. Due to its reduced complexity as compared to other body fluids, exosomes are reliable tools for early diagnosis of oral cancer and its use as a diagnostic tool may significantly improve cancer survival rates [24].

Due to its nano-scaled structure, human salivary exosomes have been identified as potential carriers for non-invasive delivery of cancer biomarkers [22]. For example, electrochemical sensing methods, such as electric field-induced release and measurement (EFIRM) approach, has been used to improve the field of salivary liquid biopsy [23]. Not least, salivary exosomes have been used to enhance the detection of human papilloma virus (HPV) positive oropharyngeal cancers [26].

The critical role of tumor-derived exosome in cancer in largely due to the presence of tumor-specific signatures within its functional cargos, which includes proteins, miRNA and mRNA (**Table 1**).

The significant physiological interaction and overlap of the blood and salivary proteome (ca. 20–30%) makes exosomal protein biomarkers attractive and many cancer-related exosomal proteins have been identified from oral cancer [23, 82, 83]. Potential proteomic biomarkers of oral cancer such as CFB, CD59, A1BG, M2b, CAT, MRP14, PFN, M2BP, ADA, S100, CFL1, IGHG, TF, IL-1B and IL-8S have been

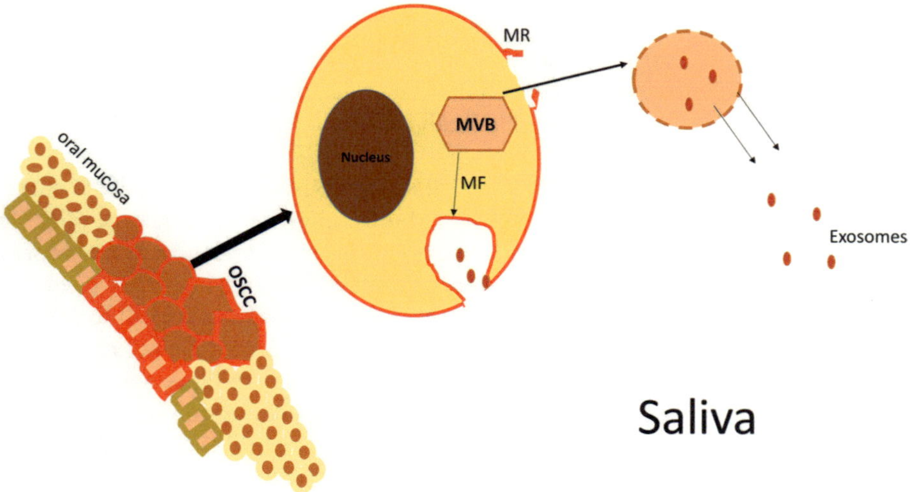

Figure 2.
Pathways for escape of exosomes into saliva. Oral squamous carcinoma cells (OSCC) may release exosomes into saliva, either by fusion of the multivesicular body (MVB) with the plasma membrane (MF) or by plasma membrane rupture (MR) and direct release through endosomal membrane.

Biomarker	Type	Sample	Methods	References
A2M, HPA, MUC5B, LGALS3BP, IGHA1, PIP, PKM1/M2, GAPDH	Protein	saliva	Mass spectrometry analysis and proteomics data analysis	Winck et al. [71]
miRNA-21	miRNA	OSCC cell line	miRNA sequencing	Li et al. [72]
miR-1246	miRNA	OSCC cell line	MicroRNA microarray	Sakha et al. [73]
miR-200c-3p	miRNA	OSCC cell line	integrated microarray	Kawakubo-Yasukochi et al. [74]
miR-34a-5p	miRNA	OSCC cell line	miRNA sequencing	Li et al. [75]
PF4V1, CXCL7, F13A1, and ApoA1	protein	serum	RT-PCR	Li et al. [76]
miR-101-3p	miRNA	OSCC cell line	Microarray analysis	Xie et al. [77]
miR-382-5p	miRNA	OSCC cell line	RT-PCR	Sun et al. [78]
miR-24-3p	miRNA	saliva	RT-PCR	He et al. [79]
miR-21-5p	miRNA	OSCC cell line	RT-PCR	Chen et al. [80]
miR-155	miRNA	OSCC cell line	RT-PCR.	Kirave et al. [81]

Table 1.
Exosome biomarker for oral cancers.

identified from whole saliva [84–88]. However, protein biomarkers such as MUC5B, A2M, LGALS3BP, HPa, GAPDH, IGHA1, PIP and PKM1/M2 have been specifically identified to be exosomal protein biomarkers of oral cancer with a classification accuracy of 90% [80, 89]. Zlotogorski-Hurvitz et al. (2016), identified CD9/−81 downregulation and CD 63 upregulation in exosomes as early diagnostic protein biomarkers of oral cancer [90]. Furthermore, salivary exosomes isolated from HPV-positive oropharyngeal cancer cell lines has been found to underexpress cyclin D1 and p53 and overexpress p16, T-cell inhibitory protein PTPN11 and E6/E7 proteins [91].

Via their interaction with mRNA, micro RNA's (miRNA) are involved in a number of physiological and disease processes (when there is aberrant expression). MiRNAs are small non-coding RNAs that mediate destabilization and/or translational repression of target messenger RNA (mRNA) molecules thereby reducing final protein output. Exosomes are a rich source of miRNA's, provides a vehicle for cell to cell transporting to alter cellular functions as well as offer protection in the extracellular environment. Exosomal miRNAs have been investigated as candidate screening tools (miR-24-3p) [92], in chemoresistance (miR-21) [81], regulating tumor progression (miR-34-5p) [93] and miR-342–3p and miR-1246 [93] and miR-382-5p [78].

In oral cancer, the intercellular transfer of molecules (such as miRNA's) by cancer associated fibroblast influences the tumor microenvironment. miR-21 represents one of the most abundant miRs transported within EV cargos secreted by oral cancer cells and is a well-established oncogenic miR whose major targets include the tumor suppressors. Its exosomal hideout contributes towards chemoresistance due to the camouflage provided by its vehicle during intercellular transfer of the oncogenic miR. It is thus also an important chemotherapeutic precision target in cancers [81]. Li et al. [94], in a study of 108 patients with OSCC, observed that tumor exosomal miR 21 was upregulated in hypoxic cancer cells as well as internalized by normoxic cells. Exosomal miR-34-5p transfer between CAF's and neighboring OSCC cells played an important role in regulating tumor progression. Sakha et al. [73], demonstrated that effect that intercellular transfer of exosomal oncogenic miRNA's (miR-342–3p and miR-1246) could be delivered were evaluated for their role in could have on cancer development and progression by influencing cell motility and invasiveness [73]. Exosomal miR-382-5p in cancer-associated fibroblast (CAF) mediated OSSC migration and invasion by evaluation of tissue samples from 47 patients who had OSSC tumor resection. The results showed that CAF's transfer miR-382-5p associated with migration and invasion [78]. The expression of exosomal miR-24-3p was found to be higher in salivary exosomes from OSCC patients compared to healthy controls. The AUC for miR-24-3p was 0.738 and could significantly distinguish OSCC patients from normal individuals with 64.4% sensitivity and 80% specificity in 49 patients with OSSC.

The functional cargos which include mRNA has been considered as potential biomarker in the diagnosis and monitoring and treatment of cancer. Valadi et al. first described the presence of mRNAs in exosomes in 2007 [95]. Subsequently, studies have shown the transfer of bioactive mRNAs (tumor suppressor genes or oncogenes) from a malignant cell to a normal cell led to a change in the phenotype and malignant transformation of the normal cell [95–97].

Few studies have identified mRNA in saliva of oral cancer patients. Li et al. identified potential mRNA biomarker which include IL8, SAT, DUSP, IL1B, OAZ1, H3F3A and S100P, in saliva from oral cancer patients [98]. The study showed that the combination of these biomarkers was highly sensitive and specific in differentiating between OSSC and healthy [98]. An in vitro study showed that oral squamous cell carcinoma cell line (PCI-13, UMSCC47) triggered significant increase expression level of IGFBP-3 mRNA and VEGF mRNA in recipient cells [99].

Even though exosomes have been widely employed to investigate head and neck squamous cell carcinomas [100–103], unraveling the biologic mechanisms and application of salivary tumor -derived exosomes is still an evolving science [67]. This emergent field of saliva-exosomics warrants further investigation.

3. Conclusions

Salivary exosomes provide viable, consistent and stable sources of cancer biomarkers. The scope of its utility as well as understanding the molecular mechanisms which underpins it, requires further investigation. Future studies refining the methodology for extracellular vesicle isolation and cleansing presents the greatest challenge that is needed to overcome the restrictions to exploring the full scope of salivary exosomes in systemic diseases including oral cancer.

Acknowledgements

H.A.A thanks the South African Medical Research Council (SAMRC) for a mid-career scientist and Self-initiated research grant; and the South African National Research Foundation (NRF) for Research Development Grant (RDG) for rated researchers. The authors thank the University Research committee (URC) of the University of Cape Town for funding this book chapter.

Conflict of interest

The authors declare no conflict of interest.

Author details

Henry Ademola Adeola[1,2], Haly Holmes[3]* and Dada Oluwaseyi Temilola[4,5]

1 Department of Oral and Maxillofacial Pathology, Faculty of Dentistry, University of the Western Cape Dental Faculty, Cape Town, South Africa

2 Division of Dermatology, Department of Medicine, Faculty of Health Sciences and Groote Schuur Hospital, University of Cape Town, Cape Town, South Africa

3 Department of Oral Medicine and Periodontology, University of the Western Cape Dental Faculty, Cape Town, South Africa

4 International Centre for Genetic Engineering and Biotechnology (ICGEB), Cape Town, South Africa

5 Integrative Biomedical Sciences Division, Faculty of Health Sciences, University of the Cape Town, South Africa

*Address all correspondence to: hholmes@uwc.ac.za

References

[1] Adeola HA, Soyele OO, Adefuye AO, Jimoh SA, Butali A. Omics-based molecular techniques in oral pathology centered cancer: Prospect and challenges in Africa. Cancer Cell International. 2017;**17**:61

[2] Olson MV. The human genome project. Proceedings of the National Academy of Sciences of the United States of America. 1993;**90**:4338-4344

[3] Collins FS, Morgan M, Patrinos A. The human genome project: Lessons from large-scale biology. Science. 2003;**300**:286-290

[4] Green ED, Watson JD, Collins FS. Human genome project: Twenty-five years of big biology. Nature. 2015;**526**:29-31

[5] Hood L, Rowen L. The human genome project: Big science transforms biology and medicine. Genome Medicine. 2013;**5**:79

[6] Wilson BJ, Nicholls SG. The human genome project, and recent advances in personalized genomics. Risk Manag Healthc Policy. 2015;**8**:9-20

[7] Cho, J., Ahn, S., Son, D. S., Kim, N. K., et al., Bridging genomics and phenomics of gastric carcinoma. International journal of cancer. Journal international du cancer 2019, 145, 2407-2417.

[8] Davatzikos, C., Rathore, S., Bakas, S., Pati, S., et al., Cancer imaging phenomics toolkit: Quantitative imaging analytics for precision diagnostics and predictive modeling of clinical outcome. J Med Imaging (Bellingham) 2018, 5, 011018.

[9] Harder N, Athelogou M, Hessel H, Brieu N, et al. Tissue phenomics for prognostic biomarker discovery in low- and intermediate-risk prostate cancer. Scientific Reports. 2018;**8**:4470

[10] Bai Y, Zhao H. Liquid biopsy in tumors: Opportunities and challenges. Annals of translational medicine. 2018;**6**:S89

[11] Temilola DO, Wium M, Coulidiati TH, Adeola HA, et al. The Prospect and challenges to the flow of liquid biopsy in Africa. Cell. 2019;**8**

[12] Jacobson, R. A., Munding, E., Hayden, D. M., Levy, M., et al., Evolving clinical utility of liquid biopsy in gastrointestinal cancers. Cancers 2019, 11.

[13] Palmirotta, R., Lovero, D., Cafforio, P., Felici, C., et al., Liquid biopsy of cancer: A multimodal diagnostic tool in clinical oncology. Therapeutic advances in medical oncology 2018, 10, 1758835918794630.

[14] Wu J, Hu S, Zhang L, Xin J, et al. Tumor circulome in the liquid biopsies for cancer diagnosis and prognosis. Theranostics. 2020;**10**:4544-4556

[15] Chen L, Chen Y, Feng YL, Zhu Y, et al. Tumor circulome in the liquid biopsies for digestive tract cancer diagnosis and prognosis. World Journal of Clinical Cases. 2020;**8**:2066-2080

[16] Bracht JWP. Mayo-de-Las-casas, C., Berenguer, J., Karachaliou, N., Rosell, R., correction to: The present and future of liquid biopsies in non-small cell lung cancer: Combining four biosources for diagnosis, prognosis, prediction, and disease monitoring. Current Oncology Reports. 2020;**22**:52

[17] De Rubis G, Rajeev Krishnan S, Bebawy M. Liquid biopsies in cancer diagnosis, monitoring, and prognosis. Trends in Pharmacological Sciences. 2019;**40**:172-186

[18] Saarenheimo J, Eigeliene N, Andersen H, Tiirola M, Jekunen A. The value of liquid biopsies for guiding therapy decisions in non-small cell lung cancer. Frontiers in Oncology. 2019;**9**:129

[19] Nair S, Tang KD, Kenny L, Punyadeera C. Salivary exosomes as potential biomarkers in cancer. Oral Oncology. 2018;**84**:31-40

[20] Cheshmi B, Cheshomi H. Salivary exosomes: Properties, medical applications, and isolation methods. Molecular Biology Reports. 2020

[21] Zlotogorski-Hurvitz A, Dayan D, Chaushu G, Korvala J, et al. Human saliva-derived exosomes: Comparing methods of isolation. The Journal of Histochemistry and Cytochemistry. 2015;**63**:181-189

[22] Han Y, Jia L, Zheng Y, Li W. Salivary exosomes: Emerging roles in systemic disease. International Journal of Biological Sciences. 2018;**14**:633-643

[23] Cheng J, Nonaka T, Wong DTW. Salivary exosomes as nanocarriers for cancer biomarker delivery. Materials. 2019;**12**

[24] Nonaka T, Wong DTW. Saliva-exosomics in cancer: Molecular characterization of cancer-derived exosomes in Saliva. Enzyme. 2017;**42**:125-151

[25] Zhan C, Yang X, Yin X, Hou J. Exosomes and other extracellular vesicles in oral and salivary gland cancers. Oral Diseases. 2020;**26**:865-875

[26] Wang ZY, Li F, Rufo J, Chen CY, et al. Acoustofluidic salivary Exosome isolation a liquid biopsy compatible approach for human papillomavirus-associated oropharyngeal cancer detection. Journal of Molecular Diagnostics. 2020;**22**:50-59

[27] A review of saliva: normal composition, flow, and function. *Humphrey SP, Williamson RT J Prosthet Dent. 2001 Feb; 85(2):162-9.*

[28] Structure and biosynthesis of human salivary mucins. Zalewska A, Zwierz K. Żółkowski K, Gindzieński A Acta Biochim Pol. 2000;**47**(4):1067-1079

[29] Saliva and dental health. Clinical implications of saliva: report of a consensus meeting. Edgar WM Br Dent J. 1990 Aug 11-25; 169(3-4):96-8.

[30] Tiwari M. Science behind human saliva. Journal of natural science, biology, and medicine. 2011;**2**(1):53-58

[31] Cove-Smith R, Defective Saliva MA. Proceedings of the Royal Society of Medicine. 1935;**29**:126-127

[32] Farnaud SJ, Kosti O, Getting SJ, Renshaw D. Saliva: Physiology and diagnostic potential in health and disease. The Scientific World Journal. 2010;**10**:434-456

[33] Humphrey SP, Williamson RT. A review of saliva: Normal composition, flow, and function. The Journal of prosthetic dentistry. 2001 Feb 1;**85**(2):162-169

[34] Holsinger F, Bui D. Salivary Gland Disorders. Berlin, Germany: Springer; 2007

[35] Pharmacokinetic principles of drug distribution in saliva. Jusko WJ, Milsap RL. Annals of the New York Academy of Sciences. 1993 Sep 20;**694**:36-47

[36] The application of saliva, sweat and tear fluid for diagnostic purposes. Haeckel R, Hänecke P Ann Biol Clin (Paris). 1993;**51**(10-11):903-910

[37] Nagarathinam AE, Kumar TD, Kumar AR, Vasanthira K, Lakshmi RS,

Jayant VS. Salivary Urea and Creatinine as a Diagnostic Marker of Chronic Kidney Disease – Review. (IOSR-JDMS). 2017;**16**:95-100

[38] Schneyer LH, Schneyer CA. Secretion of Saliva. Advances in Oral Biology. 1964;**1**:1-31

[39] Leung SW. A demonstration of the importance of bicarbonate as a salivary buffer. Journal of Dental Research. 1951;**30**:403-414

[40] Lee JM, Garon E, Wong DT. Salivary diagnostics. Orthodontics & Craniofacial Research. 2009;**12**:206-211

[41] Hundt S, Haug U, Brenner H. Blood markers for early detection of colorectal cancer: A systematic review. Cancer Epidemiology and Prevention Biomarkers. 2007 Oct 1;**16**(10):1935-1953

[42] De Seny D, Fillet M, Meuwis MA, Geurts P, Lutteri L, Ribbens C, et al. Discovery of new rheumatoid arthritis biomarkers using the surface-enhanced laser desorption/ionization time-of-flight mass spectrometry ProteinChip approach. Arthritis and Rheumatism. 2005 Dec;**52**(12):3801-3812

[43] Hodgetts A, Levin M, Kroll JS, Langford PR. Biomarker discovery in infectious diseases using SELDI. Future Microbiology. 2007;**2**(1):35-49

[44] Suzuki M, Ross GF, Wiers K, et al. Identification of a urinary proteomic signature for lupus nephritis in children. Pediatric Nephrology. 2007;**22**(12):2047-2057

[45] C. S. Buhimschi, V. Bhandari, B. D. Hamar et al., "Proteomic profiling of the amniotic fluid to detect inflammation, infection, and neonatal sepsis," PLoS Medicine, vol. 4, no. 1, article e18, 2007.

[46] De Bock M, De Seny D, Meuwis MA, Chapelle JP, Louis E. Malaise M. Fillet M. Challenges for biomarker discovery in body fluids using SELDI-TOF-MS. Journal of Biomedicine and Biotechnology: Merville MP; 2009 Dec 6. p. 2010

[47] Malamud D. PhDa,b and Isaac R. Rodriguez-Chavez, PhDc, Saliva as a diagnostic fluid. Published in final edited form as: Dent Clin North Am. 2011 January;**55**(1):159-178

[48] Campo J, Perea MA, Del Romero J, Cano J, Hernando V, Bascones A. Oral transmission of HIV, reality or fiction? An update. Oral Diseases. 2006;**12**:219-228

[49] Wei F, Yang J, Wong DT. Detection of exosomal biomarker by electric field-induced release and measurement (EFIRM). Biosensors & Bioelectronics. 2013;**44**:115-121

[50] Wei F, Lin CC, Joon A, Feng Z, Troche G, Lira ME, et al. Noninvasive saliva-based EGFR gene mutation detection in patients with lung cancer. American Journal of Respiratory and Critical Care Medicine. 2014;**190**:1117-1126

[51] Han Y, Jia L, Zheng Y, Li W. Salivary exosomes: Emerging roles in systemic disease. International Journal of Biological Sciences. 2018;**14**:633-643

[52] Hessvik NP, Llorente A. Current knowledge on exosome biogenesis and release. Cellular and molecular life sciences : CMLS. 2018;**75**:193-208

[53] Baixauli F, Lopez-Otin C, Mittelbrunn M. Exosomes and autophagy: Coordinated mechanisms for the maintenance of cellular fitness. Frontiers in Immunology. 2014;**5**:403

[54] Lai R, Yeo R, Tan K, Lim S. Exosomes for drug delivery – A novel application for the mesenchymal stem cell. Biotech Adv. 2013;**31**:543-551

[55] Zheng X, CHEN F, ZHANG J, ZHANG Q, Exosome Analysis LINJ. A promising biomarker system with special attention to saliva. The Journal of Membrane Biology. 2014;**247**:1129-1136

[56] Johnstone RM. Revisiting the road to the discovery of exosomes. Blood Cells, Molecules & Diseases. 2005;**34**:214-219

[57] Simons M, Raposo G. Exosomes - vesicular carriers for intercellular communication. Current Opinion in Cell Biology. 2009;**21**:575-581

[58] Valadi H, Ekstrom K, Bossios A, Sjostrand M, et al. Exosome-mediated transfer of mRNAs and microRNAs is a novel mechanism of genetic exchange between cells. Nature Cell Biology. 2007;**9**:654-U672

[59] Mathivanan S, Fahner CJ, Reid GE, Simpson RJ. ExoCarta 2012: Database of exosomal proteins, RNA and lipids. Nucleic Acids Research. 2012;**40**:D1241-D1244

[60] Raposo G, Stoorvogel W. Extracellular vesicles: exosomes, microvesicles. and friends. The Journal of cell biology. 2013;**200**:373-383

[61] Record M, Carayon K, Poirot M, Silvente-Poirot S. Exosomes as new vesicular lipid transporters involved in cell-cell communication and various pathophysiologies. Biochimica et Biophysica Acta-Molecular and Cell Biology of Lipids. 2014;**1841**:108-120

[62] Becker A, Thakur BK, Weiss JM, Kim HS, et al. Extracellular vesicles in cancer: Cell-to-cell mediators of metastasis. Cancer Cell. 2016;**30**:836-848

[63] Costa-Silva, B., Aiello, N. M., Ocean, A. J., Singh, S., et al., Pancreatic cancer exosomes initiate pre-metastatic niche formation in the liver. Nat Cell Biol 2015, 17, 816−+.

[64] Hoshino, A., Costa-Silva, B., Shen, T. L., Rodrigues, G., et al., Tumour exosome integrins determine organotropic metastasis. Nature 2015, 527, 329−+.

[65] Kharaziha P, Ceder S, Li Q, Panaretakis T. Tumor cell-derived exosomes: A message in a bottle. Bba-Rev Cancer. 2012;**1826**:103-111

[66] Guo Q, Jiang C. Delivery strategies for macromolecular drugs in cancer therapy. Acta Pharmaceutica Sinica B. 2020;**10**:979-986

[67] Chiappin S, Antonelli G, Gatti R, De Palo EF. Saliva specimen: A new laboratory tool for diagnostic and basic investigation. Clinica Chimica Acta. 2007;**383**:30-40

[68] Yang, J., Wei, F., Schafer, C., Wong, D. T., Detection of tumor cell-specific mRNA and protein in exosome-like microvesicles from blood and saliva. PLoS One 2014, 9, e110641.

[69] Zhou HX, Xu WR, Qian H, Yin Q, et al. Circulating RNA as a novel tumor marker: An in vitro study of the origins and characteristics of extracellular RNA. Cancer Letters. 2008;**259**:50-60

[70] Aro K, Kaczor-Urbanowicz K, Carreras-Presas CM. Salivaomics in oral cancer. Current Opinion in Otolaryngology & Head and Neck Surgery. 2019;**27**:91-97

[71] Winck FV, Prado Ribeiro AC, Ramos Domingues R, Ling LY, Riaño-Pachón DM, Rivera C, et al. Insights into immune responses in oral cancer through proteomic analysis of saliva and salivary extracellular vesicles. Scientific Reports. 2015;**5**:16305

[72] Li L, Li C, Wang S, Wang Z, Jiang J, Wang W, et al. Exosomes derived from hypoxic oral squamous cell carcinoma cells deliver miR-21 to normoxic cells to elicit a prometastatic phenotype. Cancer research. 2016 Apr 1;**76**(7):1770-1780

[73] Sakha S, Muramatsu T, Ueda K, Inazawa J. Exosomal microRNA miR-1246 induces cell motility and invasion through the regulation of DENND2D in oral squamous cell carcinoma. Scientific Reports. 2016 Dec 8;**6**:38750

[74] Kawakubo-Yasukochi T, Morioka M, Hazekawa M, Yasukochi A, Nishinakagawa T, Ono K. miR-200c-3p spreads invasive capacity in human oral squamous cell carcinoma microenvironment. Molecular Carcinogenesis. 2017

[75] Li YY, Tao YW, Gao S, Li P, Zheng JM, Zhang SE, et al. Cancer-associated fibroblasts contribute to oral cancer cells proliferation and metastasis via exosome-mediated paracrine miR-34a-5p. eBioMedicine. 2018 Oct 1;**36**:209-220

[76] Li C, Zhou Y, Liu J, Su X, Qin H, Huang S, et al. Potential markers from serum-purified exosomes for detecting oral squamous cell carcinoma metastasis. Cancer Epidemiology and Prevention Biomarkers. 2019 Oct 1;**28**(10):1668-1681

[77] Xie C, Du LY, Guo F, Li X, Cheng B. Exosomes derived from microRNA-101-3p-overexpressing human bone marrow mesenchymal stem cells suppress oral cancer cell proliferation, invasion, and migration. Molecular and Cellular Biochemistry. 2019 Aug 15;**458**(1-2):11-26

[78] Sun LP, Xu K, Cui J, Yuan DY, Zou B, Li J, et al. Cancer-associated fibroblast-derived exosomal miR-382-5p promotes the migration and invasion of oral squamous cell carcinoma. Oncology reports. 2019 Oct 1;**42**(4):1319-1328

[79] He L, Ping F, Fan Z, Zhang C, Deng M, Cheng B, Xia J. Salivary exosomal miR-24-3p serves as a potential detective biomarker for oral squamous cell carcinoma screening. Biomedicine & Pharmacotherapy. 2020 Jan 1;121:109553.

[80] Chen JH, Wu AT, Bamodu OA, Yadav VK, Chao TY, Tzeng YM, et al. Ovatodiolide suppresses oral cancer malignancy by down-regulating exosomal mir-21/STAT3/β-catenin cargo and preventing oncogenic transformation of normal gingival fibroblasts. Cancers. 2020 Jan;**12**(1):56

[81] Kirave P, Gondaliya P, Kulkarni B, Rawal R, Garg R, Jain A, et al. Exosome mediated miR-155 delivery confers cisplatin chemoresistance in oral cancer cells via epithelial-mesenchymal transition. Oncotarget. 2020;**11**(13):1157-1171 https://doi.org/10.18632/oncotarget.27531

[82] Yeh CK, Christodoulides NJ, Floriano PN, Miller CS, et al. Current development of saliva/oral fluid-based diagnostics. Texas Dental Journal. 2010;**127**:651-661

[83] Yan W, Apweiler R, Balgley BM, Boontheung P, et al. Systematic comparison of the human saliva and plasma proteomes. Proteomics. Clinical Applications. 2009;**3**:116-134

[84] Ohshiro K, Rosenthal DI, Koomen JM, Streckfus CF, et al. Pre-analytic saliva processing affect proteomic results and biomarker screening of head and neck squamous carcinoma. International Journal of Oncology. 2007;**30**:743-749

[85] Hu S, Arellano M, Boontheung P, Wang JH, et al. Salivary proteomics for Oral cancer biomarker discovery. Clinical Cancer Research. 2008;**14**:6246-6252

[86] Dowling P, Wormald R, Meleady P, Henry M, et al. Analysis of the saliva proteome from patients with head and neck squamous cell carcinoma reveals differences in abundance levels of proteins associated with tumour progression and metastasis. Journal of Proteomics. 2008;**71**:168-175

[87] Rai B, Kaur J, Jacobs R, Anand SC. Adenosine deaminase in saliva as a diagnostic marker of squamous cell carcinoma of tongue. Clin Oral Invest. 2011;**15**:347-349

[88] Elashoff D, Zhou H, Reiss J, Wang JH, et al. Prevalidation of salivary biomarkers for Oral cancer detection. Cancer Epidem Biomar. 2012;**21**:664-672

[89] Winck FV, Prado Ribeiro AC, Ramos Domingues R, Ling LY, Riaño-Pachón DM, Rivera C, et al. Insights into immune responses in oral cancer through proteomic analysis of saliva and salivary extracellular vesicles. Scientific Reports. 2015;**5**:16305

[90] Zlotogorski-Hurvitz A, Dayan D, Chaushu G, Salo T, Vered M. Morphological and molecular features of oral fluid-derived exosomes: Oral cancer patients versus healthy individuals. Journal of Cancer Research and Clinical Oncology. 2016;**142**:101-110

[91] Ludwig S, Sharma P, Theodoraki MN, Pietrowska M, et al. Molecular and functional profiles of exosomes from HPV(+) and HPV(−) head and neck cancer cell lines. Frontiers in Oncology. 2018;**8**

[92] He L, Ping F, Fan ZN, Zhang C, et al. Salivary exosomal miR-24-3p serves as a potential detective biomarker for oral squamous cell carcinoma screening. Biomedicine & Pharmacotherapy. 2020;**121**

[93] Sakha S, Muramatsu T, Ueda K, Inazawa J. Exosomal microRNA miR-1246 induces cell motility and invasion through the regulation of DENND2D in oral squamous cell carcinoma. Scientific Reports. 2016;**6**

[94] Li L, Li C, Wang S, Wang Z, et al. Exosomes derived from hypoxic Oral squamous cell carcinoma cells deliver miR-21 to normoxic cells to elicit a Prometastatic phenotype. Cancer Research. 2016;**76**:1770-1780

[95] Valadi H, Ekstrom K, Bossios A, et al. Exosome-mediated transfer of mRNAs and microRNAs is a novel mechanism of genetic exchange between cells. Nature Cell Biology. 2007;**9**:654-659

[96] Skog J, Wurdinger T, van Rijn S, et al. Glioblastoma microvesicles transport RNA and proteins that promote tumour growth and provide diagnostic biomarkers. Nature Cell Biology. 2008;**10**:1470-1476

[97] Hong BS, Cho JH, Kim H, et al. Colorectal cancer cell-derived microvesicles are enriched in cell cycle-related mRNAs that promote proliferation of endothelial cells. BMC Genomics. 2009;**10**:556

[98] Li Y, John MA, Zhou X, Kim Y, Sinha U, Jordan RC, et al. Salivary transcriptome diagnostics for oral cancer detection. Clinical Cancer Research. 2004 Dec 15;**10**(24):8442-8450

[99] Ludwig N, Yerneni SS, Razzo BM, Whiteside TL. Exosomes from hnscc promote angiogenesis through reprogramming of endothelial cells. Molecular Cancer Research. 2018;**24**:24. DOI: 10.1158/1541-7786.MCR-18-0358

[100] Xiao C, Song F, Zheng YL, Lv J, et al. Exosomes in head and neck squamous cell carcinoma. Frontiers in Oncology. 2019;**9**:894

[101] Ludwig N, Gillespie DG, Reichert TE, Jackson EK, Whiteside TL. Purine metabolites in tumor-derived exosomes may facilitate immune escape of head and neck squamous cell carcinoma. Cancers. 2020;**12**

[102] Jelonek K, Wojakowska A, Marczak L, Muer A, et al. Ionizing radiation affects protein composition of

exosomes secreted in vitro from head and neck squamous cell carcinoma. Acta Biochimica Polonica. 2015;**62**:265-272

[103] Ebnoether E, Muller L. Diagnostic and therapeutic applications of exosomes in cancer with a special focus on head and neck squamous cell carcinoma (HNSCC). International Journal of Molecular Sciences. 2020;**21**

Chapter 3

Cytopathology of Intraoral Salivary Gland Tumours and Tumour-Like Lesions: Diagnostic Challenges and Pitfalls

Jai Kumar Chaurasia and Neelkamal Kapoor

Abstract

Fine needle aspiration cytology is an important diagnostic tool in cytopathology. There are many challenges and pitfalls encountered in intraoral salivary gland cytopathology as tumours of these glands show morphological diversity and overlapping features. There are often variable solid-cystic components, metaplastic or necrotic changes, fibrosis, hyalinisation and haemorrhage accounting for heterogeneity of these tumours. The tumour profile of intraoral salivary gland is quite different from the major salivary glands and needs special attention. A low-grade malignant tumour may sometimes mimic a benign neoplasm or a non-neoplastic lesion resulting in a false negative diagnosis. Moreover, misinterpretation and failure to recognize subtle morphological and architectural patterns of cells also pose diagnostic challenges. In this chapter, we intend to highlight the key cytopathological features of intraoral salivary gland tumours and tumour-like lesions with emphasis to overcome diagnostic challenges and pitfalls to avoid misdiagnosis which will aid in planning further management and treatment.

Keywords: Challenges, Cytopathology, Intraoral, Pitfalls, Salivary

1. Introduction

Fine needle aspiration cytology (FNAC) is an important diagnostic tool for initial evaluation of salivary gland (SG) tumours. The global annual incidence for all SG tumours varies from 0.4 to 13.5 cases per 100,000 population [1]. Tumours of intraoral salivary glands (SGs) are relatively uncommon as compared to tumours of major SGs and constitutes 10–15% of all SG tumours with relative frequency varying from 0.4% to 1.52% in different part of the world [2, 3]. These tumours have a very distinct profile from tumours of major SGs with reference to tumour histological type, clinical presentation and distribution. Majority of intraoral minor SG tumours are malignant in contrast to major SG tumours where benign tumours outnumber the malignant ones [4]. While some studies documents mucoepidermoid carcinoma (MEC) as the most common malignant tumour of minor SGs, other studies documents adenoid cystic carcinoma (ADCC) or pleomorphic adenoma (PA) as the most common tumour [5–10]. This difference in frequency of these histological types may be attributed to the differences in geographic location, race and varied clinical presentation. The clinical presentation of intraoral SG tumours also range from mild pain to visible palpable mass in the oral cavity with or without ulceration leading to obstructive features such as difficulty in swallowing and deglutition. These tumours can occur at various intraoral locations such as mucosa of lips and cheeks, hard and soft palate, uvula, floor of the mouth, tongue, retromolar area and peritonsillar region. The hard palate is the most common site of occurrence [3–5]. Cytopathological evaluation of intraoral SG tumours is challenging as these tumours show heterogeneity and considerable morphological diversity and overlap [6]. The correct preoperative cytopathological diagnosis of intraoral SG tumours is essential for deciding further course of management and treatment. We here present key cytomorphological features of intraoral salivary gland tumours and tumour-like lesions with emphasis to overcome diagnostic challenges and pitfalls.

2. FNAC: a vital diagnostic tool in salivary gland pathology

FNAC is easy, minimally invasive, cost effective technique which provides a rapid initial preoperative diagnosis of SG tumours and has an impact on subsequent management and treatment [11]. The sensitivity and specificity of FNAC in diagnosing SG tumours is 85–100% and 90–100% respectively. The aspirated material obtained through FNAC can also be utilized for special staining such as Periodic acid-Schiff (PAS), Periodic acid-Schiff with diastase (PAS-D), Mucicarmine, Phosphotungstic acid-haematoxylin (PTAH), Acid fast bacilli (AFB) and Gram staining for further evaluation and diagnosis. PAS-D and mucicarmine are particularly useful for highlighting mucin containing cells in challenging cases of low-grade mucoepidermoid carcinoma (MEC). Similarly, PTAH stain can be applied on paraffin-embedded cell block preparation for identification oncocytic cells in challenging diagnosis of tumours with oncocytic differentiation. The cell blocks can also be utilized for Immunohistochemistry (IHC) for demonstrating epithelial and myoepithelial components in diagnosis of challenging tumours. The epithelial cells are positive for immunohistochemical markers such as cytokeratin and epithelial membrane antigen (EMA) and the myoepithelial cells show positivity for smooth muscle actin (SMA), calponin, p63 and S-100. Further, the aspirated material can also be used for microbiological culture, immunophenotyping and molecular analysis for confirming the cytological diagnosis. While the FNAC of palpable lesions in major SGs is relatively easy, the FNAC of intraoral SGs is challenging as many times aspirates are not cellular as these intraoral sites are often difficult to approach and sometimes inaccessible [10–12]. In such cases, radiological-guided FNAC may be advised for better yield of aspirates for subsequent cytological diagnosis. Also, while performing FNAC, there are chances of complications such as hemorrhage, nerve pain and damage and infection. There can be post FNAC induced changes in tissue such as squamous metaplastic changes, inflammation, granulation tissue formation and sometimes infarction, which may interfere with subsequent histological diagnosis. Therefore, familiarity with key cytological features with recognition of the subtle cytomorphological changes in cells is crucial for overcoming barriers and making a correct diagnosis.

3. The Milan system for reporting salivary gland cytopathology

The Milan system for reporting salivary gland cytopathology (MSRSGC) is an evidence based international classification and was developed by international consortium with the aim to standardize reporting terminology for categorizing SG lesions [13]. The intraoral SG tumour and tumour-like lesions can also be categorized according to MSRSGC. The system has advantage and impact on clinical management of the patients [13, 14]. The system consists of following six broad diagnostic categories.

3.1 Category I: non-diagnostic

It includes FNAC smears with insufficient cellular material for making a definite diagnosis.

3.2 Category II: non-neoplastic

Includes FNAC smears with benign non-neoplastic lesions such as sialadenitis, sialolithiasis, granulomatous inflammation etc.

3.3 Category III: atypia of undetermined significance (AUS)

FNAC smears with limited cellular atypia that lacks qualitative or quantitative features of a neoplasm. Smears showing reactive or reparative atypia and metaplastic changes are included in this category.

3.4 Category IV

This category is classified into:

Category IVA: Benign Neoplasm – FNAC specimens showing characteristic cytomorphological features of a benign epithelial neoplasm.

Category IVB: Salivary Gland Neoplasm of Uncertain Malignant Potential (SUMP) – This category is most challenging as it includes FNAC specimens that have diagnostic feature of a neoplasm however, the possibility of malignant neoplasm cannot be excluded.

3.5 Category V: suspicious of malignancy

FNAC specimens that have some but not all the criteria for a specific diagnosis of malignancy and yet the overall cytologic features are sugsgestive of malignancy.

3.6 Category: VI malignant

FNAC specimens that are diagnostic of malignancy. The tumours of intraoral SGs with frank features of malignancy are included in this category.

4. Overview

In this chapter, the intraoral SG tumours and tumour-like lesions are being discussed under following six headings for better understanding of these tumours and related diagnostic challenges and pitfalls.

4.1 Matrix-containing tumours

The matrix producing tumours of intraoral SGs are pleomorphic adenoma (PA), adenoid cystic carcinoma (ADCC), polymorphous adenocarcinoma (POA). Carcinoma ex pleomorphic adenoma (CEPA), epithelial-myoepithelial carcinoma (EMC) are other matrix producing tumours that can also occur in intraoral SGs.

4.1.1 Pleomorphic adenoma (PA)

Pleomorphic adenoma is the most common benign tumour of SGs. Although, majority of PA occur in parotid gland, some studies documents PA as most common neoplasm in intraoral minor SGs [2, 4]. In the oral cavity, it usually presents as a solitary nodule or mass in the palate, sometimes with obstructive clinical symptoms.

Key cytological features – Smears show variable cellularity with cells arranged in clusters and sheets, embedded in a fibrillary chondromyxoid ground substance or matrix (**Figure 1**). The majority of cells are myoepithelial which may be ovoid, spindle, plasmacytoid, epithelioid, clear or stellate shaped. The nuclei of cells are round to oval, often with eccentric nucleus with bland finely granular chromatin and inconspicuous nucleoli. The cytoplasm is pale with well-defined cell borders. Stripped naked nuclei are not seen. PA may show diverse metaplastic changes including squamous metaplasia with or without keratinisation, oncocytic, clear cell, sebaceous, lipomatous and cartilaginous metaplasia. Hyaline globules can be seen. The prototypical PA is placed in benign category (IVA) of the Milan system.

Diagnostic challenges and pitfalls – Pleomorphic Adenoma (PA)

a. Sometimes, aspirate from PA may consist of only chondromyxoid substance without presence of epithelial and myoepithelial cells. The diagnosis of a neoplasm can be suspected but reaspiration is needed to rule out the possibility of other matrix producing tumours such as adenoid cystic carcinoma (ADCC) which can also occur at various intraoral locations. Both of these tumours have fibrillar metachromatic matrix and may show formation of hyaline globules. However, the matrix in PA is fibrillar with frayed edges (**Figure 2a**) while in ADCC the matrix is in form of beaded finger-like fragments, acellular spheres and tubules with sharply defined edges (**Figure 2b**) [15, 16]. Cellular PA with scant matrix particularly may resemble solid variant of ADCC. The cells of ADCC are basaloid and careful examination of nuclear chromatin of cells reveals distinguishing features. The cells in PA have bland finely granular chromatin while the cells of ADCC have coarse nuclear chromatin, high nuclear-cytoplasmic (N:C) ratio, scant cytoplasm and nucleoli [15]. The cells of ADCC may show focal nuclear moulding. Stripped naked nuclei can be seen in ADCC but not in PA. However, in challenging cases, it is not always possible to distinguish between the two entities. Such cases may be placed in SUMP category (IVB) of the Milan system. Follow-up and excision may be advised keeping clinical context in mind.

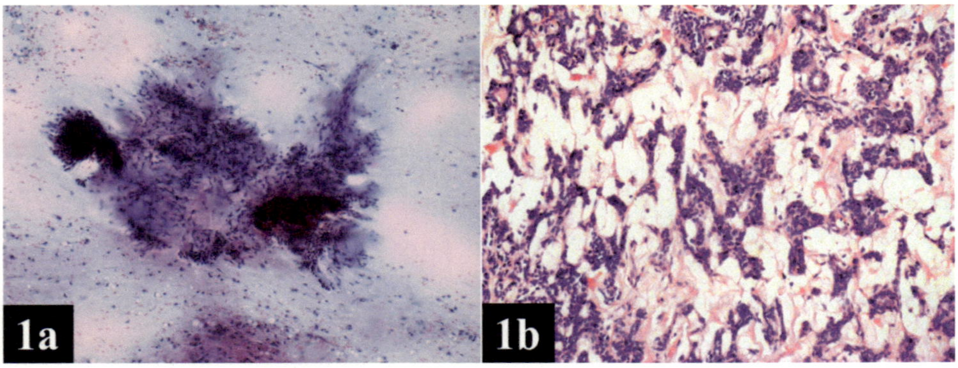

Figure 1.
1a: FNAC smear showing abundant chondromyxoid matrix with embedded cells in a case of pleomorphic adenoma (May-Grunwald Giemsa stain x 40), 1b: Corresponding histopathology showing nests, interlacing cords and strands of epithelial and myoepithelial cells in a myxoid stroma (Haematoxylin & Eosin x 40).

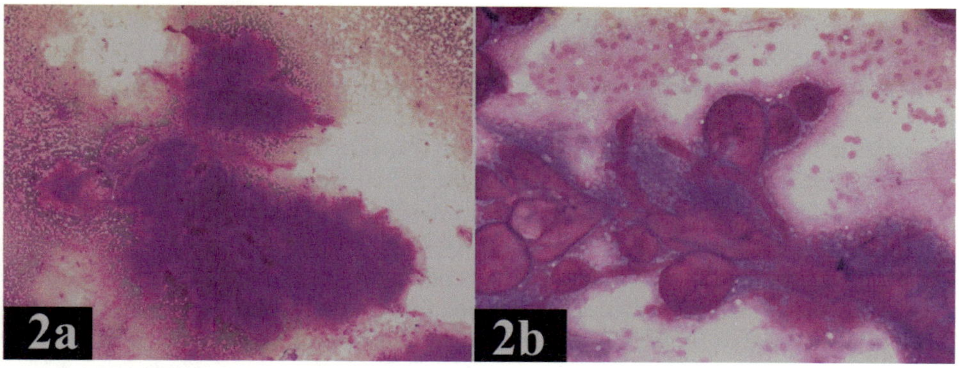

Figure 2.
2a: Smear showing abundant fibrillar metachromatic matrix with frayed edges in pleomorphic adenoma (May-Grunwald Giemsa stain x 40), 2b: Showing metachromatic matrix in form of acellular beaded, finger-like fragments and hyaline spherical globules with well-defined borders in a case of adenoid cystic carcinoma (May-Grunwald Giemsa stain x 40).

b. Cells in PA may undergo cystic and metaplastic changes. The aspirate may consist of metaplastic squamous cells with or without keratinisation (**Figure 3**) and scant or absent fibrillar metrachromatic matrix which can raise suspicion of a low-grade mucoepidermoid carcinoma (MEC) [16]. The intermediate cells of MEC in particular resemble squamous metaplastic cells of PA. However, the MEC usually have a dirty background and lacks myoepithelial cells, chondromyxoid material and keratinisation. One should also search for mucus cells, if MEC is suspected. In challenging cases, mucin containing cells of MEC can be demonstrated by using PAS-D or mucicarmine staining on cell blocks.

c. The myoepithelial cells in PA may sometimes show reactive atypia and prominent anisokaryosis which may sometimes be difficult to distinguish from malignant tumours [17]. Cells with reactive atypia can be recognized as they have bland chromatin and inconspicuous mitotic activity. The diagnostic pitfall is the occurrence of carcinoma ex-pleomorphic adenoma (CEPA). The development of CEPA in pre-existing intraoral PA is rare but few cases have been reported in literature [18]. History of long standing or recurrent PA in oral cavity with recent sudden increase in size along with cytological evidence

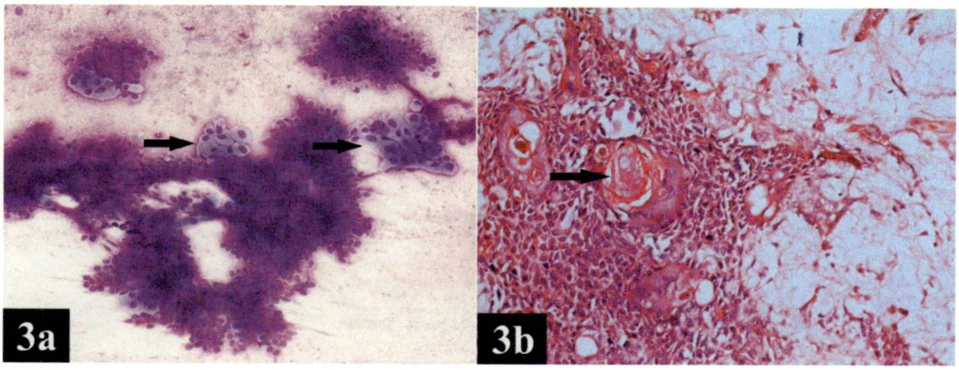

Figure 3.
3a: FNAC smear showing pleomorphic adenoma with squamous metaplasia (arrows) (May-Grunwald Giemsa stain x 4), 3b: Corresponding histology showing squamous metaplasia with evidence of keratinisation (arrow) surrounded by myxoid stroma (Haematoxylin & Eosin x 40).

of high grade atypical features in cells (**Figure 4**) and even a focal presence of areas depicting conventional PA consisting of benign cell clusters and chondromyxoid matrix (**Figure 4**), should lead to the diagnosis of CEPA [18, 19].

d. Epithelial-myoepithelial carcinoma (EMC) may sometimes also simulate a PA. It is a an unusual tumour and can also occur in minor SGs and palate [20]. This tumour can also have hyaline globules and show thin basement membrane-like metachromatic material around the clusters of cells. The predominant cell of EMC is myoepithelial. These cells are larger with abundant fragile clear delicate cytoplasm. Unlike PA, naked or stripped nuclei can be seen. Moreover, the biphasic population of epithelial and myoepithelial cells can be identified in EMC. The key cytological features and pitfalls of EMC are discussed at 4.3.1.

e. PA with predominant myoepithelial component (**Figure 5a**) may resemble other myoepithelial cell containing tumours such as myoepithelioma/myoepithelial adenoma (**Figure 5b**) in oral cavity. Myoepithelioma lacks chondroid stroma and duct cells seen of PA [21]. Distinction may not always be possible

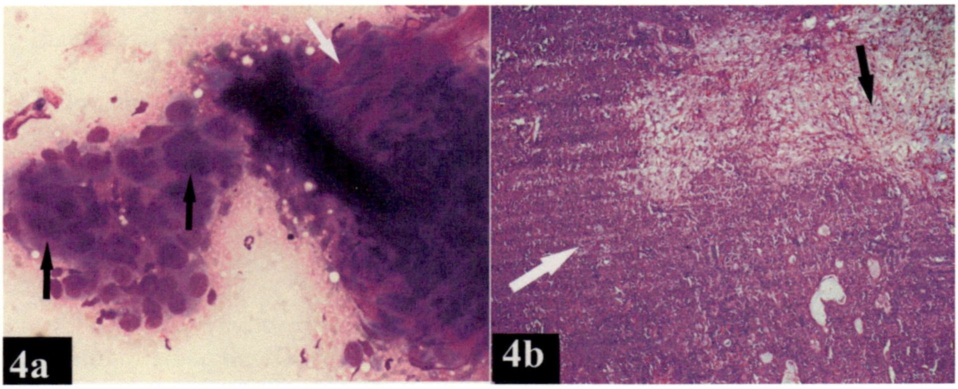

Figure 4.
4a: Showing malignant cells with high N:C ratio and hyperchromatic nuclei (black arrows) in a case of carcinoma ex-pleomorphic adenoma with evidence of metachromatic matrix of pre-existing pleomorphic adenoma (white arrow) (May-Grunwald Giemsa stain x 40), 4b: Corresponding histology showing sheet of malignant cells (white arrow) arising in background of myxoid stroma (black arrow) of pleomorphic adenoma (Haematoxylin & Eosin x 10).

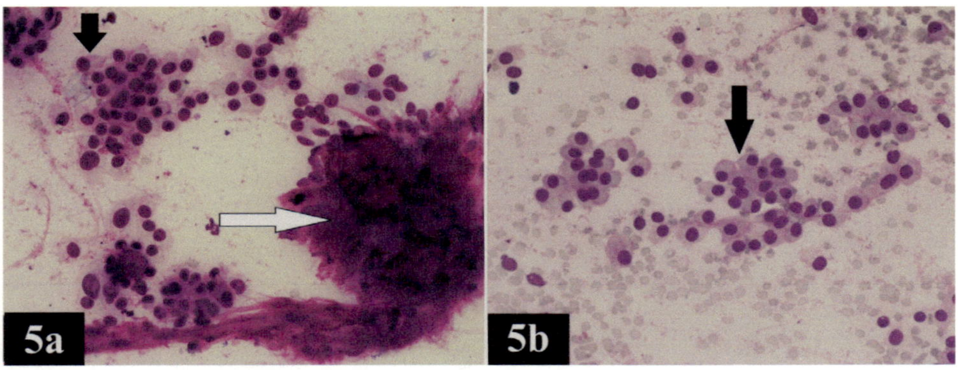

Figure 5.
5a: FNAC smear showing population of myoepithelial cells (black arrow) with metachromatic matrix (white arrow) in a case of myoepithelial predominant pleomorphic adenoma (May-Grunwald Giemsa stain x 40). 5b: Smear showing myoepithelial cells with pale to clear cytoplasm (arrow) in a case of a myoepithelioma (May-Grunwald Giemsa stain x 40).

and is not of much significance as both entities are benign (Milan system category IVA) and management is almost similar.

4.1.2 Adenoid cystic carcinoma (ADCC)

It constitutes nearly 10% of all SG tumours. Some studies suggest it to be the most common malignancy in minor salivary gland with hard palate being the most common site [22–24].

Key cytological features – Smears are cellular and cells are seen in clusters showing overlapping and multilayering. Tumour cells are also seen arranged in cup-shaped fragments and also scattered singly (**Figure 6**). The cells are basaloid with scant cytoplasm, round to ovoid hyperchromatic nuclei with coarse nuclear chromatin and nucleoli. The metachromatic matrix is in form of acellular beaded, finger like fragments, branching tubules and also forms hyaline spherical globules with well-defined borders (**Figure 2b**).

Diagnostic challenges and pitfalls – ***Adenoid Cystic Carcinoma (ADCC)***

a. PA and its distinguishing features from ADCC are discussed at 4.1.1a. However, the diagnosis of solid variant of ADCC is challenging as it lacks metachromatic matrix [25]. It can be distinguished from PA as it shows three dimensional clusters of basaloid cells with variable degree of pleomorphism. The cells are more hyperchromatic and angulated than in PA. In contrast to PA, mitosis, apoptosis and necrosis can also be seen [25]. IHC on cell blocks with CD -117 can be done in challenging cases which shows strong cytoplasmic positivity in ADCC [25, 26].

b. Sometimes, the basement membrane-like metachromatic material in EMC forms large globules resembling ADCC but the cellular compartment is entirely different in ADCC [26]. The cells of ADCC are basaloid with scant cytoplasm with round to ovoid hyperchromatic nuclei with coarse nuclear chromatin and nucleoli in contrast to myoepithelial cells of EMC with clear cytoplasm and round nuclei and vesicular chromatin [26].

c. Basal Cell Adenoma (BCA) can resemble ADCC. However, BCA arise predominantly in parotid and is extremely rare in the intraoral minor SGs [27]. It also shows metachromatic matrix and basement membrane like material and

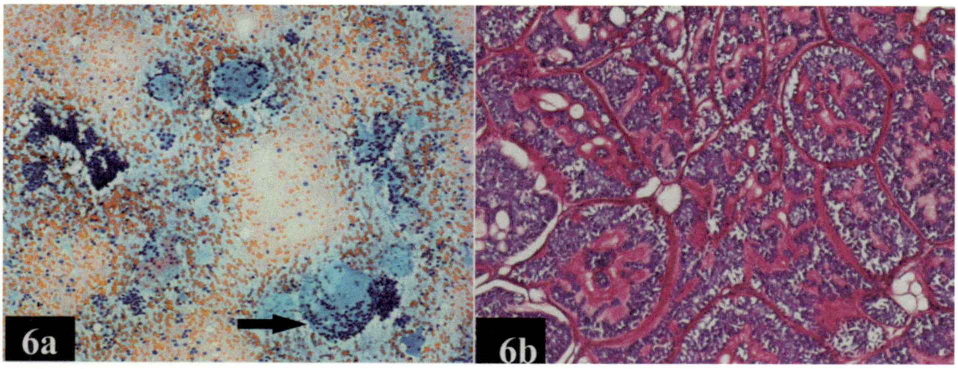

Figure 6.
6a: Smear showing large hyaline spherical globules with well-defined borders with attached tumour cells in cup-shaped fashion (arrow) and also scattered singly in a case of adenoid cystic carcinoma (Papanicolaou stain x 4). 6b: Corresponding histological section showing tumour cells surrounded by basement membrane-like metachromatic material (PAS x 40).

basaloid cells similar to ADCC but cells have granular chromatin rather than coarse nuclear chromatin seen in ADCC. The cells occasionally show peripheral palisading. Squamous morules or metaplasia can be frequently seen in BCA but not in ADCC.

d. Canalicular (CA) /Ductal Adenoma occurs in oral cavity predominantly in upper lip and buccal region [28]. It has overlapping cytological features with BCA. Cells of CA are cuboidal to columnar and are seen in clusters and cords. Unlike ADCC, the cells are monomorphic with finely dispersed chromatin and inconspicuous nucleoli.

4.1.3 Polymorphous adenocarcinoma (POA)

Previously called as polymorphous low grade adenocarcinoma, it is a low-grade matrix containing tumour occurring predominantly in intraoral minor salivary gland with palate being the most common site [29].

Key cytological features – Cells are seen in clusters, papillae, trabeculae, singly scattered and also in form of epithelial fragments attached to fibrovascular stromal cores (**Figure** 7). The cells are monomorphic with oval nuclei, open chromatin and indistinct nucleoli with moderate amount of cytoplasm. Small hyaline globules can be seen admixed with these cells.

Diagnostic challenges and pitfalls – Polymorphous Adenocarcinoma (POA). The cytological features of POA may resemble PA or ADCC [30]. The matrix of POA may be fibrillar and myxoid resembling a PA or can form hyaline globules similar to ADCC. However, the papillary architecture of cells is found in POA and its presence can distinguish it from PA and ADCC. The cells of ADCC are basaloid with coarse nuclear features rather than fine open nuclear features seen in POA [30].

4.2 Cystic tumours

Cystic tumours of intraoral SGs range from benign tumours such as sclerosing polycystic adenosis, cystadenoma, cystic PA, duct papilloma to malignant tumours such as low-grade MEC and papillary cystic variant of acinic cell carcinoma (AciCC). Evaluation and interpretation of these cystic tumours is particularly challenging as usually the aspirate of these tumours is hypocellular. This may result in false negative diagnosis particularly in a low-grade malignant cystic tumours.

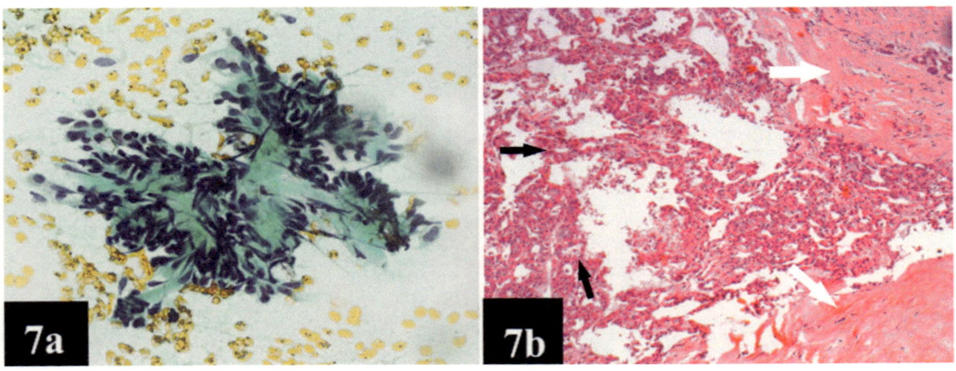

Figure 7.
7a: Smear showing monomorphic small round to oval epithelial cells attached to fibrous stromal core in a case of polymorphous adenocarcinoma (Papanicolaou stain x 40), 7b: Corresponding histology showing growth of tumour cells in glandular and acinar pattern (black arrows) surrounded by adjacent fibrous stroma (white arrows) (Haematoxylin & Eosin x 10).

Diagnostic challenges and Pitfalls – Cystic Tumours

a. **Sclerosing polycystic adenosis (SPA)** is a rare benign tumour reported in intraoral minor SGs [31]. It is predominantly cystic and shares common features with fibrocystic disease and sclerosing adenosis of the breast. The key cytological features include epithelial cells in syncytial sheets with apocrine changes with variable granular to oncocytic and vacuolated cytoplasm in a cystic background consisting of foamy histiocytes and proteinaceous material. SPA is frequently associated with intraductal proliferations. Ductal cells of SPA with vacuolated cytoplasm can resemble cells of AciCC or a low-grade cystic MEC. However, the apocrine metaplastic changes in cells is the key feature which in proper clinical context of long history of benign tumour favours a diagnosis of SPA over other carcinomas [31].

b. **Cystadenoma** is also a rare benign tumour occurring in minor SGs [32]. The tumour is multicystic and cytology reveals cuboidal to columnar cells in clusters and papillae with bland nuclear features and oncocytic cytoplasm. The cytoplasm of cells may sometimes become epidermoid and may resemble cells of low-grade MEC. Cystadenoma is indistinguishable from cystadenomacarcinoma on cytology. Histological evidence of invasion is required for diagnosis of cystadenocarcinoma [32].

c. **Duct papilloma (DP)** is a benign tumour arising predominantly from the ducts of minor SGs and characterized by intraductal proliferation of cells in form of broad papillary projections [33]. It is composed of epidermoid cells and mucous cells and can resemble a MEC. However, the papillary architecture of DP can help to distinguish it from MEC.

d. **Mucoepidermoid carcinoma (MEC)** – It is the most common malignancy of intraoral SGs in young adults and children [7–9]. Palate is the most common site of occurrence. It is composed of mucin containing cells, intermediate cells and epidermoid/squamous cells. The low-grade MEC is cystic and particularly challenging as it mimics other cystic neoplasms and non-neoplastic cystic tumour-like lesions [34]. Aspirates from low-grade MEC show mucin containing vacuolated cells in a predominantly cystic background with debris. However, it can be recognized by presence of at least few or occasional cluster or single intermediate or epidermoid cells (**Figure 8**). Intermediate

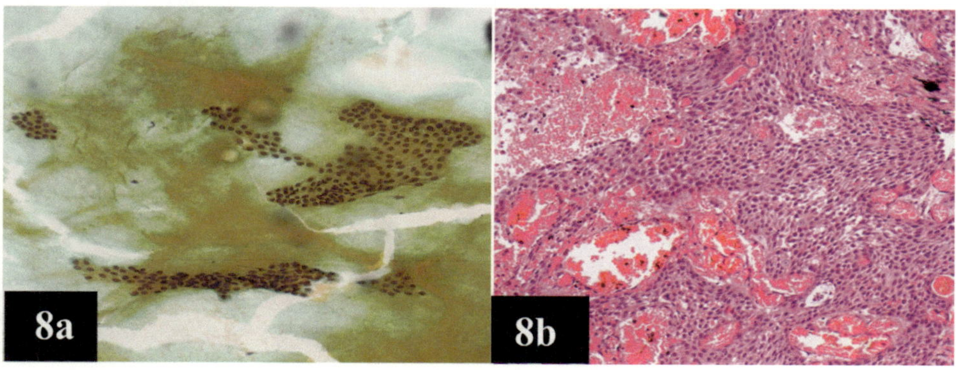

Figure 8.
8a: Showing small sheets and clusters of epidermoid cells in a cystic mucoid background in a case of low-grade mucoepidermoid carcinoma (Papanicolaou stain x 10), 8b: Corresponding histology showing sheets of epidermoid cells (Haematoxylin & Eosin x 10).

cells appear like a metaplastic squamous cell. Mucin filled cells can also be demonstrated by using mucicarmine staining on cell blocks. Sometimes, epithelial cells are not aspirated and aspirate consist of only mucoid material with few histiocytes and muciphages resembling a mucocele [35]. In proper clinical contexts, such cases should be reported with differential diagnosis of low-grade MEC and must be followed-up. High-grade MEC is predominantly solid but can have a cystic component. Smears from a high-grade MEC are cellular and are readily recognisable and shows three-dimensional clusters and sheets of atypical cells with malignant squamoid features. The cells are polygonal and have a high N:C ratio with hyperchromatic nuclei often with a prominent nucleolus. If a high-grade MEC is suspected, search should be done for mucin containing vacuolated cells. Moreover, keratinsation is not the feature of MEC which can aid in distinguishing MEC from metastatic squamous cell carcinoma [35].

e. **Cystic pleomorphic adenoma (PA)** may sometimes mimic a low-grade MEC [35]. However, identification of even a focal metachromatic fibrillary material gives clues to the diagnosis. The differentiating features of PA from MEC are discussed at 4.1.1b.

f. **Papillary cystic variant of AciCC** is another important differential in cystic SG tumours [36]. It is distinguished from other low-grade carcinomas as it shows polygonal cells with fine, abundant, delicate and vacuolated cytoplasm similar to conventional AciCC but arranged in a predominant papillary pattern consisting of a cells attached to a capillary meshwork or around a fibrovascular core (**Figure 9**) [36]. The background is cystic and can show presence of lympho-histiocytes.

4.3 Tumours with clear cell and vacuolated cell pattern

The differential diagnosis of tumours of intraoral SGs comprising of clear cells and vacuolated cell pattern include – Epithelial–Myoepithelial carcinoma (EMC), Myoepithelial tumours such as myoepithelioma (ME) and myoepithelial carcinoma (MC), clear cell carcinoma (CCC), mucoepidermoid carcinoma (MEC), acinic cell carcinoma (AciCC), secretory carcinoma (SC).

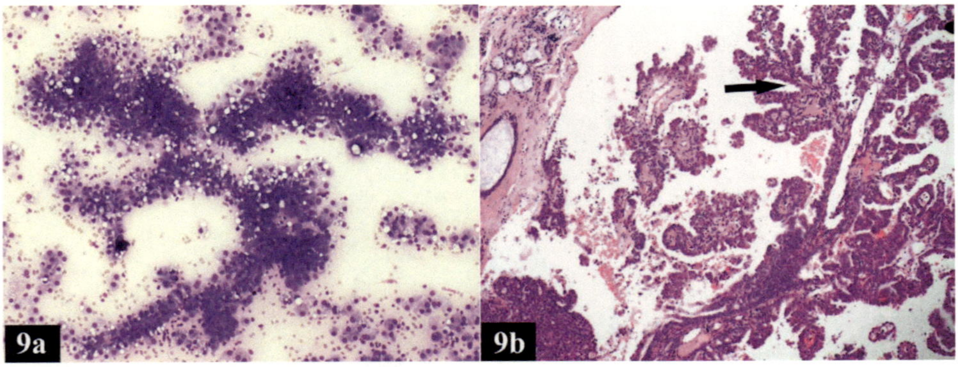

Figure 9.
9a: Showing cells arranged in a predominant papillary architecture with fine fibrovascular core in a case of acinic cell carcinoma. The cells have fine vacuolated cytoplasm (May-Grunwald Giemsa stain x 4), 9b: Corresponding histology showing branching papillae (arrow) with fibrovascular core (Haematoxylin & Eosin x 4).

4.3.1 Epithelial–myoepithelial carcinoma (EMC)

It is a an unusual tumour of major salivary gland predominantly occurring in parotid (60–80%) but can also be seen in minor SGS [20]. Palate is the most common site of occurrence and clinical presentation can be a ulcerative nodular lesion.

Key cytological features – The smears are cellular comprising of biphasic population of epithelial and myoepithelial cells. The myoepithelial cells are seen in loosly cohesive sheets, clusters and spheres with fragile, pale to clear delicate glycogen rich cytoplasm that disperses in background resulting in many naked or stripped nuclei. The nucleus of myoepithelial cells is round to oval with open chromatin and small distinct nucleoli (**Figure 10a**). Epithelial cells are seen usually in tight cohesive clusters. Sometimes mild nuclear atypia can be encountered. Hyaline stromal globules and basement membrane-like material can also be seen. The biphasic pattern of EMC can be demonstrated by using IHC on cell blocks with low molecular weight keratin and epithelial membrane antigen (EMA) for highlighting the duct cells and with smooth muscle actin (SMA), calponin, p63 and S-100 for highlighting the myoepithelial cells component [37]. Points of differentiation of EMC with other tumours with clear and vacuolated cells are discussed with each individual tumour.

4.3.2 Myoepithelioma (ME)

Myoepithelioma (ME) is a benign tumour that can occur in minor SGs with palate being the most common site. The myoepithelial cells in ME have pale to clear cytoplasm (**Figure 5b**), resembling myoepithelial cells of EMC. However, the myoepithelial cells of EMC are larger than that of ME due to presence of abundant glycogen [21]. Also, ME lacks the biphasic pattern of EMC (**Figure 10a**). ME may undergo transformation into myoepithelial carcinoma (MC). However, atypical cytological features such as nuclear pleomorphism, coarse chromatin with prominent nucleoli with background necrosis and mitotic activity seen in MC can differentiate between the two [21]. Differentiation of ME from cellular PA with predominant myoepithelial component is already discussed at 4.1.1e.

4.3.3 Clear cell carcinoma (CCC)

Clear cell carcinoma (CCC) of the SG is a rare low-grade malignancy that occurs primarily in intraoral minor salivary glands predominantly in the palate [38].

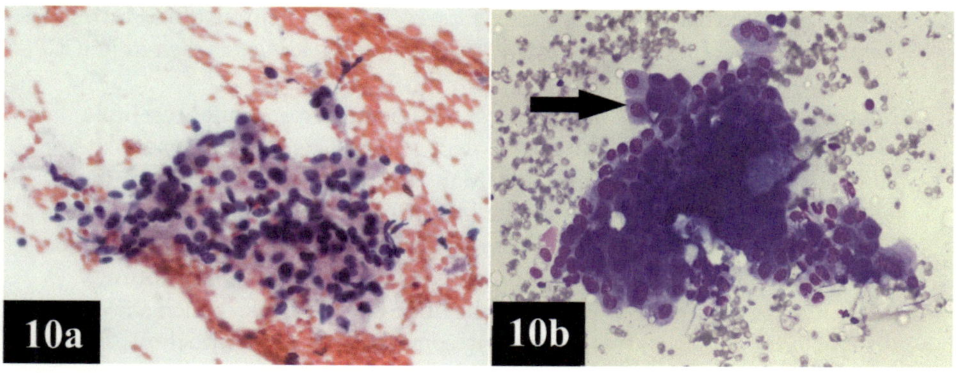

Figure 10.
10a: Smear showing admixture of dual population of cells comprising of epithelial and myoepithelial cells in a case of epithelial myoepithelial carcinoma (Haematoxylin & Eosin x 40), 10b:s Smear showing a cluster of cells with multilayering of round to polygonal oncocytic cells (arrow) with round nucleus and abundant dense granular cytoplasm in a case of an oncocytoma (May-Grunwald Giemsa stain x 40)

Epithelial cells of CCC are seen in clusters and sheets with prominent cell borders, uniform round to ovoid nuclei, granular chromatin and abundant glycogen rich clear cytoplasm. The cells of **CCC** may resemble myoepithelial cells of EMC. Unlike EMC, CCC lack evidence of either ductal or myoepithelial differentiation.

Clear cells can be encountered in MEC of minor SGs. However, identification of other accompanying cells (intermediate and epidermoid cells) in MEC gives clues to the diagnosis [34]. Mucin in cells of MEC can also be demonstrated by mucicarmine stain on cell blocks.

4.3.4 Acinic cell carcinoma (AciCC)

It is a low-grade tumour having predominantly vacuolated cell morphology. AciCC predominantly occurs in parotid (75–90%) and the remaining cases occur in intraoral minor salivary glands predominantly in buccal mucosa [39].

Key cytological features – Smears are cellular and consist of cells in three-dimensional clusters, sheets, micro-acinar groups and papillae with scant inconspicuous fibrovascular stroma. The cells are large with abundant fragile vacuolated basophilic to eosinophilic cytoplasm [40]. The nuclei are round, uniform with bland chromatin. Sometimes, the cells show oncocytic or clear cell changes. The background is clean with presence of bare stripped nuclei. The papillary cystic variant also has cells similar to conventional AciCC but the cells are arranged in a predominant papillary pattern with cells attached to a capillary meshwork or around a fibrovascular core (**Figure 9**). The cytoplasmic zymogen granules in AciCC can be demonstrated by PAS-D stain. Recent studies of IHC on cell blocks with DOG 1 reveals strong diffuse granular cytoplasmic positivity in AciCC [41].

Diagnostic challenges and pitfalls – Acinic Cell Carcinoma (AciCC)

a. Sometimes, aspirates from non-neoplastic SG tissue may resemble cells of AciCC. Single stripped nucleus of non-neoplastic SG may be difficult to distinguish from AciCC. However, cell groups and clusters of AciCC can be identified as they show three dimensional architecture with overlapping unlike the regularly arranged acini attached to duct with a thin fibrovascular core in a normal non-neoplastic SG tissue [40].

b. Sebaceous adenoma (SA) and sebaceous lymphadenoma are benign tumours and can occur in minor SGs and also have cells with vacuolated to clear cytoplasm [42]. Similarly, sebaceous carcinoma may arise rarely in intraoral SGs. The cells of these tumours contain cytoplasmic fat which can be demonstrated by oil-red O staining. PAS-D staining is negative for zymogen granules as seen in AciCC.

c. Cells of AciCC may show oncocyte like changes and sometimes resemble an oncocytoma. However, the typical cells of AciCC with finely vacuolated delicate cytoplasm can be identified. Many stripped or bare nuclei are also seen which are absent in oncocytoma [40]. Cell block preparation can be used to demonstrate periodic acid Schiff with diastase (PAS-D) positive zymogen granules in AciCC. Also, if oncocytoma is suspected, then phosphotungstic acid-haematoxylin (PTAH) stain can be done on cell blocks which shows strong positive cytoplasmic staining due to presence of abundant mitochondria.

d. AciCC may show clear cells which may resemble other tumours with clear cells such as EMC. The biphasic population of myoepithelial and epithelial cell can identified in EMC. The key cytological features of EMC are discussed at 4.3.1.

4.3.5 Secretory carcinoma (SC)

Previously called as mammary analogue secretory carcinoma, it is a new subtype of SG carcinoma and is reported to occur in minor salivary gland [43]. It also shows cells with vacuolated to clear cytoplasm.

Key cytological features – Aspirates show loosely cohesive epithelial cells arranged in small sheets, papillary fragments, acinar groups or follicular structures and also dispersed singly. The cells show variable cytoplasm ranging from granular to vacuolated and eosinophilic to clear cytoplasm. The cells show minimal or no pleomorphism. Background shows mucinous material.

Diagnostic challenges and pitfalls – The vacuolated cells may resemble cells of AciCC but lack intracytoplamic zymogen granules. Also, IHC on cell blocks is positive for markers such as mammaglobin, S-100 and vimentin and negative for DOG1 [41, 43].

4.4 Oncocytic tumours

4.4.1 Oncocytoma

Oncocytoma is a benign tumours of SG predominantly occurring in parotid. However, these tumours are also known to occur in intraoral minor SGs [44].

Key cytological features – The cells are seen in two or three dimensional and multilayered clusters. The cells are round to polygonal with oncocytic morphology consisting of dense granular abundant cytoplasm with a round nucleus and distinct nucleolus (**Figure 10b**). The background is clean without debris, fluid and lymphocytes. The oncocytic cytoplasm of cells containing abundant mitochondria can be highlighted by strong positivity for phosphotungstic acid-haematoxylin (PTAH) stain.

Diagnostic challenges and pitfalls – Oncocytic Tumours

a. The presence of oncocytes can be seen in other tumours of SGs particularly acinic cell carcinoma (AciCC) and less commonly in mucoepidermoid carcinoma (MEC) [40, 45, 46]. The distinguishing features of oncocytoma from AciCC are discussed at 4.3.5c.

b. Intraoral PA may also undergo metaplastic oncocytic change through a process known as oncocytosis. Oncocytosis is characterized by metaplastic change in SGs. Sometimes, entire salivary gland parenchyma is replaced by oncocytes mimicking an oncocytoma [45, 46]. But the typical metachromatic fibrillary matrix can usually be identified after adequate sampling in PA.

c. Oncocytic variant of mucoepidermoid carcinoma (OMEC) is a low-grade tumour and may resemble an oncocytoma as it shows bland oncocytic cells with minimal nuclear atypia [47]. However, it shows characteristic mucinous goblet cells of MEC. Also, epidermoid and intermediate cells should always be searched upon, if OMEC is suspected. Cell block can also be used to confirm mucin in goblet cells by mucicarmine staining.

d. Oncocytic carcinoma is a rare aggressive carcinoma and may develop in pre-existing oncocytoma. However, it can be distinguished from oncocytoma as it shows atypical oncocytic cells with nuclear pleomorphism. Mitosis and necrosis can also be seen.

e. Warthin's Tumour constitutes 5–15% of all salivary gland tumours. Although, it shows cohesive two or three- dimensional clusters of oncocytic cells resembling an oncocytoma but it occurs almost exclusively within the parotid gland [46]. The background is usually cystic with debris, lymphocytes and lympho-histiocytes.

4.5 Other carcinoma of intraoral salivary glands

4.5.1 Adenocarcinoma not otherwise specified (NOS)

It is an aggressive invasive tumour showing features that are not specific for any particular tumour type. It is a usually a diagnosis of exclusion. It constitutes 10–15% of all SG tumours and about 40% cases are reported in minor salivary glands with palate being the most common site [48].

Key cytological features – It shows glandular or ductal differentiation but patterns and cellular features are non-specific. The cells may be seen in nests, tubules, clusters or cords. The cellular features are variable and range from subtle low-grade tumours to a high-grade carcinoma.

Other SG carcinomas such as salivary duct carcinomas, intraductal carcinoma, lymphoepithelial carcinoma, primary squamous cell carcinoma and carcinosarcomas are rare and are reported to occur in major salivary gland and not in intraoral minor SGs.

4.6 Tumour-like lesions of intraoral salivary glands

4.6.1 Mucocele

Amongst non-neoplastic lesions, mucocele or mucous retention cyst occur in intraoral SGs and can mimic a low-grade cystic tumour. Mucocele is a pseudocyst which lack epithelial lining and contain extravasated mucin. These usually develops in minor SGs particularly on the lips and other sites such as tongue [49]. FNAC smears from mucocele are hypocellular with histiocytes and muciphages in an abundant mucoid background. Few giant cells can also be seen. Cystic consistency and mucoid background with muciphages may raise a possibility of low-grade MEC but other features of MEC such as intermediate and epidermoid cells are absent.

4.6.2 Sialadenosis (SA)

Sialadenosis (SA) is non-inflammatory and non-neoplastic enlargement of SGs predominantly occurring in parotid. However, it is also documented to occur in minor SGs in few reports in literature [50]. Aspirates from SA show plenty of acinar cells with hypertrophic changes. Sometimes, the cells may resemble cells of AciCC but in SA the architecture of normal SG tissue is maintained with regularly arranged acini instead of overlapping three-dimensional clusters, groups and sheets of acini in AciCC.

4.6.3 Sialadenitis

Inflammation of SGs may result from various causes but predominantly it occurs due to stenosis or obstruction of SG ducts because of sialolithiasis, trauma or secondary involvement by tumours [51, 52]. It may present with swelling and sometimes mimic a neoplasm.

4.6.4 Acute sialadenitis (AS)

Acute sialadenitis (AS) is usually a bacterial inflammation of the SGs and usually affects the parotid. However, it may also affect minor SGs [52]. Aspirates from AS usually shows abundant neutrophils, macrophages, few duct cells with reactive changes in a degenerating background. Sometimes, AS may occur as a part of underlying tumour. Non-regressive swelling on antibiotic treatment with abundant obscuring inflammation showing even focal evidence tumour such as chondromyxoid material or mucin laden or keratinized cells, should raise suspicion of a underlying hidden tumour and need to be followed-up by reaspiration or biopsy.

4.6.5 Chronic sialdenitis (CS)

Chronic sialdenitis (CS) can also affect minor SGs [53]. It may occur due to repeated episodes of inflammation or secondary to treatment such as radiation therapy for other cancers. Aspirates from CS are hypocellular and shows few clusters of duct cells, fragments of fibrous tissue in background showing lymphocytes. Acinar cells are usually not seen and are absent. The duct cells may undergo metaplastic squamous changes and may show reactive atypia, raising possibility of MEC. In such cases, other features of MEC like mucinous cells and frank epidermoid cells and dirty mucoid background give clues to the diagnosis. Frank atypical features of a carcinomatous cells such as hyperchromatic nuclei and high N:C ratio can be differentiated from reactive changes due to either chronic infection or treatment.

4.6.6 Granulomatous sialadenitis (GS)

Granulomatous sialadenitis (GS) can present clinically as a slow-growing mass that can mimic a neoplasm. Aspirates are usually hypocellular and consist of clusters of epithelioid histiocytes, multinucleated giant cells, lymphocytes and duct cells. Transforming or ill-formed epithelioid cells should not be mistaken for an epithelial neoplasm.

4.6.7 Lymphoepithelial sialadenitis (LESA)

Lymphoepithelial sialadenitis (LESA) primarily affects salivary and lacrimal glands and is also reported in minor SGS [54]. It is believed to be an autoimmune disorder and is associated with sjogrens syndrome and other connective tissue disorders. Aspirate shows lymphoepithelial complex comprising of clusters of cohesive duct cells infiltrated by lymphoid cells. The duct cells may show metaplastic squamous changes or reactive atypia. The background consist of abundant population of large and small lymphoid cells in various stages of maturation, plasma cells and tingible body macrophages. LESA is associated with increased risk of lymphoma particularly extranodal marginal zone lymphoma of MALT type and sometimes it is indistinguishable from it [55]. Ancillary tests such as IHC on cell blocks and immunophenotyping with flow cytometry should be done to distinguish between LESA and lymphoma. Reactive lymphnode can mimic LESA but lymphoepithelial complex is absent. Since LESA can be cystic, other pitfall includes cystic tumours showing background of lymphocytes such as AciCC and low-grade MEC which can be differentiated by presence of their other cytological features.

5. Conclusions

FNAC of intraoral SGs is challenging. There are many diagnostic challenges encountered in cytopathology of SG tumours as these tumours show morphological diversity and overlapping features with other neoplastic and non-neoplastic lesions. Careful assessment of morphological features with acquaintance of diagnostic challenges and pitfalls not only aid in avoiding misdiagnosis but also aid in planning further management and treatment.

Acknowledgements

We acknowledge Professor Vaishali Walke, Dr. Deepti Joshi, Dr. Ujjawal Khurana for contribution of images. We also thanks all the faculty of department of Pathology & Lab Medicine, AIIMS, Bhopal for their support during preparation of this chapter.

Conflict of interest

The authors declare no conflict of interest for this chapter.

Author details

Jai Kumar Chaurasia* and Neelkamal Kapoor
Department of Pathology and Lab Medicine, All India Institute of Medical Sciences (AIIMS), Bhopal, Madhya Pradesh, India

*Address all correspondence to: jai.patho@aiimsbhopal.edu.in

References

[1] Barnes L, Eveson J, Reichart P, Sidransky D. Tumours of the salivary glands. In: World Health Organization classification of tumors. Pathology and genetics of head and neck tumors. Lyon, France: IARC; 2005.

[2] Buchner A, Merrell PW, Carpenter WM. Relative frequency of intra-oral minor salivary gland tumors: a study of 380 cases from northern California and comparison to reports from other parts of the world. J Oral Pathol Med. 2007;36(4):207-214. doi: 10.1111/j.1600-0714.2007.00522.x.

[3] Venkata V, Irulandy P. The frequency and distribution pattern of minor salivary gland tumors in a government dental teaching hospital, Chennai, India. Oral Surg Oral Med Oral Pathol Oral Radiol Endod. 2011;111(1):e32-e39. doi: 10.1016/j.tripleo.2010.08.019. PMID: 21176809.

[4] Pires FR, Pringle GA, de Almeida OP, Chen SY. Intra-oral minor salivary gland tumors: a clinicopathological study of 546 cases. Oral Oncol. 2007;43(5): 463-470. doi: 10.1016/j.oraloncology. 2006.04.008.

[5] Ramesh M, Krishnan R, Paul G. Intraoral minor salivary gland tumours: a retrospective study from a dental and maxillofacial surgery centre in salem, Tamil Nadu. J Maxillofac Oral Surg. 2014;13(2):104-108. doi: 10.1007/ s12663-013-0489-4.

[6] Hughes JH, Volk EE, Wilbur DC. Pitfalls in salivary gland fine-needle aspiration cytology: Lessons from the College of American Pathologists Interlaboratory Comparison Program in Nongynecologic Cytology. Arch Pathol Lab Med. 2005;129:26-31. doi: 10.1043/1543-2165(2005)129<26:PISGF C>2.0.CO.

[7] Sarmento, Dmitry José de Santana et al. Minor intraoral salivary gland tumors: a clinical-pathological study. Einstein (Sao Paulo, Brazil) 2016;14(4):508-512. doi:10.1590/ S1679-45082016AO3749.

[8] Tian Z, Li L, Wang L, Hu Y, Li J. Salivary gland neoplasms in oral and maxillofacial regions: a 23-year retrospective study of 6982 cases in an eastern Chinese population. Int J Oral Maxillofac Surg. 2010 ;39(3):235-242. doi: 10.1016/j.ijom.2009.10.016.

[9] Singh M, Sagar N, Yadav S, Aggarwal R, Mandal S, Khurana N, Jain S, Meher R. Utility of Fine Needle Aspiration in Diagnosis of Intraoral Minor Salivary Gland Tumors. J Cytol. 2020;37(1):53-57. doi: 10.4103/JOC. JOC_62_19.

[10] Pal S, Mondal S, Bose K, Pradhan R, Bandyapadhyay A, Bhattacharyya D. Fine needle aspiration cytology of minor salivary gland tumors: A retrospective 5-year study of 42 cases in a tertiary care hospital. J Cancer Res Ther. 2019;15(3):686-689. doi: 10.4103/0973-1482.191055.

[11] Singh Nanda KD, Mehta A, Nanda J. Fine-needle aspiration cytology: a reliable tool in the diagnosis of salivary gland lesions. J Oral Pathol Med. 2012;41(1):106-112. doi: 10.1111/j.1600-0714.2011.01069.x.

[12] Netto Jde N, Miranda AM, da Silveira HM, dos Santos TC, Pires FR. Fine-needle aspiration biopsy as an auxiliary diagnostic tool on intraoral minor salivary gland adenoid cystic carcinoma. Oral Surg Oral Med Oral Pathol Oral Radiol Endod. 2008;106(2):242-245. doi: 10.1016/j. tripleo.2008.04.015.

[13] Pusztaszeri M, Rossi ED, Baloch ZW, Faquin WC. Salivary Gland Fine Needle Aspiration and Introduction of the Milan Reporting System. Adv

Anat Pathol. 2019;26(2):84-92. doi: 10.1097/PAP.0000000000000224.

[14] Rohilla M, Singh P, Rajwanshi A, Gupta N, Srinivasan R, Dey P and Vashishta RK. Three-year cytohistological correlation of salivary gland FNA cytology at a tertiary center with the application of the Milan system for risk stratification. Cancer Cytopathology. 125:767-775. doi: 10.1002/cncy.21900.

[15] Lee SS, Cho KJ, Jang JJ, Ham EK. Differential diagnosis of adenoid cystic carcinoma from pleomorphic adenoma of the salivary gland on fine needle aspiration cytology. Acta Cytol. 1996;40(6):1246-1252. doi: 10.1159/000333988.

[16] Handa U, Dhingra N, Chopra R, Mohan H. Pleomorphic adenoma: Cytologic variations and potential diagnostic pitfalls. Diagn Cytopathol. 2009;37(1):11-15. doi: 10.1002/dc.20951.

[17] Skálová A, Andrle P, Hostička L, Michal M. Pleomorfní adenom slinných žláz: diagnostická úskalí a histologické nálezy budící podezření z malignity. Pleomorphic adenoma of salivary glands: diagnostic pitfalls and mimickers of malignancy. Cesk Patol. 2012;48(4):179-183. PMID: 23121026.

[18] Reichart PA, Kalz S, Rabel A et al. Carcinoma ex pleomorphic adenoma in a minor salivary gland: report of a case. Oral Maxillofac Surg. 2010;14:59-62. https://doi.org/10.1007/s10006-009-0183-3.

[19] Sedassari BT, Dos Santos HT, Mariano FV, da Silva Lascane NA, Altemani A, Sousa S. Carcinoma ex pleomorphic adenoma of minor salivary glands with major epithelial-myoepithelial component: clinicopathologic and immunohistochemical study of 3 cases. Ann Diagn Pathol. 2015;19(3):164-168. doi: 10.1016/j.anndiagpath.2015.03.011.

[20] Mahdavi N, Ghorbanpour M. Epithelial-Myoepithelial Carcinoma of the Palate: Report of a Case and Review of the Literatures. Iran J Pathol. 2020;15(2):144-150. doi: 10.30699/ijp.2020.105039.2076.

[21] Darvishian F and Lin O. Myoepithelial cell-rich neoplasms: Cytologic features of benign and malignant lesions. Cancer. 2004:102:355-361. doi: 10.1002/cncr.20642.

[22] Coca-Pelaz A, Rodrigo JP, Bradley PJ, Vander Poorten V, Triantafyllou A, Hunt JL, Strojan P, Rinaldo A, Haigentz M Jr, Takes RP, Mondin V, Teymoortash A, Thompson LD, Ferlito A. Adenoid cystic carcinoma of the head and neck-An update. Oral Oncol. 2015;51(7):652-661. doi: 10.1016/j.oraloncology.2015.04.005.

[23] Chang CF, Hsieh MY, Chen MK, Chou MC. Adenoid cystic carcinoma of head and neck: A retrospective clinical analysis of a single institution. Auris Nasus Larynx. 2018;45(4):831-837. doi: 10.1016/j.anl.2017.10.009.

[24] Bjørndal K, Krogdahl A, Therkildsen MH, Charabi B, Kristensen CA, Andersen E, Schytte S, Primdahl H, Johansen J, Pedersen HB, Andersen LJ, Godballe C. Salivary adenoid cystic carcinoma in Denmark 1990-2005: Outcome and independent prognostic factors including the benefit of radiotherapy. Results of the Danish Head and Neck Cancer Group (DAHANCA). Oral Oncol. 2015 Dec;51(12):1138-1142. doi: 10.1016/j.oraloncology.2015.10.002.

[25] Ben Salha I, Bhide S, Mourtzoukou D, Fisher C, Thway K. Solid Variant of Adenoid Cystic Carcinoma: Difficulties in Diagnostic Recognition. Int J Surg Pathol. 2016;24(5):419-424. doi: 10.1177/1066896916642011.

[26] Nagel H, Hotze HJ, Laskawi R, Chilla R and Droese M. Cytologic

diagnosis of adenoid cystic carcinoma of salivary glands. Diagn. Cytopathol. 1999;20:358-366. doi: 10.1002/(sici)1097-0339(199906)20:6<358::aid-dc6>3.0.co;2-x.

[27] Sodhi SP, Brar RS, Singh HP, Kaur T, Dhawan R. A rare occurrence of basal cell adenoma of palate: A case report with comprehensive immunohistochemical analysis. J Cancer Res Ther. 2015;11(4):1023. doi: 10.4103/0973-1482.147391.

[28] Werder P, Altermatt HJ, Zbären P, Bornstein MM. Canalicular adenoma of a minor salivary gland on the palate: a case presentation. Quintessence Int. 2009;40(8):623-626. PMID: 19639085.

[29] Perez-Ordonez B, Linkov I and Huvos A. Polymorphous low-grade adenocarcinoma of minor salivary glands: a study of 17 cases with emphasis on cell differentiation. Histopathology. 32:521-529. doi: 10.1046/j.1365-2559.1998.t01-2-00410.x.

[30] Gibbons D, Saboorian MH, Vuitch F, Gokaslan ST, Ashfaq R. Fine-needle aspiration findings in patients with polymorphous low grade adenocarcinoma of the salivary glands. Cancer. 1999;87(1):31-36. doi: 10.1002/(sici)1097-0142(19990225)87:1<31::aid-cncr6>3.0.co;2-g.

[31] Noonan VL, Kalmar JR, Allen CM, Gallagher GT, Kabani S. Sclerosing polycystic adenosis of minor salivary glands: report of three cases and review of the literature. Oral Surg Oral Med Oral Pathol Oral Radiol Endod. 2007;104(4):516-520. doi: 10.1016/j.tripleo.2006.08.033.

[32] Tjioe KC, de Lima HG, Thompson LD, Lara VS, Damante JH, de Oliveira-Santos C. Papillary Cystadenoma of Minor Salivary Glands: Report of 11 Cases and Review of the English Literature. Head Neck Pathol. 2015;9(3):354-359. doi: 10.1007/s12105-014-0602-0

[33] Brannon RB, Sciubba JJ, Giulani M. Ductal papillomas of salivary gland origin: A report of 19 cases and a review of the literature. Oral Surg Oral Med Oral Pathol Oral Radiol Endod. 2001;92(1):68-77. doi: 10.1067/moe.2001.115978.

[34] Joseph TP, Joseph CP, Jayalakshmy PS, Poothiode U. Diagnostic challenges in cytology of mucoepidermoid carcinoma: Report of 6 cases with histopathological correlation. J Cytol. 2015;32(1):21-24. doi: 10.4103/0970-9371.155226.

[35] Pantanowitz L, Thompson LDR, Rossi ED. Diagnostic Approach to Fine Needle Aspirations of Cystic Lesions of the Salivary Gland. Head Neck Pathol. 2018;12(4):548-561. doi: 10.1007/s12105-018-0904-8.

[36] Kumar U. Acinic Cell Carcinoma Papillary-Cystic Variant: Diagnostic Pitfalls in Fine Needle Aspiration Cytology. J Clin Diagn Res. 2017;11(5):ED05-ED06. doi: 10.7860/JCDR/2017/21347.9772.

[37] Angiero F, Sozzi D, Seramondi R, Valente MG. Epithelial-myoepithelial carcinoma of the minor salivary glands: immunohistochemical and morphological features. Anticancer Res. 2009;29(11):4703-4709. PMID: 20032423.

[38] Yang S, Zhang J, Chen X, Wang L, Xie F. Clear cell carcinoma, not otherwise specified, of salivary glands: a clinicopathologic study of 4 cases and review of the literature. Oral Surg Oral Med Oral Pathol Oral Radiol Endod. 2008;106(5):712-720. doi: 10.1016/j.tripleo.2008.04.016.

[39] Triantafillidou K, Iordanidis F, Psomaderis K, Kalimeras E. Acinic cell carcinoma of minor salivary glands: a clinical and immunohistochemical study. J Oral Maxillofac Surg. 2010;68(10):2489-2496. doi: 10.1016/j.joms.2009.09.065

[40] Rodríguez MP, Martínez MJ, Hervás MN, Sanz AC, Vera-Sempere FJ. Cytological characteristics of acinic cell carcinoma (ACC) diagnosed by fine-needle aspiration biopsy (FNAB). A study of four cases. Oral Med Pathol. 2005;10:103-108. PMID: 15735541.

[41] Haq S, Kalakkunath S, Bakshi P, Verma K. Cytological Diagnosis of Acinic Cell Carcinoma. A Study of Four Cases with Emphasis on Differential Diagnosis and DOG1 Expression. J Cytol. 2020;37(3):155-156. doi: 10.4103/JOC.JOC_175_18.

[42] Gnepp DR, Brannon R. Sebaceous neoplasms of salivary gland origin. Report of 21 cases. Cancer. 1984; 53(10):2155-2170. doi:10.1002/1097-0142(19840515)53:10<2155::aid-cncr2820531026>3.0.co;2-f.

[43] Paudel D, Nishimura M, Adhikari BR, Hiraki D, Onishi A, Morikawa T, Neopane P, Giri S, Yoshida K, Sato J, Ono M, Kamino Y, Nagayasu H, Abiko Y. Secretory Carcinoma of Minor Salivary Gland in Buccal Mucosa: A Case Report and Review of the Literature. Case Rep Pathol. 2019;2019:2074504. doi: 10.1155/2019/2074504.

[44] Kanazawa H, Furuya T, Murano A, Yamaki M. Oncocytoma of an intraoral minor salivary gland: report of a case and review of literature. J Oral Maxillofac Surg. 2000;58(8):894-897. doi: 10.1053/joms.2000.8217.

[45] Verma K, Kapila K. Salivary gland tumors with a prominent oncocytic component. Cytologic findings and differential diagnosis of oncocytomas and Warthin's tumor on fine needle aspirates. Acta Cytol. 2003;47:221-226. doi: 10.1159/000326508.

[46] Paulino AF, Huvos AG. Oncocytic and oncocytoid tumors of the salivary glands. Semin Diagn Pathol. 1999;16(2):98-104. PMID: 10452575.

[47] Weinreb I, Seethala RR, Perez-Ordoñez B, Chetty R, Hoschar AP, Hunt JL. Oncocytic mucoepidermoid carcinoma: clinicopathologic description in a series of 12 cases. Am J Surg Pathol. 2009;33(3):409-416. doi: 10.1097/PAS.0b013e318184b36d.

[48] Li J, , Wang BY, Nelson M, Li L, Hu Y, Urken ML, Brandwein-Gensler M. Salivary adenocarcinoma, not otherwise specified: a collection of orphans. Arch Pathol Lab Med. 2004;128(12):1385-1394. Doi: 10.5858/2004-128-1385-SANOSA.

[49] Lewandowski B, Brodowski R, Pakla P, Makara A, Stopyra W, Startek B. Mucoceles of minor salivary glands in children. Own clinical observations. Dev Period Med. 2016;20(3):235-242. PMID: 27941195.

[50] Mignogna MD, Fedele S, Lo Russo L. Anorexia/bulimia-related sialadenosis of palatal minor salivary glands. J Oral Pathol Med. 2004;33(7):441-442. doi: 10.1111/j.1600-0714.2004.00208.x.

[51] Ben Lagha N, Alantar A, Samson J, Chapireau D, Maman L. Lithiasis of minor salivary glands: current data. Oral Surg Oral Med Oral Pathol Oral Radiol Endod. 2005;100(3):345-348. doi: 10.1016/j.tripleo.2004.12.023.

[52] Haneke E. Acute traumatic sialadenitis of the labial and buccal minor salivary glands. Dtsch Z Mund Kiefer Gesichtschir. 1986;10(4):291-293. PMID: 3482025.

[53] Burgess LP, Quilligan JJ, Lepore ML, Yim DW. Chronic sialadenitis in a minor salivary gland. Ear Nose Throat J. 1986;65(10):485-486. PMID: 3780487.

[54] Krithika C, Sreedevi J, Sivapathasundharam B, Nithya VR. Benign lymphoepithelial lesion of the minor salivary gland - A rare

presentation as a palatal swelling. J Oral Maxillofac Pathol. 2020;24 (Suppl 1): S33-S36. doi: 10.4103/jomfp.JOMFP_17_20.

[55] Carbone A, Gloghini A, Ferlito A. Pathological features of lymphoid proliferations of the salivary glands: lymphoepithelial sialadenitis versus low-grade B-cell lymphoma of the malt type. Ann Otol Rhinol Laryngol. 2000;109(12 Pt 1):1170-1175.

Chapter 4

Personalised Precision Medicine - A Novel Approach for Oral Cancer Management

Deepa Jatti Patil and Rakesh Nagaraju

Abstract

Oral Cancer is one of the most common malignancies of the head and neck region. Despite technological advancements and improvements in Oral cancer diagnosis and treatment modalities, the 5-year survival rate remains low and is associated with poor prognosis and high mortality rate especially when detected at a later stage. The empirical therapy followed for the treatment of oral cancer includes surgery, radiotherapy and chemotherapy. The treatments are not equally efficacious for all patients, are associated with side effects and poor prognosis. The need of the hour is early diagnosis and tailored treatment therapies for individual patients. With the advent of immunotherapy, the cancer treatment has moved toward personalised precision medicine which tailors' treatments to each individual. Personalised precision medicine incorporates, molecular profiling of tumours with OMICS technology, biomarkers and companion diagnostics to build databases of patients and devise tailor made treatment approaches for individual patients. This article discusses the role of precision medicine in OSCC prevention, detection, and management by reviewing our understanding of OC from both genetic and OMICS perspectives.

Keywords: Personalised precision medicine, OMICS, Genomics, Transcriptomics, Proteomics, Metabolomics, Big data, Targetted therapy, Immunotherapy

1. Introduction

Oral cancer is a type of head and neck cancer (HNC), which encompasses a wide range of tumour types that arise from a variety of anatomic structures, including the oral cavity, oropharynx, larynx, hypopharynx, and nasopharynx. Squamous cell carcinomas (OSCCs) account for over 90% of these malignancies histopathologically, with over 50% occurring in the oral cavity [1]. Tobacco usage (smoked or chewed), arecanut, excessive alcohol use, and/or human papillomavirus (HPV) infection are the most major and well-established risk factors associated with this neoplasm [2–4].

Cancer is a major public health concern around the world. According to the International Agency for Research on Cancer's GLOBOCAN project, there were approximately 14.1 million newly diagnosed cancer cases and 8.2 million deaths worldwide in 2012.Oral cancer is one of the most common cancers worldwide, accounting for 2% of all cancer cases and having a nearly 50% mortality rate [5].

Oral and pharyngeal tumours are the sixth most common cancer worldwide [6]. Internationally, South Asian countries such as Sri Lanka, India, and Taiwan have the highest rates of oral cancer, which can be attributed to high rates of cigarette smoking and areca nut use in these countries [7].

Despite technological advancements and improvements in OSCC diagnosis and treatment modalities, the 5-year survival rate remains low, hovering around 50–60%, ranging from 80% for stage I cancers to 40% for stage IV cancers. This disparity can be explained by the delay in diagnosis as well as the relatively high tumour recurrence rates found in these patients. In general, only one-third of OSCC patients have the disease in its early stages at the time of diagnosis (I and II) [8].

Treatment strategies for OSCC differ depending on the stage of the disease at the time of diagnosis. Patients with localised disease are typically treated with surgery and/or radiotherapy, which results in a high chance of long-term survival but significant morbidity. Chemotherapy and radiotherapy and recently immunotherapy are the mainstays of treatment for metastatic OSCC [9]. Despite advances in understanding the pathobiological mechanisms of OSCC, the prognosis has not improved over the last few decades. This is largely due to the high morbidity and mortality rates associated with local and regional OSCC recurrences. The clinical challenge remains in detecting regional metastasis accurately and efficiently treating second primary OSCC and recurrent tumours [10].

The practise of medicine is still primarily empirical today, with doctors relying on pattern matching to make diagnoses based on a patient's medical history, physical examination, and test data. As a result, a prescribed treatment is frequently dependent on a physician's previous experience with patients with comparable symptoms. As a result, the best drug may be given for a "typical patient" with a certain condition. The treatment decisions are made through trial and error, and patients may experience unforeseen adverse effects or poor or no efficacy for a medicine that theoretically works in some people with that disease [11].

Traditional therapeutic procedures have a poor prognosis and are associated with negative side effects. Immunotherapy adoption has moved the field of cancer treatment toward the concept of precision and personalised medicine (PPM), which tailors' treatments to each individual. For cancer treatment, there are two options: the traditional approach and the PPM model. The fundamental distinctions between the classic cancer treatment approach and the developing precision and personalised medicine (PPM) concept are compared. Traditionally, cancer has been treated with "one-size-fits-all" treatments including chemotherapy, radiation, and surgical tumour removal. These treatments have a wide range of efficacy in different people, and they frequently destroy healthy, noncancerous organs and tissues. Individualised therapy customised to specific tissues, gene alterations, and personal characteristics relevant to each unique case of cancer characterise the PPM approach [12].

This article discusses the role of precision medicine in OC prevention, detection, and management by reviewing our understanding of OC from both genetic and OMICS perspectives.

2. Why personalised precision medicine (PPM)

Traditionally Surgery, Radiotherapy and chemotherapy have been used in the treatment of OC. Some people will only need one treatment, but most people will need a combination of medicines to combat cancer's resistance. When there are solid tumours that have not metastasized and are in easily accessible places of the body, surgery can be utilised; nevertheless, many cancers do metastasis, necessitating more harsh therapies such as radiotherapy and chemotherapy. High doses of radiation and medicines are used in these methods to kill cancer cells and shrink tumours, but they often inflict additional damage to healthy cells [13]. It is stated that the given class of cancer medications is projected to be useless in up to 75% of patients The success of these treatments is influenced by a variety of factors, including the type, stage, and location of the cancer, as well as the patient's age and overall condition. This shows that before choosing a cancer treatment, various personal aspects should be examined [14]. Over the last decade, it has been increasingly obvious that no two patients' malignancies are exactly the same, and therefore generic treatments like chemotherapy and radiation may have varying outcomes. This standard cancer treatment strategy is extremely simple, resulting in ineffective, expensive treatments and unwanted side effects for patients [15]. It is well understood that a treatment's response varies across the variability of a population, including good and poor responders. Variables such as genetic predisposition, cohort heterogeneity, ethnicity, slow vs. quick metabolizers, epigenetic factors, and early vs. late stage of disease affect patient and therapy response. These variables influence whether or not a person will respond well to a certain treatment [11].

Immunotherapy, which uses a patient's own immune system to combat cancer, is another type of cancer treatment that has cleared the way for more specific and successful treatments. Monoclonal antibodies (mAbs), checkpoint inhibitors, cytokines, vaccinations, and adoptive cell transfer, most notably in the form of haematopoietic stem cell transplants (HSCTs) and chimeric antigen receptor (CAR) T-cell therapies, are examples of immunotherapy treatments [16]. Targeted therapeutics, such as cetuximab (monoclonal epidermal growth factor receptor [EGFR] antibody), bevacizumab (monoclonal vascular endothelial growth factor [VEGF] antibody), and mechanistic target of rapamycin (mTOR) inhibitors, have recently been introduced into treatment regimens or ongoing clinical trials to improve survival rate and reduce toxicity. With the advancement of immunotherapy, the Food and Drug Administration (FDA) has approved monoclonal antibodies that target programmed cell death protein-1 (PD-1), a receptor of the immune escape pathway, such as nivolumab and pembrolizumab, for recurrent and/or metastatic head and neck SCC [9]. Immunotherapy adoption has moved the field of cancer treatment toward the concept of personalised precision medicine (PPM), which tailors' treatments to each individual.

The purpose of PPM is to allow doctors to forecast the best course of action for a patient promptly, effectively, and precisely. Clinicians will require tools that are both compatible with their clinical workflow and cost-effective in order to achieve this. These techniques can make managing the biological complexity that underpins human diseases a lot easier. A PPM ecosystem is under constant development to enable the creation and refining of such tools, and it is the solution to the problem. Precision medicine emphasises the need of combining established clinical indicators with molecular profiling to provide diagnostic, prognostic, and therapeutic techniques tailored to the individual needs of each patient group. For the optimal utilisation of the PM ecosystem, accurate data interpretation is required. The PM ecosystem brings together omics and clinical data to solve problems [11].

A move from empirical treatment to PPM is now possible thanks to increased usage of Biomarkers and companion diagnostics (CDX) (the right medicine, for the right patient, at the right dose, at the right time) [17]. PPM is a more effective model that is ready to disrupt the "one size fits all" approach. Based on the measurement and manipulation of essential patient genetic and omic data, this perspective promotes the creation of customised treatments for each individual subtype of cancer (transcriptomics, metabolomics, proteomics, etc.) [12].

Based on the definition provided by the National Cancer Institute, Personalised Precision Medicine, (PPM) is "an approach to patient care that allows doctors to select treatments that are most likely to help patients based on a genetic understanding of their disease."

2.1 The PPM method and its use to cancer therapy

Patients with a cancer are enrolled randomly to prevent bias in traditional drug development, employing a "all comers" method with the assumption that the enrolled patients are nearly homogeneous. The purpose of random enrollment is to guarantee that the general population is well represented. In practise, we never conduct clinical trials on patients who are randomly chosen; instead, we apply various forms of enrichments to patients' enrolment by using particular inclusion and exclusion criteria. Despite all of the efforts to enrich the community, the population that is ultimately chosen for the study can be quite diverse in terms of drug-metabolising capacity, environmental factors (e.g., nutrition, smoking habits, lifestyle, etc.), prior medication(s) exposure, and an individual's genetic and epigenetic make-up are all factors to consider. BMs are being used to better define molecular, genetic, and environmental changes. Drug developers have been studying the epigenetic makeup of patients and attempting to take a more objective stance.

Patient stratification is used to distinguish between likely responders and non-responders. When compared to randomly selected individuals, prospective stratification can result in a smaller and shorter clinical study. At a bare minimum, stratification can expedite approval for medication candidates targeted at a subset of patients while providing room for additional testing and market development in the more heterogeneous patient group. In the best-case scenario, it can reveal an effective therapeutic agent that would otherwise be lost in the noise generated by non-responders, as was the case with trastuzumab and gefitinib. This will not only decrease the duration of the clinical trial but will also be cost effective [18].

Scientists were able to read and understand an individual's genetic code, as well as detect hereditary predispositions to particular diseases, when the Human Genome Project (HGP) was completed. This watershed moment shifted the focus of health care from reactive to proactive. Scientists are currently striving to gain a detailed understanding of the body's function at numerous omics levels, as well as characterise how environmental exposures alter genetic predispositions. When all of this data is combined, scientists and doctors will be able to better anticipate how patients will respond to a particular treatment. CDx assays patients for genetic features that determine whether or not they will respond to a specific medication. This technique has the potential to have a significant impact on the patient's care. The transformation from a clinician choosing a generic medicine that is more or less experimental for the patient to one that effectively addresses the disease with PPM is the revolution [12].

2.2 Steps in PPM

1. Acquiring PPM data

2. Developing a PPM therapy

2.3 Acquiring PPM data

2.3.1 Tools for PPM

2.3.1.1 Biomarkers

Predictive BM for immunotherapy differs from typical BM used for targeted therapies in the case of cancer immunotherapy. Because of the complexity of the tumour microenvironment (TME), immune response, and molecular profiling, a more holistic approach is required than using a single analyte BM [3]. To address this issue, researchers have developed a multiplexing strategy, in which numerous BMs are used to provide more precise patient stratification. Histological analysis now includes concomitant analysis of immuno-oncology BMs, such as PD-L1 and immune cell infiltrates (**Figure 1**), as well as more comprehensive immune and tumour-related pathways (**Figure 2**) (the "Cancer Immunogram"). Multiplexed immunoprofiling, which generates a comprehensive biomarker collection that may be associated with clinical parameters, is critical for the effectiveness of PM in cancer immunotherapy [21, 22].

A specific gene or mutation must be linked to a clinical result before a PPM treatment can be created and utilised in patients. This is a significant endeavour; discovering a therapeutically relevant phenotype or polymorphism might take years of research involving many scientists. Furthermore, determining which polymorphisms cause patients to have a good or negative therapy response necessitates additional research. Sequencing DNA from a large number of people is the first step in deciphering the genetic code. This phase is becoming easier with the improvement of sequencing technologies. The most difficult issues are in interpreting these massive data sets, which is where bioinformatics comes in.

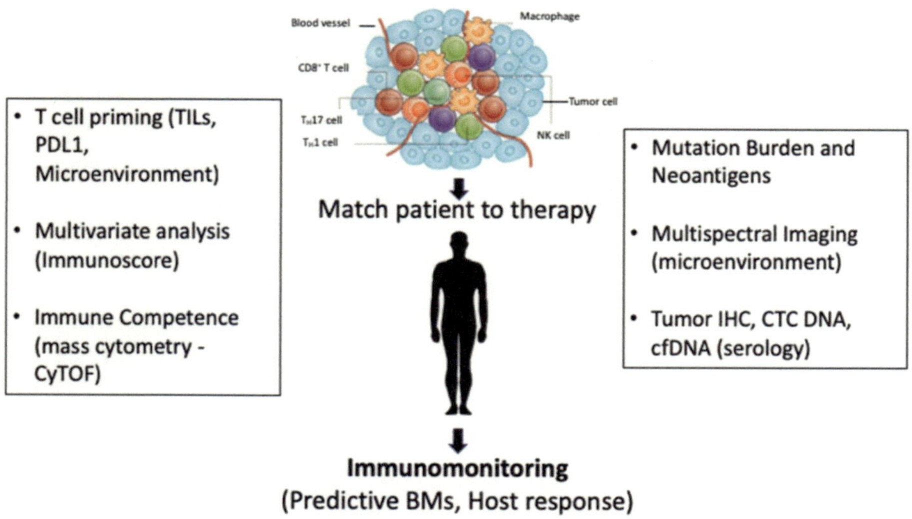

Figure 1.
Critical checkpoints for host and tumour profiling. A multiplexed biomarker approach is highly integrative and includes both tumour- and immune-related parameters assessed with both molecular and image-based methods for individualised prediction of immunotherapy response. Byassessing patient samples continuously one can collect a dynamic data on tissue-based parameters, such as immune cell infiltration and expressionof immune checkpoints, and pathology methods. These parameters are equally suited for data integration with molecular parameters. TILs: Tumour-infiltrating lymphocytes. PD-L1: Programmed cell death-ligand 1. Immunoscore: A prognostic tool for quantification of in situ immune cell infiltrates. Immunocompetence: body's ability to produce a normal immune response following exposure to an antigen (tumour drawing has been adapted from [19].

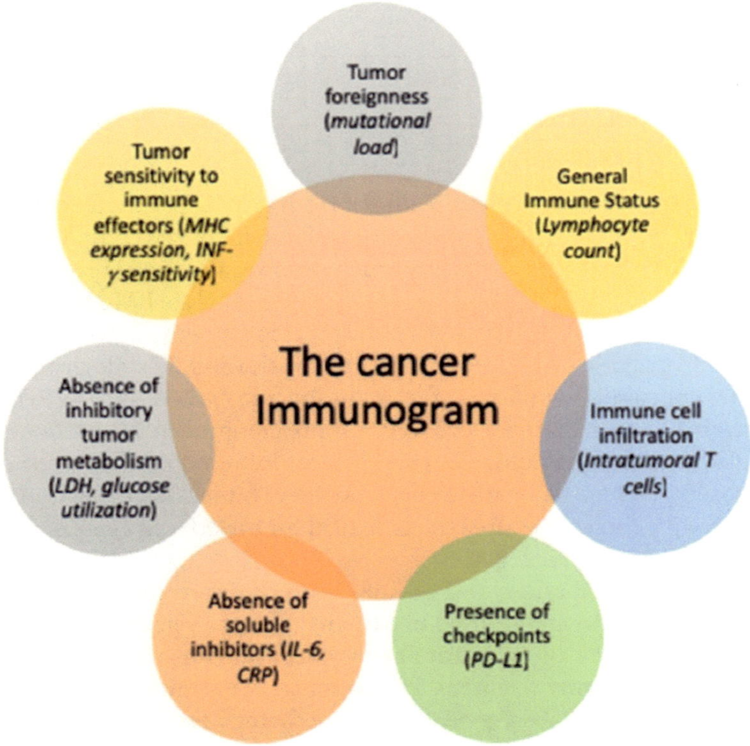

Figure 2.
The cancer immunogram. The schema depicts the seven parameters that characterise aspects of cancer-immune interactions for which biomarkers have been identified or are plausible. Italics represent those potential biomarkers for the different parameters (adapted from [20]).

Without the enormous achievement of sequencing the human genome, the discipline of PPM would not exist. From 1990 until 2003, the HGP took 13 years to complete. The International Human Genome Sequencing Consortium (IHGSC), which includes over 200 collaborators from 19 nations, was tasked with discovering new knowledge regarding the structure and organisation of the genome. The human genome has around 20,500 genes, and any two persons share 99.99 percent of their genome, implying that genetic individuality can be identified only in the remaining 0.01 percent. Long repeat sequences were also discovered in the genome, and single-base changes (single nucleotide polymorphisms [SNPs]) were found to have the potential to be distinct disease indicators. The use of bacterial artificial chromosomes (BAC) and Sanger sequencing aided in the early data collection. BAC vectors helped with the first stage of genome sequencing by determining the chromosomal location of DNA fragments recovered from a sample. Sanger sequencing, on the other hand, allowed for exact base-by-base identification of a DNA fragment. These approaches were expensive and inefficient, despite their importance in early sequencing attempts [23]. Next Generation Sequencing Technologies (NGSTs)23 have evolved as a result of years of research and development to solve these difficulties. NGSTs are a cost-effective addition to the BAC and Sanger sequencing technologies, allowing for high-dimensional and parallel sequencing [24].

Whole-genome sequencing and whole-exome sequencing are examples of genomics-related technology. There are a variety of commercial technologies for detecting gene mutations, SNPs, and copy number changes. The Cancer Genome Atlas (TCGA) is a joint project of the National Cancer Institute (NCI) and the National Human Genome Research Institute that began in 2005. In thirty-three kinds of cancer, including head and neck SCC, the TCGA has created complete, multidimensional maps of important genetic alterations. Oral and oropharyngeal SCC has two different subgroups, according to thorough genetic profiling: HPV-negative cancers that commonly develop in the oral cavity and lips; and HPV negative cancers of the oral cavity and lips in particular. The molecular changes in these two subgroups of SCC correspond to their clinical behaviour and patient prognosis. The TCGA database demonstrated that the vast majority of HPV negative OSCCs have TP53 loss-of-function mutations and CDKN2A inactivation, which is consistent with previous findings. In addition, HPV negative OSCC showed a high amount of heterogeneity, according to integrated genomic analysis [25, 26]. Whole-exome sequencing, a transcriptomics approach for sequencing all of a genome's expressed genes, revealed new mutations that had been missed in prior studies (known as the exome. NOTCH1 mutations were found in around 15% of the patients, while mutations and focal copies of NOTCH1 were found in about 15% of the cases. NOTCH1 mutations were found in about 15% of cases, and NOTCH2/3 mutations and localised copy-number changes were found in another 11% of OSCC cases [27, 28].

OSCC's incredible diversity exemplifies how precision medicine may actually help patients and enhance medical care. The Pan Cancer Analysis of Whole Genomes project (PCAWG) is now steered to reveal noncoding driver mutations, such as alternative promoter usage, splicing, expression, editing, fusion, allele specific expression, and nonsynonymous variants, as it progresses from whole-exome sequencing to whole-genome sequencing [29]. MiRNAs and long noncoding RNAs (lncRNAs) are two types of noncoding transcripts. These noncoding transcripts, including miRNAs and long noncoding RNAs (lncRNAs), have a lot of potential for clinical research [30, 31].

2.3.1.2 Omics

While genomic data is crucial for establishing a full understanding of disease progression and therapeutic effects in physiological systems, intermediate omics levels such as the transcriptome, proteome, and metabolome are used to bridge the gap between genotypic effect and phenotypic event.

2.3.1.3 Transcriptomics

The transcriptome is the total mRNA within an individual or sample. Microarray and RNA sequencing (RNA-Seq) are two modern high-throughput sequencing approaches for collecting transcriptome data. Microarray analysis measures the amount of hybridization between a sample and corresponding probe to determine mRNA expression. The quantity of fluorescence seen within each well of the array corresponding to a given probe indicates the abundance of gene expression within a sample. Microarray analysis is constrained by the fact that designing probes requires prior knowledge of the gene's sequence. This approach is similar to Sanger sequencing in that it determines the mRNA sequence by adding fluorescently tagged nucleotide bases one by one. During each loop, fluorescent pictures are recorded, and their analysis shows the exact sequence as well as its expression level. Microarray analysis takes less time to prepare samples than RNA-Seq, although RNA-Seq does not require prior knowledge of gene sequences and may handle fewer samples. Both technologies have tremendous throughput capacities, but microarray has a higher cost-value at the moment [32, 33].

Genomic profiling enables modern medication development, which often includes either microarray analysis or RNA-Seq for transcriptome profiling. Both microarray and RNA-Seq analyses allow for the identification of disease phenotype and medication effect within a system (single cell or bigger), which is crucial for the development of genome-specific therapeutics. Although RNA-Seq looks to be more advantageous for discovering novel genomic medication effects and disease characteristics, microarray analyses are less expensive and have more standardised techniques. In general, RNA-Seq results are better for clinical research since they have a lower signal-to-noise ratio than microarray results. Furthermore, as compared to microarray approaches, RNA-Seq results can be obtained from smaller sample quantities — nanogram versus microgram masses, respectively. As NGSTs become more widely used in clinical diagnostics, RNA-Seq methods are expected to become more standardised, eventually replacing microarray diagnostics [33, 34].

With transcriptomics technology, extensive attempts have been made to define OSCC at the molecular level. Reliable biomarkers are necessary to ease the prediction of clinical outcome and evaluate therapy efficacy in order to optimise therapeutic regimens for the management of OSCC. Dysregulation of several pathways (e.g., mRNA processing, cytoskeletal organisation, metabolic processes, cell cycle regulation, and apoptosis) was discovered when assessing a cohort of OSCC transcriptomes [35]. OSCC has also been recommended for molecular characterisation, similar to lung SCC [36]. Dysregulation of the KEAP1/ NFE2L2 oxidative stress pathway is one of the signalling pathways that has been impacted, SOX2 and TP63 lineage markers, as well as PIK3CA and EGFR mutations, were used differently. Different activation patterns of the EGFR pathway are linked to clinically diverse behaviours [37]. A molecular signature has also been proposed to help with OSCC treatment planning by predicting the existence of lymph node metastases using the primary tumour at the time of diagnosis [38]. Furthermore, microarray results demonstrated BGH3, MMP9, and PDIA3 upregulation in more than 80% of OSCC tumours, implying the relevance of ECM-cell receptor interactions in OSCC progression [39]. These transcriptional markers may be useful in the development of customised therapy regimens for the treatment of OSCC in the future.

2.3.1.4 Proteomics

The term "proteomics" refers to the process of identifying and cataloguing all proteins in a biological system, as well as their relationships. Protein structure, quantities, and cellular localizations, protein–protein interactions, and protein production and breakdown rates are all revealed by proteomic analysis. This data is utilised to figure out how the proteome changes throughout various biological activities and to spot disease patterns. Data on post-transcriptional alterations, or the quantity of proteins in a tissue, may be useful for illness diagnosis, progression, and treatment in the case of PPM. Mass spectrometry (MS) has been the primary instrument for gathering proteomic data for the past two decades, particularly to assess protein expression, identify protein modification sites, and analyse protein–protein interactions [40, 41].

The cellular abundance of proteins is primarily controlled by the quantity of translation, according to a landmark study published in 2011 that measured absolute mRNA and protein abundance and turnover using parallel metabolic pulse labelling [42]. Despite the fact that mRNA and protein levels are related to some extent, genome-wide protein abundance remains an important metric in determining cellular state and function. Intracellular and secreted proteins in body fluid specimens (e.g., serum, plasma, urine, and saliva) can be investigated using high-throughput total and phosphorylated protein analysis [43]. Alterations in protein expression in cell metabolism, adhesion, motility, and signal transduction have been discovered using proteomic analysis combined with in situ hybridization or immunohistochemistry [44, 45]. Promising results have been seen in studies.

Outcomes of salivary or serum proteomics in identifying OSCC and normal samples Analyses with a sensitivity and specificity of up to 90% [46, 47].

2.3.1.5 Metabolomics

The identification and analysis of metabolites, which are small-molecule intermediate products in metabolic reactions, is referred to as metabolomics. Because metabolites reflect both hereditary and environmental factors, a comprehensive metabolic examination is typically referred to as a "functional readout" of the current status of the organic system. The Human Metabolome Database (HMDB) is a freely accessible web resource that contains complete information on the human metabolome. The human metabolome is made up of peptides, lipids, amino acids, nucleic acids, carbohydrates, organic acids, biogenic amines, vitamins, minerals, and other tiny molecules found in the human body. The overall number of metabolites in HMDB 4.0 has increased dramatically from 40 153 in HMDB 3.0 to 114 100 in HMDB 4.0. This equates to approximately a fivefold increase [48].

In the context of PPM, metabolomic data could provide insight into an individual's unique physical reaction to a medicine, a technique known as metabolomics [49]. Currently, metabolomic studies of biofluids and tissues have aided in the development of PPM methods by discovering illness biomarkers that have the potential to aid doctors in diagnosis and early treatment. Because metabolites, unlike most proteins, travel throughout the body and appear in easily accessible biofluids like blood and urine one of the primary clinical advantages of metabolomics is that measurements may be conducted noninvasively [50]. Nuclear magnetic resonance (NMR) spectroscopy was commonly employed to identify metabolites in the early days of metabolomics research, but over the last decade, there has been a big movement toward MS, which offers superior resolution and sensitivity to small concentrations [51, 52].

Metabolite profiling of tissue and body fluid specimens with the purpose of biomarker discovery in OSCC research has revealed significant changes in energy metabolism pathways, according to mass spectrometry-based metabolomics analysis (eg, glycolysis and tricarboxylic acid cycle) [53]. Glycolytic metabolites (e.g., glucose) had higher amounts in OSCC patients' serum, while specific amino acids have lower levels (ie, valine, tyrosine, serine, and methionine) [54]. In OSCC tumour tissues, however, similar metabolite expression patterns are reversed, implying that this signature panel could be used as a screening tool. Early research, on the other hand, must be backed up with well-designed tests. Lipids have also been discovered as a significant class of metabolites, and abnormal cholesterol levels in the blood have been associated to a variety of cancers [55–57]. Total lipids, cholesterol, and high-density lipoprotein levels were shown to be considerably lower in OSCC patients compared to healthy controls [58, 59]. These lipidomic observations, albeit preliminary, may indicate greater usage of novel membrane synthesis by neoplastic cells and require further exploration.

These technologies will be collectively strong, with the potential to disclose molecular mechanisms and critical signalling pathways driving the disease, thanks to the rapid development of the omics tools outlined above. Furthermore, these tools have the potential to be utilised to identify new therapeutic targets as well as biomarkers that can be used to diagnose disease Cancer diagnosis, prognosis prediction, and treatment surveillance could all benefit from this technology.

2.3.1.6 Companion diagnostics (CDx)

The US FDA produced the first regulatory guideline document on CDx in 2014, and it was here that this type of assay was officially defined for the first time [60].

A CDx test is an in vitro diagnostic equipment that delivers information necessary for the safe and effective use of a related therapeutic product, according to this definition. This means that testing with this sort of assay is required and must be disclosed in both the medication and CDx assay labelling. CDx devices help clinicians provide the most effective, tailored medicines for their patients. In specific sections of DNA, relevant genetic information for defining malignancies can be identified (i.e., oncogenes). Some CDx are based on these specific oncogenes and can be used to evaluate whether or not a person will respond to a certain treatment in order to avoid sequencing the entire genome and obtaining superfluous information. Each CDx is linked to a certain medicinal treatment, which is linked to a particular genetic defect for which it is most effective [61]. Within the category of CDx products, there are a range of diagnostic procedures, each with its own role. Immunohistochemistry (IHC), fluorescent in situ hybridization (FISH), and real-time quantitative PCR (RT-qPCR) are examples of these techniques [62].

2.3.1.7 Data storage

After collecting the OMICS data, storage and analysis also poses a great challenge. The International Cancer Genome Consortium (ICGC) and The Cancer Genome Atlas (TCGA; sponsored by the National Cancer Institute and the National Human Genome Research Institute) are two large databases for oncology data. The data gateway of the International Cancer Genome Centre (ICGC) focuses on 50 tumour types and defines them on genomic, transcriptomic, and epigenomic levels across genders, mutations, tumour stage, and other factors. The TCGA portal has thorough information on genetic alterations and gene expression in 11 different types of cancer tissues and 33 different cancer subtypes. On a large number of patients, analysis is performed on high-quality tumour samples and matched normal tissue samples [63, 64].

2.4 Single nucleotide polymorphisms (SNPs)

Despite the lifestyle habits of exposure to high risk factors for oral cancer with 80% attributable risk of tobacco per se, a small proportion of the tobacco habit develop persistent premalignant lesions, and 3–8% transform to the malignant phenotype. Genomic variants, somatic mutations and epigenetic regulation play a critical role in oral cancer. SNPs are the most common genomic variants. SNPs are single base changes in a gene's exonic coding region or non-coding intronic regions that affect gene expression and function directly or indirectly in more than 1% of an ethnic population. SNPs in intronic regions may modify the three-dimensional structure of DNA, causing changes in molecular attributes such as Gibbs free energy aectLnJ stability, as well as impacting DNA polymerase activity and transcription factor activity. Binding SNPs can be found in one or both alleles, giving rise to heterozygous or homozygous genotypes. The wild-type (WT) allele is the ancestral allele, while the SNP allele is the changed allele. In a cancer case–control group, the frequency of allelotypes and genotypes differed, indicating a link between SNPs and cancer [65].

The connection of SNPs with risk propensity or susceptibility to oral cancer has been studied in several populations. In a meta-analysis research, the authors analysed SNPs in oral cancer and identified 34 SNPs in 30 genes that are strongly linked with oral cancer [66]. SNP rs1800471 in TGF- gene, with GC genotype associated with increased risk and GG genotype with lower risk in numerous studies and populations; SNP rs1048943 in CYP1A1 gene, with AG + GG genotypes resulting in increased risk and WT AA genotype resulting in decreased risk. The GSTM1 null genotype was linked to an elevated risk, while the WT genotype was linked to a lower risk. Similarly, heterozygous genotypes of SNPs rs1800870-AG in the IL-10 gene, rs11549467-GA in the HIF gene, and rs861539-CT in the XRCC3 genes were linked to an increased risk of oral cancer, while WT genotypes were linked to a lower risk. The WT genotypes rs1801133-CC in MTHFR and rs20417-GG in COX-2, on the other hand, were related with an increased risk, while the corresponding SNP homozygous genotypes TT and CC were associated with a decreased risk [67].

SNP analysis using high-throughput genomic analysis, as reported in genome-wide association studies (GWAS), and next-generation sequencing has emerged as a strong tool for identifying susceptibility loci, allowing information on thousands of SNPs to be obtained at the same time. These platforms often work with smaller samples and are more expensive, thus they must be confirmed in larger samples using alternative technology such as nucleotide sequencing and real-time PCR.SNPs investigated in various studies contribute to increased susceptibility to oral cancer, and a panel of SNPs could be used as Predictive Biomarkers to screen high-risk individuals who are prone to oral cancer due to tobacco use, providing an objective, unbiased test assay to assess oral cancer risk in individuals [66].

2.5 Developing a PPM therapy

2.5.1 The application of omics data to treatment

Establishing the link between biological data, disease, and clinical translation is a fundamental difficulty in PPM: how can we understand the data collected to make meaningful medical decisions? In the medical field, "Big Data" refers to a larger collection of medical data encompassing the tracking of various medical indicators and biomarkers across thousands of individuals (primarily clinical and omics data). Researchers may test tissues for thousands of molecular targets using high-throughput data gathering, effectively recording the response of a complex system over time.

The reconciliation of various omics components allows for the generation of prediction models of human physiology that may be employed in experimental design and clinical trial development in the field of systems biology [68].

Systems biologists and bioinformatic scientists use statistically significant trend detection approaches to link observations to biological events and phenotypes. Multivariate decomposition techniques, predictive modelling and optimization strategies, and other statistics-based tools are examples of these. Statistically understanding Big Data trends is a separate field that is required for predictive modelling, clinical decision-making, and assistance [69].

Drug discovery techniques for a number of PPM cancer products have been developed thanks to advances in omics technologies. Circulating tumour cells (CTC) and DNA detection approaches have promise not just for early diagnosis, but also for personalised patient risk monitoring and the development of effective personalised therapy. Several other cancer medicines in development take advantage of the immune system's particular power and specialisation to fight cancer. This has been the focus of research for almost a century, and it has evolved into a distinct discipline known as immunoengineering. The ultimate goal of this profession is to tailor a more particular and potent immune response, which can lead to a powerful and effective personalised cancer treatment [70].

2.5.2 Early cancer detection using CTCs and DNA

CTCs and circulating tumour DNA (ctDNA), two forms of oncological biomarkers, have emerged as the face of non-invasive cancer diagnosis using "liquid biopsy" procedures. Because research has shown that tumours release both types of biomarkers into the circulation early in cancer progression, there has been a lot of focus on their use in early detection and screening. CTCs and ctDNA are likely to become more effective in risk stratification, illness monitoring, and tailored treatment selection as research progresses and technology improves [71].

230 OSCC patients at various pathological stages of the disease and treatment modes were enrolled in a cross-sectional observational study. CTCs were obtained utilising the Onco Discover liquid biopsy method, which is based on immunomagnetic CTC enumeration and has been authorised by the Drug Controller General of India. The presence of CK18 and well-defined, DAPI-stained nuclei were found in CTCs. CTC were counted and then examined for stage, extracapsular spread (ECS), lymphovascular emboli (LVE), perineural invasion (PNI), and depth of invasion, among other clinicopathological criteria (DOI). To distinguish between early and advanced stages of dialysis, CTC cut off values were obtained. CTCs in OSCC patients were found to be associated with cancer stages (clinical and pathological) and aggressive pathological characteristics. We saw a 25–50 percent increase in CTC number when aggressive clinical characteristics were present, which frequently indicate a bad prognosis. Treatment-naive patients had a reduced number of CTCs in the early stages. The number of CTCs in advanced-stage OSCC patients was 50% greater than in early-stage OSCC patients. CTC might be considered a trustworthy measure to predict the disease outcome in oral cancer due to a positive connection of CTC number with numerous pathophysiological characteristics. The presence of CTC at all stages of the disease shows that OSCC is most likely a biologically systematic disease [72].

2.5.2.1 Organoids

Patient-derived tumour organoids, which serve as in vitro tumour models and predictors of medication responses, are one strategy now under investigation for customised cancer treatment. In vitro cancer cell lines, patient-derived xenografts, and 3D culture models are all used in traditional cancer research and therapy. Due to the diversity and variability of the tumour microenvironment, these are restricted in their ability to precisely correlate an individual tumour's response to a treatment. Organoids provide a more faithful depiction of this dynamic niche, and data suggests that the genetic and functional similarities between patient-derived tumour organoids and the real thing are striking [73].

2.5.3 Targetted mononclonal antibodies for cancer therapy

Because of their low cytotoxicity, high specificity, and scalability, mAbs have proven particularly promising for cancer therapies among the numerous molecular-based approaches (e.g., small compounds, mAbs, and vaccines). mAbs are Y-shaped proteins that can attach to a specific molecular target and are created either synthetically or by B lymphocytes. mAbs are one of the most rapidly expanding immunotherapies, with over 22 FDA-approved mAb-based oncology medicines. mAb-based therapies, in contrast to standard therapies (e.g., surgery, radiation, and/or chemotherapy), are targeted to specific molecular markers expressed by a specific tumour, and so are more likely to be effective [74]. Typically, monoclonal antibodies (e.g., cetuximab) or synthetic small molecules are used to target cancer-specific cell receptors or intracellular signalling pathways (eg, gefinitib) in OC [9]. The tested drugs include, Cetuximab (Erbitux), pembrolizumab (Keytruda) and nivolumab (Opdivo).

Anti-EGFR monoclonal antibodies (mAbs) possess an antibody-dependent cellular cytotoxicity (ADCC) and complement-dependent cytotoxicity (CDC), and antitumor activity. Mice study has shown EMab-17(Anti-EGFR mAb) may be used as an antibody-based therapy for EGFR-expressing OSCC [75].

2.5.3.1 Immune check point inhibitors

The creation of antibodies capable of blocking coinhibitory immune cell receptors, or "immune checkpoints" — T-cell surface receptors that, when activated by specific ligands, limit the T-cytotoxic cell's immunological response — is a hopeful improvement in cancer treatment. Tumour cells tend to overexpress the ligands that activate these inhibitory receptors, allowing them to evade the immunological response of T cells and proliferate freely. Despite the fact that over two dozen individual costimulatory receptors have been identified, two of them — CTLA-4 and programmed cell death 1 (PD-1), have been the focus of antibody-based immune checkpoint blockade (ICB) treatments [76].

2.5.4 Non-invasive imaging for immunotherapy

Most of the patients do not respond to immunotherapy especially the immune check point inhibitors (ICI). The traditional imaging methods only provide anatomic information and do not define the concrete representation of response or progression, especially pseudo-progression due to tumour infiltrating lymphocytes (TILs); and third, toxicities are a potential concern for the widespread use of immunotherapy, which is associated with an increased risk of cancer progression. As a result, a reliable and repeatable imaging approach is critical for identifying the patient group most or least likely to react to immunotherapy [77].

Molecular imaging, in combination with disease-specific imaging probes, can provide non-invasive, early, and dynamic information about the effects of immune cells or other cells in the tumour microenvironment (TME), as well as target

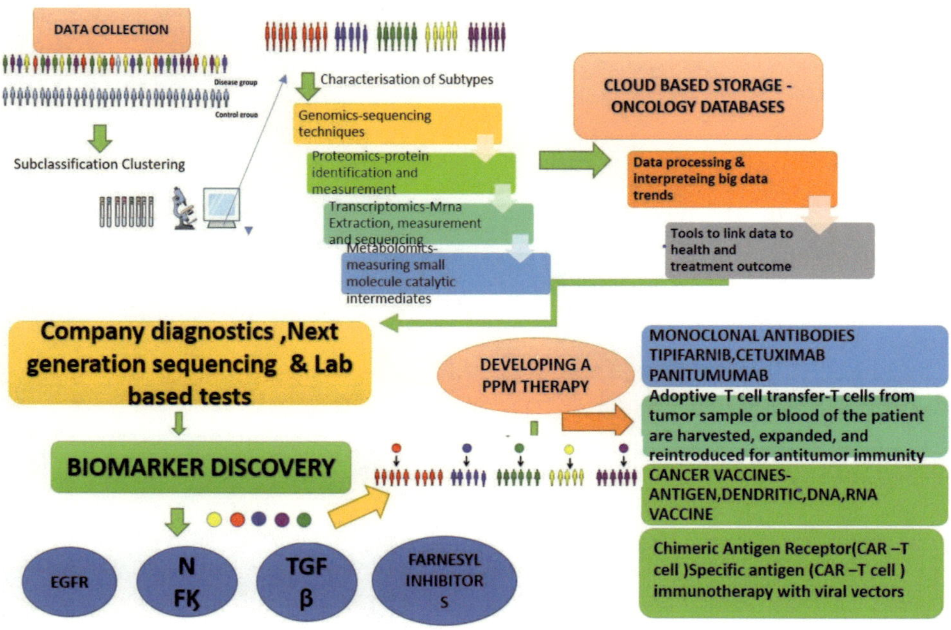

Figure 3.
Translation of PPM in to clinical practice.

expression and biodistribution of immunomodulatory drugs in the body, allowing clinicians to predict which patients will benefit most from immunotherapy. Furthermore, integrating immunotherapy with molecular imaging may improve cancer immunotherapy precision. Immunotherapies are classified into four major categories: Immune cell-based therapies, ICIs, tumour vaccines, and CAR-T cell therapy are all examples of this [78].

Figure 3 summarises the translation of PPM in to clinical practice.

3. Conclusion

This chapter has discussed the various aspects of PPM and the use of molecular and genetic profiling of tumours through omics technology for early diagnosis, formation of patient specific databases through next generation sequencing and tailored immunotherapy. Despite the advances in development technologies very few studies have been conducted in relation to OC and the research in this arena is in its budding stage. Future clinical trials on OC treatment should focus on translating the OMICs technology from bench to bedside with the use of biomarkers and CDx technologies. Tailored treatment therapies should be planned according to patients molecular and genetic profiling with consideration of individual factors. Pharma developers should create an effective medicine combining the traditional clinical data with a patient's biological profile, which includes a variety of omics-based statistics. The databases can be used to gather knowledge about disease and aid in its development more precise, safer, and better-targeted medicines for a variety of diseases in patient population.

Conflict of interest

"The authors declare no conflict of interest."

Author details

Deepa Jatti Patil[1*] and Rakesh Nagaraju[2]

1 Department of Oral Medicine and Radiology, K.M. Shah Dental College and Hospital, Sumandeep Vidyapeeth (Deemed University), Vadodara, Gujarat, India

2 Faculty of Dental Sciences, Department of Oral Medicine and Radiology, M.S. Ramaiah University of Applied Sciences, Bangalore, India

*Address all correspondence to: iafdeepa@gmail.com

References

[1] Forastiere A, Koch W, Trotti A, Sid D. Head and neck cancer. N Engl J Med. 2001;345(26):1890-900.

[2] Argiris A, Karamouzis MV, Raben D, Ferris RL. Head and neck cancer. Lancet. 2008;371(9625):1695-1709.

[3] Kreimer AR, Clifford GM, Boyle P, Franceschi S. Human papillomavirus types in head and neck squamous cell carcinomas worldwide: a systematic review. Cancer Epidemiol Biomarkers Prev. 2005;14(2):467-475.

[4] Fakhry C, Westra WH, Li S, Cmelak A, Ridge JA, Pinto H, Forastiere A, Gillison ML. Improved survival of patients with human papillomavirus positive head and neck squamous cell carcinoma in a prospective clinical trial. J Natl Cancer Inst. 2008;100(4):261-269.

[5] Ferlay J, Soerjomataram I, Dikshit R, et al. Cancer incidence and mortality worldwide: sources, methods and major patterns in GLOBOCAN 2012. Int J Cancer 2015;136: E359–E386.

[6] Torre LA, Bray F, Siegel RL, Ferlay J, Lortet-Tieulent J, Jemal A. Global cancer statistics, 2012. CA Cancer J Clin. 2015;65(2):87-108.

[7] Warnakulasuriya S. Living with oral cancer: epidemiology with particular reference to prevalence and life-style changes that influence survival. Oral Oncol 2010; 46:407-410.

[8] Braakhuis BJ, Brakenhoff RH, Leemans CR. Second field tumors: a new opportunity for cancer prevention? Oncologist. 2005;10(7):493-500.

[9] Algazi AP, Grandis JR. Head and neck cancer in 2016: a watershed year for improvements in treatment? Nat Rev Clin Oncol 2017; 14:76-78.

[10] Schmitz S, Ang KK, Vermorken J, et al. Targeted therapies for squamous cell carcinoma of the head and neck: current knowledge and future directions. Cancer Treat Rev 2014; 40:390-404.

[11] Seyhan, A.A., Carini, C. Are innovation and new technologies in precision medicine paving a new era in patients centric care? J Transl Med 2019; 17:114.

[12] Krzyszczyk P et al The growing role of precision and personalized medicine for cancer treatment. Technology Singap World Sci 2018; 6(3-4): 79-100.

[13] Morgan G, Ward R & Barton M The contribution of cytotoxic chemotherapy to 5-year survival in adult malignancies. Clin. Oncol. (R. Coll. Radiol.) 16, 549-560 (2004). [PubMed: 15630849]

[14] Personalized Medicine Coalition. The personalized medicine report. Opportunity, challenges, and the future 2017, http://www.personalizedmedicinecoalition.org/Userfiles/PMCCorporate/file/The_PM_Report.pdf

[15] Burney IA & Lakhtakia R Precision medicine: Where have we reached and where are we headed? Sultan Qaboos Univ. Med. J 2917; 17: e255–e258.

[16] Maciejko L, Smalley M & Goldman A Cancer immunotherapy and personalized medicine: Emerging technologies and biomarker-based approaches. J. Mol. Biomark. Diagn 2017;8:

[17] Seyhan AA. Biomarkers in drug discovery and development. Eur Biopharm Rev. 2010; 1:19-25.

[18] Lee HJ, Seo AN, Kim EJ, Jang MH, Kim YJ, Kim JH et al. Prognostic and predictive values of EGFR overexpression and EGFR copy number alteration in HER2-positive breast cancer. Br J Cancer. 2014; 112:103.

[19] Nagarsheth N, Wicha MS, Zou WP. Chemokines in the cancer microenvironment and their relevance in cancer immunotherapy. Nat Rev Immunol. 2017; 17:559-572.

[20] Blank CU, Haanen JB, Ribas A, Schumacher TN. The "cancer immunogram". Science. 2016; 352: 658-660.

[21] Blank CU, Haanen JB, Ribas A, Schumacher TN. The "cancer immunogram". Science. 2016; 352:658-660.

[22] Koelzer VH, Sirinukunwattana K, Rittscher J, Mertz KD. Precision immunoprofiling by image analysis and artificial intelligence. Virchows Arch. 2018. https ://doi.org/10.1007/s0042 8-018-2485-z.

[23] Chial H. DNA sequencing technologies key to the human genome project. Nat. Educ 2008;1:

[24] Goodwin S, McPherson JD & McCombie WR Coming of age: Ten years of next-generation sequencing technologies. Nat. Rev. Genet 2016; 17:333-351.

[25] Cancer Genome Atlas Network. Comprehensive genomic characterization of head and neck squamous cell carcinomas. Nature 2015; 517:576-582.

[26] Li CC, Shen Z, Bavarian R, Yang F, Bhattacharya A. Oral Cancer: Genetics and the Role of Precision Medicine. Dent Clin North Am. 2018;62(1):29-46. doi: 10.1016/j.cden.2017.08.002. PMID: 29126492.

[27] Agrawal N, Frederick MJ, Pickering CR, et al. Exome sequencing of head and neck squamous cell carcinoma reveals inactivating mutations in NOTCH1. Science 2011;333:1154-1157.

[28] Stransky N, Egloff AM, Tward AD, et al. The mutational landscape of head and neck squamous cell carcinoma. Science 2011; 333:1157-1160.

[29] Stein LD, Knoppers BM, Campbell P, et al. Data analysis: create a cloud commons. Nature 2015; 523:149-151.

[30] Wiklund ED, Gao S, Hulf T, et al. MicroRNA alterations and associated aberrant DNA methylation patterns across multiple sample types in oral squamous cell carcinoma. PLoS One 2011;6: e27840.

[31] Tang H, Wu Z, Zhang J, et al. Salivary lncRNA as a potential marker for oral squamous cell carcinoma diagnosis. Mol Med Rep 2013;7: 761-766.

[32] Lowe R, Shirley N, Bleackley M, Dolan S & Shafee T. Transcriptomics technologies. PLOS Comput. Biol 2017;13:e1005457.

[33] Kukurba KR & Montgomery SB. RNA sequencing and analysis. Cold Spring Harb. Protoc 2015, 951-969.

[34] Buguliskis JS Could RNA-Seq become the workhorse of precision medicine? Plowing through transcriptional variations by harnessing the powerful next-gen technique. Genet. Eng. Biotechnol. News 2015; 35:8-9.

[35] Severino P, Alvares AM, Michaluart P Jr, et al. Global gene expression profiling of oral cavity cancers suggests molecular heterogeneity within anatomic subsites. BMC Res Notes 2008; 1:113.

[36] Walter V, Yin X, Wilkerson MD, et al. Molecular subtypes in head and neck cancer exhibit distinct patterns of chromosomal gain and loss of canonical cancer genes. PLoS One 2013;8: e56823.

[37] Chung CH, Parker JS, Karaca G, et al. Molecular classification of head and neck squamous cell carcinomas using patterns of gene expression. Cancer Cell 2004; 5:489-500.

[38] van Hooff SR, Leusink FK, Roepman P, et al. Validation of a gene expression signature for assessment of lymph node metastasis in oral squamous cell carcinoma. J Clin Oncol 2012; 30:4104-4110.

[39] He Y, Shao F, Pi W, et al. Largescale transcriptomics analysis suggests overexpression of BGH3, MMP9 and PDIA3 in oral squamous cell carcinoma. PLoS One 2016;11: e0146530.

[40] Larance M & Lomond AI Multidimensional proteomics for cell biology. Nat. Rev. Mol. Cell. Biol 2015; 16:269-280.

[41] Han XM, Aslanian A & Yates JR Mass spectrometry for proteomics. Curr. Opin. Chem. Biol 2008;12: 483-490.

[42] Schwanhausser B, Busse D, Li N, et al. Global quantification of mammalian gene expression control. Nature 2011; 473:337-342.

[43] Malik UU, Zarina S, Pennington SR. Oral squamous cell carcinoma: key clinical questions, biomarker discovery, and the role of proteomics. Arch Oral Biol 2016; 63:53-65.

[44] Lo WY, Lai CC, Hua CH, et al. S100A8 is identified as a biomarker of HPV18- infected oral squamous cell carcinomas by suppression subtraction hybridization, clinical proteomics analysis, and immunohistochemistry staining. J Proteome Res 2007; 6:2143-2151.

[45] Hu S, Wong DT. Oral cancer proteomics. Curr Opin Mol Ther 2007; 9:467-476.

[46] Schaaij-Visser TB, Brakenhoff RH, Leemans CR, et al. Protein biomarker discovery for head and neck cancer. J Proteomics 2010; 73:1790-1803.

[47] Wadsworth JT, Somers KD, Stack BC Jr, et al. Identification of patients with head and neck cancer using serum protein profiles. Arch Otolaryngol Head Neck Surg 2004; 130:98-104.

[48] Wishart DS, Feunang YD, Marcu A, Guo AC, Liang K, Vázquez-Fresno R, *et al* HMDB 4.0: the human metabolome database for 2018. Nucleic Acids Res. 2018 4;46(D1):D608-D617.

[49] Monteiro MS, Carvalho M, Bastos ML & Guedes de Pinho P Metabolomics analysis for biomarker discovery: Advances and challenges. Curr. Med. Chem 2013;20:257-227.

[50] Roessner U & Bowne J What is metabolomics all about? Biotechniques 2009; 46:363.

[51] Everett JR, Loo RL & Pullen FS Pharmacometabonomics and personalized medicine. Ann. Clin. Biochem 2013; 50:523-545.

[52] Eckhart AD, Beebe K & Milburn M Metabolomics as a key integrator for "omic" advancement of personalized medicine and future therapies. Clin. Transl. Sci 2012; 5:285-288.

[53] Wang J, Christison TT, Misuno K, et al. Metabolomic profiling of anionic metabolites in head and neck cancer cells by capillary ion chromatography with orbitrap mass spectrometry. Anal Chem 2014; 86:5116-5124.

[54] Yonezawa K, Nishiumi S, Kitamoto-Matsuda J, et al. Serum and tissue metabolomics of head and neck cancer. Cancer Genomics Proteomics 2013;10: 233-238.

[55] Hu S, Wang J, Ji EH, et al. Targeted metabolomic analysis of head and neck cancer cells using high performance ion chromatography coupled with a Q exactive HF mass spectrometer. Anal Chem 2015; 87:6371-6379.

[56] Tie G, Yan J, Khair L, et al. Hypercholesterolemia increases

colorectal cancer incidence by reducing production of NKT and gamma delta T Cells from hematopoietic stem cells. Cancer Res 2017;77: 2351-2362.

[57] Codini M, Cataldi S, Lazzarini A, et al. Why high cholesterol levels help hematological malignancies: role of nuclear lipid microdomains. Lipids Health Dis 2016; 15:4.

[58] Acharya S, Rai P, Hallikeri K, et al. Serum lipid profile in oral squamous cell carcinoma: alterations and association with some clinicopathological parameters and tobacco use. Int J Oral Maxillofac Surg 2016; 45:713-720.

[59] Patel PS, Shah MH, Jha FP, et al. Alterations in plasma lipid profile patterns in head and neck cancer and oral precancerous conditions. Indian J Cancer 2004; 41:25-31.

[60] Papadopoulos N, Kinzler KW, Vogelstein B. The role of companion diagnostics in the development and use of mutation-targeted cancer therapies. Nat Biotechnol. 2006; 24: 985- 995.

[61] U.S. Food and Drug Administration. Mobile medical applications — Guidance for industry and food and drug administration staff (2015), https://www.fda.gov/downloads/MedicalDevices/.../UCM263366.pdf.

[62] U.S. Food and Drug Administration. List of cleared or approved companion diagnostic devices (in vitro and imaging tools) (2018), https://www.fda.gov/medicaldevices/productsandmedicalprocedures/invitrodiagnostics/ucm301431.htm.

[63] Pavlopoulou A, Spandidos DA & Michalopoulos I Human cancer databases (review). Oncol. Rep 2015;33:3-18.

[64] Kanehisa Laboratories. KEGG database (2017) http://www.genome.jp/kegg/kegg1.html.

[65] Damani Shah H, Saranath D, Pradhan S. Single nucleotide polymorphisms in transcription factor genes associated with susceptibility to oral cancer. J Cell Biochem. 2020 ;121(2):1050-1060.

[66] Multani S, Saranath D. Genotypic Distribution of Single Nucleotide Polymorphisms in Oral Cancer: Global Scene. Tumor Biol. 2016;37: 6169-6176.

[67] Multania S, Saranath D Single Nucleotide Polymorphisms and Risk of Oral Cancer: Indian Case-Control Study. J Clin Cell Immunol 2016;7: 448.

[68] Butcher EC, Berg EL & Kunkel EJ Systems biology in drug discovery. Nat. Biotechnol 2004; 22:1253-1259.

[69] McShane LM & Polley MY Development of omics-based clinical tests for prognosis and therapy selection: The challenge of achieving statistical robustness and clinical utility. Clin. Trials 2013; 10:653-665.

[70] Mackall CL Engineering a designer immunotherapy. Science 2018;359:990-991.

[71] Ried K, Eng P & Sali A. Screening for circulating tumour cells allows early detection of cancer and monitoring of treatment effectiveness: An observational study. Asian Pac. J. Cancer Prev 2017;18;2275-2285.

[72] Khandare J, Qayyumi B, Bharde A, Aland G, Jayant S, Tripathi S *et al* Correlation of CTCs with disease progression in Indian oral cancer patients. Journal of Clinical Oncology 2020 38:15 e15541-e15541.

[73] Aboulkheyr Es H, Montazeri L, Aref AR, Vosough M & Baharvand H Personalized cancer medicine: An organoid approach. Trends Biotechnol 2018;36: 358-371.

[74] Esteva FJ Monoclonal antibodies, small molecules, and vaccines in the

treatment of breast cancer. Oncologist 2004; 9:4-9.

[75] Takei J, Kaneko MK, Ohishi T, Kawada M, Harada H, Kato Y. A novel anti-EGFR monoclonal antibody (EMab-17) exerts antitumor activity against oral squamous cell carcinomas via antibody-dependent cellular cytotoxicity and complement-dependent cytotoxicity. Oncol Lett. 2020;19(4):2809-2816.

[76] Hargadon KM, Johnson CE & Williams CJ Immune checkpoint blockade therapy for cancer: An overview of FDA-approved immune checkpoint inhibitors. Int. Immunopharmacol 2018; 62:29-39.

[77] Du Y, Qi Y, Jin Z, Tian J. Noninvasive imaging in cancer immunotherapy: The way to precision medicine. Cancer Lett. 2019; 466:13-22. doi: 10.1016/j.canlet.2019.08.009.

[78] R.A. Juergens, K.A. Zukotynski, A. Singnurkar, D.P. Snider, J.F. Valliant, K.Y. Gulenchyn, Imaging biomarkers in immunotherapy, Biomarkers Canc. 2016;8:1-13.

Chapter 5

Sentinel Lymph Node Biopsy for Early Oral Cavity Squamous Cell Carcinoma

Rajith Mendis and Muzib Abdul-Razak

Abstract

Early stage oral cavity squamous cell carcinoma (OCSCC) has a significant risk of subclinical nodal metastases, which is the strongest independent prognostic factor for regional recurrence and survival. However current preoperative imaging modalities are unable to identify patients with micrometastases, and an observation strategy has been associated with inferior outcomes when compared to an elective neck dissection. Sentinel lymph node biopsy provides a safe and accurate staging procedure to select the patients who benefit from an elective neck dissection, while avoiding unnecessary surgery in the patients who are node negative. There is recent Level II evidence demonstrating equivalent oncological outcomes when compared with elective neck dissection. However, a multidisciplinary approach is required including reliable mapping of the sentinel lymph node, precise surgical technique and comprehensive histopathological analysis to ensure accurate results are obtained.

Keywords: Oral squamous cell carcinoma, oral cancer, head and neck cancer, sentinel lymph node, elective neck dissection, nodal metastases, lymphoscintigraphy

1. Introduction

Early stage oral cavity squamous cell carcinoma (T1N0 or T2N0) has a significant risk of between 20 and 44% [1–3] of harbouring subclinical nodal metastases. The presence of nodal metastases has been shown to be the strongest independent prognostic factor for predicting a poor outcome [4–6]. Current imaging techniques including computed tomography (CT), magnetic resonance imaging (MRI), positron emission tomography (PET) and ultrasound (US) cannot accurately identify micrometastases preoperatively [7, 8]. Traditionally the only way to identify this was to perform an elective neck dissection (END), however this is unnecessary in the majority (60–80%) of patients who do not harbour occult nodal metastases, and has an associated morbidity [1]. This chapter will present the histopathological factors that have been used to risk stratify patients for an END, as well as the multifaceted technique and role of sentinel lymph node biopsy (SLNB) as a staging procedure for patients with OCSCC.

2. Histopathological factors

Various parameters have been investigated to further stratify the risk of subclinical nodal metastases, including tumour thickness and depth of invasion (DOI).

Tumour thickness measures the thickness of the tumour from the deepest point of invasion to the top of the granular cell layer, or if ulcerated, the ulcer base serves as the reference point. DOI is measured from the level of the basement membrane to the deepest point of invasion, and in the case of an ulcerated OCSCC, this level is estimated by creating an imaginary line from the adjacent basement membrane [1]. This avoids under-representing an ulcerated tumour or over-representing an exophytic tumour, and has been included in staging for OCSCC in the current 8th edition American Joint Committee on Cancer (AJCC) staging manual [9]. An increased risk of subclinical nodal metastases has been associated with varying tumour thicknesses, between 2 mm to 5 mm, with thicker tumours having a risk of nodal metastases between 44 and 50% [1, 8, 10]. The anatomical sub-site of the OCSCC may also play a role with a lesion thickness > 1.5 mm on the floor of mouth being associated with a risk of nodal metastases of 35% [11]; however, this has not been a consistent finding, with another study demonstrating a 4 mm cut-off associated with an increased risk of nodal metastases regardless of sub-site [5]. This study documented rates of local control, nodal disease, and survival rates of 91%, 8%, and 100%, respectively, for lesions <4 mm thick compared with 84%, 48%, and 74% for those ≥4 mm thick ($p < .01$). Despite this there are limitations with basing management decisions on the tumour thickness or DOI, as often this may not be assessable on a biopsy alone due to the sparse amount of biopsy material, and if assessable the biopsy may not be representative of the entire tumour [12], resulting in subsequent management decisions based more on clinical assessment.

Histopathological factors predicting for sub-clinical nodal metastases in the setting of sentinel lymph node biopsy (SLNB) have also been investigated with three variables identified including grade (G1 *vs* G2/G3), presence of lymphatic invasion and mode of invasion (cohesive *vs* dissolute) [13]. Interestingly, in this study DOI and tumour thickness were not reliable predictors of nodal metastasis demonstrating the inconsistency and uncertainty in basing management decisions on histopathological factors alone.

3. Benefit of elective neck dissection

Superior outcomes have been published in a prospective randomised controlled trial (RCT) involving patients with early OCSCC (T1/T2 tumours) without clinical evidence of nodal metastases, when they underwent an END compared to observation followed by neck dissection in the setting of nodal relapse [14]. In this study 3 year overall survival was 80% for patients undergoing END compared to 67.5% for patients undergoing delayed therapeutic dissection following relapse ($p = 0.01$). Subclinical nodal positivity in the END group was 29%, while nodal relapse rates in the observation group was 45% [14].

Of note in the 'true' node negative patients in this study, which included pathological node negative patients in the END group and those who did not relapse in the observation group, *survival was equivalent.* This demonstrates that while patients with subclinical nodal metastases benefit from a neck dissection, the remaining 60–80% of patients without nodal metastases do not experience a survival benefit by undergoing a neck dissection (see **Figure 1**). It is also important to consider that even patients with a pathologically negative neck following END have a rate of regional failure up to 5–10% [3, 15].

This benefit of END has been reported in a previous observational study where patients with early (T1/T2) OCSCC had significantly improved outcomes undergoing END (median survival 12 years) compared to observation (median survival 4.1 years), with the majority (11/12) of recurrences in the observation group

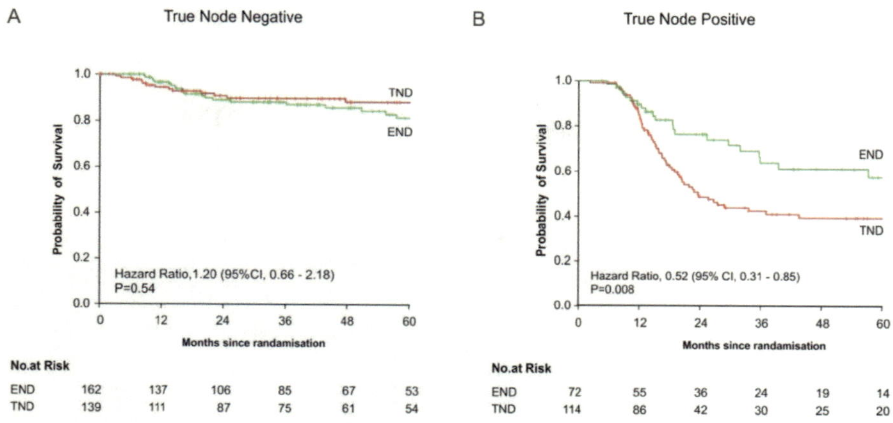

Figure 1.
Overall survival in 'true node negative' and 'true node positive' patients [14].

occurring as regional failures [2]. This benefit is selectively achieved in patients undergoing SLNB, as patients with a positive sentinel lymph node (SLN) undergo a completion neck dissection while the morbidity of the neck dissection is avoided when the SLNB is negative.

4. Technique of sentinel lymph node biopsy

There is marked heterogeneity in the published data assessing the role of SLNB in OCSCC including preoperative investigations, technique of identifying the SLN and the pathological assessment of the specimens [16]. The GETTEC (Groupe d'Etude des Tumeurs de la Tête et du Cou) guidelines [17] have attempted to standardise the technique in performing SLNB with recommendations for lymphoscintigraphy, surgery and pathological analysis. Of note, they recommend a median of three SLNs to be sampled, with a single SLN node considered insufficient to accurately determine the nodal pathological status.

SLNB for OCSCC presents unique challenges in relation to both the complex anatomy of the head and neck, in addition to the short distance between the primary lesion and the draining nodal basin, particularly for lesions located in the floor of mouth. This is due to the high activity at the adjacent injection site, which can be easily overlooked by planar lymphoscintigraphy and intraoperative gamma probes [18]. Intraoperatively, the close relationship between the primary lesion and the draining lymph nodes can result in so called 'shine through' of the radioactive tracer from the primary site with difficulties in identifying the SLN if it is in an adjacent nodal basin, particularly the submental (IA) and submandibular (IB) basins. Composite single photon emission computed tomography (SPECT) with concurrent CT combines functional and anatomical imaging to enhance topographic orientation and diagnostic sensitivity, with more SLNs being detectable than by planar lymphoscintigraphy alone, as well as providing more detailed anatomical information to assist with intraoperative localisation [19]. **Figures 2** and **3** demonstrates the lymphoscintigraphy result and composite SPECT/CT for patients with unilateral and bilateral lymphatic drainage respectively. The SPECT/CT provides detailed anatomical information to assist with identification of the SLN.

Another consideration that may impact on the accuracy of lymphoscintigraphy is the choice of radiotracer. These have different molecular characteristics as

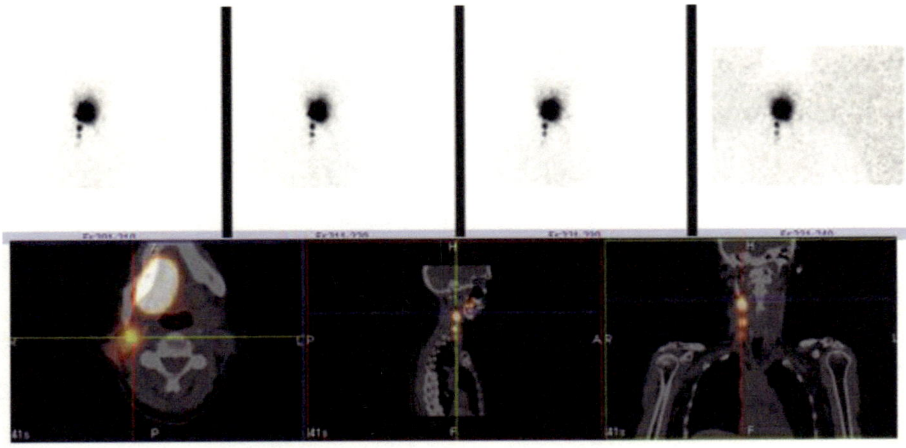

Figure 2.
Lymphoscintigraphy and SPECT/CT demonstrating ipsilateral level 2 sentinel lymph node.

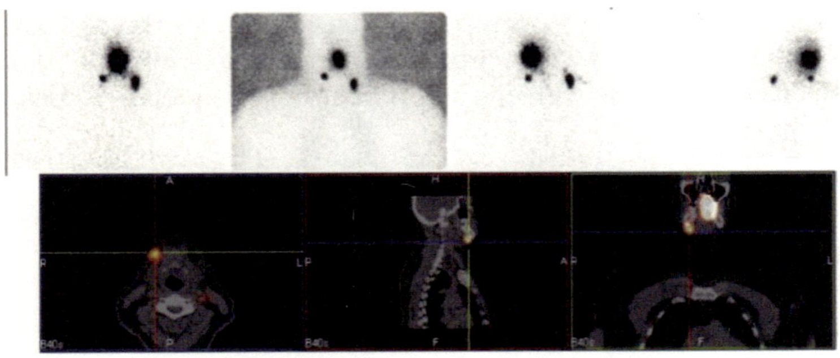

Figure 3.
Lymphoscintigraphy and SPECT/CT demonstrating bilateral drainage from a lateralised tumour.

summarised in **Table 1**, which impacts the drainage characteristics, and this may be utilised to counteract the 'shine through' effect. The potential of [^{99m}Tc]Tilmanocept is of particular interest as it has a small molecular size of 7 nm facilitating rapid injection site clearance, and targets the CD206 receptor found on the reticuloendothelial cells in lymph nodes to promote accumulation within the SLN while reducing drainage to second tier nodes [21, 22]. A study assessing [^{99m}Tc]Tilmanocept in the setting of both OSCC and head and neck cutaneous SCC demonstrated a SLN detection rate of 97.6%, with a false negative rate of 2.56% [22]. This study included

Agent	Mean Particle size (nm)
Sulphur Colloid	100–220
Antimony trisulphide	3–30
Suphide nanocolloid	10–50
Nanocolloidal albumin	5–80
Rhenium sulphide nanocolloid	50–200
ICG-99mTc-Nanocolloid	5–80
Tilmanocept	~7

Table 1.
^{99m}TC labelled radiotracers [20].

20 patients with floor of mouth OSCCs, where [^{99m}Tc]Tilmanocept may be of particular use, and a SLN was successfully identified in all cases without any false negatives [22]. A recent comparison study between [^{99m}Tc]Tilmanocept and [^{99m}Tc] Nanocolloid found that [^{99m}Tc]Tilmanocept had higher rates of clearance from the primary injection site but also had reduced accumulation within the SLN, with a similar SLN to injection site ratio of radioactivity between the two radiotracers [23].

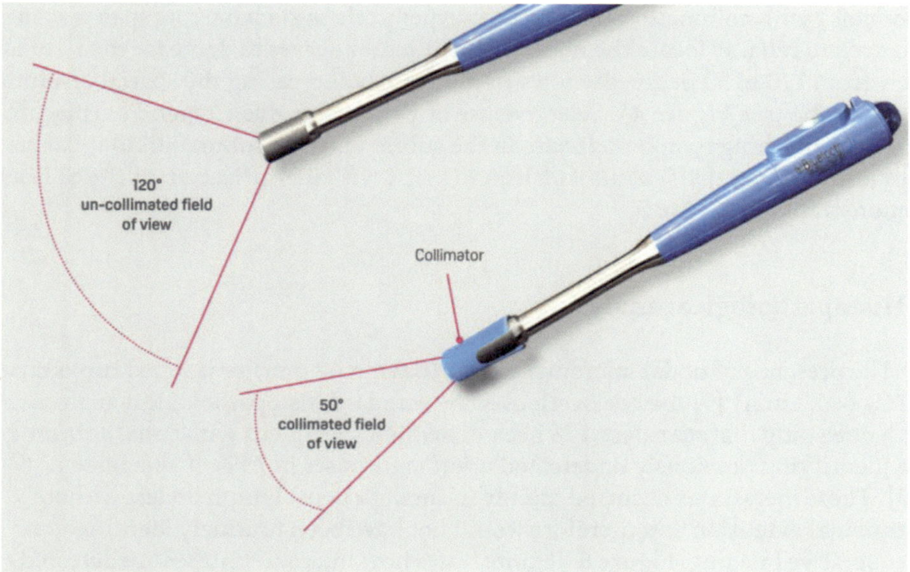

Figure 4.
Focused field of view with use of collimator. (This image is © 2021 Devicor Medical Products, Inc.; used with permission).

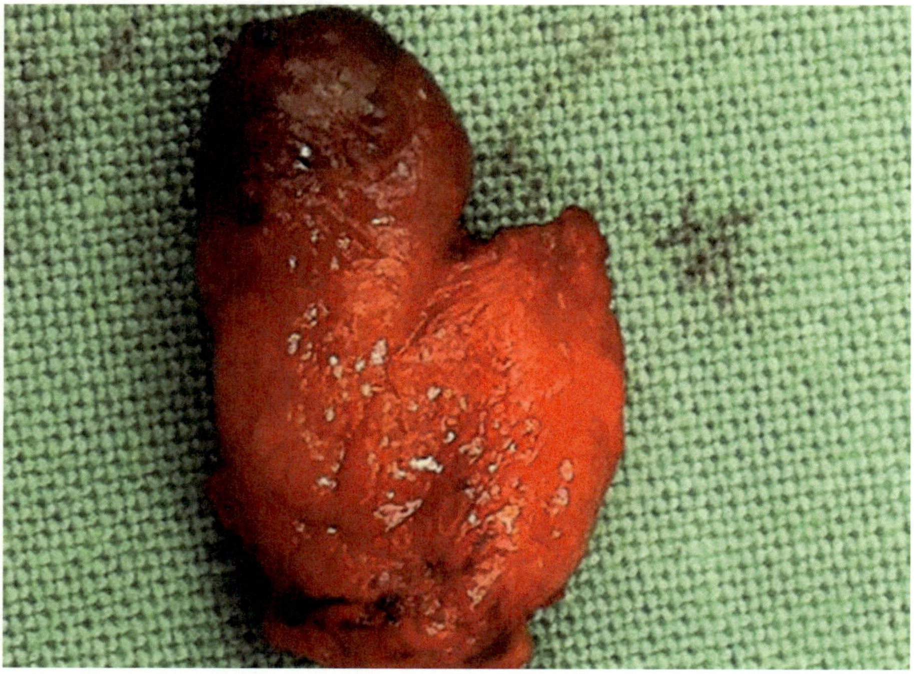

Figure 5.
Sentinel lymph node with blue dye on one surface facilitating visual identification.

This study demonstrated a high degree of agreement in the identification of SLNs between each radiotracer, however it is difficult to draw definitive conclusions with a small sample size, and further studies are required.

Specific surgical techniques can be employed to counteract the 'shine through' effect, including mobilisation of the fat pad between the submandibular gland and anterior belly of digastric to reflect the tissue, allowing for careful analysis with the handheld gamma probe while avoiding radiation from the primary tumour injection site [24]. A probe with an angled head (Neoprobe, Devicor Medical Products) with collimator attached is indispensable in such narrow spaces as in the neck to reliably locate the node. The collimator serves to decrease the field of view from 120 to 50 degrees while simultaneously increasing the spatial resolution of the probe (see **Figure 4**). Selective use of patent blue dye (Aspen Pharmacare) when the draining lymph nodes are in the submental and submandibular basins provides additional visual information to assist with identification of the SLN as demonstrated in **Figure 5**.

5. Histopathological analysis

The presence of nodal micrometastases (0.2 mm–2 mm) or isolated tumour cells (ITC) (<0.2 mm) [9] may be overlooked by standard histopathological analysis, with one study that reanalysed 76 neck dissection specimens with serial sectioning identifying previously undetected micrometastases in 7.9% of specimens [25]. These metastases occurred mainly in small (<1 cm) lymph nodes, without extranodal extension and therefore would not have been routinely identified on preoperative imaging. **Figure 6** demonstrates how micrometastases are detected more reliably by performing serial sectioning. Another smaller prospective study analysed 34 neck dissection specimens with serial sectioning and immunohistochemistry (IHC) in addition to standard haematoxylin–eosin staining (HES) and found that 3 patients (8.8%) were upstaged by the additional analysis, with two cases of micrometastases and one patient harbouring ITC [26]. Importantly the identification of these micrometastases did not warrant further treatment beyond the neck dissection which had already been performed [25]. However, the revised findings of node positivity has both a staging and prognostic impact on patients.

In another study in the setting of SLNB, serial sectioning and IHC upstaged 5 of 27 (19%) patients with nodal metastases [8], and a retrospective review of 272

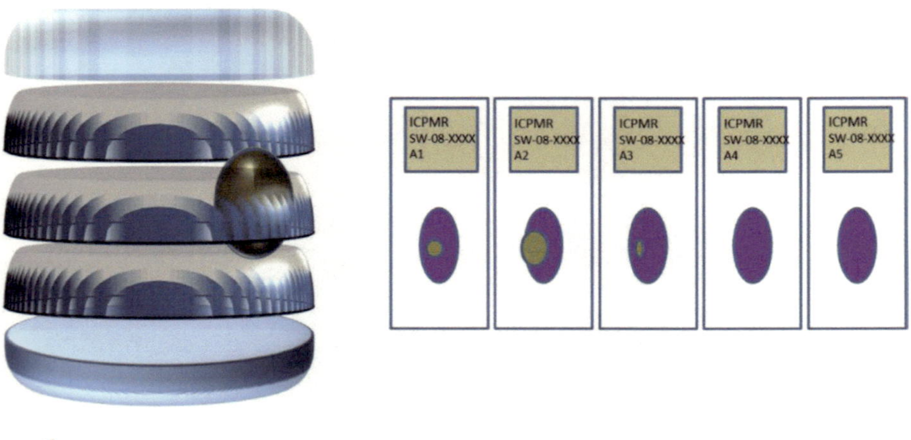

Figure 6.
Serial sectioning a lymph node.

patients undergoing SLNB found that 51.7% of their positive sentinel lymph nodes were only detected following serial sectioning and IHC [27]. The addition of IHC to standard HES increases both the sensitivity and negative predictive value of SLNB [16, 28, 29] and has now become part of the standard pathological assessment of SLNs in most institutions.

Performing serial sectioning and IHC (cytokeratin – AE1/AE3) is both labour and time intensive for the pathologist. By performing a SLNB, the detailed examination can be focused on the most likely lymph nodes which might harbour micrometastatic disease for each individual patient, providing the most precise staging and prognostic information.

6. Accuracy in predicting neck status

The Sentinel European Node Trial (SENT) was a large multicentre European study investigating SLNB in 415 patients with early OCSCC, of which subclinical nodal metastases were identified in 26% of the study population. The findings demonstrated the procedure to be safe, reliable and accurate with a SLN identified in 99% of cases, with 86% sensitivity, 95% negative predictive value and 14% false negative rate [30]. These results have been replicated in other similar studies, albeit with lower false negative rates of 2.56% [22] and 9.1% [31], and with higher rates of contralateral drainage (23–40%) [31, 32].

SLNB allows for identification of unexpected lymphatic drainage patterns, and the SENT trial found that bilateral drainage was identified in 10% of lateralised tumours, and 2.4% had exclusive contralateral drainage. The patients with contralateral drainage, 7 of 49 had positive SLNs, with 5 of the patients draining exclusively contralaterally [30]. The rate of contralateral drainage for lateralised tumours has been documented in other studies to be as high as 23–40% [31, 32].

The detection of contralateral drainage is a major benefit of performing a SLNB as it allows accurate mapping of the lymphatic drainage for each individual patient, and for patients with lateralised tumours with contralateral drainage, these nodes will not be addressed if they undergo a unilateral END. If there were undetected subclinical nodal metastases in these nodes, these patients would then be at risk of a contralateral nodal failure.

The accuracy of SLNB has been further investigated by a systematic review/meta-analysis assessing the performance of SLNB as a staging procedure for OCSCC and documented it to be reliable with a sensitivity of 88% and specificity of 99%. However, when assessing covariates, performing IHC on the SLN significantly improved the sensitivity to 93% [29]. In addition to the differences in processing of specimens, there was a degree of heterogeneity in the articles in relation to measurement of failure with a combination of END and clinical follow up to detect potential false negatives. Despite this the review demonstrated that SLNB is highly accurate across several different institutions, with an improvement in quality of life including pain, shoulder mobility and scarring when compared to END [29].

7. Outcomes following sentinel lymph node biopsy

A systematic review assessing outcomes in patients with early OCSCC managed with either a SLNB or END found no significant difference in overall survival or disease free survival between the two approaches [33]. This study analysed 5 separate studies with a total of 560 patients and reported 10 more neck recurrences per 1000 patients undergoing the SLNB strategy compared with END, although this was not statistically significant. Conversely SLNB avoided the need for a neck dissection in 64% of patients. While this did demonstrate robust outcomes for patients treated with SLNB, none of the included studies were randomised and as such the overall quality of the evidence was considered low.

Two RCTs have been subsequently published comparing SLNB and END for early OCSCC with both demonstrating equivalent oncological outcomes, and their findings are summarised in **Table 2** and **Figure 7**. The Senti-MERORL trial was a multi-centre RCT with 307 patients that documented a 25% rate of SLN positivity, with these patients proceeding to a neck dissection [15]. There was a mean follow up of 4.95 years, and rates of nodal recurrence were 10.1% in the neck dissection group and 9.3% in the SLNB group, which was not a statistically significant difference. Equivalent locoregional disease control, disease specific survival and overall survival were demonstrated at 2 and 5 years [15]. When looking at the nodal recurrences in patients initially classified as pathologically node negative (pN0), there were 11 patients (10% of the 109 pN0 patients) in the END group and 8 patients (8% of the 99 pN0 patients) in the SLNB group, demonstrating similar rates of nodal staging failure between the two strategies.

A Japanese RCT compared 137 patients in the neck dissection arm and 134 patients in the SLN arm. They found a 34% rate of SLN positivity, and regional recurrence rates were 9.5% and 11.2% in the END and SLNB groups respectively.

	Garrel et al. [15]		Hasegawa et al. [34]	
	SLNB (n = 140)	**END (n = 139)**	**SLNB (n = 134)**	**END (n = 137)**
Age	60.8 (mean)	59.1 (mean)	63 (median)	63 (median)
Sex				
Male Female	88 (63%) 52 (37%)	101 (73%) 38 (27%)	89 (66%) 45 (34%)	90 (66%) 47 (34%)
Site of primary				
Oral Tongue	124 (89.2%)	119 (85.6%)	109 (81.3%)	114 (83.2%)
Floor of mouth			13 (9.7%)	14 (10.2%)
Lower gingiva			7 (5.2%)	6 (4.4%)
Buccal mucosa			5 (3.7%)	3 (2.2%)
Oropharynx	15 (10.8%)	20 (14.4%)		
T1	88 (63%)	91 (66%)	26 (19%)	25 (18%)
T2	52 (37%)	48 (35%)	108 (81%)	112 (82%)
Positive lymph nodes	35 (25%)[a]	30 (22%)	46 (34%)	34 (25%)
Frozen section/ Imprint cytology	21 (15%)		32 (24%)	
H&E/IHC	12 (9%)		14 (10%)	
Adjuvant treatment				
Radiotherapy Chemoradiotherapy	23 (16%) 10 (7%)	28 (20%) 6 (4%)	4 (3%) 0	3 (2%) 3 (2%)
Nodal recurrence	13 (9%)	14 (10%)	15 (11%)	13 (10%)
Follow up (months)	56.9 (mean)	59.4 (mean)	37 (median)	37 (median)
Overall Survival	82.2% at 5 y	81.8% at 5 y	87.9% at 3 y	86.6% at 3 ys

[a]*Includes 2 positive cases out of 8 undergoing END due to localization failure.*

Table 2.
Comparison of two RCTs.

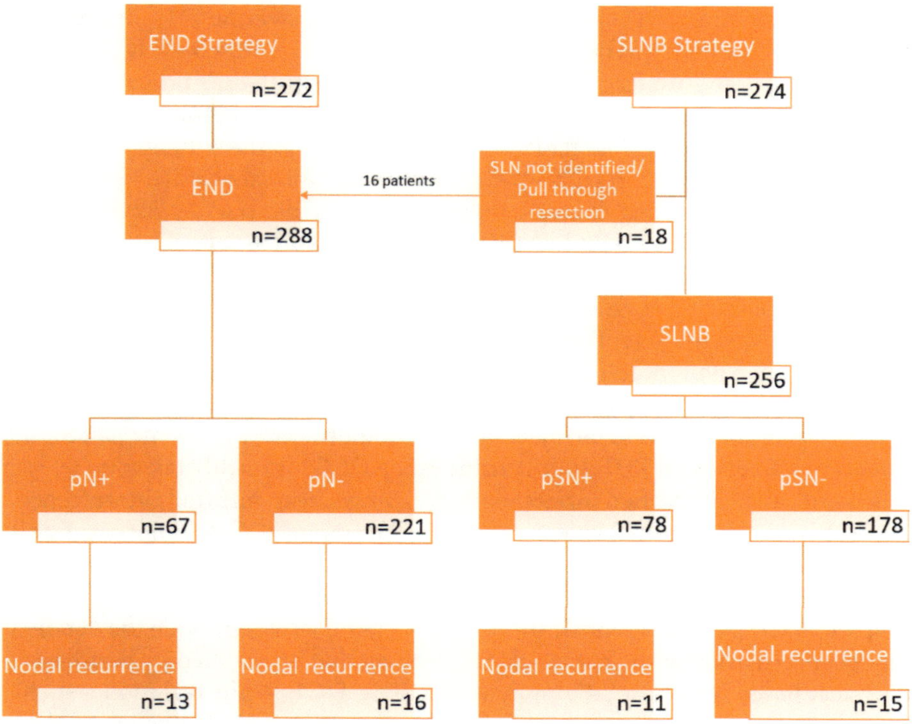

Figure 7.
Combined RCT outcomes of nodal recurrence. (Adapted from Garrel et al. [15], Hasegawa et al. [34]).

This study demonstrated equivalent 3 year overall survival and disease free survival between the END group (87.9% and 81.3%) and the SLN group (86.6% and 78.7%) [34]. Both studies demonstrate high-level evidence to support the use of SLNB as a staging procedure for patients with early T1 or T2 OCSCC.

END has an associated morbidity including shoulder dysfunction, pain and contour changes [16]. Comparison of morbidity associated with SLNB or a neck dissection demonstrates low rates of morbidity overall, however, in one study all the morbidity occurred following neck dissection, with no cases of shoulder dysfunction in the SLNB group [6]. Quality of life assessments demonstrate improved tactile sensitivity and reduced pain sensitivity in the SLNB group, with no significant difference in the presence of lymphoedema although there was trend towards improved symptoms in the sentinel lymph node biopsy group [35]. Functional outcomes were also assessed in the two RCTs, with the Senti-MERORL study finding an initial functional difference between the two groups favouring SLNB at 6 months, however this resolved by 12 months [15]. Hasegawa reported that the END group had persisting inferior scores at 12 months post operatively, when assessing neck stiffness and shoulder dysfunction compared to the SLN group [34].

8. Future directions

It is widely accepted that macrometastases and micrometastases should undergo a completion neck dissection, however management of ITC remains uncertain without a clear consensus. This is a significant issue as the incidence of ITC ranges between 14 and 27% of positive SLNs [27, 30, 36] and the two RCTs managed this subgroup with differing strategies. The Senti-MERORL trial treated ITC with observation, and in those 11 patients there were no nodal recurrences [15]. Conversely the Japanese RCT treated ITC with a completion neck dissection [34], however subgroup outcome data was not published. A retrospective Dutch study analysing outcomes for patients undergoing SLNB for OCSCC found a SLN positivity rate of 22% (107/488 patients) and of these patients, 15 (14%) had ITC, 31 (29%) had micrometastases and 61 (57%) had micrometastases. 13 of the patients with ITC underwent a neck dissection with 1 patient having additional positive lymph nodes, and the other 2 patients had adjuvant radiotherapy, and did not develop regional recurrence during follow up [36]. While ITC is considered to represent node negative disease in the setting of breast cancer [9], management of these patients remain uncertain in the setting of OCSCC and further data is required to clarify both the natural history and management outcomes for this subset of patients.

Intraoperative lymphoscintigraphy is a developing technique which has particular utility in the management of oropharyngeal or laryngeal SCC with a SLNB. These tumours are unable to be injected with a radiotracer in an awake patient for a preoperative assessment [37]. Indocyanine green (ICG) is readily taken up by lymphatics and can be identified intraoperatively using a near-infrared fluorescence camera to locate the sentinel lymph node [38]. The use of ICG does not cause any staining of the primary site as seen with use of patent blue dye, and also provides an immediate result, which offers obvious benefits in the setting of intraoperative sentinel lymph node identification. However, it does not provide the detailed drainage information with anatomical referencing that is provided by performing radiotracer based lymphoscintigraphy with a SPECT/CT. While techniques such as skin compression have been described to identify lymphatic drainage and the SLN before making a skin incision [37], often the skin flaps need to be raised to comprehensively assess the nodal basins [39]. In addition, the ICG signal spreads rapidly with time and thus second tier lymph nodes can be hard to distinguish from the true sentinel lymph node [40]. The use of hybrid tracers which assemble ICG with a radiocolloid to increase the retention time in the sentinel lymph node has been described [38], and may have an increasing future role, along with the use of intraoperative SPECT scanners, to counteract the disadvantages of using ICG alone. However, this is an exciting new tool which can be utilised to expand the utility of the SLN technique.

9. Conclusion

Early OCSCCs have a risk of subclinical nodal metastases to the draining cervical lymph nodes, which has a negative impact on the patient's prognosis and survival. The subclinical nature limits the ability to identify these with current imaging techniques including a PET scan. Despite this, there is recent high quality evidence demonstrating that treating this disease surgically has superior survival outcomes compared with an observation strategy. However, the patients *without* subclinical nodal metastases (up to 80%) do not gain any benefit by undergoing a neck dissection.

SLNB technique represents a minimally invasive technique allowing treatment de-intensification without compromising the oncological efficacy. SLNB has been demonstrated to provide an accurate and safe staging procedure to assess for subclinical nodal metastases with added benefits over an END including identification of out-of-field drainage, as well as a more detailed pathological assessment of the SLN However, a high quality multidisciplinary approach is required including accurate preoperative lymphoscintigraphy, precise surgical technique and detailed pathological assessment to ensure reliable results and good patient outcomes.

Acknowledgements

We would like to thank Professor Michael Veness, MD, for providing support with preparation of this chapter.

Conflict of interest

The authors declare no conflict of interest.

Author details

Rajith Mendis* and Muzib Abdul-Razak
Westmead Hospital, Sydney, Australia

*Address all correspondence to: rajith.mendis@health.nsw.gov.au

References

[1] Pentenero M, Gandolfo S, Carrozzo M. Importance of tumor thickness and depth of invasion in nodal involvement and prognosis of oral squamous cell carcinoma: A review of the literature. Head Neck 2005; 27: 1080-1091.

[2] Ebrahimi A, Ashford BG, Clark JR. Improved survival with elective neck dissection in thick early-stage oral squamous cell carcinoma. Head Neck 2012; 34: 709-716.

[3] Ferris RL, Kraus DH. Sentinel lymph node biopsy versus selective neck dissection for detection of metastatic oral squamous cell carcinoma. Clin Exp Metastasis 2012; 29: 693-698.

[4] Gurney BAS, Schilling C, Putcha V, et al. Implications of a positive sentinel node in oral squamous cell carcinoma. Head Neck 2012; 34: 1580-1585.

[5] O'Brien CJ, Lauer CS, Fredricks S, et al. Tumor thickness influences prognosis of T1 and T2 oral cavity cancer - But what thickness? Head Neck 2003; 25: 937-945.

[6] Murer K, Huber GF, Haile SR, et al. Comparison of morbidity between sentinel node biopsy and elective neck dissection for treatment of the n0 neck in patients with oral squamous cell carcinoma. Head Neck 2011; 33: 1260-1264.

[7] Stoeckli SJ, Haerle SK, Strobel K, et al. Initial staging of the neck in head and neck squamous cell carcinoma: A comparison of CT, PET/CT, and ultrasound-guided fine-needle aspiration cytology. Head Neck 2012; 34: 469-476.

[8] Ross GL, Soutar DS, MacDonald DG, et al. Improved staging of cervical metastases in clinically node-negative patients with head and neck squamous cell carcinoma. Ann Surg Oncol 2004; 11: 213-218.

[9] Amin MB, Edge S, Greene F, et al. *AJCC Cancer Staging Manual*. 8th ed. 2017.

[10] Yuen APW, Lam KY, Lam LK, et al. Prognostic factors of clinically stage I and II oral tongue carcinoma - A comparative study of stage, thickness, shape, growth pattern, invasive front malignancy grading, Martinez-Gimeno score, and pathologic features. Head Neck 2002; 24: 513-520.

[11] Mohit-Tabatabai MA, Sobel HJ, Rush BF, et al. Relation of thickness of floor of mouth stage I and II cancers to regional metastasis. Am J Surg 1986; 152: 351-353.

[12] Bundgaard T, Bentzen SM, Wildt J. and Clinical Parameters in the Prognostic Evaluation of Squamous Cell Carcinoma of. 1996; 142-152.

[13] Goerkem M, Braun J, Stoeckli SJ. Evaluation of clinical and histomorphological parameters as potential predictors of occult metastases in sentinel lymph nodes of early squamous cell carcinoma of the oral cavity. Ann Surg Oncol 2010; 17: 527-535.

[14] D'Cruz AK, Vaish R, Kapre N, et al. Elective versus Therapeutic Neck Dissection in Node-Negative Oral Cancer. N Engl J Med 2015; 373: 521-529.

[15] Garrel R, Poissonnet G, Plana AM, et al. Equivalence randomized trial to compare treatment on the basis of sentinel node biopsy versus neck node dissection in operable T1-T2N0 oral and oropharyngeal cancer. J Clin Oncol 2020; 38: 4010-4018.

[16] Yang Y, Zhou J, Wu H. Diagnostic value of sentinel lymph node biopsy for cT1/T2N0 tongue squamous cell carcinoma: a meta-analysis. Eur Arch Oto-Rhino-Laryngology 2017; 274: 3843-3852.

[17] Garrel R, Poissonnet G, Temam S, et al. Review of sentinel node procedure in cN0 head and neck squamous cell carcinomas. Guidelines from the French evaluation cooperative subgroup of GETTEC. Eur Ann Otorhinolaryngol Head Neck Dis 2017; 134: 89-93.

[18] Wagner T, Buscombe J, Gnanasegaran G, et al. SPECT/CT in sentinel node imaging. Nucl Med Commun 2013; 34: 191-202.

[19] Meerwein CM, Sekine T, Veit-Haibach P, et al. Multi-slice SPECT/CT vs. lymphoscintigraphy and intra-operative gamma ray probe for sentinel node mapping in HNSCC. Eur Arch Oto-Rhino-Laryngology 2017; 274: 1633-1642.

[20] Giammarile F, Schilling C, Gnanasegaran G, et al. The EANM practical guidelines for sentinel lymph node localisation in oral cavity squamous cell carcinoma. Eur J Nucl Med Mol Imaging 2019; 46: 623-637.

[21] Wallace AM, Hoh CK, Vera DR, et al. Lymphoseek: A molecular radio-pharmaceutical for sentinel node detection. Ann Surg Oncol 2003; 10: 531-538.

[22] Agrawal A, Civantos FJ, Brumund KT, et al. [99mTc] Tilmanocept Accurately Detects Sentinel Lymph Nodes and Predicts Node Pathology Status in Patients with Oral Squamous Cell Carcinoma of the Head and Neck: Results of a Phase III Multi-institutional Trial. Ann Surg Oncol 2015; 22: 3708-3715.

[23] den Toom IJ, Mahieu R, van Rooij R, et al. Sentinel lymph node detection in oral cancer: a within-patient comparison between [99mTc]Tc-tilmanocept and [99mTc]Tc-nanocolloid. Eur J Nucl Med Mol Imaging 2021; 48: 851-858.

[24] Stoeckli SJ, Huebner T, Huber GF, et al. Technique for reliable sentinel node biopsy in squamous cell carcinomas of the floor of mouth. Head Neck 2016; 38: 1367-1372.

[25] Ambrosch P, Kron M, Fischer G, et al. Micrometastases in carcinoma of the upper aerodigestive tract: Detection, risk of metastasizing, and prognostic value of depth of invasion. Head Neck 1995; 17: 473-479.

[26] Majumdar KS, Rao VUS, Prasad R, et al. Incidence of Micrometastasis and Isolated Tumour Cells in Clinico-pathologically Node-Negative Head and Neck Squamous Cell Carcinoma. J Maxillofac Oral Surg 2020; 19: 131-135.

[27] King C, Elsherif N, Kirwan R, et al. Serial step sections at narrow intervals with immunohistochemistry are required for accurate histological assessment of sentinel lymph node biopsy in oral squamous cell carcinoma. Head Neck.

[28] Chone CT, Aniteli MB, Magalhães RS, et al. Impact of immunohistochemistry in sentinel lymph node biopsy in head and neck cancer. Eur Arch Oto-Rhino-Laryngology 2013; 270: 313-317.

[29] Mallo Magariños M, Suárez Ajuria M, Marichalar Mendía X, et al. Diagnostic yield of sentinel lymph node biopsy in oral squamous cell carcinoma T1/T2-N0: systematic review and meta-analysis. *Int J Oral Maxillofac Surg*. Epub ahead of print 2021. DOI: 10.1016/j.ijom.2021.01.020.

[30] Schilling C, Stoeckli SJ, Haerle SK, et al. Sentinel European Node Trial (SENT): 3-year results of sentinel node biopsy in oral cancer. Eur J Cancer 2015; 51: 2777-2784.

[31] Miura K, Hirakawa H, Uemura H, et al. Sentinel node biopsy for oral cancer: A prospective multicenter Phase II trial. Auris Nasus Larynx 2017; 44: 319-326.

[32] Abdul-Razak M, Chung H, Wong E, et al. Sentinel lymph node biopsy for

early oral cancers: Westmead Hospital experience. ANZ J Surg 2017; 87: 65-69.

[33] Crocetta FM, Botti C, Pernice C, et al. Sentinel node biopsy versus elective neck dissection in early-stage oral cancer: a systematic review. Eur Arch Oto-Rhino-Laryngology 2020; 277: 3247-3260.

[34] Hasegawa Y, Tsukahara K, Yoshimoto S, et al. Neck Dissections Based on Sentinel Lymph Node Navigation Versus Elective Neck Dissections in Early Oral Cancers: A Randomized, Multicenter, and Noninferiority Trial. J Clin Oncol 2021; 39: 2025-2036.

[35] Schiefke F, Akdemir M, Weber A, et al. Function, postoperative morbidity, and quality of life after cervical sentinel node biopsy and after selective neck dissection. Head Neck 2009; 31: 503-512.

[36] Den Toom IJ, Boeve K, Lobeek D, et al. Elective neck dissection or sentinel lymph node biopsy in early stage oral cavity cancer patients: The dutch experience. Cancers (Basel) 2020; 12: 1-13.

[37] Yokoyama J, Hasegawa Y, Sugasawa M, et al. Long term-follow-up multicenter feasibility study of icg fluorescence-navigated sentinel node biopsy in oral cancer. Mol Clin Oncol 2020; 13: 1-8.

[38] Van Den Berg NS, Brouwer OR, Klop WMC, et al. Concomitant radio- and fluorescence-guided sentinel lymph node biopsy in squamous cell carcinoma of the oral cavity using ICG-99mTc-nanocolloid. Eur J Nucl Med Mol Imaging 2012; 39: 1128-1136.

[39] Peng H, Wang SJ, Niu X, et al. Sentinel node biopsy using indocyanine green in oral/oropharyngeal cancer. World J Surg Oncol 2015; 13: 1-7.

[40] Honda K, Ishiyama K, Suzuki S, et al. Sentinel lymph node biopsy using preoperative computed tomographic lymphography and intraoperative indocyanine green fluorescence imaging in patients with localized tongue cancer. JAMA Otolaryngol - Head Neck Surg 2019; 145: 735-740.

Chapter 6

Way to Cure Oral Squamous Cell Carcinoma with Theranostics and Nanoparticular Approaches

Sankha Bhattacharya

Abstract

One of the most prevalent forms of oral cancer is oral squamous cell carcinoma (OSCC), a major cause of morbidity and mortality worldwide. Following a definite oral cancer diagnosis, OSCC is typically treated with a multidisciplinary approach including surgery, chemotherapy, and radiation. In contrast, conventional chemotherapy medicines may be ineffective and have a range of side effects. Many techniques have been proved and authorized for treatment and diagnostics of different types of oral cancer, while others are currently being investigated in clinical trials. This book chapter is aimed to explain the current preclinical status of nano-based techniques to successfully diagnose and treat OSCC. This book chapter would also emphasize recent theranostics approaches utilized to cure OSCC. Nanotechnology also improved cancer biomarker detection, making them faster and more sensitive. To overcome these constraints and improve *in situ* drug delivery, various nanoparticles have been employed as innovation drivers.

Keywords: squamous cell carcinoma (OSCC), matrix metalloproteases (MMPs), magnetic nanoparticles (MNPs), HSC-3 cells, vital protein endothelial growth factor (VEGF), C-reactive protein (CRP)

1. Introduction

According to the World Health Organization (WHO), cancer would take the lives of 10.3 million people globally by 2020, and patients with oral cancer would have a five-year survival rate of just 50% globally. Oral cancer is a challenging disease that affects about 600,000 individuals worldwide each year and is linked to a high rate of morbidity and mortality [1–4]. Mouth cancer is a group of tumors that may affect any area of the mouth, including the pharynx and salivary glands, as well as the surrounding tissues [5]. This term, on the other hand, is often interchanged with oral squamous cell carcinoma (OSCC), the most common malignant epithelial tumor of the oral cavity. OSCC is thought to be responsible for more than 90% of all oral neoplasms [6]. According to the current study results, year survival rates for OSCC range from 50 to 60%, depending on a number of factors such as the patient's lifestyle, the timing of diagnosis, and the location of the primary tumor [7, 8]. As a consequence, OSCC is linked with a poor prognosis in the medical community. Patients with OSCC who get conventional therapy have a significant recurrence rate of the illness, regardless of when treatment started (18–76%). The use of biopsy or histology testing to diagnose OSCC is time intensive, resulting in a delay in treatment initiation, and as a result, a shorter overall survival time period is obtained [9]. Early-stage cancer detection is critical in determining the most suitable treatment for the patient, which has an impact on their total survival, as stated in the previous paragraph. According to recent research studies, the development of cancer is related to the molecular level of particular indicators in tumor tissue and bodily fluids. Molecular biomarkers, which are categorized as genomic, proteomic, and metabolomic profiles of body specimens, are used to identify the existence or absence of a certain malignancy, as well as its spread and recurrence, among other things. Science and technology focused on extremely small objects, and nanoscience and nanotechnology are providing innovative methods to cancer treatment and detection. Site-specific chemoprevention/therapy using nanoparticles for local drug delivery has recently gained popularity. It is a novel method for treating cancer that aims to overcome and minimize the limits of current cancer treatment and diagnostics. It can detect a single cancer cell *in vivo* and administer drugs straight to it. Nanotechnology has also improved the detection of cancer biomarkers [10–12]. Oral cancer is often treated with a multidisciplinary approach that involves surgery, chemotherapy, and radiation. However, conventional chemotherapy medicines may be ineffective and have side effects. Many nanoparticles have been employed as technological drivers of innovation to overcome these constraints. The present book chapter seeks to highlight developments in the use of new methods in the detection and treatment of oral cancer due to the significance of OSCC as a widespread public health issue. The purpose of this book chapter is to describe the current preclinical state of nano-based methods for oral cancer detection and therapy. This review also discussed (a) oral squamous cell carcinoma, (b) OSCC diagnosis using serum and saliva biomarkers, (c) nano-based OSCC biomarker detection, (d) OSCC therapy methods, and (e) nanotechnology techniques for OSCC treatment or diagnostic.

2. Squamous cell carcinoma of the oral cavity

Oral cancers are a group of cancers that develop in different parts of the mouth, each with its own set of risk factors, incidence, and treatment options [13]. Understanding the mechanisms of cancer initiation and progression may aid us in selecting the most appropriate therapeutic strategy at the appropriate time. Despite advances in therapeutic methods, the morbidity and mortality ratios for squamous cell carcinoma of the oral cavity have remained unchanged for the past 30 years. After a carcinogenic insult to the oral cavity, it occurs in several steps, resulting in various molecular changes that disrupt cellular growth, proliferation, and differentiation. The latter is marked by cellular transformation and carcinogenesis. Oral carcinogenesis follows the same pattern as other cancers, starting with a precursor lesion and progressing to localized and metastatic disease [14]. The histological grade of dysplasia indicates how far the disease has progressed from normal to hyperplasia. The most common cellular events discovered in these examinations are changes in nuclear size and shape, enlarged cells and nuclei, enhanced mitotic picture, and increased nucleus/cytoplasm ratio. Elevated cellular density, dyskeratosis, hyperplasia of basal cells, bulbous drop-form of rete pegs, and secondary nodules on rete tips are pathological features of tissues in the later stages of squamous cell carcinoma.

3. Biomarkers in oral squamous cell carcinoma (OSCC)

Early detection of OSCC improves life quality while lowering the cost and side effects of medical treatments. Because OSCC has such a high recurrence rate, early detection is crucial in determining the disease's prognosis [15]. OSCC remains a significant challenge due to the disease's nature, despite recent advances in this area. As a result, as discussed in this book chapter, monitoring the level of biologic markers with high specificity and sensitivity is a promising diagnostic tool for both primary and recurrent oral cancer detections. According to the National Institutes of Health, biomarkers are indices of normal or pathological conditions that can be reliably and precisely measured [16]. Mutated DNA, mRNA, metabolomes, secreted proteins, and small molecules are examples of biomarkers [17, 18]. A cancer biomarker is a molecule that is secreted by a tumor or produced in response to the onset or progression of cancer. In addition, the ideal biomarker should be a noninvasive method with high-positive and high-negative predictive values that reflect the stage of cancer. As a result, the marker can be used to predict treatment efficacy, diagnosis, and prognosis in cancer patients.

3.1 OSCC salivary biomarkers

Saliva collection is easy and painless, making it a promising biomarker discovery tool. The changes in the saliva genome and protein profile after the onset of cancer or as the disease progresses in oral cancer have been studied in several studies [19, 20]. When collecting, processing, and storing saliva, however, some acquaintances should be considered. Cross-validation is required before extrapolating biomarkers into clinical applications. Different data collection, processing, and analysis techniques could explain the wide range of results seen in studies looking for salivary oral cancer biomarkers. As a result, more research is needed to standardize the aforementioned techniques as well as reference levels in order to obtain valid biomarkers.

3.2 Salivary RNA-base biomarkers

In the mouth, salivary RNAases were supposed to break down RNA. These alluring biomarkers, on the other hand, are obstinate, being carried in apoptotic bodies or actively liberated from cellular vesicles such as exosomes. Oral cancer patients have been found to have low levels of miRNA 200a and miRNA 125a, but significantly higher levels of miRNA 31. Upregulated miRNA 184 and downregulated miRNA 145 have also been linked to malignant oral cancer.

3.3 Salivary protein-based biomarkers

Cancer biomarkers could include oxidative stress markers. Carbonylation causes irreversible protein damage, which leads to cell toxicity. In OSCC patients, the infiltration of reactive radicals into the oral epithelial cells results in a significant increase in salivary carbonyls. Matrix metalloproteases (MMPs) are enzymes that degrade a wide range of proteins. During OSCC, which is highly invasive and metastatic, different types of MMPs have been shown to be significantly altered. MMP-2 and MMP-9 expression in oral cancer patients has been linked to a poor prognosis in the wild. The immune system produces proteins called interleukins (IL). In cellular signaling cascades, naturally occurring proteins play a variety of roles, some of which are critical in cancer. Interleukin-6 (IL-6) and interleukin-8 (IL-8) are two different types of interleukin-6. The prevalence of OSCC has been reported to be on the rise. The cytokeratin fragment 21–1 is a squamous tumor marker (Cyfra 21–1).

4. Serum biomarkers

During tumor development, the release of synthesized markers into the circulation results in an increase in markers in cancer patients' serum, which can be used to predict the development of the cancer itself. The secreted origins of tumor-specific or tumor-associated serum biomarkers are known. Taking regular measurements of these biomarkers could provide valuable insight into how patients respond to anticancer treatments in the long run. Both the progression of the disease and its treatment are discussed in detail. Adiponectin is a protein hormone that can be found in the bloodstream and performs a number of different functions. It aids in the digestion of glucose and fatty acids in the bloodstream. Guo et al. discovered that the levels of adiponectin were higher. The incidence of tongue squamous cell carcinoma (TSCC) has dropped significantly. Hypoadiponectinemia has also been associated with lymphoma in some studies. The prognosis for TSCC metastasis is abysmal. Another protein, hemoglobin (Hb), being associated with an increased risk of oral cancer in the opposite direction. Reduced hemoglobin levels and anemia have been linked to increased tumor oxygenation and lymph node metastasis, and Hb corrections have been shown to improve prognosis in cancer patients.

Low hemoglobin levels indicate advanced OSCC, especially in larger tumors requiring more radial treatment. Pro-inflammatory cytokines are a group of small proteins that play a role in inflammation. Oral cancer is the most common link. In a prospective study, Schiegnitz et al. looked at the role of IL-6, 8, soluble IL-2 receptor (SIL-2R), MHC class I polypeptide-related sequence B (MICB), and tumor necrosis factor alpha (TNF-a) in OSCC. According to their findings, all of these biomarkers showed an upward trend in serum samples from oral cancer patients. Promising OSCC prognostic indicators have been identified as IL-6 and SIL-2R. Chang et al. also discovered a link between oral cancer clinical manifestations and blood levels of 12 cytokines. However, the results of a different study refuted these assertions. Individual or panels of serum cytokines are not appropriate oral cancer biomarker candidates due to these discrepancies and heterogeneous literature searches. However, it has been suggested that some inflammatory and immune system-related proteins are self-contained. Oral cancer metastasis indicator C-reactive protein (CRP), for example, is an IgG analog that stimulates the release of pro-inflammatory cytokines. CRP is an inflammatory marker that has been linked to a variety of diseases and cancers. Previous research has looked into the relationship between OSCC size, stage, and subsequent survival and CRP serum levels. Elevated serum CRP has been proposed as a predictor of poor prognosis and a low survival rate in oral cancer patients. The soluble protein Decoy receptor 3 (Dcr3) prevents programmed cell death. It is a member of the TNF receptor family. Several cancers have been found to have a high rate of cell death and amplification. According to estimates, when lymph node metastasis occurs at the same time as OSCC, the prognosis is worsened. In this context, serum MMPs have also been investigated. Liu et al. investigated the link between MMP-9 and pathological manifestations in oral cancer patients in a survey. A higher level of this factor was discovered to be linked to a shorter life expectancy. On the other hand, some of these serum proteins have been suggested as potential biomarkers for OSCC diagnosis but not prognosis prediction. For example, MMP-3 levels have not been linked to OSCC clinicopathological features. As potential biomarkers, different levels of growth factors in the serum of oral cancer patients have been proposed. Vascular. In various tumor propagation processes, the vital protein endothelial growth factor (VEGF) is thought to induce angiogenesis. Nodal metastasis and advanced OSCC have been linked to higher levels of this factor. Furthermore, in a 6-month cumulative survival study, the results of a 12-month study OSCC serum insulin-like growth factor (IGF) and survival were found to be strongly linked.

5. OSCC treatment strategies based on nanomaterials

Low levels of cancer biomarkers in tumor tissue or body fluids, a narrow margin between non-cancerous and cancerous samples, and the sensitivity of measurement assays are all major roadblocks to precise cancer biomarker detection. As a result, the ideal biomarker is one that can detect even the tiniest tumor cells using specific biomarkers before cancer progresses and clinical symptoms emerge. Previously, a variety of methods for measuring multiple biomarkers were developed, with immunoassays like ELISA becoming the most popular technique for protein detection due to low detection limits. However, this area has some limitations, including a long detection time, high costs, and a small sample size. Some novel approaches are currently being used. Polynucleotide barcodes, multiplexed bead platforms, and microarrays, for example, have superior limits of detection but are costly and require technical expertise. They are widely available in clinics and are efficient and cost-effective methods for detecting cancer biomarkers, despite scientists' attempts to put in place some quick and sensitive measures. Nanotechnology, for example, is gaining popularity among scientists in this field. In a study by Sungyub et al., gold nanoparticles were used to conjugate with DNA probes in oral cancer salivary samples. S100 calcium-binding protein P (S100P) mRNA was found to have a detection limit of 3 nM as a potential OSCC biomarker. The use of nanotechnology in the *in vitro* treatment of oral cancer is demonstrated in **Figure 1.**

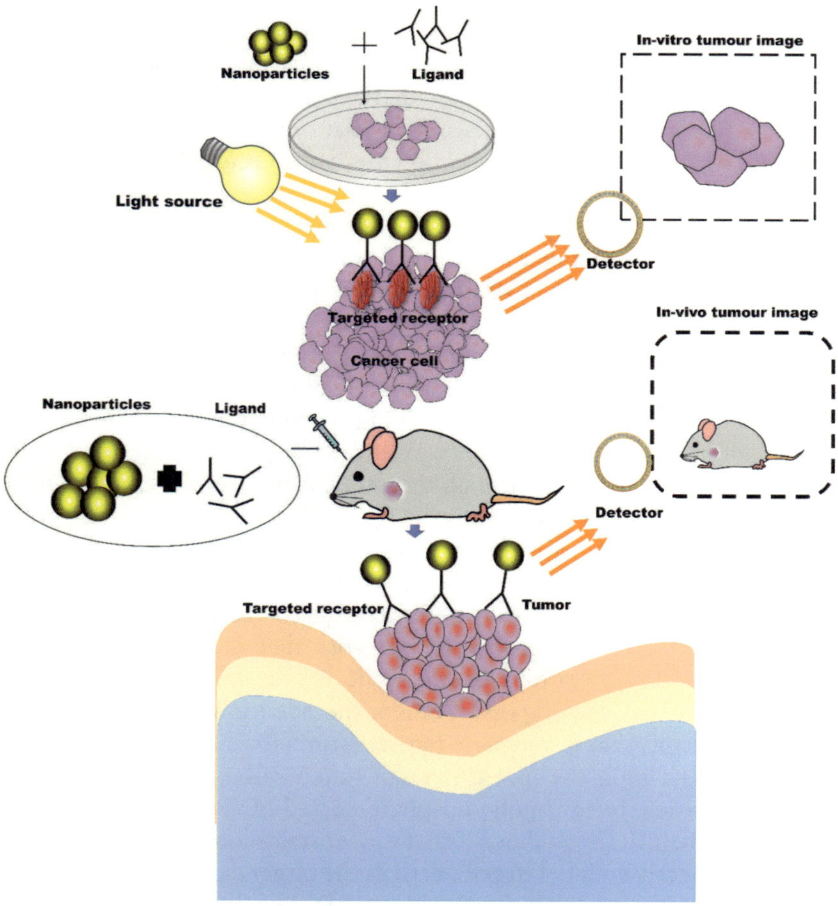

Figure 1.
In vitro *and* in vivo *imaging of oral cancer using nanotechnology has been demonstrated.*

6. OSCC treatment strategies based on nanomaterials

Traditional therapeutic approaches to treating OSCC are associated with a number of side effects that can be both temporary and permanent. Oral carcinogenesis has been shown to respond well to novel treatment approaches. This group could include therapeutic molecules such as siRNAs and various active targeting ligands. Several natural products have also shown promise in the treatment of oral cancer by interfering with various cell signaling pathways such as free radical scavenging, inhibiting the formation of DNA adducts, and regulating the properties of apoptosis-related genes. However, these compounds' low bioavailability and solubility have limited their clinical application. As a result, it is critical to improve preventative and therapeutic strategies. For the development of drug delivery systems, the time of drug contact with oral tumor cells is an important consideration. As a result, a sustained and targeted mucoadhesive drug delivery system into the oral cavity has been developed. The residence time of nanoparticles can improve drug mucus interaction and result in better results. The studies also revealed that local delivery of nanoparticles can be used for site-specific chemoprevention and therapy. Nonspecific drug uptake is reduced by cells to improve drug targeting into the oral cancer site. The reticuloendothelial system (RES) and improved plasma half-life, which result in lower drug dosage, are two other advantages. The aspects of cancer therapy are based on nanoparticles. According to scientific reports, various types of nanoparticles have been tested for cancer therapy. Some of the most recent nanoparticles that have been tested for the treatment of drug-resistant cancer cells include magnetic nanoparticles (MNPs), liposomes, polymeric nanoparticles, gold (Au) nanoparticles, and nano-diamonds. Various nanotechnology approaches can be used to selectively target cancer biomarkers and cancer cells. The use of specific crosslinkers against cancer cells, such as antibodies or aptamers, can also facilitate the development of early detection methods. **Figure 2** summarizes the potential therapeutic approaches.

Oral oncogenesis is a type of cancer that starts in the mouth and spreads to the rest of the body. Nanocarriers are also being developed that are functionalized with various targeting agents (ligands, tumor-associated proteins). Antigens, antibodies, and aptamers have shown promise in improving the cancer cell delivery of a specific target. In a variety of main cancer immunotherapy or target drug/gene delivery pathways, this strategy can use a single agent or a combination of agents. It can be viewed as a primary strategy involving specific interactions between the nanocarrier and receptors on the target cancer cell, which could promote nanocarrier internalization endocytosis through receptors. A basic understanding of cell biology, tumor biology, and immunology is required for the rational design of NPs for cancer therapeutics, and advances in nanotechnology will be heavily reliant on advances in cancer biology. Magnetic nanoparticles (MNPs) are one of the most researched nano-delivery systems in cancer treatment. The MNPs showed high efficiency and ideal drug loading when coated with oleic acid and embedded with anticancer agents such as doxorubicin and paclitaxel, according to the reports. Various researchers have investigated them for therapeutic approaches such as hyperthermic therapy, that is, magneto hyperthermia (MHT). The toxicity of this method was reduced while the specific lysis of tumor cells was increased. Candido et al. investigated the effects of polyphosphate-coated MNPs on human OSCC (UM-SCC14A). Their findings showed that cancer treatment with magneto hyperthermia can be effective related to cell death in the target cancer tissue According to the authors, there were two main findings from MNP-based magneto hyperthermia treatment: a high level of apoptosis and fibrosis, as well as an inhibition effect on cell proliferation. As a carrier for anticancer drug delivery, polymeric nanoparticles

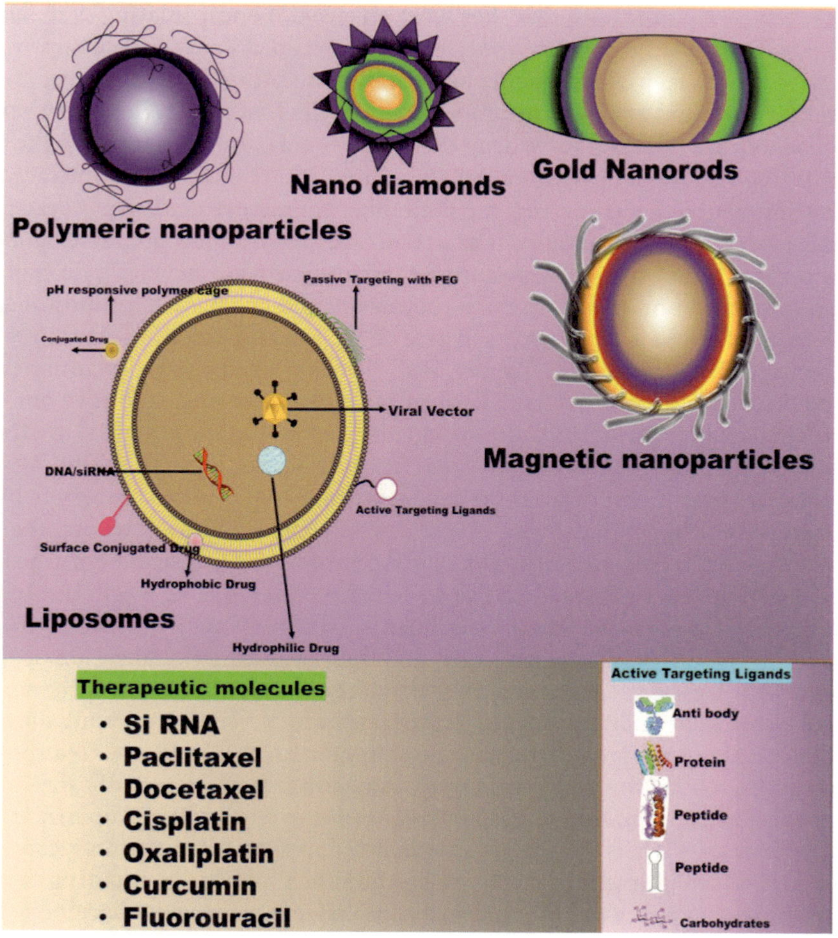

Figure 2.
There have been advancements in the treatment of oral cancer. A wide range of drugs and/or therapeutic molecules are used to treat oral cancer. Nanocarriers show promise in the development of effective oral oncology therapy, in addition to active targeting ligands.

have been shown to be impactful. It is one of the most widely used nanoparticles *in vitro* and *in vivo*. However, before they can be used in clinical trials, they must overcome a number of challenges. In addition to low molecular weight drugs, polymeric nanoparticles have demonstrated the ability to transport macromolecules such as proteins and genes. Hydrophilic polymers, such as polyethylene glycol (PEG), aid in the stabilization of nanoparticles, which improves drug targeting into cancer sites by reducing nonspecific drug uptake by cells, according to the studies. These nanoparticles are less toxic, have a higher level of stability, and have a higher loading capacity, according to reports. Because of the properties of drugs that are not soluble in water, the use of biodegradable polymers has increased dramatically in recent years, such as increased plasma half-life and reticuloendothelial system inhibition of fast clearance (RES). Biodegradable linkages can be used as a backbone to assist in the formation of high-surface-area nanoparticles. In the case of apoptosis induction in SCC-9 human OSCCs, PCL nanoparticles with curcumin were coated with chitosan, which showed promising outcomes of this research. When Sulfikkarali et al. used the nanoprecipitation method to create naringenin-loaded polymeric (Eudragit E) nanoparticles and tested their anticancer activity in hamster carcinogenesis, they discovered that they had a significant anticancer effect. The prepared nanoparticles (with an average size of 90 nm) had an encapsulation efficiency of 88%, indicating that they were effective at encapsulating their surroundings. They discovered that a polymeric drug-loaded nanoparticle improved the anticancer efficacy of naringenin and had better antilipid peroxidative, antiproliferative, and antioxidant properties than the free drug. When developing controlled-release mucoadhesive drug delivery systems, the time at which the drug comes into contact with oral tumor cells is an important factor to take into account. The development of a long-acting, targeted mucoadhesive drug delivery system for the oral cavity may be advantageous as a result. To create a mucoadhesive patch of methotrexate (MTX)-loaded liposomes for targeted delivery in OSCC, Jin et al. used the thin film hydration method, which they developed in-house. The liposomes that were prepared had a mean particle size of 105 nm and a loading efficiency of 54%, respectively. Using an MTT assay, HSC-3 cells were utilised to examine the cytotoxicity of the liposomes that had been generated. The mucoadhesive buccal patches had appropriate bioadhesive qualities as well as the potential to offer sustained MTX release, according to the scientists. According to their findings, oral mucoadhesive patches for oral cancer can be utilised as a primary strategy to bypass the constraints of targeted delivery in oral cancer chemotherapy, lowering the required dose while reducing drug toxicity. According to the researchers' findings, the nanoparticles they prepared had a pro-oxidant effect in HSC-3 cells due to the high levels of ROS present in their experiments. Due to the ease with which they can be prepared, their high biocompatibility, and their ideal functionalization properties, gold (Au) nanoparticles are gaining attention in the field of cancer therapy. It is possible that their ability to conjugate with other biomolecules without altering their biological properties will prove to be a very useful option for the treatment of oral cancer, having the ability to conjugate a wide range of mucoadhesive substances. The combination of biopolymers and the outstanding properties of Au nanoparticles, such as their non-cytotoxicity, has resulted in their widespread application, which is used in a variety of biomedical applications and drug delivery systems to treat a variety of oral cancer cells of different types. Furthermore, these nanoparticles are one of the most well-known cancer nanoparticles due to their surface plasmon resonance, which is a property of surface plasmon resonance. The importance of early detection cannot be overstated. In order to improve the early detection of diseases such as cancer, as previously stated, many studies are being conducted and expanded. For bio-imaging and diagnostic applications, nano-diamonds have attracted considerable attention due to their low toxicity, ideal surface properties, and stable fluorescence that does not fade when exposed to ultraviolet light. These nanoparticles can also be used to immobilize proteins, making them excellent candidates for local drug delivery into oral diseases such as oral cancer.

7. Conclusion

Oral cancer is a type of cancer that primarily affects oral epithelial cells, but it can also spread to other parts of the body and be fatal. The most common type of cancer is OSCC, which accounts for more than 90% of all oral cancers. OSCC remains a serious public health concern despite extensive research because of its poor prognosis . Novel chemoprevention technologies are becoming increasingly important as traditional therapeutic methodologies are frequently insufficient. Nanotechnology has proven to be extremely beneficial in this case. Nanoparticle-based diagnostic methods for OSCC detection and diagnosis are capable of providing real-time, appropriate, and cost-effective diagnoses. They can show molecular-targeted imaging, nano-scale biomarker analysis, and post-treatment OSCC prediction. Bioconjugate nanoparticles have a wide range of applications for amplified transduction of biomolecular recognition events, as demonstrated by the studies described above. Because of their optical and electrochemical applications, such nanoparticle labels serve as the foundation for ultrasensitive protein and nucleic acid assays. This book chapter summarized the most recent advances in nanoparticles for oral cancer diagnosis and treatment. Nanoparticles have been studied for their unique physicochemical properties, such as their ultrasmall size, high reactivity, and ability to be functionalized. It has been demonstrated that accurate and timely oral cancer diagnosis tools, as well as highly effective oral cancer treatment strategies, exist. Nanoparticles can be used to visualize oral cancer, deliver therapeutic agents to tumors selectively, and destroy tumors by using a variety of therapeutic techniques. Hybrid systems, in particular, will garner more attention because they provide nanoparticles with a flexible platform for achieving bio-multifunctionality. The use of nanomedicine in the modern diagnosis and treatment of oral cancer is very exciting. Despite the fact that nanoparticles have a wide range of potential applications in the treatment and prevention of diseases, the nanomedicine field is currently limited in its use of nanoparticle technologies in the prevention and treatment of oral cancer. The studies in this collection focused on therapeutic activities, which were mostly conducted *in vitro* or in preclinical oral cancer models. Because of the complex pathophysiology of oral cancer, such as abnormal hemodynamics, the pharmacokinetics and biodistribution of therapeutic agents can vary, leading to misleading results. Because of the high sensitivity of the new nanoparticle-based sensing protocols, they can detect disease markers, biothreat agents, and infectious agents that are not detectable by traditional methods. Methods of the past early disease detection or terrorist attack warnings could be provided by such highly sensitive biodetection schemes. Although the use of nanoparticle tags for protein detection is still in its early stages, the lessons learned in ultrasensitive DNA detection should be useful. Nonspecific adsorption issues, which frequently limit bioaffinity assay detectability, must be carefully considered for the successful implementation of the new signal-amplify cation strategies. Proper washing and surface blocking steps should be used to avoid amplifying the cation of background signals (associated with non-specific adsorption of the nanoparticle). Although there were *ex vivo* studies of tissue and saliva samples, as well as *in vivo* training in animal models, more experiments must be applied before these strategies can be implemented. In the near future, nanobiosensors are expected to play a larger role in electroanalytical science. For clinical applications, protocols for the synthesis and functionalization of nanoparticles must be developed. Early disease detection, genetic mutations, and bio-targets appear to have the greatest implications. Nanomaterial-based biosensors offer quick, simple, and sensitive cancer detection systems that could be useful in anticancer biosensor research.

Acknowledgements

The authors like to acknowledge the help and motivation of Prof. R.S. Gaud, Director, Pharmacy & Technology Management, SVKM's NMIMS Deemed-to-be University, for providing excellent research facilities and profound inspiration while drafting this book chapter.

Competing interests

The author declares that the author has no competing interests.

Author details

Sankha Bhattacharya
Department of Pharmaceutics, School of Pharmacy and Technology Management, SVKM'S NMIMS Deemed-to-be University, Shirpur, Maharashtra, India

*Address all correspondence to: sankhabhatt@gmail.com

References

[1] Wei R, Qiu H, Xu J, et al. Expression and prognostic potential of GPX1 in human cancers based on data mining. Ann Transl Med. 2020;8(4):124. doi:10.21037/atm.2020.02.36

[2] Liu Q, Li S, Dupuy A, et al. Exosomes as New Biomarkers and Drug Delivery Tools for the Prevention and Treatment of Various Diseases: Current Perspectives. Int J Mol Sci. 2021;22(15): 7763. Published 2021 Jul 21. doi:10.3390/ijms22157763.

[3] Van DN, Van LP, Tien HN, Van ND, Le Van Q. Multidisciplinary Therapy Management for Locally Advanced Minor Salivary Gland Cancer in Oral Cavity: A Case Report and Literature Review [published online ahead of print, 2021 Jul 19]. Ear Nose Throat J. 2021;1455613211031026. doi:10.1177/01455613211031026.

[4] Al-Jamaei AAH, van Dijk BAC, Helder MN, Forouzanfar T, Leemans CR, de Visscher JGAM. A population-based study of the epidemiology of oral squamous cell carcinoma in the Netherlands 1989-2018, with emphasis on young adults [published online ahead of print, 2021 Mar 24]. Int J Oral Maxillofac Surg. 2021;S0901-5027(21)00101-6. doi:10.1016/j.ijom.2021.03.006

[5] RaziyehsadatRezvaninejad H. Evaluation of Relationship between ABO bloods with Oral Cancer and Compared with Healthy Individuals. Annals of the Romanian Society for Cell Biology. 2021 Jul 16;25(6):17712-20

[6] Vassiliou LV, Acero J, Gulati A, et al. Management of the clinically N0 neck in early-stage oral squamous cell carcinoma (OSCC). An EACMFS position paper. J Craniomaxillofac Surg. 2020;48(8):711-718. doi:10.1016/j.jcms.2020.06.004.

[7] Wushou A, Wang M, Yibulayin F, et al. Patients With cT1N0M0 Oral Squamous Cell Carcinoma Benefit From Elective Neck Dissection: A SEER-Based Study. J Natl Compr Canc Netw. 2021;19(4):385-392. Published 2021 Jan 29. doi:10.6004/jnccn.2020.7632.

[8] Jardim JF, Galvis MM, Fabelo IR, Soares FA, Pinto CA, Kowalski LP. Intratumoral lymphatic vascular density is an independent factor for disease-free and overall survival in advanced stage oral squamous cell carcinoma. Oral Surgery, Oral Medicine, Oral Pathology and Oral Radiology. 2021 Jul 21.

[9] Narayanan MS, Kassim NK, Liszen T, Abdullah B, Omar J, Hairon SM, Lazim NM. The Utility of Beta 2 Microglobulin (B2M) as an Initial Diagnostic Tool for Oral Squamous Cell Carcinoma (OSCC): Evidence from a Malaysian Scenario. Bangladesh Journal of Medical Science. 2019 Aug 30;18(4):729-35.

[10] Singhal J, Verma S, Kumar S, Mehrotra D. Recent Advances in Nano-Bio-Sensing Fabrication Technology for the Detection of Oral Cancer. Mol Biotechnol. 2021;63(5):339-362. doi:10.1007/s12033-021-00306-x.

[11] Fang Z, Zhao J, Xie W, Sun Q, Wang H, Qiao B. LncRNA UCA1 promotes proliferation and cisplatin resistance of oral squamous cell carcinoma by sunppressing miR-184 expression. Cancer Med. 2017;6(12):2897-2908. doi:10.1002/cam4.1253

[12] Durgalakshmi D, Rishvanth R, Mohanraj J, Aruna P, Ganesan S. A Roadmap of Cancer: From the Historical Evidence to Recent Salivary Metabolites-based Nanobiosensor Diagnostic Devices. Current Metabolomics and Systems Biology Formerly: Current Metabolomics. 2021 Mar 1;8(1):27-52.

[13] Barrett TF, Mazul AL, Stepan KO, Wood CB, Paniello RC, Zevallos JP, Massa S, Jackson RS, Schmitt NC, Zenga J, Kang SY. The role of age in treatment decisions for oral cavity squamous cell carcinoma: Analysis of the National Cancer Database. Oral Oncology. 2021 Jul 1;118:105330.

[14] Johnson DE, Burtness B, Leemans CR, Lui VWY, Bauman JE, Grandis JR. Head and neck squamous cell carcinoma. Nat Rev Dis Primers. 2020;6(1):92. Published 2020 Nov 26. doi:10.1038/s41572-020-00224-3

[15] Capote-Moreno A, Brabyn P, Muñoz-Guerra MF, et al. Oral squamous cell carcinoma: epidemiological study and risk factor assessment based on a 39-year series. Int J Oral Maxillofac Surg. 2020;49(12):1525-1534. doi:10.1016/j.ijom.2020.03.009

[16] Durham JS, Brasher P, Anderson DW, et al. Effect of Fluorescence Visualization-Guided Surgery on Local Recurrence of Oral Squamous Cell Carcinoma: A Randomized Clinical Trial. JAMA Otolaryngol Head Neck Surg. 2020;146(12):1149-1155. doi:10.1001/jamaoto.2020.3147

[17] Loktionov A. Biomarkers for detecting colorectal cancer non-invasively: DNA, RNA or proteins?. World J Gastrointest Oncol. 2020;12(2):124-148. doi:10.4251/wjgo.v12.i2.124.

[18] Huda MN, Nafiujjaman M, Deaguero IG, et al. Potential Use of Exosomes as Diagnostic Biomarkers and in Targeted Drug Delivery: Progress in Clinical and Preclinical Applications. ACS Biomater Sci Eng. 2021;7(6):2106-2149. doi:10.1021/acsbiomaterials.1c00217.

[19] Buzalaf MAR, Ortiz AC, Carvalho TS, et al. Saliva as a diagnostic tool for dental caries, periodontal disease and cancer: is there a need for more biomarkers?. Expert Rev Mol Diagn. 2020;20(5):543-555. doi:10.1080/14737159.2020.1743686.

[20] Campanati A, Martina E, Diotallevi F, et al. Saliva Proteomics as Fluid Signature of Inflammatory and Immune-Mediated Skin Diseases. Int J Mol Sci. 2021;22(13):7018.

Chapter 7

Radiotherapy in Oral Cancers: Current Perspective and Future Directions

A.S. Kirthi Koushik and Ram Charith Alva

Abstract

Oral cancers form one of the most common malignancies seen worldwide, with a steady increase in number over time. Surgery with the addition of adjuvant therapy forms the cornerstone of therapeutic management for these cancers. Despite excellent surgical management, loco-regional recurrences have always been of concern. This has expanded the role of radiotherapy, with concomitant therapies, allowing to establish an effective management protocol. Over the last two decades, there have been huge strides taken towards understanding these specific aspects and providing insight into the most fruitful application of radiotherapy in these patients. In this chapter, we have presented the oncologists perspective to dealing with the non-surgical aspects of oral cancer management. We have elaborated on the chronological order with which radiotherapy has evolved and provided the contemporary aspects of decision making, essential for current practice. The evidence-based approach will address all components of radiotherapy workflow from basic understanding of patient's anatomy, planning & evaluation during therapy to the outcomes & toxicity profiles to be expected in day-to-day clinics. Established guidelines have been incorporated into the graphical representations to ensure scenario-based understanding. Future perspectives, essential for identifying the possible direction of therapy & potential improvements in outcomes, have also been addressed.

Keywords: Oral cancers, Radiotherapy, Adjuvant, Definitive, Brachytherapy, Chemotherapy

1. Introduction

Oral cancers are one of the most well described & clearly detailed cancers in history, since the times of ancient Egyptian and Ayurveda (Sushrutha) systems. Globally, as per the data released from International Agency for research on cancer (IARC), oral cancer occurs most commonly in middle- & low-income countries with worldwide incidence of 377,713 cases with 177,757 deaths seen in 2020 [1]. The worldwide incidence rate is 4.1 cases per 100,000.

Since the evolution of modern contemporary management for oral cavity cancers, radiotherapy has played a pivotal role along with surgery and recently with chemotherapy in improving patient outcomes. After the milestone discovery of x-rays by Wilhem Roentgen in 1898, utility of radiation in various cancers was established. The role of radiotherapy in oral cancers specifically, developed between the two world wars, as the morbidity was less troublesome and was easier to deliver in community hospitals [2]. However, as surgical processes got more flexible and easier to execute and the survival rates of patients receiving radiation alone were not very encouraging, radical surgery resurfaced as the primary modality for oral cancers mid-century. Also, concerns of long-term radiation morbidity affecting patient's quality of life, in those receiving conventional radiation as a sole modality came to the fore. Keeping this in mind, towards the end of the 20th century, development of newer technology was directed towards minimising these particular issues. Also, optimum and effective combinations between surgery & radiotherapy with or without the addition of chemotherapy, were slowly established as standards of care which have been thoroughly reviewed in this chapter.

In order to keep the options simple and to make the life of an oncologist simpler, one can divide oral cancers as early, locally advanced and metastatic disease. In this chapter, we will give an overview of the current understanding for the choice of treatment in these different categories with insight into the specific therapeutic aspects of both external & internal radiation therapy. We will also dwell upon the advances in recent research related to oral cancer management as well as the possible future directions from the prism of the new age radiation oncologist.

2. Basic aspects in oral cavity cancers

2.1 Anatomy from an oncologist perspective

In order to understand a disease, one needs to be well versed with the anatomy of the area and since we want to know the way this would influence a radiation oncologist's outlook, the following section will address anatomy from a radiation oncologists' perspective (**Figure 1**).

Oral cavity includes lips, buccal mucosa, gingivobuccal sulcus, superior and inferior alveolar ridges, teeth & mandible, oral tongue, floor of mouth (FOM),

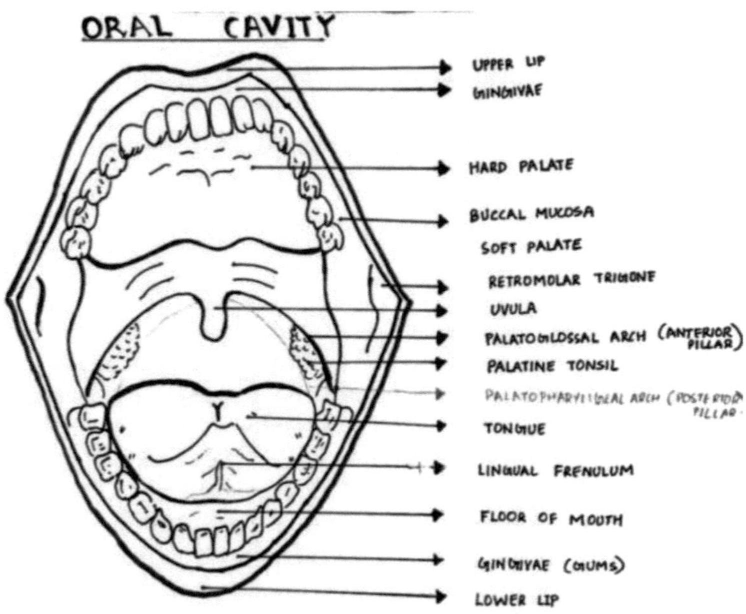

Figure 1.
Anatomical aspects of oral cavity.

DOI: http://dx.doi.org/10.5772/intechopen.99557

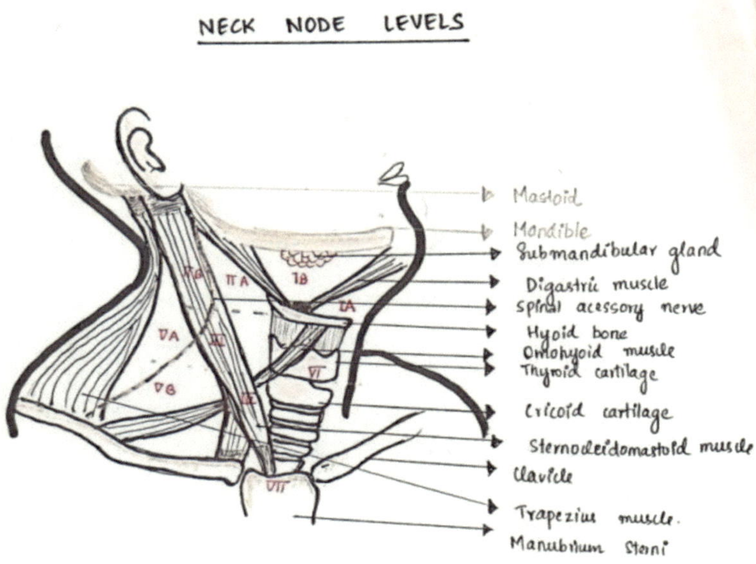

Figure 2.
Description of various nodal levels in the neck.

retromolar trigone (RMT) and hard palate [3]. One needs to know a few terminologies like buccal mucosa which means mucosal surface of lips and cheek, whereas gingival mucosa means mucosal lining of teeth, alveolar arches and gums. The area of maximum incidence of squamous cell carcinoma is at the gingivobuccal sulcus which is the junction of buccal mucosa to gingival mucosa. Floor of mouth is the U-shaped sling formed due to joining of two mylohyoid muscles to a fibrous median raphe. Oral tongue also known as Anterior 2/3rd of tongue includes the tip, lateral border and body which consists of intrinsic and extrinsic muscles. It is imperative to know the muscles as their involvement can upstage the disease, which will be discussed later in the chapter. Intrinsic muscles have no bony attachment and are divided into longitudinal, transverse and vertical groups. Extrinsic muscles do have a bony attachment and originate outside the tongue, and are made up of four paired bundles - genioglossus, hyoglossus, styloglossus and palatoglossus. These can be appreciated well on a CT scan and an MRI scans.

The most important feature of neoplasia is the potential for spread and the most common route of spread in oral cavity tumours is the lymphatic spread (**Figure 2**). Since radiotherapy is a branch which tackles locoregional disease it becomes imperative to have a thorough knowledge of the lymphatic drainage. In order to understand this better, we are dividing the lymphatic channels as functional pathways:

1. Main lymphatic pathway: submental ➔ submandibular ➔ anterior jugulodigastric ➔ middle and lower deep cervical nodal groups ➔ jugular collecting trunk

2. Posterior accessory pathway: posterior part of jugulodigastric group ➔ middle and deep posterior cervical groups

3. Anterior lymphatic pathway: submental and jugulo-omohyoid ➔ lower internal jugular nodes.

4. Superficial lateral pathway: occipital and mastoid group.

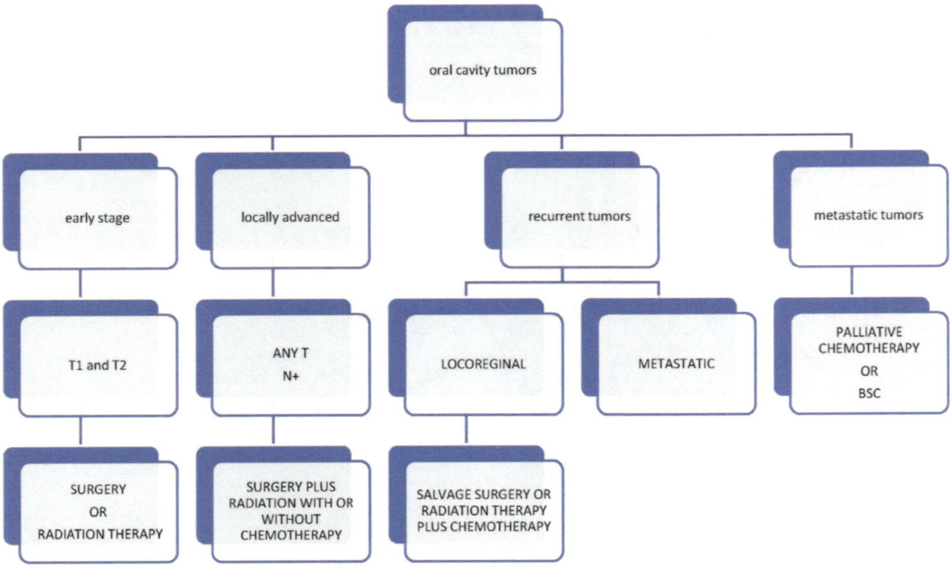

Figure 3.
Overview of management of Oral cancers.

2.2 Basic principles of treatment and broad guidelines

Radiotherapy is loco-regional form of treatment just like surgery. In oral cavity cancers one needs to keep in mind the functionality and cosmesis when deciding on the management, hence it requires a multidisciplinary team to take a call. For management and prognosis reasons, these tumours are divided in to early stage, locally advanced and metastatic tumours. The flow chart provides concise & definitive steps on how to manage oral cavity tumours (**Figure 3**).

For any malignancy there are only three weapons and they are surgery, radiation therapy and systemic therapy. The sequencing and need of each therapy are a point of debate. However, in oral cavity tumours, mostly all modalities are required and sequencing is usually pre-determined and rationale is also established.

2.2.1 Early stage

As per TNM this group includes cT1 and cT2, which means localised tumours only. This group is usually tackled by surgery or radiation therapy and role of systemic therapy is limited (**Table 1**).

	Surgery	Radiation therapy	Rationale
Lip	Yes	Yes	Cosmetically better
Buccal mucosa	Yes	Yes	If localised and margins are clear
Tongue	Yes	No	Usually aggressive and depth can be better made out on hpe than mri
FOM	No	Yes	As organ preservation is better
RMT	No	Yes	As posterior margin will not be an issue

Table 1.
Rationale for application of radiotherapy in early oral cancers.

	Surgery +/− Radiation therapy	Rationale
LIP	Surgery followed by Radiation +/− Chemotherapy	As locally advanced one modality will not be able to achieve cure.
BUCCAL MUCOSA	Surgery followed by Radiation +/− Chemotherapy	Locally advanced diseases tend to recur locally
TONGUE	Surgery followed by Radiation +/− Chemotherapy	Usually aggressive and tend to recur locally as well as systemically
FOM	Radiation and chemotherapy	As organ preservation is better
RMT	Radiation and chemotherapy	As posterior margin will not be an issue

Table 2.
Rationale for combined modality therapy in advanced oral cancers.

2.2.2 Locally advanced disease

As per TNM this group will include cT1-4 and N+ disease. Basically, it means that the disease has spread to nodes and or direct extension to surrounding structures. This group has to be addressed by combined modality therapy and there will always be some amount of deliberation to be had about the sequencing of the three modalities (**Table 2**).

Recurrent tumours: a tumour can be suggested to have recurred if there is disease recurrence after a period of documented complete remission and usually it is taken as 2 follow-ups of 6 weeks apart with a period of 6 months post primary therapy. Based on this they can be:

1. Locally recurrent: the plan of treatment will depend on the primary therapy received and also the operability. Usually, it is important to reassess the disease to take a call on treatment. If the disease is operable, salvage surgery gives best results. If more than 2 years has elapsed post primary therapy, then radiation can also be advised based on site of recurrence.

2. Locoregionally recurrent: if the duration post primary therapy is more than 2 years and if operable then both salvage surgery with radiation can be offered or else based on the status the treatment can be tailored.

3. Metastatic: these are usually managed with palliative systemic therapy and role of radiation is limited to palliation to relieve the symptoms such as bleeding, pain or dysphagia.

In the following section we are going to address the basis of radiation, how it is delivered and what are the relevant toxicities encountered.

2.3 Basis for radiation

2.3.1 What is radiation?

One needs to remember that discovery of many great things happened by accident. Same thing holds good for practice of radiotherapy, as its use was established when Henry Becquerel left 200 mg of Radium in his vest pocket for 6 hours and later noted ulceration along the adjacent skin. This event opened the eyes of the scientific community towards the clinical effects of radiation & radioactive sources. From then on, there were many experiments done to establish the role of radiation in treatment of malignancy.

Radiation is nothing but energy in the form of waves or stream of particles which can be explained by emission, propagation and absorption of energy. In the present day, most common form of radiation in use is X-rays though there are utilisation of gamma in brachytherapy and proton in particle therapy but in order to restrict ourselves to common terminologies we are not going in detail about them. This form of radiation is considered to have the ability to produce ions in the cells of tissues it passes through, by dislodging the electrons from atoms, and hence it is commonly called as ionising radiation.

If one needed to know the most basic principle about radiation, it would be that - "radiation is effective only on dividing cells". There are 5 phases that each cell goes through from G0 ➔ G1 ➔ S ➔ G2 ➔ M. Among these G2 & M phases are the most radiosensitive and S phase is the most radioresistant phase. The knowledge of these help in deciding on combination therapy and use of radiosensitisers. Radiation is usually delivered in a fractionated manner and it would be paramount to have the knowledge of the 4R's of radiation therapy to understand the basis for this fractionation:

- Repair: differential rate of repair between tumour & normal tissue cells, is what is utilised in fractionation

- Repopulation: this helps in normal tissues such that if one cell dies, then due to compensatory mechanisms other cells divide rapidly to replace this loss.

- Reoxygenation: oxygen is the most important component for both cell survival and also for effective action of radiation.

- Redistribution: as cell death happens there will be redistribution, making the cells in less radiosensitive phases to move to more radiosensitive phases, thus making radiation very effective and forms another basis for fractionation.

2.3.2 How is it delivered?

One can divide this based on technology, based on setting and based on type. The following flowchart will briefly describe about it (**Figure 4**).

Description of these commonly employed terminology are as follows

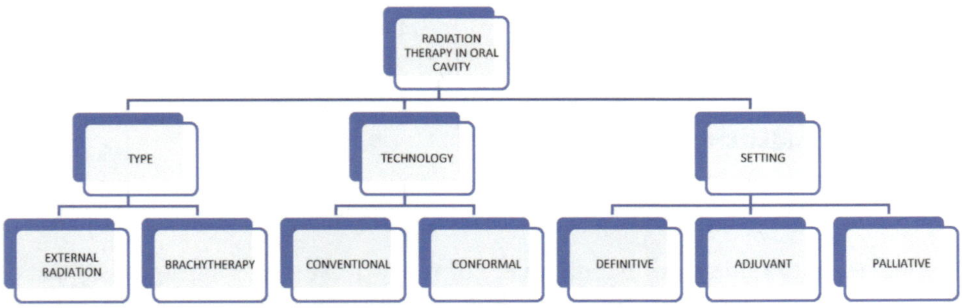

Figure 4.
Aspects of radiotherapy in Oral cancers.

1. External radiation: radiation delivered from a distance away from the body is called external radiation and the unit that's commonly employed for this are known as linear accelerators. There are different types of radiation that are used such as X-rays, gamma rays and particle therapy like protons.

2. Brachytherapy: delivery of radiation in close proximity to or within the target tissue is known as brachytherapy. The usual sources used are Iridium192 and Cobalt60.

3. Conventional: it is the traditional way of radiation delivery, where the dose is delivered without much conformity and is based mainly on bony landmarks.

4. Conformal: it is a contemporary form of radiation delivery where in the conformity is good and avoidance of normal structures can be achieved.

5. Definitive: it means radiation is the main modality of treatment and it is used with an intent to cure.

6. Adjuvant: it means radiation is delivered post-surgery in order to mop up the most probable microscopic disease that is present.

7. Palliative: as the name indicates is to only tackle the symptoms and give relief.

3. Evidence based review on current management concepts in oral cavity cancers

3.1 Risk factors for locoregional recurrence

3.1.1 Risk factors which have been utilised traditionally

Oral cavity cancers are commonly managed with single modality treatment in early stages and a combined modality approach in advanced stages. Radical, oncologically-sound surgical approaches form the backbone of early cancers with a meticulous assessment of the histopathological specimen. Even with appropriate excisions, local and regional recurrences are an extremely concerning aspect which can alter the eventual outcomes in these cancers.

Many retrospective studies and single institution prospective trials demonstrated the benefit of adding radiation adjuvantly for oral cancer patients who have undergone radical surgery. Cooper et al. collated data from RTOG #85-03 & #88-24 to retrospectively sort into 3 risk groups of presumed progressive risk to enable adjuvant treatment decisions [4]. Group I included fewer than 2 involved nodes, no ECE & negative surgical margins. Group II included at least 2 involved nodes or presence of ECE of tumour with uninvolved margins. Group III included microscopically involved surgical margins. Accordingly, comparing outcomes in groups I to III, the loco-regional recurrence rates at 5 years was 17%, 27% & 61% and median survival was 5.6 yrs., 2.6 yrs. and 1.5 yrs. respectively.

Langendijk et al. used the Classification and Regression Tree(CART) or the Recursive Partitioning Analysis(RPA) method to construct homogenous subgroups of well-known prognostication parameters to be able to identify locoregional recurrence risk [5]. Accordingly, 801 patients were divided into RPA 1 group (Intermediate risk) which included no ECE and free surgical margins; RPA 2 (High Risk) which included T1,T2 and T4 tumours with close or positive surgical margins or one positive node with ECE and RPA 3 (Very High Risk) which included T3 tumours with close or positive margin, N3 neck or multiple nodes with ECE. The 5-year LRC was 92%, 78% and 58% and OS rates were 67%, 50% and 36% for the three RPA classes respectively.

Salama JK et al. used pooled multivariate analysis to give a consensus statement on use of adjuvant therapy in head and neck cancers [6]. They divided patients into two groups to identify their risk for developing loco-regional recurrences based on pathological features. High risk group included those with involved surgical margins and extranodal spread. Low risk group included other adverse features such as T3/4 tumours, perineural invasion, lymphovascular space invasion, multiple nodal involvement and lower neck adenopathy. They advised for postop radiotherapy alone for patients with low-risk features and addition of concurrent chemotherapy for those with high-risk features. They also suggested postop radiotherapy dose of upto 63Gy for high-risk features and 57Gy for those with low-risk disease.

Perineural Invasion (PNI): There is no standardised definition of this entity, but the most accepted one is when tumour cells are present in any one of the three layers of the nerve sheath & when tumour cells are in close proximity to the nerve & involves more than one-third of circumference. Bur et al. identified an incidence of PNI in literature of between 3 and 52% [7]. Though many authors have not been able to assign prognostic significance to presence of PNI, some features such as multiple foci of PNI, involvement of large nerves (>1 mm) and higher maximum extent of PNI were associated with increased local failure and reduced disease specific survival.

In the systematic review collated data from 13 retrospective studies, they identified local recurrence rates of 4.4% - 22.9%, regional recurrence rates of 12.3% - 30.8% and 5-yr overall survival estimates of 48–89.6% in those patients with presence of PNI [7]. In two studies from this review, where neck dissection was conducted, regional failure rates were 12.3% and 17.6% which undermines the fact of ineffective salvage options after this. However, the authors suggest that in the absence of any prospective trial to assess the impact of PNI on loco-regional recurrence or survival, it would be imperative to discuss the options of treatment in detail in those patients where positive PNI is the only risk factor post radical surgery.

Depth of Invasion (DOI): Tumour thickness or depth of invasion has been consistently identified as a predictor for cervical lymph node metastasis in oral cavity cancers. Oral cavity cancers have occult nodal metastases of up to 40% in clinically negative neck, which is usually managed with elective nodal dissection as opposed to just observation. Huang et al. in their meta-analysis, have tried to address this aspect and have concluded that the optimal cut-off point for DOI is 4 mm, to consider for neck management [8].

In another study, Liao et al. followed-up patients who underwent surgery of early-stage oral cavity cancers(pT1-2 N0) to identify poor prognostic features and suggest for adjuvant therapy [9]. They found that poorly differentiated tumours and DOI of 4 mm and above were both independent poor prognostic factors, and when present together accounts for 2-yr regional failure of 42%. Hence, they suggest for the use of PORT in this subset of early OC cancers.

Bulbul et al. conducted a meta-analysis of 8 studies (1427 patients), which used frozen section (FS) evaluation to define margin status in early(T1/2N0) oral cavity cancers [10]. They compared positive/close FS margins which was cleared by further resection (R1 – R0), positive margin not cleared (R1) to those with negative margins upfront (R0). They found that patient with R1-R0 had poorer local recurrence free survival (LRFS) when compared to R0, regardless of clearance which was statistically significant. Furthermore, R1-R0 patients showed almost equal LRFS to that of R1, though the trend to worse result was with R1 patients. They concluded that upfront positive/close margin was a marker of a locally aggressive disease regardless of re-resection & correction. They also indicated that there should be standardisation of the FS sampling method too.

3.2 Surgery followed by radiotherapy

The value of postoperative radiotherapy (PORT) for advanced head & neck cancers, was established in 1970's with few well researched studies [11]. Marcus et al. suggested doses for OC cancers of 6500Rads to achieve high local control and up to 7000rads for those with positive surgical margins [12].

Outcomes in locally advanced cancers are suboptimal with primary failure being loco-regional relapses. Hence combined modality treatments have been employed to counter this aspect as well as to ascertain if they added to overall survival patterns too. Lavaf et al. retrospectively analysed data from the Surveillance Epidemiology End Results (SEER) data base to collate results on 8795 lymph node positive cases of advanced head and neck cancers [13]. They found addition of adjuvant radiotherapy in these patients improved 5 yr. overall survival rates (43.2% vs. 33.4%; $p<0.001$) and cause specific survival rates (50.9% vs. 42.1%).

Kao et al. did a similar SEER group analysis of advanced cancers of head and neck region and specifically tried to address benefit of RT with respect to various nodal stages and specific sites of disease [14]. Subset analysis found that all nodal stages, including N1 Disease, has improved survival with the addition of adjuvant RT. Also, in multivariate analysis, addition of RT in node positive oral cavity tumours improved overall survival [HR, 0.84; 95% CI, 0.73–0.98; $p = 0.025$], though it was not as significant as compared to the other head and neck sites.

Another population-based study done by Shrimeet al, tried to specifically address the benefit of PORT in early-stage primary oral cavity cancers (pT1/T2N1) with single ipsilateral node without extracapsular spread and being <3 cm in size [15]. For all patients, adjuvant RT was associated with superior 5 yr. overall survival [52.4% vs. 41.4%($p<.001$)]. Survival advantage was statistically significant in T2 cases, with a trend to significance in T1 cases. When individual sub-sites were analysed, PORT significantly improved survival in patients with cancers of oral tongue [52.3% vs. 37.9%($p=.002$)] and floor of mouth [39.9% vs. 17.7%($p=.003$)].

Addition of Chemotherapy to Radiation in post-op setting: Several retrospective and small prospective trials had showed improvement in outcomes of advanced head and neck cancers by adding chemotherapy (adjuvant or concurrent) to post-operative radiotherapy, especially in those with high-risk features such as inadequate margins, presence of extracapsular nodal spread and multiple involved nodes. Single institution trials by Bachaud and Smid, revealed improved loco-regional control rates and superior DFS/OS rates in combined modality group at a slightly higher rate of complications [16, 17].

Lacas & Pignon et al. (MACH-NC) in their updated meta-analysis of chemotherapy in head and neck cancer have studied the effect of concurrent chemotherapy use along with radiotherapy (upfront & post-surgery) [18]. Out of 107 studies (19,805 patients), 71 studies (10,680 patients) were on concomitant chemotherapy with a median follow up of 9.2 years. There was an absolute benefit in overall survival & event free survival of 6.5% & 5.8% at 5 years and 3.6% & 3.1% at 10 years with significant reduction in LRF rates [sub-HR = 0.71; $p < 0.0001$]. The study also showed that concurrent chemotherapy outcomes were better than induction chemotherapy and also that platin based chemotherapy gave maximum benefit, however there was no significant difference between weekly or three-weekly chemotherapy protocols in terms of outcomes or toxicity.

Bernier et al. (EORTC 22931) conducted a multi-institutional prospective study in 334 patients and found that addition of chemotherapy to adjuvant radiotherapy showed a benefit in 5 yr. PFS rates [47%(CMT) vs. 36%(RT)] and OS rates [53% (CMT) vs. 40%(RT)] & reduced the 5-year risk of death in combined modality from 43–27% [19]. Cooper et al.(RTOG 9501) did a similar study in 459 patients and showed significantly improved local/regional control as well as disease free survival (10% absolute benefit at 2 years) in the combined modality group after 45.9 months follow up [20].

As both these studies had few differences in their definition of high-risk disease, a pooled analysis was done to get some clarity and this concluded that outcomes for patients with ECE and/or involved surgical margins was significantly better with CMT [21]. Also, there was a trend to improved outcomes in patients with clinically enlarged level IV/V nodes with oral cavity/oropharyngeal primaries and perineural infiltration.

Three weekly high dose cisplatin (100 mg/m^2) is the standard systemic chemotherapy regimen given concurrently with radiation in high-risk oral cavity cancers. However, due to compliance issues low dose regimens have been applied in clinical practice without any prospective evidence to support the same. Szturz et al. conducted a meta-analysis to compare the standard three weekly regimen (100 mg/m^2; 3 doses) with the low dose weekly regimen $\leq$50 mg/m^2; $\geq$6 doses) [22]. Though there were no prospective comparative studies till date, 52 studies with 4209 patients were included and it showed no difference in the efficacy indices such as overall survival or response rates. In the definitive treatment setting, weekly regimen was more compliant and significantly less toxic with respect to myelosuppression, severe nausea/vomiting and nephrotoxicity. In the post-op setting, the two approaches were similar with the weekly arm causing more grade 3/4 dysphagia and weight loss.

JCOG1008 was a multi-institutional phase II/III non-inferiority trial comparing 3 weekly cisplatin with weekly schedule (40 mg/m^2) as a concurrent chemotherapy option in post-operative high-risk H&N cancers [23]. After enrolling 261 patients and a median follow up of 2.2 years, the trial was stopped as the non-inferiority criteria was reached. The 3-year OS (76.1% vs. 59.1%; HR of 0.69) &RFS (64.5% vs. 53%; HR of 0.71) was favouring the weekly arm as against the 3 weekly arm, confirming the non-inferiority of the lower dose weekly regimen.

3.3 Definitive radiotherapy (with or without chemotherapy)

There are no prospective trials which have directly compared primary surgery vs. primary radiotherapy in oral cavity cancers specifically. Two case series comparing these two modalities suggested a lower loco-regional control with primary radiotherapy compared to a surgical approach.

First was Studer et al., who assessed 58 consecutive oral cancer patients referred for either adjuvant or definitive radiotherapy [24]. They found local control rates were highest in the surgery followed by post-op IMRT group (92% LC at 2 yr), followed by patients treated with surgery alone or those receiving post-op 3DCRT (70–80% LC at 2 yr) and least in the definitive radiotherapy group treated with IMRT (40%LC at 2 yr) or 3DCRT (30% LC at 2 yr).

Murthy V. et al. studied 1180 oral cancer patients treated with PORT or definitive RT, by dividing them into 2 groups – Group 1 included gingiva-alveolar-buccal complex, lip and hard palate sites and group 2 included tongue and floor of mouth sites [25]. The 3 yr. LC, LRC and DFS for those treated with PORT was 74%, 65% % 60% respectively. And for those treated with definitive RT it was 34%, 31% & 30%

respectively. Also, they found Group 1 patients had significantly better LC, LRC and DFS than group 2 patients.

Cohen et al. did a retrospective review of 4 multi-institutional phase II trials dealing with primary chemo-radiotherapy for T4 oral cavity tumours [26]. In all 39 patients were assessed, 42% of them having bone involvement. Median dose of RT given was 74Gy. Five-year OS, PFS and LC were 56%, 51% & 75% respectively suggesting definitive chemoradiation to be a reasonable option in these tumours.

Hosni et al. retrospectively analysed all oral cancer patients (108 patients) treated with IMRT (with no surgical intervention) [27]. The cases had 63% cT3/T4 disease, 35% cN2/3 and 35% received concurrent chemotherapy. After a median follow up of 52 months, the 5-year local, regional and distant control rate was 78%, 92% & 90% respectively. The 5-year DFS, OS and CSS were 42%, 50% & 76% respectively justifying definitive non-surgical chemoradiation as a meaningful alternative in appropriately chosen cases.

Updated MACH-NC results showed the benefit of concomitant chemotherapy was due to its effect on deaths related to head and neck cancer (absolute benefit of 9.8% in 5 years) [18]. Addition of chemotherapy showed a significant reduction in loco-regional failure (sub-HR = 0.71; $p<0.0001$) with a non-significant effect on distant failure.

The first Meta-Analysis of Radiotherapy in Head and neck cancer (MARCH) in 2005 and clearly showed an advantage of altered fractionation radiotherapy over conventional radiotherapy in terms of overall and progression free survival. The updated analysis of this study was conducted by Lacas et al. in 2017 by including 34 trials and 11,969 patients and extended the comparison to benefit of concomitant chemoradiotherapy over altered fractionation schemes [28]. They reiterated that altered fractionation was superior to conventional RT alone schemes in all disease indices and also that hyperfractionation schemes were better than accelerated RT plans especially when nodal disease was higher. The comparison between concomitant chemoradiation and altered fractionation revealed a clear benefit for CMT with an absolute benefit of 5.8% and 5.1% at 5 & 10 years respectively.

Combining altered fractionation RT schemes with chemotherapy in head and neck cancers have been studied in the following two trials. GORTEC 99–02 did a three-arm study comparing standard chemoradiation, accelerated radiotherapy-chemotherapy and very accelerated radiotherapy alone [29]. Progression free survival were 37.6%, 34.1% & 32.2% respectively with acute grade 3/4 toxicity of 76–84% in the altered fractionation arms. The RTOG 0129 trial did a direct head on comparison between standard fractionation chemoradiotherapy and accelerated chemotherapy-radiotherapy in 743 patients [30]. At a median follow up of 7.9 years, there were no differences in OS, PFS, LRF or DM rates between the two arms. Both these studies concluded that addition of chemotherapy to altered fractionation radiation schemes in locally advanced head and neck cancers provided no benefit in terms of outcomes.

3.4 Time factor in PORT

Two aspects of timing with regards to radiotherapy has been shown to be important for eventual outcomes in head and neck cancer management – overall treatment duration of radiotherapy as well as total time of both surgery and radiotherapy in CMT. Prolongation of both these indices seems to negatively impact the outcomes. Ang et al. conducted a multi-institutional study including 288 patients and found that in high-risk H&N cancers, there was a trend towards higher LRC and survival rates when PORT was delivered in 5 rather than 7 weeks [31]. Also, a prolonged interval between surgery and PORT of >6 weeks or a total duration of surgery and PORT of >13 weeks significantly impacted outcomes negatively.

Huang et al. in their meta-analysis involving 46 studies dealing with this aspect found that in the combined analysis the rates of local recurrences were significantly higher among patients who received PORT more than 6 weeks after surgery (OR = 2.89; 95% CI) [32].

Fast tumour cell repopulation has been postulated as the reason behind why prolonging overall treatment time (OTT) can negatively impact local control and survival in cancers. González Ferreira et al. in their review of literature found prolongation of OTT resulted in an average loss of LRC ranging from 1 to 1.2%per day to 12–14% per day, requiring an average increase of 0.6–0.8Gy/day to compensate for it [33]. Also, they postulated that the lag period for the accelerated repopulation to be initiated was between 21 and 28 days.

Graboyes et al. conducted an institutional review to study this aspect and found that starting PORT > 6 weeks post-surgery resulted in decreased OS rates in both multivariate and propensity score-matched subsets [34]. They also found that increasing delay beyond 6 weeks resulted in small, progressive survival decrements [aHR 1.09, 1.10, 1.12 for 7–8 wks, 8–10 wks and >10wks respectively].

Zumer et al. did a retrospective analysis to identify the relationship between time before treatment intervention and tumour growth kinetics on treatment outcomes in those undergoing definitive radiotherapy with or without chemotherapy in 273 head and neck cancer patients [35]. There was no significant association between loco-regional control or survival indices and time to treatment intervention. They also found that the median tumour volume relative increase rate & tumour volume doubling time was 3.2%/day and 19 days respectively, but both had no impact on outcomes.

3.5 Dose & volumes considerations for radiation in oral cancers

As a principle in radiotherapy, at least for oral cavity squamous cell carcinomas, the dose needs to be delivered in the desired fractionated regimen without unnecessary interruptions and in the shortest time possible with no reduction in dose below that what is tolerated by late responding normal tissue.

This means that the total dose is important to prevent local recurrences and the factors that need to be kept in mind are [36].

- Dose
- Dose per fraction
- Overall treatment time
- Normal tissue toxicity

Radiotherapy in oral cavity tumours is associated with lot of acute as well as chronic toxicities which will be dealt separately. In order to minimise this, there are several steps taken and one of them is the use of highly conformal Intensity modulated radiotherapy (IMRT), and there is lot of data to support its use in head and neck cancers. Before starting radiation therapy all patients undergo a detailed examination by a dental surgeon and this is known as dental prophylaxis. The dental surgeon will assess the area of treatment and also estimate the dose that would probably be delivered to the surrounding bony structures as well as ascertain the status of the teeth and score it as per DMF (Decayed, Missing, Filled) index.

Based on this, treatment is advised and appropriately followed. By doing this exercise, the chances of osteoradionecrosis & soft tissue related long-term toxicities can be reduced or even eliminated. IMRT involves simulation and planning for which the most basic step is immobilisation by thermoplastic facemask attached to a base plate indexed to the treatment table. After the planning CT scan is done the volumes are outlined on them as per the guidelines [37].

3.5.1 For definitive radiation therapy

GTV or gross tumour volume is defined as the visible tumour along with the nodes which are abnormal. HRCTV [High Risk Clinical Target Volume] includes the margin around the GTV and also the first echelon group of nodes which will be level IB to level II. For LRCTV [Low Risk Clinical Target Volume] one would include level III, IV, supraclavicular and IA. Usually bilateral neck is to be treated, based on institutional protocol. PTV [Planning Target Volume] would be 5 mm around the CTV trimmed from skin, but based on institutional protocol, it could range from 3 mm to 10 mm (**Figures 5** and **6**).

3.5.2 For postop radiation therapy

HRCTV encompasses the area of the tumour bed [if features such as margin positivity, node positivity with extracapsular extension, peri-neural invasion and soft tissue extension is present]. IRCTV [Intermediate Risk Clinical Target Volume] would include the involved nodes without ECE & uninvolved adjacent nodal levels.

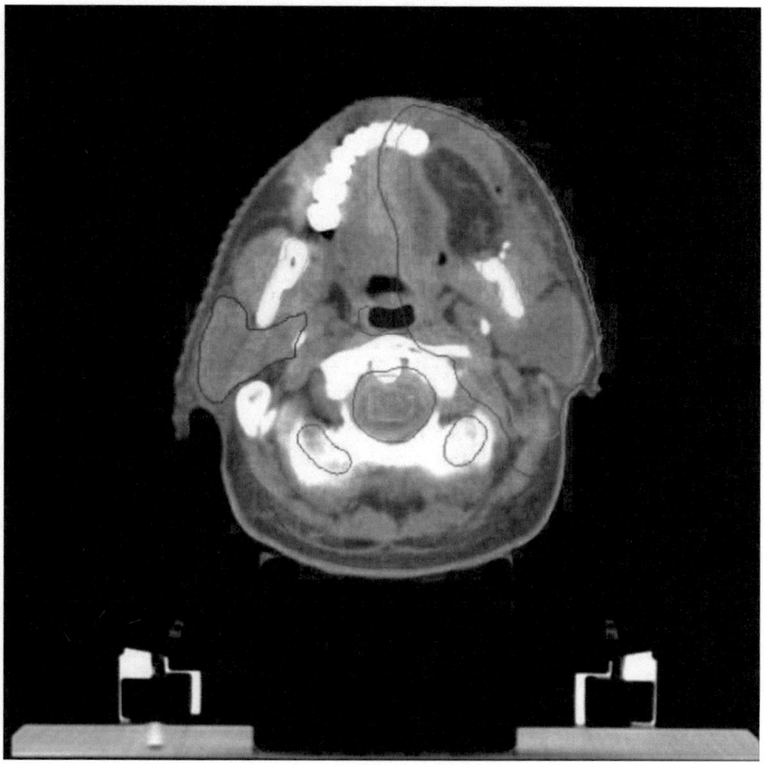

Figure 5.
Contouring of target volumes & organs at risk(OAR) for a case of carcinoma Oral tongue post surgery [pT3N1M0]; Orange – clinical target volume; Red – planning target volume; Cyan – mandible; brown – right parotid; green – spinal cord; pink - constrictor.

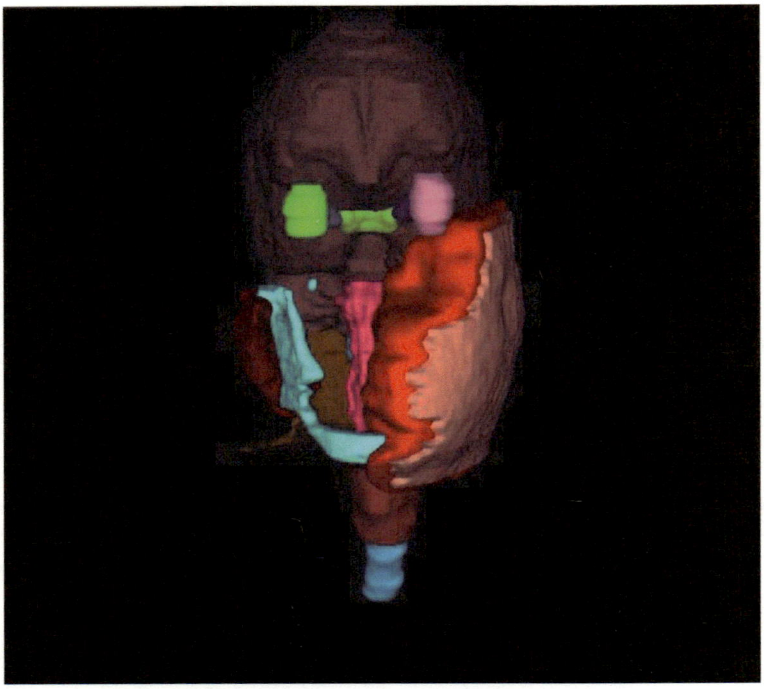

Figure 6.
3-dimensional projection of target & normal tissues contoured.

LRCTV would include rest of the nodal levels based on the risk stratification and bilateral neck is treated if risk is higher. PTV would be 5 mm around the CTV trimmed from skin, but based on institutional protocol, it could range from 3 mm to 10 mm (**Figure 5**).

As far as dose and dose per fraction is concerned there are multiple regimens and multiple doses available with their pros and cons. The following table depicts the usual practice with some insight on hypothesis (**Tables 3** and **4**).

3.6 Radiation related toxicity in oral cancer management

Radiotherapy is an essential part of multi-modality treatment for oral cancers. However, several uninvolved organs in the vicinity of these cancers like the skin, salivary glands, oral mucosa, masticatory apparatus, dentition and jaws receive significant doses of radiation during treatment. This could result in moderate to severe adverse effects during and after completion of treatment and also affect the patient's quality of life. The effects may be acute such as dermatitis, mucositis and hyposalivation or chronic and long-term such as xerostomia, radiation caries, trismus and osteoradionecrosis [38].

As many of these effects are dose-limiting, introduction of newer radiation techniques and schedules have minimised late effects to a large extent. Nutting et al. were able to demonstrate 50% reduction in subjective xerostomia rates with IMRT by keeping mean dose to contralateral parotid gland at 26Gy [39]. Parotid sparing IMRT was achieved by avoiding the contralateral parotid, upper parapharyngeal space as well as giving a tight constraint for the anterior oral cavity [36, 40].

A more problematic late effect is osteoradionecrosis, which is the process of bone and soft tissue necrosis, arising as a result of radiation induced hypocellularity, hypoxia and hypovascularity, resulting in a non-healing region [41]. As spontaneous ORN is dose dependent (>60Gy), IMRT is able to reduce the maximum

Post operative disease			
R1-Microscopic Disease 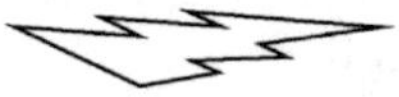	R0 Resection 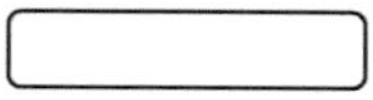	R0 & N0 Disease	Volumes are applicable for conformal therapy. These volumes are subjective based on dose/fraction. Surgery to radiation interval should be </=6 weeks
NODE +, ECE/PNI + 	NODE +, No ECE/PNI 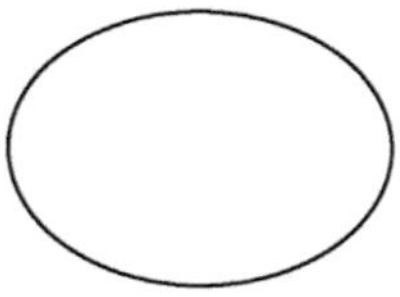	ELECTIVE ONLY 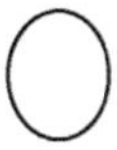	
RISK OF RELAPSE – >30%	RISK OF RELAPSE – 15–20%	RISK OF RELAPSE – 5–10%	
VOLUME – CTV-HR (PRIMARY)	VOLUME - CTVIR (PRIMARY) CTV IR(NODES)	VOLUME -CTVLR (NODES)	
DOSE – 66Gy–70Gy at 2Gy per fraction	DOSE – 60Gy at 2Gy per fraction	DOSE – 50Gy at 2Gy per fraction	

Table 3.
Dose & volume consideration for post-op adjuvant radiotherapy.

Definitive radiotherapy			
MACROSCOPIC DISEASE 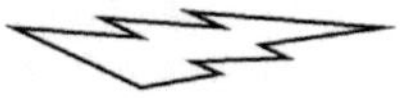	MARGIN AROUND THE GTV	NODE NEGATIVE, BUT DRAINAGE NODAL AREA	Volumes are applicable for conformal therapy. These volumes are subjective based on dose/fraction.
NODE + WITH ECE 	PRIMARY ECHELON 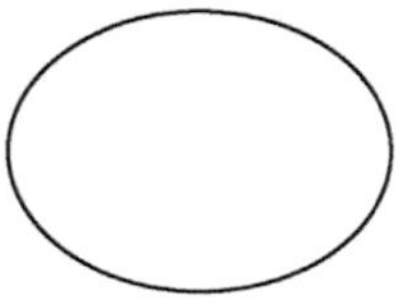	ELECTIVE ONLY 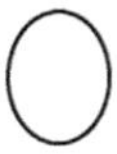	
VOLUME – GTV or CTVHR	VOLUME- CTVIR (PRIMARY) CTV IR(NODES)	VOLUME- CTVLR(NODES)	
DOSE – 66Gy–70Gy at 2Gy per fraction	DOSE – 60Gy at 2Gy per fraction	DOSE – 50Gy at 2Gy per fraction	

Table 4.
Dose & volume consideration for definitive radiotherapy.

dose received by the mandible as well as volume of mandible covered by 50-55Gy isodoses. The reported ORN rates in IMRT series is 5–6%.

Chen et al. found that IMRT also helped reduce dysphagia related complications in oral cancer patients undergoing radiotherapy [42]. Those receiving IMRT had significantly lesser moderate (grade 2) and severe(grade 3) dysphagia when compared to those receiving conventional radiotherapy (21% vs. 59%; $p = 0.02$) [42].

3.7 Targeted therapy, current bio-markers and future perspectives for oral cancers

Epidermal growth factor receptor (EGFR) regulates many cellular functions crucial for tumorigenesis. Huang et al. studied 160 oral cancer patients using immunohistochemistry for EGFR protein over-expression and fluorescence in situ hybridization for copy number [43]. EGFR overexpression was noted in 46.88% and 31.25% had increased gene copy numbers. They also found 100% concordance rate between EGFR gene amplification and protein overexpression. EGFR overexpression was associated with poor prognosis, both in terms of DFS and OS.

Cetuximab, an EGFR antibody has shown good results in head and neck cancers, in combination with definitive radiation [44]. The RTOG 0920 trial (Ongoing) is trying to address outcomes with addition of cetuximab to PORT in intermediate-risk oral cancers.

The development of PD-1/PD-L1 inhibitors (pembrolizumab & nivolumab) & other immune checkpoint inhibitors (ICI) has changed the systemic management of HNSCC [45, 46]. PD-L1 expression in pre-treatment biopsies have been associated with good prognosis. Preclinical data suggests synergy between anti-PD1 inhibitors and radiation, making it a potential therapeutic option for high-risk oral cancers in the future [47]. Several phase II studies addressing these agents in combination with standard therapy or as a neoadjuvant/adjuvant option are in the works [48].

Tumour mutational burden (TMB) as a biomarker of ICI response has shown mixed response in HNSCC, with KEYNOTE-012 trial showing a positive correlation while using a cut-off of ≥102 mutations per exome [49].

Other aspects being studied are tumour immune microenvironment and oral/gut microbiome as regulating mechanisms having implications for response of HNSCC to immune therapies. Oral microbiome has also shown an effect on toxicity profile of patients undergoing concurrent chemoradiation [50]. Cell therapy-based options such as the use of activated cytotoxic T-Lymphocytes (CTL's) to result in tumour cell death has also been attempted in HNSCC [51]. Chimeric antigen Receptor T cells are one such example being used in advanced oral cancers.

4. Brachytherapy

Brachytherapy is the delivery of radiation therapy using sealed sources placed within or close to the site to be treated. Oral cavity cancers with their ease of accessibility and better visibility had provided the best sites for use of this therapy for improved local control and outcomes in the past. With its ability to give high doses to tumour and very minimal dose to the surrounding tissues, brachytherapy could be considered the most ideal conformal therapy. However, in recent times the technological advancements associated with external beam therapy, improved imaging and surgical techniques and lack of appropriate knowledge or expertise in invasive implants has relegated brachytherapy to be used in very specific and not so common indications of these cancers. Modern brachytherapy too has evolved to allow for acceptable dose and fractionation schedules, image guidance, dose optimization and better radiation protection mechanisms.

Common cancer sites where brachytherapy can be used in oral cavity are mobile tongue, lip, buccal mucosa, floor of mouth and palate [52, 53]. Indications for use of brachytherapy presently is

- Small localised T1 squamous cell cancers as primary treatment
- In combination of external beam radiotherapy as a boost modality
- As a re-irradiation modality in previously treated sites or development of second primaries

Disadvantages for brachytherapy are primarily due to lack of expertise and need for an initial learning curve which is usually lacking other than in bigger institutes, ease of modern conformal external radiotherapy techniques, competition with modern surgical techniques and concerns of radiation protection. Some relative contraindications to this procedure in oral cavity tumours would be compromised mouth opening, difficult naso-tracheal intubation & those having large defects requiring flap reconstructions in post-op setting.

Usually, the procedure followed is a single implant with multiple treatment fractions over nearly a week. Procedure is done under general anaesthesia with the help of nasotracheal intubation and dental separators to allow for proper visualisation. An interstitial implant is done following the principles of the Paris technique (**Figures** 7 and **8**). A CT-scan based planning is done and the oncologist will delineate the tumour and organs at risk on the treatment planning system. Doses delivered are between 3-4Gy in 10–12 fractions delivered six hours apart over

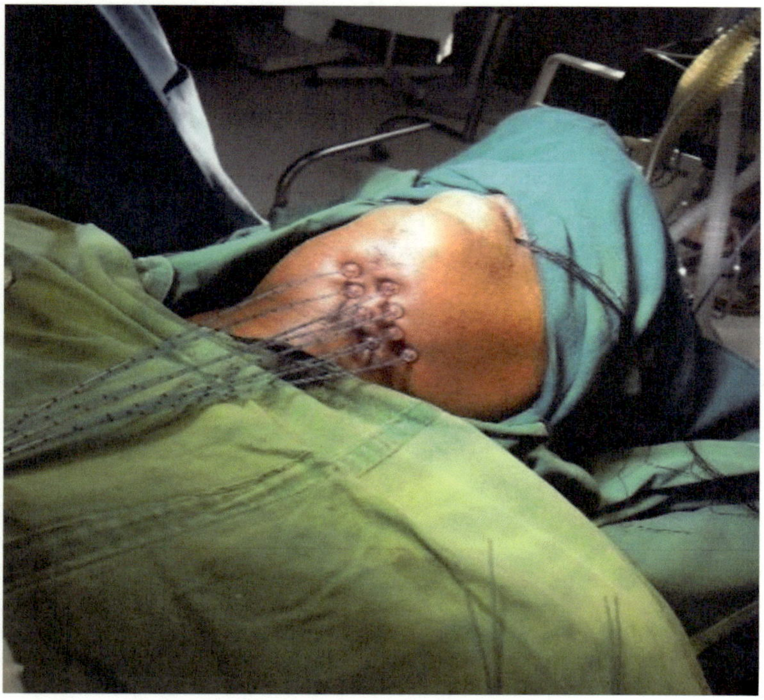

Figure 7.
Brachytherapy of tongue.

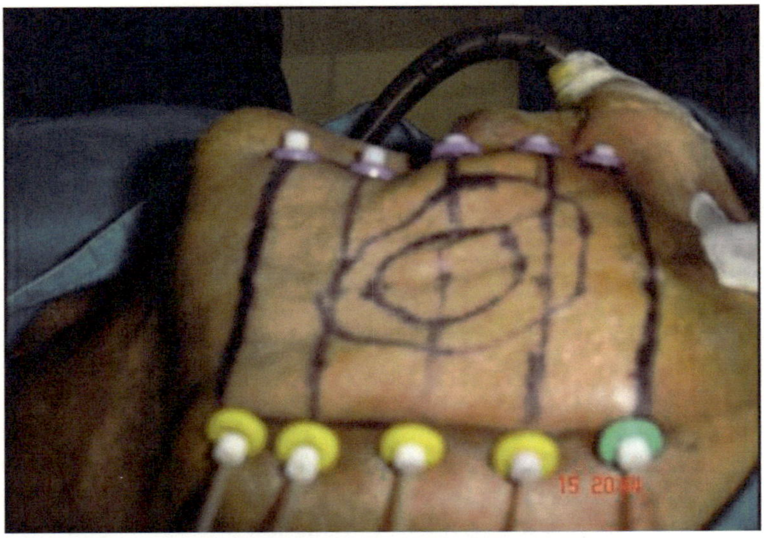

Figure 8.
Brachytherapy of buccal mucosa.

5–6 days in the primary treatment setting and 3-4Gy in 6–8 fractions over 3–4 days in the boost setting.

Acute complications of brachytherapy could be haemorrhage, infection, airway compromise & sialadenitis. Long term side effects could be soft tissue necrosis, telangiectasia and rarely osteoradionecrosis.

5. Conclusions

Oral cavity cancers are a diverse group of tumours which are known for its aggressive behaviour and higher chances of recurrences, which can lead to extremely difficult & cumbersome management decisions. This current review denotes the various available options for treatment for different categories of these tumours, to provide us a glimmer of hope to not only manage the disease well but also give good results in terms of locoregional control, long-term survival and at the same time ensuring cosmetically acceptable outcomes. As the primary focus of this chapter was on aspects of use of radiotherapy in oral cancers, the specific nuances on current evidence-based practice have been elaborated upon. Though most of the general details on use of external & internal radiation in oral cancers have been described, the detailed specific site-based & technique-based points have not been elaborated as they are beyond the scope of this chapter.

Available potential therapeutic options being currently investigated to ascertain possible benefit in oral cancers have also been described in this chapter. The future advances in use of radiation therapy should focus on recognising & refining the most appropriate indications for its application, strategic use of higher end technology like modulated arc therapy/stereotactic radiation & proton therapy, better amalgamation of radiation with newer concomitant systemic therapy agents as well as a well-rounded approach in inculcating genomic attributes of oral cancers in identifying the future standard of care for these tumours.

DOI: http://dx.doi.org/10.5772/intechopen.99557

Author details

A.S. Kirthi Koushik* and Ram Charith Alva
Ramaiah Medical College and Hospital, Bengaluru, India

*Address all correspondence to: kirthi.koushik@gmail.com

References

[1] World Health Organization. Oral Health. 2020. Available online. https://gco.iarc.fr/today/data/factsheets/cancers/1-Lip-oral-cavity-fact-sheet.pdf. (Accessed on 11th July, 2021)

[2] Petrosyan V, Kane G, Ameerally P. Oral Cancer Treatment Through the Ages: Part 2. J Oral Maxillofac Surg. 2019 Jul;77(7):1484-1489. doi: 10.1016/j.joms.2019.01.024. Epub 2019 Jan 28. PMID: 30794811.

[3] Fred J. Laine, Wendy R.K. Smoker. Oral cavity: Anatomy and pathology, Seminars in Ultrasound, CT and MRI, Volume 16, Issue 6, 1995, Pages 527-545, https://doi.org/10.1016/S0887-2171(06)80024-7

[4] Cooper JS, Pajak TF, Forastiere A, Jacobs J, Fu KK, Ang KK, Laramore GE, Al-Sarraf M. Precisely defining high-risk operable head and neck tumors based on RTOG #83-03 and #88-24: Targets for postoperative radiochemotherapy? Head Neck 1998;20:588-94

[5] Langendijk JA, Slotman BJ, van der Waal I, Doornaert P, Berkof J, Leemans CR. Risk group definition by recursive partitioning analysis of patients with squamous cell head and neck carcinoma treated with surgery and postoperative radiotherapy. Cancer 2005;104:1408-17

[6] Expert Panel on Radiation Oncology-Head and Neck, Salama JK, Saba N, Quon H, Garg MK, Lawson J, McDonald MW, Ridge JA, Smith RV, Yeung AR, Yom SS, Beitler JJ. ACR appropriateness criteria® adjuvant therapy for resected squamous cell carcinoma of the head and neck. Oral Oncol 2011;47:554-9

[7] Bur AM, Lin A, Weinstein GS. Adjuvant radiotherapy for early head and neck squamous cell carcinoma with perineural invasion: a systematic review. Head Neck 2016;38 Suppl1: E2350-7

[8] Huang SH, Hwang D, Lockwood G, Goldstein DP, O'Sullivan B. Predictive value of tumor thickness for cervical lymph-node involvement in squamous cell carcinoma of the oral cavity: a meta-analysis of reported studies. Cancer. 2009;115:1489-1497.

[9] Liao CT, Lin CY, Fan KH, Wang HM, Ng SH, Lee LY, et al. Identification of a high-risk group among patients with oral cavity squamous cell carcinoma and pT1-2N0 disease. Int J Radiat Oncol Biol Phys. 2012;82:284-90.

[10] Bulbul MG, Tarabichi O, Sethi RK, Parikh AS, Varvares MA (2019) Does clearance of positive margins improve local control in oral cavity cancer? A meta-analysis. Otolaryngol Head Neck Surg 161:235–244.

[11] Fletcher GH, Evers WT. Radiotherapeutic management of surgical recurrences and postoperative residuals tumors of the head and neck. Radiology 1970:95:185-8. 57.

[12] Marcus RB Jr, Million RR, Cassissi NJ. Postoperative irradiation for squamous cell carcinomas of the head and neck: analysis of time-dose factors related to control above the clavicles. Int J Radiat Oncol Biol Phys 1979;5:1943-49

[13] Lavaf A, Genden EM, Cesaretti JA, Packer S, Kao J. Adjuvant radiotherapy improves overall survival for patients with lymph node-positive head and neck squamous cell carcinoma. Cancer 2008;112:535-43. 60.

[14] Kao J, Lavaf F, Teng MS, Huang D, Genden EM. Adjuvant radiotherapy and survival for patients with node-positive head and neck cancer: an analysis by primary site and nodal stage. Int J Radiat Oncol Biol Phys 2008;71:362-70

[15] Shrime MG, Gullane PJ, Dawson L, Kim J, Gilbert RW, Irish JC, Brown DH, Goldstein DP. The impact of adjuvant radiotherapy on survival in T1-2N1 squamous cell carcinoma of the oral cavity. Arch Otolaryngol Head Neck Surg2010;136:225-8

[16] Bachaud JM, Cohen-Jonathan E, Alzieu C, David JM, Serrano E, Daly-Schveitzer N. Combined postoperative radiotherapy and weekly cisplatininfusion for locally advanced head and neck carcinoma: final report ofa randomized trial. Int J Radiat Oncol Biol Phys. (1996) 36:999–1004.doi: 10.1016/S0360-3016(96) 00430-0

[17] Smid L, Budihna M, Zakotnik B, Soba E, Strojan P, Fajdiga I, et al. Postoperative concomitant irradiation and chemotherapy with mitomycinC and bleomycin for advanced head-and-neck carcinoma. Int J RadiatOncolBiol Phys. (2003) 56:1055–62. doi: 10.1016/S0360-3016(03)00207-4

[18] Lacas B, Carmel A, Landais C et al. Meta-analysis of chemotherapy in head and neck cancer (MACH-NC): An update on 107 randomized trials and 19,805 patients, on behalf of MACH-NC Group. Radiother Oncol. 2021 Mar;156: 281-293. doi: 10.1016/j.radonc.2021 .01.013. Epub 2021 Jan 27. PMID: 33515668

[19] Bernier J, Domenge C, Ozsahin M, Matuszewska K, Lefèbvre JL, Greiner RH, et al. Postoperative irradiation with or without concomitant chemotherapy for locally advanced head and neck cancer. N Engl J Med. 2004; 350:1945-52.

[20] Cooper JS, Pajak TF, Forastiere AA, Jacobs J, Campbell BH, Saxman SB, et al. Postoperative concurrent radiotherapy and chemotherapy for high-risk squamous-cell carcinoma of the head and neck. N Engl J Med. 2004;350: 1937-44

[21] Bernier J, Cooper JS, Pajak T, Van Glabbeke M, Bourhis J, Forastiere A, et al. Defining risk levels in locally advanced head and neck cancers: a comparative analysis of concurrent postoperative radiation plus chemotherapy trials of the EORTC (# 22931) and RTOG (# 9501). Head Neck (2005) 27:843–50. doi: 10.1002/hed.20279

[22] Szturz P, Wouters K, Kiyota N, Tahara M, Prabhash K, Noronha V, Castro A, Licitra L, Adelstein D, Vermorken JB. Weekly Low-Dose Versus Three-Weekly High-Dose Cisplatin for Concurrent Chemoradiation in Locoregionally Advanced Non-Nasopharyngeal Head and Neck Cancer: A Systematic Review and Meta-Analysis of Aggregate Data. Oncologist. 2017 Sep;22(9):1056-1066. doi: 10.1634/theoncologist.2017-0015. Epub 2017 May 22. PMID: 28533474; PMCID: PMC5599190

[23] Naomi Kiyota, Makoto Tahara, Hirofumi Fujii, Tomoko Yamazaki, Hiroki Mitani, ShigemichiIwae, Yasushi Fujimoto, Yusuke Onozawa, NobuhiroHanai, Takenori Ogawa, Hiroki Hara, NobuyaMonden, Eiji Shimura, Shujiro Minami, Takashi Fujii, Kaoru Tanaka, Takeshi Kodaira, JunkiMizusawa, Kenichi Nakamura, Ryuichi Hayashi, and Head and Neck Cancer Study Group of Japan Clinical Oncology Group (JCOG-HNCSG). Phase II/III trial of post-operative chemoradiotherapy comparing 3-weekly cisplatin with weekly cisplatin in high-risk patients with squamous cell carcinoma of head and neck (JCOG1008).Journal of Clinical Oncology 2020 38:15_suppl, 6502-6502

[24] Studer G, Zwahlen RA, Graetz KW, Davis BJ, Glanzmann C. IMRT in oral cavity cancer. Radiat Oncol. 2007;2:16.

[25] Murthy V, Agarwal JP, Laskar SG, Gupta T, Budrukkar A, Pai P, et al. Analysis of prognostic factors in 1180

patients with oral cavity primary cancer treated with definitive or adjuvant radiotherapy. J Cancer Res Ther. 2010;6: 282-9.

[26] Cohen EE, Baru J, Huo D, Haraf DJ, Crowley M, Witt ME, Blair EA, Weichselbaum RR, Rosen F, Vokes EE, Stenson K. Efficacy and safety of treating T4 oral cavity tumors with primary chemoradiotherapy. Head Neck. 2009;31:1013-21

[27] Hosni, Ali et al. "Non-operative management for oral cavity carcinoma: Definitive radiation therapy as a potential alternative treatment approach." Radiotherapy and oncology : journal of the European Society for Therapeutic Radiology and Oncology vol. 154 (2021): 70-75. doi:10.1016/j.radonc.2020.08.013

[28] Lacas B, Bourhis J, Overgaard J, Zhang Q, Grégoire V, Nankivell M, Zackrisson B, Szutkowski Z, Suwiński R, Poulsen M, O'Sullivan B, Corvò R, Laskar SG, Fallai C, Yamazaki H, Dobrowsky W, Cho KH, Beadle B, Langendijk JA, Viegas CMP, Hay J, Lotayef M, Parmar MKB, Aupérin A, van Herpen C, Maingon P, Trotti AM, Grau C, Pignon JP, Blanchard P; MARCH Collaborative Group. Role of radiotherapy fractionation in head and neck cancers (MARCH): an updated meta-analysis. Lancet Oncol. 2017 Sep;18(9):1221-1237. doi: 10.1016/S1470-2045(17)30458-8. Epub 2017 Jul 27. Erratum in: Lancet Oncol. 2018 Apr;19(4):e184. PMID: 28757375; PMCID: PMC5737765.

[29] Bourhis J, Sire C, Graff P, Grégoire V, Maingon P, Calais G, Gery B, Martin L, Alfonsi M, Desprez P, Pignon T, Bardet E, Rives M, Geoffrois L, Daly- Schveitzer N, Sen S, Tuchais C, Dupuis O, Guerif S, Lapeyre M, Favrel V, Hamoir M, Lusinchi A, Temam S, Pinna A, Tao YG, Blanchard P, Aupérin A. Concomitant chemoradiotherapy versus acceleration of radiotherapy with or without concomitant chemotherapy in locally advanced head and neck carcinoma (GORTEC 99-02): an open-label phase 3 randomised trial. Lancet Oncol 2012;13: 145-53

[30] Nguyen-Tan PF, Zhang Q, Ang KK, Weber RS, Rosenthal DI, Soulieres D, Kim H, Silverman C, Raben A, Galloway TJ, Fortin A, Gore E, Westra WH, Chung CH, Jordan RC, Gillison ML, List M, Le QT. Randomized phase III trial to test accelerated versus standard fractionation in combination with concurrent cisplatin for head and neck carcinomas in the Radiation Therapy Oncology Group 0129 trial: long-term report of efficacy and toxicity. J Clin Oncol 2014;32:3858-66.

[31] Ang KK, Trotti A, Brown BW, Garden AS, Foote RL, Morrison WH, Geara FB, Klotch DW, Goepfert H, Peters LJ. Randomized trial addressing risk features and time factors of surgery plus radiotherapy in advanced headand-neck cancer. Int J Radiat Oncol Biol Phys 2001;51:571-8

[32] Huang J, Barbera L, Brouwers M, Browman G, Mackillop WJ. Does delay instarting treatment affect the outcomes of radiotherapy? a systematic review. J Clin Oncol 2003;21:555-63

[33] González Ferreira JA, JaénOlasolo J, Azinovic I, Jeremic B. Effect of radiotherapy delay in overall treatment time on local control andsurvival in head and neck cancer: review of the literature. Rep Pract Oncol Radiother2015;20:328-39.

[34] Graboyes, E.M., Garrett-Mayer, E., Ellis, M.A., Sharma, A.K., Wahlquist, A. E., Lentsch, E.J., Nussenbaum, B. and Day, T.A. (2017), Effect of time to initiation of postoperative radiation therapy on survival in surgically managed head and neck cancer. Cancer, 123: 4841-4850. https://doi.org/10.1002/cncr.30939

[35] Žumer, B., PoharPerme, M., Jereb, S. et al. Impact of delays in radiotherapy of head and neck cancer on outcome. Radiat Oncol **15,** 202 (2020). https://doi.org/10.1186/s13014-020-01645-w

[36] Daly ME, Le QT, Kozak MM, Maxim PG, Murphy JD, Hsu A, Loo BW Jr, Kaplan MJ, Fischbein NJ, Chang DT. Intensity-modulated radiotherapy for oral cavity squamous cell carcinoma: patterns of failure and predictors of local control. Int J Radiat Oncol Biol Phys. 2011 Aug 1;80(5):1412-22. doi: 10.1016/j.ijrobp.2010.04.031. Epub 2010 Aug 2. PMID: 20675073.

[37] Merlotti A, Alterio D, Vigna-Taglianti R, Muraglia A, Lastrucci L, Manzo R, Gambaro G, Caspiani O, Miccichè F, Deodato F, Pergolizzi S, Franco P, Corvò R, Russi EG, Sanguineti G; Italian Association of Radiation Oncology. Technical guidelines for head and neck cancer IMRT on behalf of the Italian association of radiation oncology - head and neck working group. Radiat Oncol. 2014 Dec 29;9:264. doi: 10.1186/s13014-014-0264-9. PMID: 25544268; PMCID: PMC4316652

[38] Basu T, Laskar SG, Gupta T, Budrukkar A, Murthy V, Agarwal JP. Toxicity with radiotherapy for oral cancers and its management: a practical approach. J Cancer Res Ther. 2012 Jan;8 Suppl1:S72-84. doi: 10.4103/0973-1482.92219. PMID: 22322736.

[39] Nutting CM, Morden JP, Harrington KJ, Urbano TG, Bhide SA, Clark C, et al. Parotid-sparing intensity modulated versus conventional radiotherapy in head and neck cancer (PARSPORT): A phase 3 multicentre randomised controlled trial. Lancet Oncol 2011;12:127-36

[40] Bhide SA, Ahmed M, Newbold K, Harrington KJ, Nutting CM. The role of intensity modulated radiotherapy in advanced oral cavity carcinoma. J Cancer Res Ther. 2012;8 Suppl1:S67-71.

[41] Eisbruch AH, Garden A, et al. Phase II Multi-institutional Study of IMRT for Oropharyngeal Cancer (RTOG 00-22): Int J Radiat Oncol Biol Phys 2006;66 Supplement.

[42] Chen WC, Hwang TZ, Wang WH, Lu CH, Chen CC, Chen CM, et al. Comparison between conventional and intensity-modulated post-operative radiotherapy for stage III and IV oral cavity cancer in terms of treatment results and toxicity. Oral Oncol. 2009; 45:505-10

[43] Huang SF, Cheng SD, Chien HT, Liao CT, Chen IH, Wang HM, et al. Relationship between epidermal growth factor receptor gene copy number and protein expression in oral cavity squamous cell carcinoma. Oral Oncol. 2012;48:67-72

[44] Bonner, J.A.; Harari, P.M.; Giralt, J.; Azarnia, N.; Shin, D.M.; Cohen, R.B.; Jones, C.U.; Sur, R.; Raben, D.; Jassem, J.; et al. Radiotherapy plus cetuximab for squamous-cell carcinoma of the head and neck. N. Engl. J. Med. 2006, 354, 567–578

[45] Muzaffar J, Bari S, Kirtane K, Chung CH. Recent Advances and Future Directions in Clinical Management of Head and Neck Squamous Cell Carcinoma. Cancers (Basel). 2021 Jan 18;13(2):338. doi: 10.3390/cancers13020338. PMID: 33477635; PMCID: PMC7831487.

[46] Herbst, R.S.; Soria, J.C.; Kowanetz, M.; Fine, G.D.; Hamid, O.; Gordon, M. S.; Sosman, J.A.; McDermott, D.F.; Powderly, J.D.; Gettinger, S.N.; et al. Predictive correlates of response to the anti-PD-L1 antibody MPDL3280A in cancer patients. Nature 2014, 515, 563

[47] Twyman-Saint Victor C, Rech AJ, Maity A, Rengan R, Pauken KE, Stelekati E, et al. Radiation and dual checkpoint blockade activate nonredundantimmune mechanisms in

cancer. Nature (2015) 520:373–7.doi: 10.1038/nature14292

[48] Kirtane K, Rodriguez CP. Postoperative Combined Modality Treatment in High Risk Resected Locally Advanced Squamous Cell Carcinomas of the Head and Neck (HNSCC). Front Oncol. 2018 Dec 4;8: 588. doi: 10.3389/fonc.2018.00588. PMID: 30564559; PMCID: PMC6288294.

[49] Seiwert, T.Y.; Burtness, B.; Mehra, R.; Weiss, J.; Berger, R.; Eder, J.P.; Heath, K.; McClanahan, T.; Lunceford, J.; Gause, C.; et al. Safety and clinical activity of pembrolizumab for treatment of recurrent or metastatic squamous cell carcinoma of the head and neck (KEYNOTE-012): An open-label, multicentre, phase 1b trial. Lancet Oncol. 2016, 17, 956–965

[50] Pierce, C.M.; Hogue, S.; Paul, S.; Hong, B.Y.; da Silva, W.V.; Gomez, M. F.; Giuliano, A.R.; Caudell, J.J.; Weinstock, G.M. Abstract 3326: Mucositis, candidiasis, and associations with the oral microbiome in treatment naive patients with oropharyngeal cancer. Cancer Res. 2019, 79

[51] Ohtani, T.; Yamada, Y.; Furuhashi, A.; Ohmura, Y.; Nakamura, S.; Kato, H.; Yoshikawa, K.; Kazaoka, Y. Activated cytotoxic T-lymphocyte immunotherapy is effective for advanced oral and maxillofacial cancers. Int. J. Oncol. 2014, 45, 2051–2057

[52] Mazeron JJ, Ardiet JM, Haie-Méder C, Kovács G, Levendag P, Peiffert D, Polo A, Rovirosa A, Strnad V. GEC-ESTRO recommendations for brachytherapy for head and neck squamous cell carcinomas. Radiother Oncol 2009;91:150-6

[53] Nag S, Cano ER, Demanes DJ, Puthawala AA, Vikram B; American Brachytherapy Society. The American Brachytherapy Society recommendations for high-dose-rate brachytherapy for head-and-neck carcinoma. Int J Radiat Oncol Biol Phys 2001;50:1190-8

Medicine in the frail elderly

Medicine in the frail elderly

A problem-oriented approach

Roy A Fox
Division of Geriatric Medicine, Camp Hill Medical Centre, Dalhousie University, Halifax, Nova Scotia, Canada

and

John A H Puxty
St. Mary's of the Lake Hospital and Queen's University, Kingston, Ontario, Canada

Edward Arnold
A division of Hodder & Stoughton
LONDON BOSTON MELBOURNE AUCKLAND

First published in Great Britain 1993

Distributed in the Americas by Little, Brown and Company
34 Beacon Street, Boston, MA 02108

British Library Cataloguing in Publication Data

Fox, Roy A.
Medicine in the Frail Elderly:
Problem-oriented Approach
I. Title II. Puxty, John
618.97

ISBN 0–7131–4564–1

Whilst the advice and information in this book is believed to be true and accurate at the date of going to press, neither the author nor the publisher can accept any legal responsibility or liability for any errors or omissions that may be made. In particular (but without limiting the generality of the preceding disclaimer) every effort has been made to check drug dosages; however, it is still possible that errors have been missed. Furthermore, dosage schedules are constantly being revised and new side effects recognized. For these reasons the reader is strongly urged to consult the drug companies' printed instructions before administering any of the drugs recommended in this book.

Typeset in 10/11pt Baskerville by Anneset. Printed and bound in Great Britain for Edward Arnold, a division of Hodder and Stoughton Limited, Mill Road, Dunton Green, Sevenoaks, Kent TN13 2YA by St Edmundsbury Press, Bury St Edmunds, Suffolk and Hunter & Foulis Ltd., Edinburgh.

Preface

One of the most rewarding aspects of the practice of geriatric medicine is to see frail, ill patients get better and reach a level of health or wellness that they thought was unattainable. When first entering this field we asked ourselves 'How is this done?'. As we watched our colleagues at work we realised that a great deal was being achieved by treating the whole patient and paying attention to all the problems. Demoralised patients unable to cooperate in rehabilitation were quietly transformed into therapeutic successes as their unmet needs were managed. The main approach to teaching the skills necessary for such therapy was the master/apprentice model and practice approaches were transferred by 'osmosis'.

It appeared to us difficult to conceptualize therapeutic strategies and the complexity of the patients always proved intimidating to students and learners at all stages. Geriatric medicine like other disciplines and specialities can be easily taught, and the vision of this therapeutic strategy can be handed on to quite junior inexperienced students. The key rests in pattern recognition and identifying a common approach to many functional problems. Students at all levels need to be able to handle information overload, to sort it and to develop a therapeutic approach that all members of the team can handle. As we thought of this further we realised that the only rational approach was to identify each problem and to adopt the problem oriented approach put forward by Lawrence Weed. However this would need to be altered to accommodate the frail elderly.

Out of these thoughts this book was born. We have attempted to deal with the common geriatric problems of dysfunction in the first chapters of the book. There are many pathophysiological problems that can give rise to such dysfunction and these are dealt with in the later chapters. As we progress through the book we move to higher levels of definition from the pathophysiological to the etiological.

The book is not modelled on conventional textbooks of medicine and there are not exhaustive reference lists. We have tried to outline approaches to problems. Each patient represents a unique challenge often with problems that have not been met before. If the patients has inflammatory bowel disease as part of their illness then information can be gathered from standard textbooks and treatment will only need to be modified in so far as there are other interacting pathological and functional problems. We have tried to capture the uniqueness of geriatric medicine and to conceptualize the approach so that it can be taught. The book has been several years in the process of being written since the early discussions in Hope Hospital, Salford, and many things have changed in our lives. However we feel that we have achieved much of what we set out to do and hope that you will gain new knowledge that will help you in your management of ill frail elders, and that all will find the paths to wellness challenging and rewarding.

Contents

List of Contributors

William H. Barker, Department of Community and Preventive Medicine, University of Rochester Medical Center, Rochester, New York, USA
Geriatrics internationally

David B. Hogan, Division of Geriatric Medicine, Foothills Hospital, Calgary, Alberta, Canada
Medical education and geriatrics

Michael A. Horan, Department of Geriatric Medicine, Withington Hospital, Manchester, UK
Abnormalities of water, sodium and potassium; abnormalities of pH; abnormalities of serum calcium; drug prescribing and iatrogenic disease in the elderly

Graham P. Mulley, Department of Medicine for the Elderly, St James's University Hospital, Leeds, UK
Rehabilitation of the elderly

D. Gwyn Seymour, Senior Lecturer in Geriatric Medicine, University of Wales College of Medicine, Cardiff, UK
The elderly surgical patient

Ruth M. Seymour, Senior Registrar in Geriatric Medicine, University of Wales College of Medicine, Cardiff, UK
The elderly surgical patient

1

Geriatrics and the problem solving approach

Geriatrics is the study of the medical aspects of old age and the application of knowledge related to the biological, biomedical, behavioral and social aspects of aging, to prevention, diagnosis, treatment and care of older persons. Within the field of geriatrics are two medical specialties, namely geriatric medicine and geriatric psychiatry. In this book we deal with a problem orientated approach to geriatric medicine.

Geriatric medicine has often been defined as an age described specialty, like pediatrics, dealing with the problems of all those over a certain age. Chronological age has been arbitrarily set at 65 by most, but by others as 60 for females and 65 for males. There are however a number of limitations to a purely age-related approach. The majority of seniors, especially the 'young-elderly', are healthy and when they become ill can be well cared for within traditional internal medical units. The specialty of geriatric medicine is better utilized if targeted towards those with multiple, complex, interacting problems brought on by disease or aging, resulting in disability, functional impairment and dependency. Such patients are not simply old but are complex because of the interacting psychosocial and physical problems. This group is often referred to as the frail elderly.

This book has come about because of our awareness of challenges in helping such patients, and in an attempt to assist practitioners of this emerging discipline. We present an approach to geriatric medicine wherein the patient's problems are identified so that predisposing and precipitating factors can be identified for which there are treatments and solutions. We suggest logical pathways from presentation through to successful management.

1. Presentation of illness in old age

It is important to remember that disease or illness in the elderly can present in the same way as in younger age groups (Table 1.1). The patient has the typical signs or symptoms of single system disease. For the most part such patients do not need a specialist geriatric approach. However the very old although presenting initially with a single system problem, are extremely susceptible to iatrogenic disease from a variety of sources including: polypharmacy, inactivity, failure to adopt preventive and restorative rehabilitation principles. For this reason a geriatric consultation may become desirable with advice and assistance in the prevention and management of important complications like loss of mobility, decubiti, incontinence of urine with catheterization, fecal loading and impaction, and inappropriate fostering of dependency.

Table 1.1 Presentation of illness in old age

1. Typical (classical symptoms and signs) – usually single system disease
2. Atypical or geriatric presentation:
   decompensation with onset of one or more of the major geriatric problems
   - confusion, memory failure, psychosis
   - postural instability and falling
   - immobility
   - incontinence of urine
   - fecal loading, impaction and incontinence
   - social crisis
3. Silent presentation
   diagnosed very late or at autopsy
4. Pseudosilent or missed presentation
   manifestation of ageism

The pathophysiological changes of aging modify the *milieu interieur* and the body's reaction to disease. Age changes usually manifest themselves as degenerative conditions, and people vary in the degree and type of infirmity that may develop. In fact one important characteristic of aging is the increased diversity of presentation and reaction to stress. Coupled with this increased diversity is the other major characteristic of aging, namely the loss of functional reserve of organs and systems (Fig. 1.1). The reduced functional reserve may be asymptomatic during health and normal lifestyle activities, but the onset of acute illness produces additional stress with symptomatic decompensation of several organs and systems. Thus pneumonia may precipitate cardiac failure and renal failure in a predisposed elderly individual.

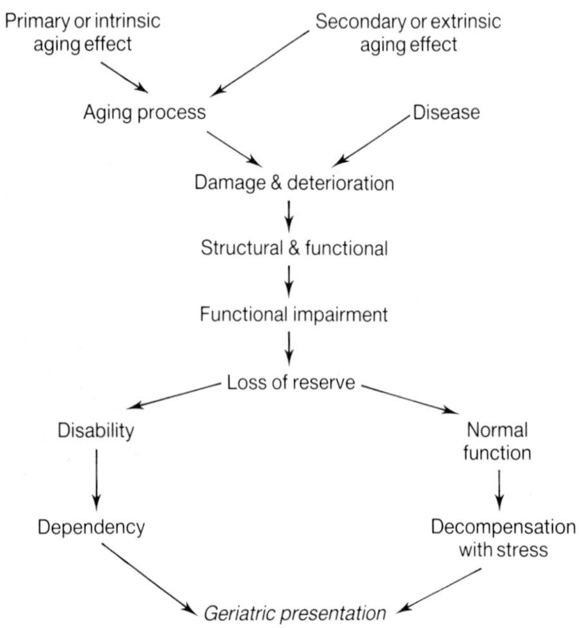

Fig. 1.1 Loss of reserve with advancing age.

Pathophysiological changes which occur with aging therefore are likely to modify the presentation of disease which needs to be recognized in order to ensure appropriate assessment and treatment. This is particularly common when preexisting disability and dependency are present. Co-existing chronic diseases are also not uncommonly present and complicate the picture. The onset of a new illness or additional problem, may not be associated with the typical signs and symptoms of that particular problem and there is in fact a masking of the features ('the atypical presentation'). The exact reasons for the loss of acuity are not fully understood but are related to changes in homeostatic mechanisms, the waning inflammatory response, decreases in visceral sensation and the decreased pain appreciation which have been recorded with aging. The phenomena of acute disease being masked but precipitating functional impairment in other areas, is a common feature of patients seen within a geriatric program (Fig. 1.2). A problem such as peritonitis may thus present with minimal abdominal pain and tenderness but other features such as delirium, falls and incontinence may be prominent.

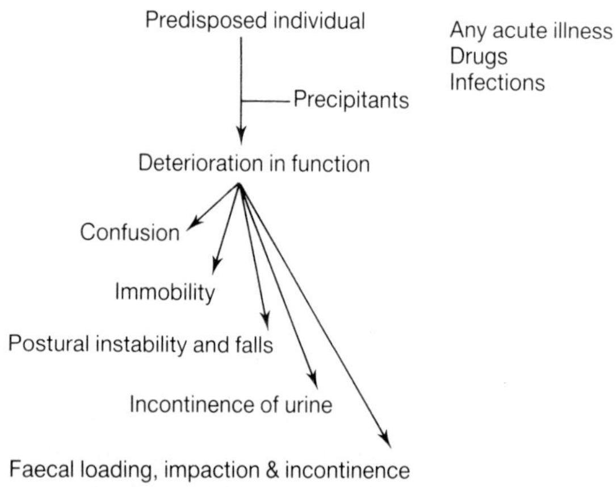

Fig. 1.2 Geriatric presentation.

The common geriatric presentations include:

- Confusion
- Loss of Mobility (confinement to a chair or bed)
- Postural Instability with Falls
- Incontinence of Urine
- Bowel Dysfunction with Loading
- Impaction or Incontinence
- Social Crisis.

Thus the onset of confusion and incontinence of urine may well be the first signs of illness and disease in areas remote from the geriatric 'problem'. These features indicate that the patient is ill and that in addition to management of these problems there is a need for a careful assessment aimed at identifying significant and treatable precipitating factors.

The functionally impaired or disabled elderly patient is often dependent upon others for various aspects of their care. When the 'geriatric presentation' occurs there is usually an increase in dependency. For example, much more care is required for the immobile or incontinent patient, or for the mildly forgetful who now is awake disturbing the household throughout the night. The apparent reason for bringing the patient to the attention of the physician is a 'social crisis'. The care providers finding the increased demands for care an unacceptable strain and seek help. Thus the social crisis that is often present is in fact related to care provider strain or sometimes to the absence of an appropriate care provider. It is inappropriate therefore to use terms such as 'social problem' or 'social admission' in this situation. These terms are prejudicial and do not encourage a careful diagnostic approach to identify remedial conditions which are often present.

The challenge to the physician when presented with a 'geriatric presentation' is therefore considerable. An essential component of the response is the recognition of the need for careful assessment looking for remedial components and avoidance of premature 'labelling'. When dealing with confusion and memory failure it is of course imperative to obtain the history from a third party. This should be done for most patients since many elderly patients tend to underplay their problems.

It is important to remember that there is usually more than one pathological process present at any time. Although the apparent problem may be related to a single disease entity, recovery and treatment are often modified by other diseases. There is often a delicate balance between health and disease. The equilibrium is easily disturbed which makes iatrogenic disease common. The physician needs to assess the whole patient. Predisposing and precipitating factors need to be identified, diagnoses made and treatments instituted.

When the symptoms and signs are extensively dampened down then presentation as an 'acute illness' may not occur and the diagnoses made only by chance. This is referred to as a silent presentation. This is quite common and missed diagnoses, made at autopsy, appear to increase with age.

Finally, diagnoses may be missed because the physician does not enter into a diagnostic approach. The patient's ailments and change in status are falsely attributed to aging or social problems. Legitimate concerns are disregarded and problems that need medical treatment are responded to with social measures, such as referral for institutional care. This is often a reflection of ageism and is referred to as a pseudo-silent or missed presentation.

2. Predisposing factors

In each of the chapters on the major geriatric problems the predisposing age changes, due to aging effects or disease, will be discussed. It is important to understand predisposing changes since they may be modifiable and further deterioration may be prevented. When specific diseases are identified early on in their course it is obvious that treatment may be instituted with the idea of preventing irreversible damage. This is also true for the aging effects – if these are found to be secondary, then it might be possible to modify the external factors and prevent the change. Although in individual patients it might not be possible to change the damage that has already occurred, this might be important in prevention for other individuals.

Aging affects everyone and all parts of the human body. However there is a great deal of variation between different tissues in the same body, and there is great variation between different individuals. Whatever 'aging' is due to, the term has been used to describe the wide array of processes of accruing maturity with the passage of time. One of the best definitions is that of Makinodan, 'aging is an age dependent process that finally results in an impaired capacity of the intact organism to respond to external stimuli, which is associated with an increased mortality rate'. These changes occur after sexual maturation is complete and form the basis of the progressive decline in the efficiency of homeostasis and the increased probability that a reaction to injury of various types will not be successful, leading to acute and chronic illness and an increase in the probability of death over a given period of time.

3. Precipitating factors

The individual who is predisposed to one or more of the common geriatric problems because of the changes of aging or disease, may well function adequately for a long period of time. Although there is loss of reserve, function remains adequate when the stress is low. Failure or decompensation occurs when there is additional stress. Failure can be precipitated by many things, but in the setting of the failing elderly patient, the two most common precipitants are drugs and infections (Fig. 1.2). For example, the 85 year-old patient is doing well at home, although she needs some help with excursions outside the home for grocery shopping and some assistance with house cleaning. The level of care required goes up when the patient becomes incontinent and confused. Careful inquiry reveals that this has been precipitated by the use of a potent diuretic – frusemide.

Although drugs and infections are the most common precipitants there are many others, in fact we conclude that the list is nigh infinite. It is of little value for the physician to have a checklist or a mnemonic as an *aide-mémoire*. Using this approach identification of precipitants will be lacking and important diseases missed. Omission is minimized by the use of a logical approach with a comprehensive assessment.

It should be clear that precipitants include acute diseases, iatrogenic causes, metabolic disturbances and psychiatric illnesses. The physician is consulted to identify the precipitants with a view to modifying by specific treatment. This is the major role of the physician in the health care team for geriatric assessment. When a problem is identified, establishing an etiological diagnosis (or sometimes a pathophysiological diagnosis) is in effect identifying the precipitant.

As diagnosis is being pursued some problems will need to be treated. The problems with impaired function will need to be managed immediately, and in the very old this may take on a preventive aspect. For example dealing with poor mobility by the use of physiotherapy – in many instances this may be reconditioning but for some this is preventing deconditioning whilst other problems are being dealt with. Full identification of the precipitants or in other words diagnosis may not be achieved before treatment of the other interacting problems is started.

4. Diagnostic approach

The taking of a history and a careful physical examination allows the development of a problem list. It has been noted that in old age the manifestations of acute illness may be attenuated, therefore the initial assessment of a patient presenting with any of the geriatric problems would not be considered complete without certain investigations. The results of these tests expand the data base. All patients should have a complete (full) blood count and measurement of erythrocyte sedimentation rate (ESR). A standard biochemical profile would include electrolytes, urea, creatinine, calcium, phosphorus, uric acid, total protein, albumin, glucose, bilirubin, alkaline phosphatase, gamma glutamyl transpeptidase (or another enzyme or isoenzyme to determine site of origin of alkaline phosphatase), lactate dehydrogenase and a transaminase (aminotransferase). Thyroid function (serum T4 and TSH) should be routine. The measurement of serum B12 and folate should be done only if there is an indication from the data base. A clean specimen of urine is required for analysis as well as for microscopy and culture. Chest radiograph is often helpful and should be mandatory.

With this data base a problem list is generated and it is the rule that patients in geriatric practice have multiple problems. Successful treatment of some of the problems commonly leads to eradication of others. Several management plans may be pursued at the same time and although the major geriatric problems of impaired function will need to be identified, all may not need further investigation. For example, confusion may lift with treatment of the cardiac or respiratory failure or urinary incontinence may be transient and clear with eradication of the fecal loading. If such problems of dysfunction persist then further investigation and treatment is indicated. It is important therefore to keep a problem list under active review.

Although the objective is to make as accurate an assessment as possible, unnecessary investigation should be avoided. It needs to be remembered that with multiple pathology and with multiple degenerative conditions that there is often no shortage of physical signs. There may be features which mislead, some of these are known and will be discussed in the appropriate chapters. The clinician needs to be able to recognize the normative changes of aging, and therefore non-diagnostic, as well as the signs of disease.

Clinical pointers will allow the logical use of further investigations. These patients frequently need access to high technology medicine for investigation and treatment. This is one of the reasons why assessment units are best located in modern acute hospitals. Iatrogenic problems are kept to a minimum by restricting checklists and pursuing logical investigational pathways. Accurate diagnosis encourages correct management of major problems. The result is less dependency, less iatrogenic disease, earlier discharge from hospital and reduced readmission rate.

5. Assessment

The recognition that elderly patients have different problems to younger patients and that their care is often much more complex has been long in coming. The health care systems in most developed countries have not been designed to deal with these problems. In this chapter we have stressed an approach to the elderly patient where all the problems are identified, because all may need to be addressed. Failure to attend to the whole patient and his or her needs has resulted in inappropriate care – a social response to medical problems, with resulting high rates of institutionalization; or responding medically to what are in fact psychosocial problems.

To deal with this complexity of health care problems health professionals need to collect and organize a variety of clinically relevant information. This process is referred to as the comprehensive geriatric assessment. It usually implies a multidimensional evaluation to demonstrate a variety of problems and disabilities which have to be put into the context of available social networks. The results of such assessments are then used to generate coordinated care plans which attempt to focus relevant interventions. Comprehensive geriatric assessment usually includes evaluations of the mental, physical, functional, social, and economic status.

Each individual professional discipline brings its own orientation and perceptions to the method of assessment, interpretation, and treatment of problems. Collaboration is necessary when two or more health professional are involved in common assessment and therapeutic manoeuvres. Mechanisms must exist for sharing of information, mutual common interpretation and consensus of responses. The reality of the complexity and chronicity of the problems often implies a need for re-evaluation. A team mechanism therefore often becomes necessary to facilitate the process of communication and coordination.

The geriatric team

A variety of team models may exist, each may have its own merits in different situations. The intradisciplinary approach reflects the subspecialization within a discipline. The generalist seeks advice regarding a component of the care process. The interaction may not be comprehensive or prolonged, indeed the individuals may function independently approaching the issue from their own perspective and addressing care within the context of their own speciality.

A multidisciplinary approach necessarily implies that participants come from different professions or disciplines. Individuals conduct assessments and interpretation independently, develop care regimens and evaluate outcomes from the perspective of their discipline. Communication occurs but it remains within their professional boundaries. The approach has the merit of recognizing the complex, multidimensional nature of illness in the elderly and enabling multiple skills to be utilized in resolving them. Inherent in the approach is the potential for duplication of effort, possibility of diverse contradictory approaches and potential for conflict.

The interdisciplinary approach differs in the multidisciplinary in the extent of interaction of the professional disciplines. The team work on common problems, communicating freely and bringing their pooled expertise to resolving the issue. Cross referral and type and extent of direct involvement is based on the patients problem profile not from administrative need. Necessarily the team must achieve consensus on individual roles, assessment interpretations, problem definition and goals of further assessments and treatments.

The transdisciplinary approach implies a system where no firm boundaries exist between the disciplines where knowledge and skills are truly synthesized.

The different models of team working may each have applications to health care responses towards the elderly. A transdisciplinary team approach would be appropriate for a first-contact where a multidimensional screening assessment might be desired for the purpose of problem identification and triage. Individuals may within the same team function in an interdisciplinary manner by cross-referring to each other in specific instances. Referrals from the screening team may be made to services utilizing a multidisciplinary/interdisciplinary approach where although common goals are established, specific discipline assessment and treatment skills may be indicated. The results of such assessment within a discipline may indicate the need for more refined assessment resulting in an intradisciplinary referral. The assessment of the elderly therefore often requires the use of a hierarchial approach of different team models if service uses are to be rationalized.

Members of the geriatric team

The physicians involved as nucleus or core members of the team are the patient's family physician (general practitioner) and the specialist geriatrician. For medicolegal reasons in most places the physician is responsible for the patient, for admitting and discharge and supervision of treatment. For these reasons the leadership role commonly rests with the physician, although in the setting of the team conference, the chairmanship or facilitator role can be taken up by other members. The family physician can make important contributions with continuity of care of the patient. In many instances, however, there are barriers in terms of time commitment, remuneration and formal training. Thus the leadership role usually rests with the geriatrician or at least with the physician who is working full-time with the team.

The other members of the team may be considered in three ways

1. the nucleus or core group
2. the support group
3. the consultation group (Table 1.2)

The different team members commonly change from one group to another depending upon the nature of the patient's problems. However, when resources are scarce and when programs are developing the core members are essential for a viable program to develop. It is our experience that assessment teams tend to rapidly become busy and the escalating workload tends to overload the members. Most teams function in a multidisciplinary manner but with good communication and understanding of each disciplines roles a more interdisciplinary model tends to develop where team members assessments and roles blend and overlap. The common nucleus or core discipline's in addition to medicine are nursing, physiotherapy, occupational therapy and social work. Each discipline will need to perform their own assessment but with the use of common assessment tools unnecessary duplication can be avoided and time saved. All disciplines contribute to the master problem list kept at the front of the chart.

Table 1.2 The assessment team

1. *Nucleus/core disciplines*	
Medicine:	Geriatric medical specialist
Nursing:	Nurses at different levels within various in-patient units, day hospital and ambulatory care, nurse specialists, liaison nurses, community nurses
Physiotherapy	
Occupational therapy	
Social work	
2. *Support disciplines*	
Medicine:	Family physician, psychiatrist
Dietary	
Psychology	Neuropsychological and behavioural
Pharmacy	
Speech therapy	(pathology)
Pastoral care	
Chiropody (podiatry)	
Recreational therapy	(recreology)
3. *Other disciplines available for consultation*	
Medicine:	*All sub-specialties usually available within acute care hospital*
Dentistry	

The nursing role varies with the site whether it be an in-patient unit, a geriatric day hospital, institutional consult or at home. In most of these settings the nurse will be responsible for day-to-day care, ensuring that treatment is given and monitoring activities of daily living. The emphasis being to ensure that the environment is safe and conducive to enabling the patient to do as much as possible for themselves. The essential communication link between the nurse and rehabilitation therapists ensures continuation of a consistent rehabilitative approach throughout the 24-hour period (see Chapter 33). Assessment is a vital component of the nursing role and normally adopts a holistic approach including measures of mood, cognition, functional abilities, nutrition, skin integrity, bowel and bladder function, social networks and general well-being. It is important to recognize that the nurse has wide-ranging responsibilities in the overall care of the patient and their role in the team is not to simply focus on 'bowels and bladders'.

Restoring mobility with improvements in function, endurance and independence are major roles of physiotherapy. Assessment is a crucial part of their activity and will build upon data from the medical and nursing assessments. This will include an emphasis on the locomotor system, neurological and cardiopulmonary status in relation to functional ability. Not uncommonly further medical assessments will be indicated as a result of the physiotherapists findings. The use of physical techniques to reduce pain are invaluable in permitting more effective restorative rehabilitation. The physiotherapist will set guide lines for the patients daily routines in terms of: range of joint movements; exercise programs to restore and maintain strength and endurance; safe routines for transfers and ambulation; and appropriate use of walking aids.

Occupational therapy has a number of roles including; assessments and training in activities of daily living, assessment and training in sensorimotor activities, design and modification of aids and adaptations to facilitate independence, fabrication and application of splints and braces, developing individual and group psychosocial intervention and promoting therapeutic activities in the form of crafts and games. The occupational therapist will often carry out a home visit to assess the environment and any need for modification, and this may well include a kitchen assessment to determine safety and adequacy of meal preparation.

The roles of physiotherapy and occupational therapy may overlap, particularly when it comes to improving the function of the individual to rise from the sitting position, to transfer, ambulate and carry out self-care activities. In this situation the two often work together to the benefit of the patient, by increasing the time period of rehabilitation and ensuring a consistency of approach.

The social worker gathers information that is important in understanding the patient within their previous social and environmental backgrounds. Such information is invaluable in deriving effective solutions. It will often clarify the minimal requirements of the family care providers – what level of function can they cope with, what supports can they access, and at what stage institutionalization may need to be considered? As the patient is completing assessment and rehabilitation the social worker maintains a current appreciation of the social support network status. Final recommendation regarding care support structures and possible need for long term care must await the patient attaining optimal function. Early decisions are often incorrect and inhumane and result in excessive demands for care including institutionalization.

The social worker, with other members of the team may also assist the patient and the family in coping with the profound changes that are occurring or that have already taken place, helping them with the losses that they experience. Counselling of the client, family and other care givers are important roles.

The nucleus or core members meet together on a regular basis to ensure that all members of the team are informed of the details of assessment, to develop and update goals and specific treatment plans that can be followed by all members of the team. In the case of nursing it is usually only possible for two or three members to be present at the conference. Those present need to document the discussion and ensure that decisions and treatment plans are accurately communicated to the other nurses involved in care. Depending upon the size of the unit, team conferences may not be completed in one sitting. Conferences are necessary for the following functions:

1. to ensure a smooth system of communication between the disciplines
2. to correlate the individual assessments and to formulate plans
3. to monitor progress
4. to make discharge plans
5. to ensure a team feeling of participation.

Discussion should be patient focused and a convenient way of ensuring this is to work from the master problem list. During the initial conference the master problem list is agreed upon, each problem can then be followed at subsequent conferences. Problems are usually a mixture of diagnoses and functional disabilities or handicaps. In many instances all members of the team contribute to discussion on the various problems being defined. For example, as the problem of falls is increasingly defined, predisposing and precipitating factors are identified such as aspiration pneumonia (physician), orthostatic hypotension (nurse), foot drop (physiotherapist), environmental hazards (occupational therapist), and poor illumination due to financial distress (social worker).

Our own personal experience of assessment units indicates that the physicians, nurses and social workers are involved in all patients. Physiotherapists in 90 per cent, and occupational therapists in 75 per cent.

As suggested above there are a number of key disciplines which provide a support group to the geriatric team. They will commonly attend group conference and play supportive roles in the form of information resources, participation in problem resolution discussions and may carry out second-level assessments when indicated. Based on our own experiences they will be actively involved in assessments in about a third of cases. They include psychiatrist and psychologist (30–40 per cent), speech therapy (10–12 per cent), dietary (40 per cent) and pharmacy (25 per cent). Other disciplines are variable and depend upon the availability.

The assessment site

Geriatric assessment is a process that can take a variable length of time to complete depending upon the nature of the patient's problems. In the context of geriatric practice the process begins with the initial consultation and determination of the problems that need treatment and ending with the patient attaining a plateau of optimal function. The assessment is multidimensional involving a team of health care professionals.

The initial consultation, or contact with the physician can occur in various places – the patient's home, a nursing home, a hospital ward or the doctor's office (Fig. 1.3). The site being determined by the needs of the patient. It has been claimed that all patients should be seen in their own home prior to admission. This is clearly not practical in most circumstances. There is little objective data to support the claims that it is beneficial to management or that it improves outcome. Home consultation should be done for the benefit of the patient when it is clearly impossible for the patient to access a doctor's office or hospital. Home visits do provide valuable information which help in the assessment of the patient. However such information can be obtained from care providers and family members by various members of the assessment team. Home visits are often essential when decisions are being made about when to return home and when environmental changes are indicated to make this possible.

At the time of this consultation, particularly within the hospital setting, information may be available from other health professionals such as nursing, physiotherapy and occupational therapy. In this situation the geriatrician needs to determine if the patient is at optimal function or if there is the need for further treatment. Recommendations may be made on the available evidence if it is concluded that there is no potential for further improvement. Recommendations may include living arrangements on discharge, nursing home or home with social supports, or even further investigations and treatment before discharge. When seen in a hospital setting it is often possible to influence management without needing to transfer.

If it is determined that the patient is functionally impaired and has the potential for further treatment and rehabilitation, and that this cannot be done at the present site then the patient will need to be admitted to a geriatric program. Such a decision indicates the need for a full assessment and a trial of treatment. The most accomplished geriatrician cannot determine the true potential of patients for rehabilitation with one hundred per cent accuracy. One of the purposes of more complete assessment is to determine the impact of a full rehabilitation and treatment program. This implies that some patients inevitably fail to live up to expectations and continue to function at a lower level than thought at first. It is for this reason that an appropriate exit route from the assessment program is considered and that contingency plans are available for the worst scenario.

For full assessment by a geriatric team there are two major sites that are available – the geriatric day hospital and the geriatric inpatient assessment unit. In both such sites there will be a full team of health professionals. The major factors that determine which is the appropriate site are the degree of functional impairment, the extent of the support network within the community and the accessibility of the service to the patient. Accessibility and transportation are the common determinants of whether the day hospital is a practical option. Otherwise patients need to be admitted to the inpatient unit.

Geriatric assessment units (GAU) are often within an acute care hospital, with access to diagnostic and therapeutic facilities and the availability of consultants in the different medical disciplines. Although such units have been located in geriatric hospitals and isolated buildings this is much less desirable. Studies have shown that such units are less efficient with longer lengths of stay.

The patient (targeting)

Patients admitted to a GAU have an average age of about 80 years, have multiple problems and only the minority (<10 per cent) have no evidence of functional impairment. The majority (>50 per cent) have moderate to severe functional impairment. Patients have varying degrees of acuity and a mortality rate of between 8 and 14 per cent is usual.

There have been various attempts to define the

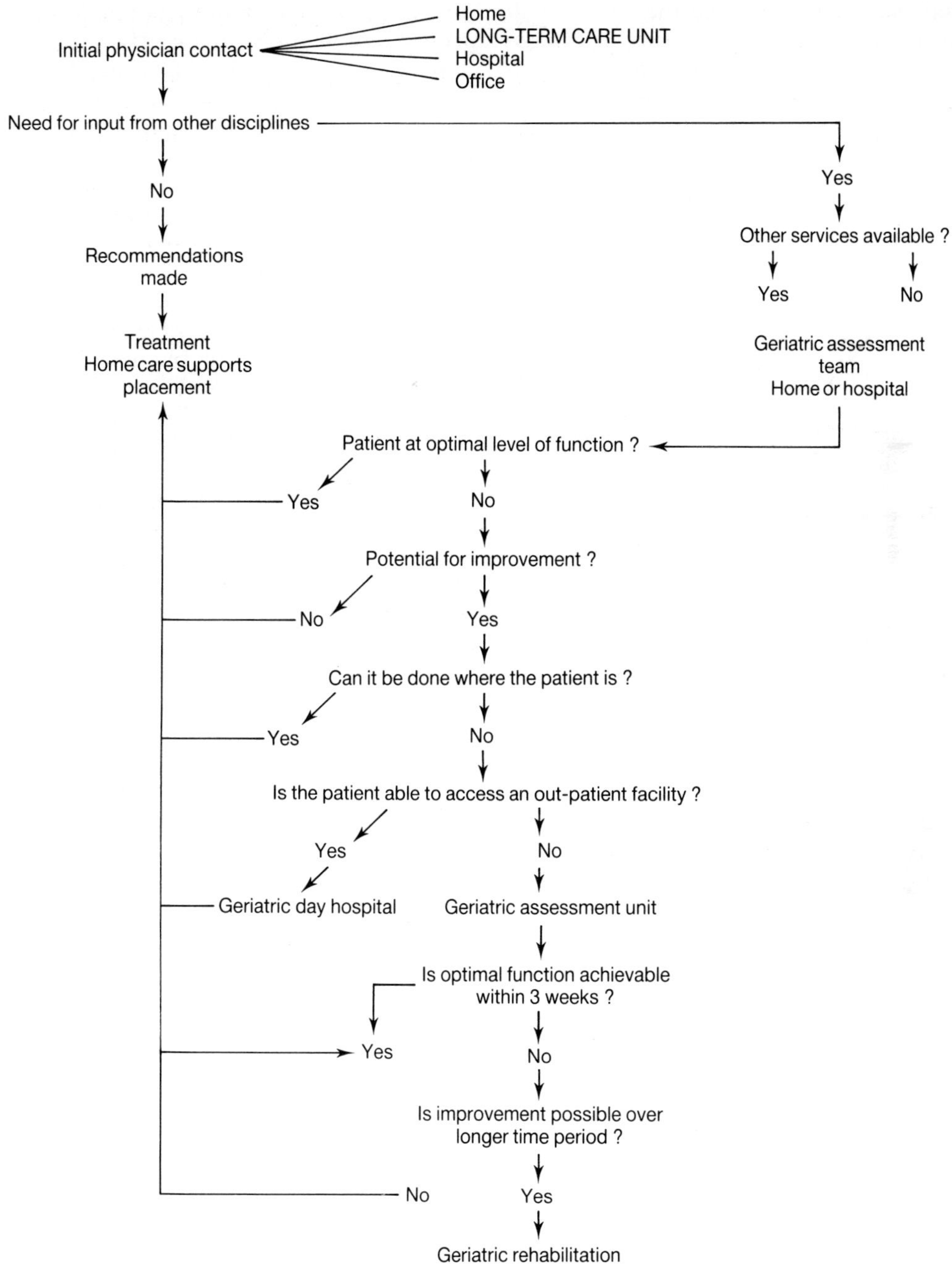

Fig. 1.3 The process of assessment.

patients that are appropriate for a geriatric service. Chronological age does not define the patient that needs geriatric medical expertise. By using age the impact of geriatric care upon those that need it is diminished, there is also the probability that the care of the young old with single system disease is less than optimal. Geriatric care needs to be targeted towards those who are functionally impaired, and those who as a result of aging have diminished reserve and therefore the potential for further deterioration and functional impairment as a result of hospitalization (Table 1.3). Patients in categories 3 and 4 have been shown to benefit from geriatric intervention in the acute care hospital setting. These are the patients in whom it is most likely to demonstrate benefit from geriatric assessment and rehabilitation.

Patients in group 2 may have functional impairment in one major system in an area that requires geriatric expertise but are unlikely to require full geriatric assessment. However, patients in groups 2 may require some intervention in hospital by a geriatric team under certain circumstances. The extremely old confined to bed may be precipitated into immobility, postural instability and falling. New surroundings and medications may precipitate confusion. Loss of mobility may precipitate incontinence of urine. Fecal loading may result from immobility and medications. Hospital admission leads to infection and precipitation of the various functional problems already outlined. With advancing age iatrogenic or nurisgenic problems become more likely. It is for these reasons that the very old may require input from a geriatric assessment team with expertise in dealing with these problems and the knowledge to prevent their progression.

Table 1.3 Geriatric functional status scale

1. *Healthy*
   Independent function – no evidence of functional impairment. No problems with mobility, ADL or elimination.
   Scores >8 on MSQ
2. *Mild impairment of function*
   Problems with distance, Architectural Barriers
   Independent in ADL
   Incontinence only rarely (<1 per day)
   MSQ 7–8
3. *Moderate impairment* (one or more)
   Mobility – uses walker or wheelchair and/or is housebound
   ADL – utilizes mechanical aid
   Incontinence – 1 day
   MSQ 5–6
4. *Moderately severe* (one or more)
   Mobility – requires assistance with transfer
   ADL – requires personal assistance with two of – grooming, bathing, feeding
   Incontinence – >1/day
   MSO >5
5. *Severe impairment*
   Requires assistance in all areas but two of four are complete dependency
   Mobility – immobile, bed to chair lift
   ADL – dependent
   Incontinence – total
   MSQ – <3
6. *Totally dependent*
   Dependent in all four areas
7. Terminally ill and likely to die within 30 days

Usually individuals within groups 5–7 are not felt to be suitable for in-patient geriatric assessment units. The patients in groups 5 and 6 are less likely to show benefit from geriatric intervention. It is however, important that the care given is appropriate to the patient. Individuals involved in their care must be aware of a range of ethical issues and be at ease with dealing with multiple interacting problems in the dependent ill elderly. It has been recognized that these patients need to have appropriate limits set upon the type of technological intervention that is used. This is discussed in Chapter 30 on long-term care. The terminally ill, group 7, may be found within geriatric units since sudden decline may be the presenting feature of a malignancy and the reason for assessment. It may be appropriate for many of these patients to be looked after in the long-term care institution in which they reside or within special palliative care units and it is here that assessments need to be carried out.

Geriatric medicine is defined dynamically by the patients which benefit from the services. The patients are defined by functional impairment and disease burden and not by age. Individuals who enter the specialty need to be aware of this. It is inappropriate to sidetrack the geriatrician by looking after young elderly with single system problems – even if that is what the geriatrician wants to do. If this is happening then training needs to change, and the trainers need to emphasize this. The younger elderly and those with single system problems can continue to be looked after by the sub-specialists and the general internists (general physicians) to the benefit of all.

6. The tools of assessment

The search for a universal assessment tool in geriatric medicine is a little like the search for the Holy Grail in the middle ages. A universal assessment tool appears to be elusive and perhaps in the context of geriatric medicine inappropriate and unnecessary.

There is no doubt that assessment tools bring objectivity into clinical practice. It has already been mentioned that geriatric assessment is a dynamic process. Assessment therefore often continues over a period of time until optimal function is attained. It is necessary to consider assessment tools under the headings of *cognition, depression, activities of daily living, behavioral assessment,* and *qualities of life.*

After reviewing a number of short mental status assessment instruments there are two examples we routinely use. We suggest that the Mini Mental State Examination of Folstein is an appropriate instrument for case finding in the geriatric assessment setting. It is reported as having excellent sensitivity and specificity, with data available in a variety of geriatric populations and settings. Although, recognizing the relative wealth of literature concerning its use in Canadian and American populations, some concerns can be expressed about the brevity of instructions particularly in relating to scoring of the assessments. The instrument could also be said to suffer from the problem of missing mild cases. Another useful screening tool for cognitive function is the 10 point Mental Status Questionnaire (MSQ) which has been validated in Europe and North America. This is a useful and sensitive screening tool, and takes only a few moments to perform (Table 1.4).

A variety of instruments have been described and used in the assessment of depression in the elderly. The Yesavage Geriatric Depression Scale is a reasonable instrument and has been validated in North American populations. The available data would suggest that the shortened 15-question version is as reliable as the longer version and is improved by its brevity.

The areas that need to be assessed under *activities of daily living* (ADL) include self-care (feeding, bathing, grooming, dressing of upper and lower

Table 1.4 Mental status questionnaire

Remember these three objects, I will ask you about them later:
door, envelope, car (repeat them)

1. What year is it?
2. What day of the week is it?
3. What is the name of this place?
4. What is your home address?
5. What is the capital of Canada? (or country of domicile)
6. What year were you born in?
7. Who is the prime minister? (or president)
8. What were the three objects that I asked you to remember?
9. When did World War I (or II) start?
10. Subtract 3 from 20 and keep going.

Total score: normal expectation is 9 or 10, except in illiterate patients when one more wrong answer is acceptable.

body), mobility (transfers from sitting to standing, bed to chair, toilet and bathtub, walking on the level and negotiating stairs) and continence. The parameters commonly measured under *instrumental activities of daily living* (IADL) commonly include food preparation, grocery shopping, housekeeping, laundry, telephone use, administration of medications and finance, and the use of public transport.

A large number of ADL Scales have been described. The three commonly considered are the modified Barthel Index, Rapid Disability Rating Scale, and the Philadelphia Geriatric Physical Centre Maintenance and Instrumental Activities of Daily Living Scale of Lawton. Each instrument has different merits depending upon the actual need. The Barthel is brief and has been shown to be predictive of prognosis in stroke rehabilitation but has the disadvantage of insensitivity to change in some ADL parameters. The Rapid Disability Scale is simple and includes several additional parameters but its main use is in measuring care level needs in the stable situation. The Lawton ADL Scale, although taking longer and requiring more standardization, is more useful in measuring change within a rehabilitation program.

The assessment of caregiver burden has been relatively neglected. The Zarit Family Burden Scale was developed for use of caregivers of clients with an Alzheimer type dementia. The scales measure feelings about health, psychological well being, financial and social life and relationship with a patient. Validation against a caregiver's perceptions has been attempted. An alternative group of patients caregivers is considered in the Robinson's Caregiver Training Index which reports to measure the impact of caring for seniors in the community after hospitalization. It is difficult at the moment to therefore recommended any one instrument since choices are limited, but either of the two above could be considered in the appropriate situation.

Quality of life scales suffer from similar problems to burden indexes. Two possible instruments for consideration are the Quality of life index of Spitzer, and the Philadelphia Geriatric Centre Morale Scale of Lawton. The Philadelphia Geriatric Centre Morale Scale is designed to measure dimensions of emotional adjustment in persons aged 70–90. It is claimed to be applicable both to community residents and to people in institutions. There is reasonable data to suggests that it is a reliable and consistent instrument. The Spitzer Quality of Life Index measures the general well-being of patients with cancer and other chronic diseases.

It was originally intended to evaluate the effects of treatment and supporter programs. The instrument is practical, brief and easy to administer yet broad in scope. It has been acceptable to clinicians and clients and used in a wide range of populations and cultures. It seems particularly relevant to an ill elderly population which makes it perhaps relevant to the geriatric assessment purpose. The advantage of it over the Lawton instrument is its relative brevity requiring only 5 items compared to 22 of the Philadelphia Geriatric Centre Morale Scale of Lawton.

Table 1.5 Activities of daily living

Barthel's Self-care	Self	Assistance requ.		Unable to do
1. Drinking from a cup	4		0	0
2. Eating	6		0	0
3. Dressing upper body	5		4	0
4. Dressing lower body	7		4	0
5. Putting on brace or artificial limb	0	−2		0
6. Grooming	5		0	0
7. Washing or bathing	6		0	0
8. Controlling urination	10	5		0
9. Controlling bowel movements	10	5		0
	53			
Mobility Index				
10. Getting in and out of chair	15		7	0
11. Getting on and off toilet	6		3	0
12. Getting in and out of tub or shower	1		0	0
13. Walking 25 ft on the level	15		10	0
14. Walking up/down 1 flight of stairs	10		5	0
15. If not walking, propelling wheel chair	5		0	0

Best score is 100; worst score is 0

Table 1.6 Modified Lawton's Scales

Instrumental activities of daily living	*Assistance codes*
Food preparation	0 = not assessed
Grocery shopping	1 = independent
Housekeeping	2 = modified independence
Laundry	3 = supervision required
Finances	4 = assistance required, patient contributes to task
Telephone use	
Medications	5 = dependent and accepting assistance
Transportation	
Outdoor maintenance	6 = dependent, refuses assistance or neglects task
	8 = not applicable
Activities of daily living	*Assistance codes*
Feeding	0 = not assessed
Bathing	1 = independent
Grooming	2 = independent with aids and adaptations
Dressing	
Toileting	3 = requires supervision
	4 = minimal physical assist of one person
Transfers sit-stand	
bed-chair	5 = moderate assistance, helper assisting most of time
Toilet	
bathtub	6 = total physical assistance patient rarely contributes climb
Ambulation (50 yds on level)	
Stairs (1 flight)	8 = not applicable

7. Conclusion

The problem oriented medical record helps the physician in the medical approach, and challenges him or her to take problem solution to its highest level. Benign neglect is discouraged. It will also assist the physician in identifying those problems that cannot be changed so that realistic plans of management can be set forth. At the same time communication within the health care team is encouraged. The use of a common, Master Problem List is invaluable in fostering communication and identifying common goals between members of the geriatric team. The use of appropriate assessment tools is also useful in this regard. All members can then focus on the problems that need to be addressed at the same time as pathophysiological diagnosis is being achieved and other treatments or investigations are underway.

It is unfortunate that in many cases the diagnostic process for each problem is not entered into, the significance of the geriatric presentation is not recognized. The social crisis is identified but responses are directed towards social supports or institutionalization rather than diagnostic. The predisposing age changes may be identified but no precipitants are recognized and therefore the patient is left untreated. This is the pseudo-silent presentation that has been mentioned. Patients that require full geriatric assessment are complex and present formidable challenges in diagnosis and management. Without an appropriate framework and training background the physician may find the task too daunting and retreat into a social response and benign neglect. An act of omission rather than commission. The approach in this book is aimed at overcoming this and assisting the physician in dealing effectively with the problems at hand.

Suggested reading

Cape, R. D. T. (1972). A geriatric service. *Midland Med. Rev.* **8**: 21–30.

Droller, H. (1964). *Age with a Future: Evaluation of Medical Needs of Older People*. Copenhagen, Monksgaard.

Exton Smith, A. N. (1977). Functional consequences of ageing: clinical manifestations. In: Exton Smith, A. N. and Grimley Evans, J. (eds) *Care of the Elderly: Meeting the Challenges of Dependency*. Academic Press, London.

Isaacs, B. (1964). *Current Achievements in Geriatrics, Morbidity in Elderly Hospital Patients*. Cassell, London.

Isaacs, B. (1981). Is geriatrics a speciality? In: Arie, T. (ed.) *Health Care of the Elderly*, Croom Helm, London, ch. 14, p. 224.

Kane, R. A. and Kane, R. L. (1981). *Assessing the Elderly*. Lexington Books, D.C. Heath, Lexington, Mass. & Toronto.

Puxty, J. A. H. and Andrews, K. (1986). The role of chest radiography in the evaluation of the geriatric giants. *Age and Ageing*, **15**: 174–6.

Weed, L. L. (1969). *Medical Records, Medical Education and Patient Care*. Case Western Reserve University Press. Year Book Publishers, Chicago.

2

Confusion

Confusion, a syndrome comprising temporal and spatial disorientation with impairment of intellectual functioning, is one of the most common problems associated with a geriatric presentation. It presents one of the most difficult challenges to the clinician. Inappropriate assessment can lead to misdiagnosis, failure to correct reversible elements and long-term care at an inappropriate level. An inappropriate label of dementia can modify the responses of relatives and the caring professionals to that individual, often in a detrimental fashion.

A number of different terminologies have arisen to apply to conditions which involve disturbance of cognition. One commonly used classification is the division into organic and functional brain syndromes. In this book the term 'functional' is used in a different context to refer to complex functions such as thought, mobility or posture. Organic brain syndrome is a term that is often applied more loosely than dementia and for some implies a diagnosis. For this reason we will refer to these cognitive disturbances as acute confusional states (or delirium) and dementia (or chronic confusional states).

1. Acute confusional state (delirium)

An acute confusional state occurs when there is abrupt onset of disorientation and global impairment of intellectual function which includes difficulties in appropriate focusing and maintaining of attention. This state is also referred to as delirium and there are many other synonyms. The diagnostic criteria for Delirium from the American Psychiatric Association are shown in Table 2.1. In the DSM-IIIR criteria the only reference to duration is of hours or days. It is important to know in the course of clinical practice when an acute confusional state becomes chronic. It seems to us that there is no set time limit for this, although when the problem has been present for 7 days the chances of reversal seem to be significantly reduced. Any confusional state

Table 2.1 Diagnostic criteria for delirium

A. Reduced ability to maintain attention to external stimuli (e.g. questions must be repeated because attention wanders) and to approximately shift attention to new external stimuli (e.g. perseverates, answers previous question).
B. Disorganized thinking as indicated by rambling, irrelevant or incoherent speech.
C. At least two of the following:
   1. reduced level of consciousness, e.g. difficulty in keeping awake during examination
   2. perceptual disturbances: misinterpretations, illusions or hallucinations
   3. disturbance of sleep-wake cycle, with insomnia or daytime sleepiness
   4. increased or decreased psychomotor activity
   5. disorientation to time, place or person
   6. memory impairment, e.g. inability to learn new material, such as the names of several unrelated objects after five minutes, or to remember past events, such as history of current episode of illness.
D. Clinical features that develop over a short period of time (usually hours to days) and tend to fluctuate over the course of a day.
E. Either 1 or 2 below:
   1. evidence from the history, physical examination or laboratory tests of a specific organic factor judged to be etiologically related to the disturbance
   2. in the absence of such evidence, an etiologic organic factor can be presumed if the disturbance cannot be accounted for by any non-organic mental disorder, e.g. manic episode accounting for igitation and sleep disturbance.

that has been present for over a month should be referred to as chronic. For the in between period patients should be looked at in the same way as Acute Confusional States for diagnostic and therapeutic approach but may simply be referred to as 'confusional states' – this avoids over optimism for reversal if considered acute and also prevents the early labelling of dementia.

The clinical features are outlined in Table (2.1) and need not be repeated at this stage. This is a common problem and the frequency depends upon the age and the type of patients that one looks at. For example for people over the age of 75 admitted to hospital as medical emergencies approximately one-quarter experience an acute confusional episode during hospitalization. A variety of studies of the over 65 year-olds report a frequency of between 10 and 50 per cent. The outcome of the acute confusional state obviously depends upon the nature of the precipitating problems, but between one-quarter and one-third will die within the first few months of the occurrence. Of the rest the condition of about three quarters is reversible, but about one-quarter are left with permanent cognitive impairment. It should be emphasized that recognition is important since there is evidence that the longer the period of time before reversing the less likely are the chances for full recovery and the greater the chance of permanent cognitive impairment.

The concept of diminishing reserve with age has already been discussed. With aging there is decline in the ability of the brain and its 'function' to withstand stress. Under normal circumstances the brain functions adequately, any decline that occurs is almost imperceptible and if it has occurred may well be compensated for by a spouse or significant other. With a sudden change in circumstances and the addition of stress, the brain may be precipitated into failure. The failure is manifest as an acute confusional state. We need to consider the changes that predispose the individual to confusion and the events that precipitate.

Predisposing factors

The brain that has undergone change with advancing age so that there is loss of reserve can be considered to be predisposed. The deterioration can be considered under three main headings:

a) Intrinsic aging of the central nervous system (CNS)
b) Disease – intrinsic to CNS
c) Disease – extrinsic to CNS

a) Changes within the brain with age have been the subject of study for a long time. Changes have been observed in two ways. First of all structural or physical change. It has been noted for a long time that the size of the brain decreases with age. Shrinkage is most obvious in the front half of the cerebral hemispheres with the sulci becoming more prominent and the ventricles larger. On histological examination there is lipofuscin deposition throughout and this is thought to represent wear and tear. The presence of senile plaques, neurofibrillary tangles and granulovacuolar degeneration have also been described in 'normal' brains. There appears to be general acceptance that there is neuronal fallout with age, although the extent and etiology are not clearly defined. It should be emphasized that these changes have been obtained from the study of postmortem material and that it is not possible to do appropriate longitudinal studies in humans. However with the introduction of computerized tomography scans it has become clear that the finding of a small brain with prominent sulci is not indicative of disease.

It is claimed that these structural changes are accompanied by changes in function. There have been many studies done by psychologists and others measuring different aspects of brain function. It should be noted that much of this work was done in cross-sectional studies and interpretation of differences as a true aging effect is difficult because of the many other factors such as cultural and educational differences. It is generally accepted that there is decline in fluid intelligence with age. This would mean a decreasing ability to solve fresh problems and to meet new challenges. On the other hand, crystalline intelligence which depends upon previously acquired information such as vocabulary does not deteriorate but if anything improves. There is some evidence to suggest that distractibility is increased so unless new memories have relevance or are reinforced, it appears there is some decline in the ability to create them.

b) Disease – intrinsic to CNS

A variety of pathological states or conditions serve to make the elderly person more vulnerable to acute confusional states. Conditions such as Alzheimer's disease and multi-infarct dementia may have a presymptomatic period these individuals will have limited adaptability and are therefore predisposed to acute confusional episode. Individuals with impaired cognition (dementia) may well get an acute confusional state on top of overt memory failure. Focal brain deficits from lesions in the frontal or temporal lobes which interfere with attention span and registration may present with acute confusional states with appropriate precipitants. Sensory or language dysfunction may limit the available accurate information about the environment and so make misinterpretation likely.

c) Disease – extrinsic to CNS

Sensory deprivation is particularly common in the elderly and increase the likelihood of misinterpretation of environmental stimuli and reduces accessibility to reassurance. Sleep disturbance predisposes to confusion, as well as being a feature of it. Some sleep disturbances are more obvious such as anxiety, pain or noise; less obvious may be restlessness resulting from visceral stimuli due to fecal loading or bladder distension.

Changes in the environment, such as admission to hospital, for an individual with already impaired sensory input can also add to the predisposing factors. With hospitalization may come attempts at physical restraint which will only add to anxiety and feed delusions of persecution. In the setting of hospital such environmental influences are often most important at night.

Precipitating factors

Almost any illness can precipitate delirium in a predisposed individual. Probably the most common causes are infections and adverse drug reactions. Other common problems would include those conditions that reduce oxygenation either from cardiac or respiratory problems or from local ischemia due to stroke. Another important group of causes are metabolic disturbances such as hyponatremia or hypercalcemia, which may only become clear from the laboratory investigation.

In the confused patient the major aim of history taking and examination is to identify the precipitants so that specific treatment can be commenced. The algorithmic approach, outlined in Fig. 2.1., will allow the uncovering of the majority of the precipitants.

Subjective

An accurate clinical history which has been corroborated (or provided) by friends, relatives or other care providers is essential. The duration of confusion, the premorbid state of the individual and the relationship to other events are crucial in evaluation. It may not be possible to obtain as full a history as desired at first but the clinician should try to determine if this state is definitely new or whether there is a background of dementia. This issue is important when potential reversibility is being considered and also the options for discharge. Onset following surgery may suggest the possibility of pain, infection, a metabolic disturbance or adverse reaction to drugs. A nocturnal pattern may indicate the important role of sensory deprivation or alternatively the use of a hypnotic drug. An episodic history of confusion following periods of loss of consciousness may suggest a transient ischemic attack or epileptiform seizures. Periods of hypoxia or hypercapnia result in confusion and cardiorespiratory disease should be asked about.

If the history suggests fluctuating levels of consciousness over a period of several days following an injury or fall then a diagnosis like subdural hematoma needs to be considered. A more rapid decline after injury might favor the possibility of extradural hematoma.

The etiology of confusion is often multifactorial and it is therefore of importance to inquire in all areas. In considering common causes, a proper drug history is vital. Because of age changes in pharmacokinetics drugs can accumulate and have an effect on cognition long beyond the normal quoted half life. All drugs should be brought in to be examined and inquiry should be made as to who is supervising and the reliability of the patient in monitoring her medications. A patient with failing memory may well be consuming incorrect amounts if unsupervised at home. Any drug should be considered to have the potential to cause confusion but certain ones are more likely to (Table 2.2).

The features of infection are dealt with in Chapter 23. In the presence of confusion these features may be difficult to elicit.

The dietary history may well be important. Avitaminoses may present with confusion and be made worse by infection for example. Nutrition may contribute to anemia which in turns leads to confusion. It is important to inquire into alcohol use and to look for features of alcohol abuse.

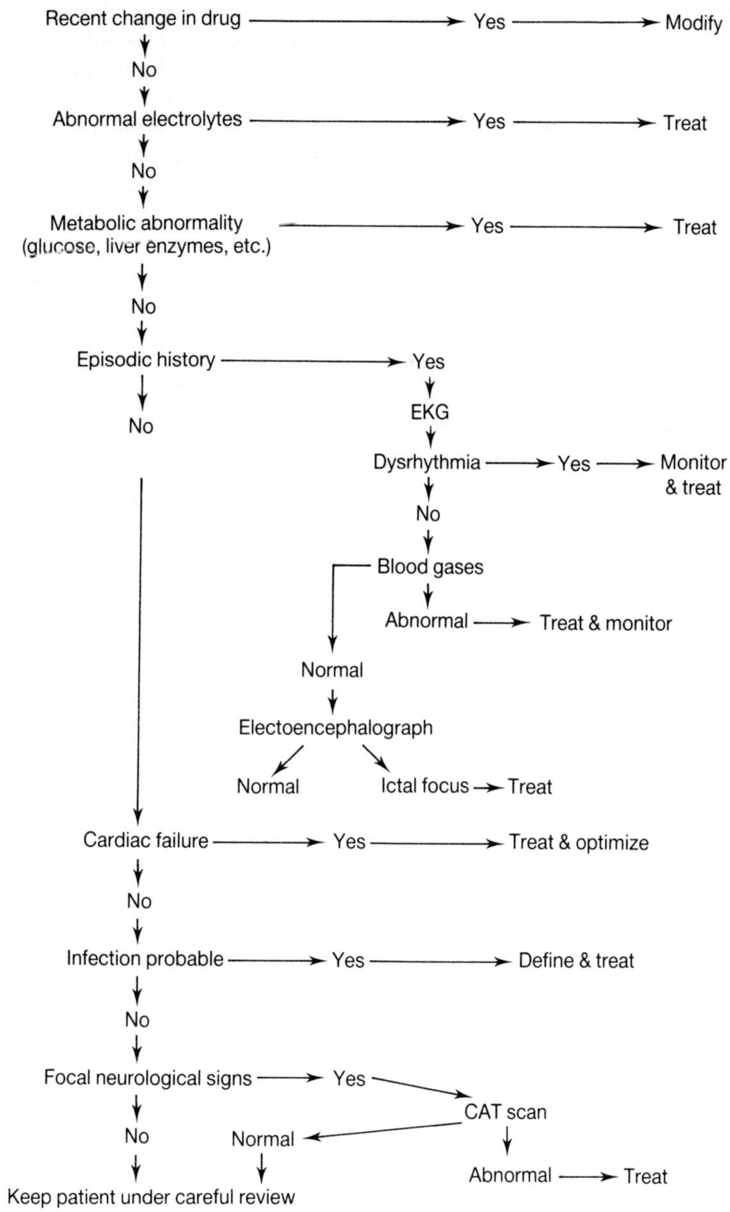

Fig. 2.1 Algorithm for delirium (acute confusional state).

Although toxic poisoning is uncommon it should be considered.

It is important to seek a clear history of previous disease. A history of cardiac disease may give a valuable clue to a number of cardiac etiologies to acute contusional states. Associated symptoms such as thirst or polyuria may suggest endocrine or metabolic disturbance such as hyperglycemia or hypercalcemia.

Objective

A thorough examination may be very difficult in the presence of confusion, particularly when the

Table 2.2 Drugs often implicated in confusion in the elderly

Neutroleptics
Tri-cyclic antidepressants
Benzodiazepines
Hypnotics
Antiparkinsonian medications: L-dopa Bromocryptine Anticholinergic
Cimetidine
Digoxin
Anticonvulsants
Hypoglycemic agents

patient is anxious and aggressive. The examination serves two purposes:

1. To document that confusion is present and to identify the different features to this.
2. To try and identify the predisposing and precipitating factors so that appropriate treatment can be commenced.

The patient needs to be observed and the behaviour noted. Questions of a non-threatening, general nature may reveal much about the state of mind of the patient. It will become apparent whether the patient is aware of what is happening and is oriented. It is usually possible to administer a formal mental status questionnaire (Chapter 1) which may confirm the presence of confusion and will also be useful in monitoring the progress of the patient. As a result of this examination the physician should have established the presence of an acute confusional state.

Examination needs to be thorough, following up any clinical pointers that become apparent. It needs to be remembered that typical features may be occult or will need to be searched for very closely.

Acute confusional states are often multifactorial in origin. For example patients may have an acute illness like pneumonia but will also be fecally impacted, this will also need to be treated. At the first visit, the examination might not be possible to complete and it will be necessary to complete over several assessments. This is particularly so for neurological examination. Often careful observation will give clues to the presence of problems such as visual field defects, sensory inattention or agnosia.

Any feature that is out of keeping with a normative age change, should be considered a clinical pointer and followed up. For example, vitamin or nutritional deficiencies may be revealed by skin changes. This would include clues picked up on a home visit such as the empty liquor bottles or multiple medicine containers. Olfactory as well as visual clues are important (Table 2.3).

Table 2.3 Olfactory clues to causes of confusion

Smell	Condition
Acetone	Diabetes mellitus
Alcohol	Alcohol intoxication
Ammonia	Uremia
Musty fish	Liver failure
Wet leaves	Pulmonary TB
Feculent	Anerobic infection
Garlic	Arsenic poisoning

Assessment

Once the information is gathered there is usually a clear idea of the likely precipitants so that further diagnosis and appropriate treatment can be started.

Assessment includes consideration of other conditions. It is important to determine if the patient is acute on chronic confusion – a decompensated dementia. The same approach is necessary and the same urgency pertains. Inappropriate handling may allow the decompensated state to continue with a permanent lowering of the level of function.

There may be other important features on examination that allow problem definition to be taken to a higher level. For example Wernicke's encephalopathy includes behavioral change in association with extraocular movement disorders and ataxia. There is usually a degree of memory loss present but when this is a dominant feature the label of Korsakoff's psychosis is applied. It is a well appreciated situation in the alcoholic but other groups are at risk such as the severely malnourished. A precipitating factor may be infection or the injudicious use of parenteral glucose in the patient with thiamine avitaminosis. The condition is readily reversible in the very early stages by parenteral administration of thiamine.

Intermittent episodes of bizarre behavior may be labelled as confusion when in fact they are manifestations of temporal lobe epilepsy. The important clues to the diagnosis are the episodic nature, the presence of an aura, a loss of contact with the environment and automatisms. The aura may be of a specific type depending upon the focus for example gustatory or olfactory sensation (uncus), a change in perception such as déjà vu, euphoria or doom (cingulate cortex), butterflies in the stomach (insular cortex), photophobia (amygdala), auditory or visual hallucinations (temporal associated areas).

Another rare entity that needs to be considered is transient global amnesia. During an attack a patient may appear confused or disorientated but the problem is an amnestic syndrome without global intellectual impairment. This is usually seen in elderly men with a history of vascular disease. The patient will often have insight into their memory disturbance. Episodes are usually self-limiting but amnesia for the period persists.

Dysphasia, following a stroke, may also be mistaken for confusion. Sometimes the two occur together.

Plan

a) Diagnostic

The appropriate screening investigations have been discussed (Chapter 1) and more definitive investigations will depend upon the findings. Thoughtless application of a battery of tests in addition to being expensive often only add to the bewilderment and anxiety of the patient. The algorithm (Fig. 2.1) provides a guide to the application of resources. If one follows this approach it will be seen that an examination like computerized axial tomography (CAT scan) is only done when there are definite indications. It is also worth emphasizing that investigations are only done when they may make a difference, tests that are unlikely to change management or influence outcome should not be performed.

b) Management

Management of the confused patient should start at the moment of presentation to the clinician. The two main aims of management being the control of symptomatic distress or hyperactivity, and treatment of the precipitating problems. Unfortunately the environments in which patients with acute confusipn are managed often add to the disorientation and agitation. Hospitals are often noisy with a great deal of activity, patients may get moved around frequently. In order to manage confusion effectively the environment should be as calming as possible. Illumination should be appropriate for the aged eye. There should be a clear identification of areas such as the patient's room, bathrooms or day rooms. Noise should be kept to a minimum with the elimination of unnecessary noise from television or radio. The approach by staff should be consistently reassuring and non-threatening. Confrontation needs to be avoided but patients should be supplied information about the environment and what is happening. When patients are wandering they can often be steered back towards reality by diverting attention and supplying further information. Recognizing that many elderly patients have hearing difficulty appropriate aids may be used if indicated, and carers should speak slowly and clearly.

Patients should not be restrained if at all possible. Interventions that restrict the patient should be kept to a minimum – for example, the patient should be managed as 'normally' as possible with avoidance of unnecessary bladder catheterization or intravenous therapy.

There should be careful review of all medications which might be contributing to the situation. When all this has been done one may be left with a patient who remains extremely anxious and very difficult to manage. Agitation and psychic stress may need to be controlled pharmacologically.

Drugs that are used in this situation should be given in doses that are appropriate for control. In other words, over-sedation needs to be avoided, but under treatment is also bad. This means regular monitoring and the avoidance of 'p.r.n.' orders. Drug regimens should be reviewed daily. In order to calm patients commonly used drugs are haloperidol, loxapine or thioridazine. Loxapine is the most specific for the psychomotor agitation. All may over-sedate, haloperidol may immobilize from parkinsonian side effects, thioridazine is more likely to have cardiac side effects or hypotension. Haloperidol is usually started at a dose of 0.5 mg every 4 to 6 hours, thioridazine at 10 mg every 4 to 6 hours, and loxapine 5 mg two to four times a day. Dosage is increased or decreased as required. Occasionally patients will have a paradoxical reaction to haloperidol and one should immediately switch to an alternative. Once the confusion is brought under control the drug should be reduced to a level that will alleviate the anxiety and not produce undue sedation. We have found that doses of haloperidol as low as 0.5 mg every 8 hours may suffice. It is usually possible to get the patients off such drugs altogether unless there is not complete reversal and the patient has developed a dementia.

If the patient is not sleeping properly, which is a common problem, then a hypnotic drug should be used to induce sleep. This should be short acting with no after effects. Our choice is to use either chloral hydrate, temazepam or triazolam. With chloral hydrate the usual starting dose is 500 mg at night. If this does not induce sleep then the dose is doubled. If still insufficient then 500 mg should be given at approximately 7 pm, followed by 1000 mg at bedtime. This is usually effective in inducing sleep. These drugs need to be constantly monitored to be sure that they are not making matters worse and that they are really necessary. All too often patients are put on a drug and left on it and the cumulative effect may take days to clear once stopped.

In addition to symptomatic management any identifiable precipitant is of course treated appropriately. Those patients who do not return to their premorbid level and remain cognitively impaired need to be treated as dementia which is discussed in the next section.

2. Dementia

Dementia is the preferred clinical term to describe a syndrome in which there is progressive mental deterioration with impairment of orientation, memory, comprehension, calculation, learning capacity, judgement and all aspects of cognitive function with the resultant inability to carry out activities of daily living. Other terms which are frequently used include chronic organic brain syndrome, chronic brain failure or chronic confusional state. It is important to remember that many patients who present have potentially remediable elements and are functioning at a suboptimal level. If patients are identified from a screening program before they present for 'crisis intervention' as many as 40 per cent have conditions such as avitaminosis or anaemia which are having a detrimental effect on their cognitive function.

There are a number of different conditions which play an etiological role in the development of dementia. Some are important to recognize because of the potential for treatment and reversibility (Table 2.4). It needs to be emphasized, however that in present day geriatric practice when patients present with a history of change over months or years the potential for reversibility is extremely low. In most surveys of patients referred with established dementia, Alzheimer's disease and multiinfarct dementia account for 80–90 per cent of cases. Unless brain tissue is obtained for histology the diagnosis of Alzheimer's disease is one of exclusion, although there are well established criteria which render the diagnosis probable.

Table 2.4 Etiology of dementia

Primary cerebral degeneration:
Alzheimer's disease (AP)
Parkinson's disease
Jakob–Creuzfeldt disease (?secondary)
Pick's disease
Huntington's chorea
Secondary cerebral degeneration:
Multi-infarct-dementia (MID)
Anoxic (Post-cardiopulmonary arrest)
Post-traumatic
Normal pressure hydrocephalus
Metabolic:
B12 deficiency
alcohol induced
hepatic encephalopathy
Neurosyphilis

Pathophysiology

Alzheimer's disease is characterized morphologically by cortical atrophy with widening of the sulci, and histologically there are senile plaques, neurofibrillary tangles, granuolovacular degeneration and amyloid deposition. The senile plaques are found in abundance in the brain in Alzheimer's disease, and are composed of a core of amyloid surrounded by astrocytes and degenerating neurites. The gene for amyloid is carried on chromosome 21, the same chromosome which carries the gene for familial Alzheimer's. There is astrocytosis surrounding the areas of amyloid deposition of degeneration and there is neuronal loss with a poverty of dendritic branches. The changes which have been described appear to start within the area of the hippocampus, the nucleus basalis of Meynert, and then to spread throughout the brain mainly to the frontal and temporal lobes. A deficiency of the cholinergic neurotransmitter system has been consistently demonstrated.

In multi-infarct dementia (MID) pathological examination reveals multiple small infarcts or lacunae. The damage resulting from cerebrovascular disease can occur in any area of the brain and often includes corticobulbar and corticospinal disease.

Another cause of dementia, normal pressure hydrocephalus, was first described in 1965. This may be secondary to lesions that produce a communicating or obstructive hydrocephalus, or may be idiopathic of unknown etiology. The result is a dilated ventricular system with consequent cortical atrophy, although the cerebrospinal fluid pressure is often normal.

Parkinson's disease may be associated with a subcortical memory deficit picture. Nearly half have features of bradyphrenia, problems of memory retrieval and difficulty in changing mind sets which respond to dopamine replacement therapy. In about 10 per cent the changes persist and a subcortical dementia exists.

Memory failure with other features of dementia may occur in individuals with alcoholism. In some the features are typical of Korsakoff's psychosis which has become chronic. It may be difficult to determine if the cortical atrophy is secondary to alcohol damage or whether there is a coincident process such as Alzheimer's disease.

There are other important types of dementia such as Pick's disease but the importance of identifying this as a separate entity is not clear. An increasing number of older people are surviving major trauma as the result of motor vehicle accidents and a proportion of these are cognitively impaired needing similar considerations as other types. This would also apply to the survivors of resuscitation from cardiopulmonary failure, and anoxic brain damage is a significant etiological factor for dementia.

A proportion of patients with dementia do not fit clearly into one group and at autopsy are found to have mixed etiology, most frequently Alzheimer's disease and multi-infarct state. A proportion of patients die with diagnostic labels of an Alzheimer's-type dementia but are found to have pathologically normal brains.

Subjective

The length of time that the cognitive impairment has been present is of extreme importance in deciding that the problem is dementia and not an acute confusional state (delirium). However the use of this term has an air of finality about it and in early problem definition it might be better to use terms such as chronic confusional state. If cognitive impairment has been constantly present, without reversible features, for at least a month then a dementia syndrome may be present (this does not preclude reversibility and does not preclude going on to the next question).

When patient's present with dementia the problems have usually been developing over several months or years. It may be that decline has occurred but has not been appreciated by those around the patient. The deficits are brought to the attention of others by a significant change such as the death or hospital admission of a spouse who has been protecting the patient and taking over various functions. The patient may appear to be presenting with an acute confusional state but on close questioning and discussion changes are reported over a period of time.

A gradual onset, stretching over months, favors the diagnosis of Alzheimer's disease (AD). In MID the decline is likely to be more stepwise, with confusion accompanying a stroke. This usually occurs several times, with episodes of deterioration followed by slight improvement until the patient is functioning at a much lower level.

Whatever the etiology of the memory failure the patient is likely to have increasing difficulty in relationship to complex household chores, for a woman this is likely to be cooking. The house may become dirty and accidents in the kitchen by burning utensils are commonplace. There is usually loss of interest in hobbies because of decreasing ability to participate. Eating patterns may change, most patients being less able to prepare food and therefore losing weight. Food may be allowed to spoil within the refrigerator. Some patients over-eat and have a constant craving, gaining excessive amounts of weight. Individuals become less able to manage their financial affairs, some losing considerable sums. Because of forgetfulness money may be lost or misplaced and then false accusations made. A history of problems with vehicle driving such as getting lost or recent accidents are not uncommon early presenting features of AD.

As these changes occur the personality of the individual changes, although with MID there is often preservation of the personality until the end which is a marked contrast to AD. Patients with MID may have marked emotional lability due to the bulbar damage (Table 2.5). Failing intellect is often noted by others rather than the patient, although many patients do recognize the changes and may become depressed as a result of it.

The decline in the subject's personal standards

Table 2.5 Hachinski ischemia score

Feature	Score
Abrupt onset	2
Stepwise deterioration	1
Fluctuating course	2
Nocturnal confusion	1
Preservation of personality	1
Depression	1
Somatic complaints	1
Emotional incontinence	1
History of hypertension	1
History of strokes	2
Evidence of associated atherosclerosis	1
Focal neurological symptoms	2
Focal neurological signs	2

are distressing to friends and relatives, and the individual is often very resistant to efforts to clean up and change clothes. They will often become extremely combative at these times. Changes in sleep pattern seem to be more of an issue with AD and nocturnal hyperactivity or wandering may disturb the sleep of others. At night visual cues decrease and confusion often increases with associated anxiety and often aggression. As the dementia progresses the individual may become euphoric and unaware of the difficulties, cheerfully denying any problems.

In AD and MID there may be deterioration of other aspects of neurological function so that patients may experience gait difficulties and fall frequently. Many patients retain full mobility and may wander. In a cold climate this is an important problem and may lead to significant problems from exposure. There are of course other hazards, such as traffic.

These patients are predisposed to decompensation in the form of an acute confusional state (delirium) and are extremely susceptible to the adverse effects of medications. The patients may insist in maintaining control over their own drugs so that adverse effects are common.

As the disease progresses incontinence of urine and feces occurs. The development of urinary incontinence and gait abnormalities early on in the course of the disease is said to favour normal pressure hydrocephalus, although in our experience this condition is rarely identified in geriatric practice.

If the dementia is part of Parkinson's disease this should be obvious from the history. Patients will have had Parkinson's disease for a number of years since this tends to be a late feature of the disease. It should also be recognized that AD can and does occur coincidentally with Parkinson's disease. The family history should be inquired into. Other degenerative problems like Huntington's disease may be identified. Some patient's with AD have a strong family history of this disease.

There is no way to identify Pick's Disease during life and there are no significant features in the history. In the case of Jakob–Creuzfeldt's disease this is identified by a rapid deterioration and the association of other features such as those of Parkinson's disease or motor neurone disease and the onset of myoclonic jerks.

Objective

A variety of conditions may mask as a memory disturbance and need to be excluded. Fatigue or drowsiness can obviously interfere with intellectual functioning. Anxiety or depression will interfere with attention and memory registration and retrieval. Sensory and language deficits may result in miscommunication. There may be evidence of widespread cortical damage which can be found in any type of dementia (Table 2.6).

It is important to develop a hypothesis as to the likely etiology since this will determine reversibility. The focus of examination will be to look for any features that point to etiology, for example focal neurological signs or evidence of raised intracranial pressure. Physical examination needs to be complete, although it may be difficult due to agitation or resistance by the patient. One should look for features of hypothyroidism, pernicious anaemia or vitamin deficiency for example. Patients with AD usually have a paucity of physical findings, apart from the cognitive impairment, which has led some to conclude that they are healthier than age matched controls. As part of this initial evaluation a low serum thyroxine with a raised thyroid stimulating hormone may be found. This will need to be treated and may indicate a possible etiology, however this is likely to be disappointing. The hypothyroidism may be corrected but the patient remains demented.

A very important area to be explored is the mood of the patient. It is important to consider whether depression is present but this is often very difficult to decide. Occasionally treatment of an individual with a dementia syndrome with depressive features results in an apparent 'cure' of the cognitive problems. On follow-up though many of these individuals subsequently present with a dementia syndrome which is not reversible. It is probable that

Table 2.6 Signs of diffuse cortical dysfunction

Sign	Elicited by	Positive response
Suck reflex	Placing an object between the lips	Puckering or sucking motion
Snout reflex	Brief pressure on the lips	Puckering movement
Grasp reflex	Stroking the palm	Grasping or closing hand
Palmomental reflex	Firm stimulation of thenar eminence	Nonfatiguing contraction of ipsilateral mentalis muscle
Glabellar reflex	Light tapping on Glabellar region	Nonfatiguing blinking
Nuchocephalic reflex	Turning shoulders to right or left	Head moves in bloc with no delay
Paratonia (gegenhalten)	Failing to relax with passive movement of arms or legs	Inconsistent and irregular resistance
Motor impersistence	Look to side (examiner's finger)	Moves away in under 30 seconds
Limb placement	Hold patient's arm and ask to relax	Arm stays in place
Visual tracking	Ask to hold head still and follow finger with eyes	Irregular, hesitant or jerking saccades
Conjugate gaze	To follow finger with eyes up and down	Limitation of gaze Up – <5 mm Down – <7 mm

the depression was precipitating an early cognitive decline and once removed the dementia became preclinical and unable to be detected by our relatively insensitive measures of cognitive decline.

The important clues to the presence of treatable causes of dementia are summarized in Table 2.7.

In looking at the consequences for the patient there is a great deal of assessment that will need to be done. However, the physician will be gathering information about it at this stage.

Note should be made as to whether there are signs of malnutrition and neglect? Is there evidence of any kind of physical abuse? Other areas that need to be addressed are those of competency of the patient and will be discussed in the next section.

Assessment

In assessing the patient with dementia the physician is attempting to answer three questions:

Table 2.7 Clues to 'treatable' causes of dementria

Disease	Findings	Diagnostic test
Depression Hematoma	Flat affect; psychomotor slowing Fluctuating symptoms; drowsiness	Past history of depression; Subdural brain scan/CAT
Neoplasm	Focal neurological signs	CAT scan
Drug toxicity	Depends on drug	Drug level; trial off drug;
Deficiency	Anemia; neuropathy	serum B12; Schilling's;
Hypothyroidism	Signs of myxedema	low T4; high TSH
Normal pressure hydrocephalus	Gait disorder incontinence of urine	
Hepatic encephalopathy	Signs of liver disease/failure	Liver function Tests, EEG
Neurosyphilis	Other neurological signs	Serology

1. Is dementia present?
2. What are the consequences for the patient, in other words what is the severity (mild, moderate or severe)?
3. What is the likely etiology?

The criteria for diagnosing dementia are well described in the DSM IIIR. Clearly, a consistent memory loss, associated with other cognitive impairments, in a fully conscious patient, which interferes with their social/occupational function without reversibility is necessary for the diagnosis to be substantiated.

At this stage the physician should have a good idea as to the nature of the patient's problems. The features will help to determine the extent of further investigation that is necessary and also the treatment that is indicated. The findings from history and examination are the most important part of the whole procedure.

Plan

Diagnostic

In addition to the tests that all patients receive, these patients should have serum B12 measured and syphilis serology performed. Other tests depend upon the clinical features (Fig. 2.1). It can be seen that those with a typical onset of gradual decline over a period of months or years need limited examination and CAT scan is not indicated. However detailed examination by a neuropsychologist helps in defining Alzheimer's disease as the probable diagnosis, for example the finding of dysphasia and perceptual problems with widespread changes, early on in the course of the disease.

It is important to determine the level of competency that a patient has, since this has a profound influence on future care. There are several areas that should be addressed:

1. *Decision making with regard to treatment*. This is something that has to be considered early on. The physician needs to assess what the patients contribution is with regard to consent, and so on. Does a surrogate decision-maker need to be identified and does there need to be a legal guardian?
2. *Judgement in self-care*. This will involve observation of the patient and usually occupational therapy assessment. It is important to know if it is safe for the patient to be left on their own unsupervised for periods of time or whether constant supervision is necessary.
3. *Financial competency*. Does the patient understand what assets they have and are they capable of handling money. Psychiatric consultation may be necessary in some of these patients. If the patient appears to be incompetent then families need to be advised to apply for guardianship.
4. *Ability to drive a motor vehicle*. Many patients who present with dementia are still driving motor vehicles. This aspect needs to be considered and if the assessment by the physician, occupational therapist and neuropsychologist is that driving would be dangerous then this needs to be brought to the attention of the patient, the guardian and the licensing authority.

There are other areas of competency that one looks at including the ability to execute a will and being able to serve as a juror in court. These will not be considered further here.

Management

If a reversible cause is identified this should of course be treated. This is a rare event in geriatric practice. Although patients with low B12 or with hypothyroidism are often identified and treated, it is unusual to see major improvement in cognitive function. Associated problems which may be contributing to a reduction in level of function are frequently found. Any problem should be corrected if it is thought that it will benefit the patient's well-being.

Patients with persisting cognitive impairment require management in a similar manner to those with acute confusional states which has been discussed. Patients do better in familiar surroundings so that it is important to maintain them at home for as long as possible. One needs to be aware of the considerable strain that care providers are under and should be helped by appropriate education and with respite care.

Psychotropic or hypnotic drugs should be avoided as far as possible but can be extremely useful in some situations. For example with the induction of sleep or calming aggressive behaviour. This was discussed with acute confusional states and the dosage schedules apply. Other pharmaceutical agents have been recommended to replace impaired neurotransmitter function with claims of beneficial effect. At the present time the evidence does not exist to allow the recommendation for general use of these agents.

Patient education

There is much to be done here in helping families and others cope with the strain of caring for a patient with dementia. Information needs to be provided with regards to what help is available. Care providers need to be warned of the significance of a change in level of function of the patient – that this often indicates the development of an intercurrent problem for which medical help should be sought. Patients and their families usually need follow up to help with future decisions about care when it is becoming too heavy at home.

Suggested reading

Katzman, R. and Terry, R. D. (1982). *The Neurology of Aging*. F. A. Davis, Philadelphia, Pennsylvania.

Lipowski, Z. J. (1983). Transient cognitive disorders (delirium, acute confusional states) in the elderly. *Amer. J. Psych.*, **140**: 1426–36.

Rabins, P. V. and Folstein, M. F. (1982). Delirium and Dementia: Diagnostic criteria and fatality rates. *Brit. J. Psych.*, **140**: 149–53.

3

Immobility

1. Introduction

Immobility is an inability, either partial or complete of the patient to move. It is one of the most common forms of impaired function in elderly patients. The patient may be described as having difficulty in their movements, and be restricted within their normal range of environments, for example block-bound, house-bound, room-bound, chair-bound or bed-bound. The presentation may be even less specific and which may be loosely described as failure to thrive.

At the age of 90, it is suggested half of seniors will experience some major impairment of independence relating to mobility. The individuals normal expectations and lifestyle will often determine the stage at which they will present. A previously active senior may be reluctant to accept difficulties in accessing public transport and restrictions of mobility to their immediate environment. In such a case an early presentation might be seen. Conversely a sedentary senior may only complain at the extent of being room-bound or even chair-bound. In such cases the problems contributing to the mobility difficulty may have been present for a considerable length of time. A variety of adaptive mechanisms may have occurred such as the use of ambulatory aids, modifications of the environment and assistance from formal and informal services.

2. Predisposing factors

The factors that predispose to immobility are multifactorial and often poorly understood. They can be loosely linked under three main subheadings of problems in tolerance and endurance, locomotor systems and postural control.

Problems of reduced tolerance and endurance

The individual's previous expectations and lifestyles will determine what they consider to be normal ranges of mobility. Such expectations may change due to a variety of factors. Some may be understandable such as cyclic variations in the weather, others may be less easily understood and reflect abnormalities of mood and motivation. Depressive symptomatology has a reported prevalence as high as 20 per cent in community residing seniors. Adverse major life events such as bereavement, isolation, loss of autonomy and major illness are common. The increase in dependency resulting from immobility may in itself foster depression and so contribute to further dependency.

The individual's tolerance to exertion may be impaired over a long period. This may reflect disease processes affecting the cardiovascular and respiratory system presenting over a number of years. Hematological abnormalities such as anemia may present with apathy and reduced mobility. A variety of endocrine metabolic disorders may reduce tolerance. Multiple medications may interact or act singly to interfere with the individual's endurance and tolerance.

Reduced tolerance and activity in itself predisposes to further immobility. The cardiovascular responses to reduced activity included orthostatic hypotension, increased heart rate with exertion, reduced stroke volume and impaired oxygen utilization. Changes in the respiratory system include increased physiological dead space, abnormal ventilation perfusion ratios and predisposition to aspiration pneumonia. Locomotor changes include predisposition to osteoporosis, reduced range of movements of joints and articular cartilage degeneration.

Locomotor Problems

Locomotor changes are common with increase in age. The bones tend to undergo demineralization with resulting increase in osteopenia. Osteopenia increases the likelihood of fracture should injury occur. Increasing curvature of the spine result in abnormalities of gait and inefficiency of the locomotor process. Wedge fractures may occur producing pain and worsening mobility. Some degree of degenerative arthritis is common with increase in age. These changes are seen in a majority of people in the seventh and eighth decades on radiographs of the cervical spine. In the majority they appear asymptomatic. It can be demonstrated, however, that the energy expenditure by an elderly person for the same level of activity is increased compared to a younger person suggesting that perhaps that some of these abnormalities may make the locomotor system less efficient.

Changes in the muscular system are common with age. There is a generally observed decrease in lean body mass, with particular loss of fast reacting muscle fibers. These changes may not be an inevitable consequence of aging, but may reflect changes in nutrition, activity and disease. Regardless, they tend to render the musculoskeletal system less efficient. For example, perhaps 80 per cent of the knee, hip, pelvic and trunk musculature are required for an old person to stand up from a chair, compared to only 40 per cent for a young person.

Posture Control Problems

Impairment of postural control is not an uncommon change with age. Characteristically, the older patient feels insecure in the upright position. Changes in gait even in the absence of disease have been reported in seniors (see falls). The postural and gait changes in all ages are complex and a variety of diseases can also contribute and exacerbate such changes.

3. Precipitating Factors

A number of elderly patients with problems with immobility already had evidence of reduced mobility prior to this and so are predisposed to further immobility as indicated above. In a previously independent mobile senior, the precipitating factors which produce immobility are often more severe. A gradual or sudden decline into immobility can be precipitated by a variety of disease states.

Neurological conditions such as stroke or Parkinson's disease are not uncommon precipitating factors. Cardiovascular and respiratory disease can present atypically as falls and decrease in mobility. In fact falls with or without obvious injury may result in immobility. Anxieties following falls, trauma, or physical abuse may result in adoption of abnormal gait, inappropriate restriction of activity and eventual immobility. The fear of falling is not an uncommon precipitant of progressive immobility.

Arthralgia and arthritis often present with some degree of restricted mobility. Pain and/or stiffness may be a major factor in this and may be intermittent in severity. Joint disruption and bony deformity may seriously interfere with a normal range of movement. A fracture may present as immobility in the demented, elderly where symptom reporting and localizing may be poor.

Conditions such as polymyalgia rheumatica, and polymyositis may present as immobility. Abnormalities of metabolism and endocrine systems such as hypothyroidism, hyponatremia and poorly controlled diabetes mellitus may also present with reduced mobility.

Social and psychological factors are known to precipitate immobility. Sudden bereavement with reactive depression can result in loss of motivation, decrease in activity and therefore both predisposition and precipitation of immobility.

Subjective

The duration and nature of onset of the reduced mobility is important to clarify. A gradual onset with initially some restriction in distance travel, progressing to dependency on assistance of holding on to someone else or furniture, is often associated with multiple predisposing factors. Not uncommonly, such a gradual onset of difficulties in mobility is associated with failure in other activities of daily living such as home care, self care, food preparation activities and continence control.

A sudden onset of immobility or rapid acceleration should always serve as a hallmark of illness. A previous history of falls is often relevant as discussed under fears of falling. Infection, cardiac failure, metabolic and endocrine disorders should be suspected when problems of tolerance or motivation are seen. Focal limb weakness or instability should raise the possibility of cerebral vascular events, acute joint or bony pathology. Complaints of pain need to be actively sought but may be vague or masked by disorientation. A drug history is always imperative particularly in relation to the onset of the problem of mobility.

Evidence of major anxiety or depressive states need to be sought. Depressive symptoms may be overlooked and attributed to 'aging'.

Objective

Careful inspection for evidence of injury must be undertaken since fractures can be surprisingly pain free. Unexplained bruising or hematoma should always raise suspicion of fracture. Local tenderness requires explanation.

The hydration status of the patient should always be carefully assessed as dehydration may be difficult to appreciate and present only as apathy and retardation.

The neurological examination should include a careful search for evidence of focal signs which may give clues to possible etiology. In particular, evidence will be sought for signs of pyramidal or extrapyramidal disease, peripheral neuropathies or autonomic neuropathies and evidence of anterior horn disease.

The careful examination of medications should include the containers and methods of self-application. Inappropriate use of medications or polypharmacy may only become apparent when multiple tablets are found within a single bottle.

If the immobility is secondary or has been present for some time, then other relevant features should be sought. Evidence of muscle wasting may explain an inability to get from a sitting to standing position. In an elderly individual who uses perhaps 70 to 80 per cent of the musculature to stand when healthy, relatively short periods of bedrest, of the order of 14 days, may result in loss of 20–30 per cent of muscle bulk making it a physical impossibility for that individual to stand. Contractures may form with prolonged immobility. Immobilized joints develop capsular adhesions and articular cartilage degeneration with secondary arthritis. The individual who has been in the recumbent position for several days will suffer problems with orthostatic hypotension when sitting up. If nursed in a reclining chair, such an individual will have difficulty in maintaining the vertical position and will tend to fall backwards when standing.

The examination is not complete until the patient has transferred themselves from bed to chair and demonstrated their ability to stand. Stability of standing and sitting should be noted. It should be repeated with the eyes closed and open. The patient's gait should be observed and they should be asked to walk heel-to-toe. Evidence of footdrop, poor foot clearance, festinant gait, broad-based gait, and so on, may give valuable clues as to possible etiological factors in the individual's immobility. Often the assistance of a nurse or other physician is necessary to safely assess such gait patterns.

Assessment and Plan

Diagnostic

Mobility problems are common in a variety of elderly patients presenting with diverse diagnostic problems. In many instances the secondary immobility of disease is avoidable, and prevention of this problem in the ill, hospitalized elderly cannot be overemphasized. Very few conditions require complete bedrest for more than a day or two. The simple action of spending several hours in a chair with standing and transferring to a commode or bathroom will prevent many of the hemodynamic, respiratory and locomotor changes of immobility. Many ill elderly are themselves suffering from a variety of chronic disorders and so even more predisposed to immobility. There are many possible consequences of immobility which can be prevented by early attention to this problem (Table 3.1).

It is important to list mobility problems as a diagnostic challenge and enter into a search for definite treatable causes. In the short-term, it may require more paramedical staff time to allow the patient with Parkinson's disease to stand, transfer and toilet themselves by restricting themselves to supervision, prompting or minimal assistance. The

Table 3.1 Sequelae of reduced mobility

Immobility
Deconditioning
Impaired balance
Orthostatic hypotension
Reduced exercise tolerance
Osteoporosis
Contractures
Decubiti
Rhabdomyolysis

alternative however, of lifting the person on and off a commode or keeping them in bed and using bed pans or diapers will rapidly create a dependent, heavy care individual. This will ultimately be far more expensive in manpower terms and result in needless human suffering.

Management

The management of the elderly individual with reduced mobility is four-fold (Table 3.2). First of all precipitating factors once identified need appropriate treatment. For example, the pain of degenerative arthritis must be controlled. The second phase is avoidance of secondary immobility, and restoration of former activity by regular activity, encourage appropriate posture and avoid abnormal positioning of limbs to prevent development of contractures. Skin care is optimized. The third phase is optimization of the environment in such a manner as to minimize handicap. This may involve the provision of walking aids, bars in the bathroom, raised beds and high back chairs with a solid base. The fourth phase which may not be applicable in all patients is to improve upon the former level of function by ongoing rehabilitation.

Table 3.2 Management of reduced mobility

1. Identify and treat precipitants
2. Avoid secondary immobility and restore function
3. Optimize environment to minimize handicap
4. Increase strength and endurance

The therapist will need to focus on two aspects of rehabilitation, strength and endurance. Patients with reduced mobility, particularly following hospitalization, are inevitably deconditioned. The weakness of muscle groups can be identified on physical examination and improvement can be objectively measured. Regular resistive exercise can increase in strength in a short period of time and patients can be rehabilitated to a functional level. It has become clear that in many frail elders the reduction in activity has occurred over a long time period. The goal in many of these patients should be higher than simply restoration of function. Optimal function may be achieved by strengthening exercises and activities to increase endurance over a longer time period. Such exercise programs can be achieved in the setting of a day hospital, for example. In this way, the risk of reduced mobility in the future may be reduced.

The overall objective of this assessment and management is to allow the individual to live at an independent level. The individual's premorbid state, level of activity and motivation to improve will dictate realistic goals and objectives. One has to also accept the realities of the reduced life-span of the elderly population compared to more traditional rehabilitation programs. It may be more realistic to accept adaptive posture and gait rather than strive for the perfect results one might ideally wish for. Necessarily, treatment options aimed at improving ambulation must take into consideration the need for independence in other activities of daily living. Clothing and foot wear are necessary for maintenance of dignity but also for optimization of gait.

Patient Education

Motivation and tolerance problems need appreciation and treatment as separate problems. Necessarily, fatigue will be experienced by the patient, who has for some weeks been immobile, after relatively short periods of exertion. Education of the patient and relatives may be necessary. The importance of avoiding attitudes and actions on their part which encourage dependency has to be stressed. Relatives may perceive the risk of falling as serious and request restraints and avoidance of ambulation. The dangers of this to the patient in impairing mobility further, predisposing to infection, pressure sores and more serious injuries are obvious.

Complications of immobility such as contractures and pressure sores may require prolonged treatment which in itself is painful. These options need to be carefully explained to the patient and relatives. It is also necessary to establish these principles with the nursing staff and other care providers, particularly when new programs are being established.

Suggested reading

Cheshire, C. M. and Cummings, W. J. K. (1985). The Musculoskeletal System – Skeletal muscle. In: Testbook of Geriatric Medicine and Gerontology. Brocklehurst Third Edition. Churchill Livingstone.

Lewis, C. B. (1989). Improving Mobility in Older Persons. A Manual for Geriatric Specialists. Aspen Publishers Inc.

Steinberg, F. U. (1980). The Immobilized Patient. Plenum Medical Book Company.

4

Falls

Introduction

Falls are often poorly defined in the literature and this explains some of the problems in interpreting the available data. We will use the term fall for 'an involuntary event producing a change in posture resulting in the individual adopting an unplanned supine position'. A trip refers to a similar event but where some corrective maneuvers results in maintenance of an erect posture.

There have been several community surveys which indicate a prevalence of one-third to one-half of the elderly population in the community having problems with falls. The incidence of the falls increases markedly with age.

Falls have a particularly bad prognosis resulting in much long term morbidity and some lethal complications. In a study of falls in the home treated at a community hospital 42 per cent were admitted to hospital, nearly two-thirds with fractures. The average duration of stay was 27.3 days and 9 per cent of the patients died. In a study of an institutionalized population 65 per cent of the residents who had 6 or more falls died within the 2.2 years of the study. It has been reported that three-quarters of fatal accidents due to falls in a residential home involve those over the age of 65.

In the classical study of Sheldon one-third of the falls were accidental in nature and about one-third of these occurred on the stairs. Nevertheless, most falls are regarded as being due to ill health of one sort or another. Fallers are more likely to have other mobility problems, difficulties with daily living function and associated serious disease such as stroke or heart disease.

Predisposing Factors to Falls

Increasing age, female sex, isolation and illness appear to be associated with increased frequency of at least clinically significant falls. It is suggested that falls occur in the presence of such factors in the absence of often clinically detectable causes. A number of factors have been implicated as predisposing the elderly to falls (Table 4.1). Much of the work investigating falls has concentrated on their relationship to sway. There is an increase in the amount of sway as age advances. This inability to control sway in advancing years is likely to increase the risk of falls. Fallers typically sway more and the speed of sway is greater than non-fallers. Sway is a relatively crude assessment of the function of balance and a variety of organ systems may undergo pathological change and contribute to it. In simple terms, finding increased sway informs us that there is a problem with balance and that further analysis is required.

Standing from the sitting position has been studied using a Kistler force platform and healthy elderly subjects need more time to stabilize the

Table 4.1 Predisposing factors to falls in the elderly

Changes in center of gravity
Reduced proprioceptive input
Reduced visual cues
Retarded corrective movements to postural change
Anxiety
Previous falls
Drugs
Other conditions affecting gait, e.g. parkinson's disease
Inappropriate walking aids
Environmental hazards

antero-posterior sway in the standing-up motion and the grade of sway is greater in females than males. The center of force in females is located more posteriorly.

Pathological changes in gait have been recorded in the elderly since ancient times. Specific gait abnormalities may be associated with disease processes which are reversed with treatment of the underlying condition and rehabilitation. Examples are those following fracture of the lower limb, stroke and Parkinson's disease. Ataxic, hemiplegic, spastic, equine and many other gaits are readily recognized clinically.

Even healthy old people show slower walking speeds, shorter step length and lower frequency of stepping, though little change in stride width when compared to younger people. Although the velocity of walking has been shown to decrease slightly with advancing age, this was found to be dependent more on associated pathology than on age itself.

Environmental hazards such as poor illumination, steps, scatter mats, pets, and so on are unfortunately common in the homes of many seniors, so trips are not uncommon. Any change that reduces postural stability, or impairs the ability to correct a trip will predispose the older person to falls. Some of the changes described are secondary to an identifiable disease state. For others no single pathology can be defined, and it is thought that the changes (for example sway) are secondary to the 'aging process'. Although further studies are likely to show that these 'age changes' are after occult disease which have the potential for modification or even prevention.

Precipitating Factors to Falls

The causes of falls are numerous. In addition to accidents resulting from age related predisposition such as impaired vision and multiple interacting environmental factors, there are a number of pathological conditions to be considered (Table 4.2). Any condition that reduces 'well being', increases sway, reduces judgement, and so on may precipitate a fall. The most common problems are adverse reactions to drugs, infections and metabolic diseases. These conditions impair many functions, increasing the chance of falling whilst the actual event occurs secondary to a trip.

The adverse drug reaction may precipitate a fall by different pathophysiological effects – for example one of the most frequent would be orthostatic hypotension. This may be induced by any number of drugs, perhaps the most common being hypotensive agents including diuretics (Table 4.2).

Table 4.2 Conditions associated with falls

Stroke
Cerebral ischemia
Epilepsy
Syncope
Transient ischemic attack (TIA)
Hypovolemia (shock)
Carotid hypersensitivity
Postural hypotension
Adverse drug reactions
Cardiac arrhythmia
Aortic stenosis
Vestibular dysfunction
Anemia and polycythemia
Vertigo
Infection
Ataxia

It can be seen that vertebrobasilar insufficiency is not included in Table 4.2. This is a diagnosis often made, however, there is usually little to support it. Most elderly individuals have cervical spondylosis and significant degenerative changes on radiograph. Arteriosclerosis is almost universal. Many of these patients fall when they turn their head, yet close inquiry most often reveals that the individual had a slow, 'protective' gait and the head turn represents a loss of concentration or focus, rather than true vertigo.

As with other areas of impaired function there may well be more than a single contributing factor. It is a commonly observed clinical picture that a series of falls often commence after one major fall. The patient becomes increasingly anxious and prone to hold onto furniture and reach out in panic. By so doing they adopt abnormal postures and predispose to a vicious cycle of increasing falls. A temporary transfer to a 'safe' environment such as a hospital ward with reassurance and patience often results in the relief of 'fear of falling' and the falls cease. Unless the 'hostile' environment is modified in some way the situation often reoccurs. Forty per cent of admissions to a Manchester teaching hospital with fracture of the neck or femur had presented on at least one occasion to the accident and emergency department in the preceding three months. Less than 25 per cent of them had been referred for some investigation of their falls and most returned to the same environment.

Subjective

It is vital to determine the circumstances that surround the fall(s). The 'pre' fall condition of the patient must be determined. It is important to document the normal level of activity and independence of the patient, as well as the activity at the time of the fall.

If possible the patient should be asked to relate the sequence of events, and their interpretation. It may not be possible to obtain a history from the patient. Care providers will be interviewed as a matter of course, the information may be particularly valuable if the fall has been observed. Common questions to be asked include:

1. Do the falls occur in similar circumstances, e.g. on micturition?
2. Were there any associated symptoms at the time?
3. Specifically did the patient lose consciousness?
4. Were there any changes in pulse preceding the event, or the presence of palpitations?
5. Were there features of syncope, anginal chest pain or an epileptic aura?

All of these questions are important to ask, in order to define the pathophysiological change and probable etiology (Table 4.2). A careful history should be taken of present and previous medical conditions. A previous history of disorders of locomotion such as a stroke may be relevant in explaining abnormalities of gait and predisposition to falls. The presence of significant foot-drop may predispose the individual to trips on stairs and steps. A history of diabetes mellitus makes autonomic neuropathy resulting in orthostatic hypotension a possibility.

A variety of drugs may be relevant in contributing to falls. Hypnotics, sedatives, or psychotropic drugs may depress the individuals sensorium producing clumsiness and risk of falling. Antihypertensive medication may produce postural hypotension. Drugs with an anticholinergic property may cause visual blurring and increase likelihood of falling.

Enquiring about postfall sequela may be useful in the assessment of the fall. A history of drowsiness and/or associated incontinence of urine may be suggestive of an ictal phenomenon. Focal weakness after the fall may imply a post-ictal phenomenon, TIA, or frank stroke depending on the duration of the deficit. Symptoms of palpitation, cardiac chest pain or shortness of breath suggest a cardiac etiology. The presence of tachypnea, pyrexia, and respiratory distress raises the possibility of chest infection. Hypotension raises the possibility of hypovolemia or a cardiogenic source.

It is important to determine whether the fall was associated with a period of loss of consciousness. If this is the case and there is also a history of pallor, feeling cold and sweaty, and faint one should consider syncope as being present. The presence of involuntary movements associated with loss of consciousness could raise the possibility of an ictal event.

The complaint of a sudden fall to the ground without loss of consciousness, associated with inability to stand, which is corrected when this person is assisted into the upright position raises the possibility of a drop attack. Sometimes the subjects themselves spontaneously volunteer that they learn to abort the period of lower limb weakness by pushing on an arm chair or wall.

A perforated abdominal viscus sometimes initially presents with a little more than a sudden fall and post-fall confusion with vague abdominal tenderness, so should always be considered.

A history of previous falls is relevant. Not uncommonly an individual presenting with one fall has had other falls in the past. Sometimes anxiety and apprehension about such falls makes the individual more prone to falling by their shaking, jerky panic when reaching out for furniture, and soon, to support themselves.

Objective

The first priority for the physician is to identify any immediate physical injury resulting from the fall which includes assessment of conscious level, airway patency and circulatory status (see Chapter 10, Disturbance of Consciousness). The next priority is then to ascertain the extent of any injuries to soft tissues, skeletal structures, and underlying viscera. It is suggested that perhaps as many as 25 per cent of all falls are complicated by some physical injury. Colles' fractures are more often seen in women with a peak around the second decade after the menopause. Fractures of the neck of femur are seen more commonly after the age of 75 and again more commonly in females.

In the determination of the presence and severity of injury certain factors have to be appreciated. Pain may not be complained of or may be poorly localized. Disorientation may mask the presence of pain. Hypothermia is an important complication of falls and requires identification, but may mask other complications. Even relatively short periods of lying in one position may impair skin integrity such that pressure sores rapidly develop.

Injuries to the shoulder girdle and upper limb are usually possible to detect on pure clinical grounds because of the overt deformity and crepitus. Fractures of the hip may be more difficult and not necessarily associated with external rotation and shortening of the affected limb. Any history of head injury particularly associated with periods of unconsciousness necessarily require sequential estimations of conscious level to exclude significant subdural or extradural hematomas.

The underlying etiological factors may result in other complications requiring immediate attention. A myocardial infarction may necessitate treatment of severe left ventricular failure. A fall from hypovolemia secondary to gastrointestinal bleed may necessitate transfusion. Infections not uncommonly present with falls in the elderly and rapid decline can occur if treatment is withheld.

Having determined that the immediate situation is stable the examination can then be directed towards assessing factors contributing to the falls.

An assessment of mental state is obligatory including measurement of conscious level and mood. Individuals with chronic confusional states are more likely to fall. Acute delirium is not uncommonly associated also with an excess of falls. Anxiety will render the individual vulnerable to falling and interfere with rehabilitation.

The subject's sensory apparatus requires assessment. Visual impairment may be the result of underlying ocular disease and also possibly arise from readily correctable factors such as inappropriate spectacles. The subject's hearing should be assessed and any hearing aid be reviewed so as to optimize communication. Evidence of peripheral neuropathies and perceptive impairment may explain a falling tendency. Cortical sensory problems with neglect may explain episodes of walking into objects and tripping.

The feet should be examined carefully. Evidence of bunions, ingrown toe nails, and ulcers should be sought. Painful conditions of the feet may explain the individual's instability. The appropriateness of footwear in both size and state of repair should be determined. Attention should also be paid to the condition of the remainder of the patient's skin and a careful examination made for the evidence of pressure sores and ammonia rashes.

The individual's blood pressure should be measured particularly in relation to changes in posture. Examination of the cardiovascular system should be directed towards determination of significant arrhythmias or valvular heart disease.

The abdomen should be examined for evidence of tenderness or absent bowel sounds suggesting a perforated viscus. The presence of a pulsatile mass should raise the possibility of a ruptured aortic aneurysm. The presence of faecal masses and/or hard feces on rectal examination should raise the possibility of faecal impaction with impairment of cognition and therefore predisposition to falls.

A careful neurological examination should follow to assess for evidence of a cerebrovascular event. The presence of an Akinetic Rigidity Syndrome such as Parkinson's disease and progressive supranuclear palsy should be sought. Disturbances of coordination and ataxia suggestive of cerebellar disease should be tested for. Involuntary movements should be noted.

The individual's sitting balance, ability to stand from sitting, standing balance, posture, and gait should be carefully assessed. Gait abnormalities resulting from abnormal posture and deformities such as kyphosis or scoliosis are usually easy to detect. The shortening of a leg on account of an old femoral fracture or severe osteoarthrosis of the hip may cause an abnormal gait. Unstable and peculiar gaits in which both legs are markedly and externally rotated may be due to bilateral osteoarthrosis of the hip. Marked hip stiffness resulting from osteoarthrosis may produce a gait with small limited rocky movements. The lateral instability of a grossly disorganized knee such as that seen in severe osteoarthritis will sometimes result in an unsteady wobbling gait. Hopping gaits are a result of painful feet and limping may be due to bone pain of various causes or intermittent claudication. A foot drop may be readily noted. Broad based stomping steps may be suggestive of a peripheral neuropathy with absence of proprioceptive input.

Assessment

As a result of the history taking and examination the physician should have taken the problem solution beyond 'fall'. The predisposed senior is more likely to fall and the statistical evidence supports this. Close scrutiny of a fall may lead the clinician to the conclusion that it is a simple trip in a predisposed individual. It is hoped that predisposing factors will be identified. These then take on their own identity as problems, some of which are modifiable, for example an exercise program to improve gait and muscle strength. Advice may also be offered in terms of reducing environmental risk. Those falls not identified as simple trips may be classified as medical, and a search is made for the condition(s) which has precipitated the fall.

The precipitant(s) may be identified and any problems are defined so that each can be treated.

Laboratory investigations will be required to complete the assessment of seniors presenting with falls. Initial assessments should include a comprehensive screen as discussed in Chapter 1. Evidence of local contusion, tenderness or deformity should be taken as indicators for further local radiographic examination.

In specific instances other investigations such as CAT scan, abdominal ultrasound, electroencephalogram, and arterial studies may be indicated depending upon the clinical pointers.

Plans

Diagnostic

This has been discussed under 'Assessment'.

Management

The management of the falling elderly individual requires removal or modification of predisposing factors, treatment of precipitating factors, and optimization of the environment. The sensory apparatus should be assessed and optimised wherever possible. Appropriate foot care and foot wear should be provided.

Medications, if thought to be contributory, should be appropriately adjusted. The specific management of stroke, Parkinson's disease, arthralgia, fractures, and so on will not be discussed here as they are discussed in detail in other chapters. One point worth emphasizing is that pain and anxiety are not uncommon contributors to falls so require treatment in their own right. Often milder analgesia can be used if given on a regular basis rather than when required. Reassurance, supervision, and provision of a walking aid can go a long way to remove an anxiety which may be contributing to the falling tendency. Sometimes in the absence of contraindications to their use a small dose of a betablocker such as Propranolol at 10 mg twice daily can block the peripheral manifestations of panic attacks which may be seen in individuals with multiple falls. Often such a beta blockade can be discontinued after several days.

The management of fractures necessarily involves a close cooperation between geriatrics and orthopedics. The orthopedic procedure should be directed towards making it possible to rapidly mobilize the individual. The geriatrician's role being the management of any previous medical problems, advice about medications, and direction of appropriate rehabilitation.

Not infrequently an individual after admission to hospital with some adjustment in medications and treatment of underlying conditions will no longer suffer falls. However, on discharge back to the previous environment, not uncommonly the falls recommence. Environmental modification is often neglected in discussions on falls, and environmental manipulations to make the living space safer for the impaired elderly is of great value. Information from medical examination and gait analysis can only be properly evaluated in the context of the individuals immediate environment. The value of a predischarge home assessment with the patient present cannot be over-stressed. These assessments are usually done by an occupational therapist. Suggested schedule for evaluation of the environment is included in Table 4.3.

Therapists have often noted that different floor surfaces may have apparently different effects on gait. The use of a standard walker for example being more difficult on a carpeted surface. Often simple measures such as appropriate removal of hazards, for example mats and loose carpet edges, and the clearing of a cluttered room will go a long way towards reducing the likelihood of further falls. Appropriate furniture of a suitable height and design may make it much easier for the individual to stand. Walking aids such as canes and walkers may be of value. The type of walking aid must however be appropriate for the environment with sufficient space available for its use. Rails in the vicinity of the bath and toilet may be of great assistance. The provision of electronic devices to enable aid to be summoned in the event of a fall may considerably relieve the anxiety of the subject and care givers. Their use has to be restricted to the cognitively intact. Those individuals suffering even mild cognitive decline cannot handle them.

Part of the rehabilitation of falls is training and instruction in appropriate measures to take in the event of further falls. The individual should attempt to keep themselves warm and have accessible methods of summoning aid. Training in methods of getting up once the person has fallen may be of value.

Table 4.3 Possible environmental hazards in relation to falls

1. *Rugs:* loose, corner(s) turned up, etc., including rugs on stairs, scatter rugs, and broadloom.
2. *Furniture:* cluttered, obstructing walking pathways, unsafe furniture for person's functional level, i.e. furniture on wheels, rocking chair, furniture that is too low.
3. *Stairs:* too steep, no hand rail/or loose hand rail, too deep, step length too short, poor lighting, loose rug on stairs, stairway open on one/or both sides.
4. *Floor surfaces:* slippery, wet, inside or outside, scattered objects on floor.
5. *Exposed cords:* telephone, cablevision, etc., in walking path.
6. *Reaching ability:* to high and low places, e.g., cupboards, floor.
7. *Emergency systems access:* difficulty in accessing emergency systems should the need arise . . . telephone alert system. It also surveys the ability to physically exit the dwelling in the event of an emergency.
8. *Previous accidents:* evidence of burn marks – rugs, furniture, pots, etc.
9. *Electrical:* poor lighting, inaccessible or broken light switches, unsafe electrical wiring, overloading of circuits unsafe use of appliances (stove, iron, heating pad, electric heater).
10. *Judgement:* poor judgment re: safe living (impaired mental status, refusal of necessary support systems).
11. *Alcohol:* abuse of alcohol.
12. *Medications:* unsafe use of medications polypharmacy abuse, over/under medicating, use of over-the-counter (OTC) drugs, using other peoples medications.
13. *Other:* mobility aid, footwear, impaired vision or hearing.

Suggested reading

Cape, R. (1978). In: Cape, R. (ed). Aging: It's Complex Management. Maryland, Harper, Row, pp. 113–36.

Cummings, S. R., Nevitt, M. C. and Kidd, S. (1988). Forgetting Falls in the Elderly. *JAGS* **36** (7): 613–16.

Drachman, D. A. (1972). An Approach to the Dizzy Patient. *Neurology* **22**: 323–33.

Kapoor, W. N. (1987). Evaluation of Syncope in the Elderly. *JAGS* **35** (8): 826–8.

Radebaugh, T. S., Hadley, E. and Suzman, R. (eds). (1985). Clinics in Geriatric Medicine, Symposium on Falls in the Elderly: Biologic and Behavioural Aspects, 1:3. Philadelphia, Saunders, WB.

Rowe, J. W. Falls (1982). In: Rowe, J. W. and Besdine, R. W. (eds). Health and Disease in Old Age. Boston, Little, Brown pp. 393–98.

Rubenstein, L. Z., Robbins, A. S., Shulman, B. L., Rosado, J., Osterweil, D. and Josephson, K. R. (1988). Falls and Instability in the Elderly. *JAGS* **36** (3): 266–78.

Sheldon, J. H. (1960). On the Natural History of Falls in Old Age. BMJ December 10: 5214.

Solomon, D. H. (1988). Intensive Course in Geriatric Medicine and Board Review, Syllabus. Beverley Hills, California, Regents of the University of California at Los Angeles (UCLA) pp. 75–84.

Tinetti, M. E. (1987). Factors Associated with Serious Injury During Falls by Ambulatory Nursing Home Residents. *JAGS* **35** (7): 644–8.

Tinetti, M. E., Speechley, M. and Ginter, S. F. (1988). Risk Factors For Falls Among Elderly Persons Living in the Community. *New Engl. J. Med.*, **319**: 1701–7.

Tinetti, M. E. and Speechley, M. (1989). Prevention of Falls Among The Elderly. *New Engl. J. Med.*, **320**: 1055–9.

Venna, N. (1987). Dizziness, Falling, and Fainting: Differential Diagnosis in the Aged – Part I. Modern Medicine of Canada: **42** (12): 884–95.

Venna, N. (1988). Dizziness, Falling, and Fainting: Differential Diagnosis in the Aged – Part II. Modern Medicine of Canada: **43** (2): 128–41.

5

Urinary incontinence

1. Introduction

Urinary incontinence can be defined as the involuntary loss of urine, which is a social or hygienic problem and is objectively demonstrable.

Incontinence should be considered to be either established (true) or transient. When incontinence is being seen for the first time and it is not known if it has been present for a long period of time it should be treated as transient. This will ensure that the treatable, more easily reversible problems will be dealt with, before advancing to more complicated investigational approaches such as cystometry or urological consultations.

2. Predisposing Factors

With advancing age the combined effects of aging and disease predispose many elderly individuals to incontinence of urine. There is an age-related increase in the prevalence of urinary incontinence in both sexes. Community surveys have suggested a prevalence of 10–20 per cent in women and 5–15 per cent in males over 65 years of age. A number of surveys of institutionalized elderly suggest a prevalence usually between 25 and 40 per cent. There is some correlation between cognitive status and mobility in determining the prevalence of incontinence. The prevalence, for example, in residential homes has been reported as 17 per cent and in psychogeriatric patients to be as high as 89 per cent. A variety of age-associated changes have been described which include decreased bladder capacity, increased residual urine, a tendency to uninhibited bladder contraction, decreased maximal urethral pressure and prostatic enlargement.

With advancing age nocturia becomes more frequent, the majority of healthy elderly individuals will pass urine from one to three times a night. At the same time the 'safe time' between awareness of a full bladder, and the time to empty decreases. Most people adjust to this and recognize that they cannot suppress the urge to urinate as they could when younger.

3. Precipitation of Incontinence

These changes described above predispose the elderly to incontinence when the system is stressed. Anything that decreases awareness, inhibits access or increases the 'load' (the volume of urine produced) may result in incontinence (Table 5.1). Conditions which interfere with orientation, and or sensory input will be associated with incontinence of a short duration which is exacerbated by changes in environment. A number of conditions interfering with mobility such as stroke, fracture, arthritis, and so on, particularly in the presence of urgency, readily precipitate incontinence. Problems with dexterity and clothing may contribute to incontinence and are often readily manipulable. Hyperosmolar urinary conditions such as with diabetes mellitus, polyuria from impaired tubular function and use of diuretics may result in frequency and incontinence particularly if associated with any of the other problems.

The problems which have been described will usually precipitate transient incontinence for the first time, but in some it remains even after the initial precipitants are reversed. This is referred to as established incontinence. There are four major types that should be considered (Table 5.2).

Incontinence is frequently found in those with advanced dementia. The cortical failure results in the patient being unaware that the bladder is distended. It may well be that these patients also have a bladder problem such as detrusor instability, but the cognitive impairment dominates the picture.

Hyper-reflexive (unstable bladder, detrusor instability) is one of the most common causes of incontinence in a geriatric population. It is characterized by involuntary loss of urine, often with some desire to void and usually associated with partial or complete uninhibited bladder contraction. The presence of detrusor instability, often explains why relatively small changes in mobility and dexterity result in incontinence. The individual may be able to tolerate only relatively small bladder volumes of the order of 50–100 mls but this can be consistent with continence if toileting is possible every 2–3 hours.

Overflow incontinence may be of two types: that due to an outlet obstruction (mechanical or dyssynergism), or a result of an atonic bladder secondary to neuropathy or spinal cord lesion. In both cases a significant residual urine will result, with predisposition to infection, back-flow effects and overflow of urine.

Stress incontinence is a condition found in females and is not usually found in younger age groups. It is characterized by the loss of small amounts of urine frequently. Such losses are precipitated by movement, straining, coughing or laughing.

Subjective

A description of the type of incontinence, frequency and its duration is necessary. The pattern of incontinence should be ascertained; as to whether it occurs throughout the 24-hour period or just at specific times. The relationship of the incontinence to drug administration should be sought. A careful history of bladder function should be obtained and include documentation of the number of micturitions during the night, frequency of micturition by the day, the presence or absence of urgency, dysuria, and dribbling incontinence. The presence or absence of these symptoms, together with their duration, is an essential guide to the differentiation of the diagnosis of incontinence.

From the information obtained it can usually be determined if the incontinence is transient or

Table 5.1 Precipitants of transient incontinence

		Mechanism
Loss of awareness	Disorientation confusion	Drugs Infection
Increased urinary flow	Diuresis	Drugs Diabetes Hypercalcaemia
Urinary overflow and obstruction	Outlet obstruction Atonia	Drugs Constipation Tumour Prolapse Surgery
Accessibility	Confusion Impaired dexerity	Frailty Multiple geriatric problems

Table 5.2 Causes of established incontinence

1. *Cognitive Impairment:* Involuntary loss of urine occurring because of cognitive impairment, disorientation in space, mobility limitations or dexterity problems.
2. *Hyperreflexive* (unstable bladder, detrusor instability): Involuntary loss of urine usually associated with a desire to void and usually associated with partial or complete uninhibited bladder contraction.
3. *Overflow* a) *Outlet obstruction* – mechanical (prostate, etc.)
– dyssynergia
involuntary loss of urine associated with a significant residual urine even after micturition.
4. *Stress incontinence:* Involuntary loss of urine occurring when the intravesical pressure exceeds the maximal urethral pressure in the absence of a bladder contraction.

established. If it is thought to be of short duration and transient, then questions need to be asked with regard to the common precipitants (Table 5.1).

It should be apparent if the patient has advanced dementia and whether there is awareness that the bladder is full. Patients with milder degrees of cognitive impairment should be asked directly if they know when their bladder is full.

An attempt should be made to distinguish between true stress incontinence and that which occurs with uninhibited bladder contractions of detrusor instability. The association of such episodes of incontinence with coughing, raised intra-abdominal pressure, standing, and so on. and the volumes of urine usually produced should be sought. When the volume loss is large, the patient being unable to stop the flow once started, then detrusor instability or hyper-reflexive bladder is the likely diagnosis. True stress incontinence is characteristically small volume losses. With detrusor instability there is also usually an urgent desire to micturate.

When there is outflow obstruction there is a history of incontinence of small volumes of urine, often with a poor stream. In certain situations such as dyssynergia, the greater the straining, the lower the rate.

A bowel history should be taken to seek evidence of constipation and possible fecal impaction. The presence of conditions such as diabetes mellitus, treated heart failure, previous strokes, other central nervous system disease and spinal cord pathologies should be sought. Symptoms of urgency, poor stream, and post-voiding dribbling which are suggestive of prostatism in a male should be sought. A gynecological history in the female should be obtained particularly in terms of multiple pregnancies and prolonged labour.

Objective

The clinical examination of the incontinent patient should include inspection of the vulva and urethra and digital examination of the rectum. The abdomen should be carefully assessed for evidence of urinary retention. Evidence of fecal loading should be sought. Abnormalities of kidneys should be noted.

The presence of neurological signs in the form of changes in sensation and reflexes in the legs, and presence of extensor plantar reflexes should be noted. An assessment should be made of the subject's comprehension, orientation and awareness of bladder filling.

An assessment of ambulation and dexterity, particularly with the manipulation of clothing is essential. The ability to transfer to and from a commode or lavatory is important to note and the effect of adjusting seat height and providing wall rails.

Assessment

The initial assessment should include the screening investigations described in Chapter 1. A careful chart of periods of continence and incontinence should ideally be kept. The chart should indicate not only the time of incontinence, but also the time of any visit to the lavatory, whether or not incontinence was present prior to the visit, and whether urine was passed on each occasion. It is useful to have such a chart maintained at 2-hourly intervals during the day and 4-hourly at night. Such objective recordings can be both a valuable diagnostic guide and act as a baseline to monitor treatment responses.

The incontinence monitoring record of Ouslander has been found to be practical, providing maximal information (Ouslander et al, 1986).

Plans

Diagnostic

It is paramount to exclude or treat a transient cause of incontinence such as infection, constipation and side effects of drugs. Urine is cultured in the usual way to look for the presence of infection. Once this is done and any infection located, further investigation is indicated. The individual's orientation, ambulation and dexterity should be optimized.

A urodynamic assessment is not essential at this stage. The general approach to assessment of established incontinence is to:

1. Exclude local urogenital causes such as prostatic enlargement and atrophic vaginitis. Rectal and/or vaginal examination is essential.
2. If the main symptom is leaking on coughing and the leaking can be seen to coincide with coughing, pelvic floor exercise should be prescribed as the probable cause is stress incontinence due to pelvic floor weakness.
3. If the main symptoms is urge incontinence, with or without stress incontinence, then there is an 80 per cent probability of detrusor instability. The individual should be toileted at regular 2-hourly intervals during the day. The frequency should be reduced to 4-hourly during the night.

The active toileting itself re-establishes a normal routine and plays an essential part of the rehabilitation program of an immobile patient. Males should be encouraged to micturate in the standing position. The chart is carefully reviewed and in those patients who remains incontinent residual urine is measured, preferably on two occasions.

A trial of bladder training, together with anticholinergic drugs, if not contraindicated by the finding of a residual greater than 100 cc, may be undertaken for 2 to 4 weeks. If the problem fails to improve then urodynamic studies should be considered.

4. In the situation of established incontinence where acute exacerbating conditions have been excluded, and the individual fails to show significant improvement within 10 to 14 days of a toileting regimen, then cystometry should be carried out.
5. In patients with residuals of greater than 100 cc a urology consultation and urodynamic studies are indicated.

It should be appreciated that often causes of incontinence are multiple. There are often transient factors such as reduced mobility and confusion present, which exacerbate an underlying tendency to established incontinence. Prostatic enlargement may coexist with detrusor instability so that prostatectomy may not cure the associated incontinence. Stress incontinence may occur with detrusor instability and this should be considered when large volumes of urine are passed with elevation of intra-abdominal pressure.

Management

Underlying conditions which may predispose or aggravate incontinence should be dealt with. The need for diuretics should be carefully reviewed. Fluid intake particularly at night should be monitored. Beds and chairs should be at an optimal height and type. Mobilization should be optimized and clothing should be appropriate to the individuals dexterity.

A regular toileting regimen should be initiated with careful charting to document improvements. Where possible underlying abnormalities of the urogenital system amenable to surgery should be dealt with.

In some instances, drug medication should be considered. These fall into the three main categories – estrogens, anti-diuretic drugs and drugs to diminish or increase bladder excitability. The beneficial effects of estrogens on urinary incontinence in old people was first stated by Wilson in 1948 using Stilbestrol cream in the treatment of senile vaginitis. It is generally felt that if after vaginal smear, atrophic changes are shown, a month's course of treatment with oral estrogen should be considered. In some women, there will be reduction of their incontinence and in this group, treatment should be repeated twice a year.

Antidiuretic drugs like vasopressin have been claimed to be beneficial with nocturnal frequency. These drugs, however, have limited use and are contraindicated in the presence of ischemic heart disease and hypertension.

The use of an antiparasympathomimetic drug to produce a pharmacological blockade of the uninhibited sacral micturition reflex is well documented. Many of these drugs unfortunately have profound anticholinergic side effects of confusion, blurred vision, dry mouth and constipation. Imipramine started at small doses of perhaps 10 mg at night and increased slowly up to an effective dose is usually well tolerated. Doses above 50 mg are rarely required. The antidepressant properties of the drug may also have worthwhile mood elevating effects. Oxybutynin (Ditropan) may also be considered but for the frail elderly is started at a low dose of 2.5 mgs. daily to be increased every 3 days to a maximum of 5 mgs 3 times daily, or when side effects preclude further increase. These drugs should only be continued if they can be seen to benefit.

Two other groups of drugs have been assessed for their ability to diminished uninhibited bladder contractions. Prostaglandin inhibitors have been shown in some studies to produce useful improvement, although not without side-effects. The calcium antagonists appear to have an effect on the bladder, possibly by preventing the release of calcium into the microtubule necessary to initiate muscle contraction. Their use in women with unstable bladders has been described.

A variety of other drugs have been used which may effect the autonomic nervous system. Alpha-adrenergic drugs such as Ephedrine have been known to produce side effects of urinary retention. This side effect has been used in patient's of with non-urogenic stress incontinence and in post-prostatectomy incontinence.

Alpha-adrenergic blocking agents such as Prazosin have been used for conditions in which the bladder smooth muscle does not relax synchronously with the detrusor contraction (detrusor dyssynergia). Cholinergic drugs (Bethanechol) have been used in the management of recurrent retention of urine when there is no physical obstruction to the flow.

Genuine stress incontinence due to pelvic floor weakness may be treated by physiotherapy, the use of a pessary, use of estrogens or by gynaecological surgery. The importance of an accurate diagnosis and exclusion of an underlying uninhibited bladder, cannot be over stressed. In the absence of any significant degree of uterine descent, pelvic floor exercises should be taught by a physiotherapist and practised several times a day. If the woman is able to understand and cooperate then the physiotherapy may be an important form of treatment. In the event of a failure of such physiotherapy, a vaginal pessary may be considered and possibly gynaecological operation.

When incontinence is established, and toilet training and other approaches have failed, the use of incontinence aids is often appropriate. In many situations, the frequency of incontinence and the amount expelled can be reduced so that the wearing of, for example, marsupial pants with absorbent pads may make a relatively normal social life possible. In the case of the male, condom catheters may be considered although they may cause local skin reactions, pressure effects and have a high incidence of infection.

The use of an indwelling catheter is the last step in the management of urinary incontinence. It should be avoided in cases of transient incontinence and only indicated where there is a need to carefully monitor fluid status or in the unconscious patient. The individual with significant residual urine may require catheterization because of discomfort and or deteriorating renal function. In post-operative patients with overflow incontinence intermittent catheterization may be necessary. This can often be decreased and eventually discontinued, particularly when retraining is occurring in conjunction with parasympathomimetic drugs. Some patients require intermittent catheterization on a permanent basis and age is no contraindication to self-catheterization. In some instances with intractable incontinence, catheterization may make it possible for the individual to lead a more normal social life and avoid the stigma of the condition. It should be appreciated, however, that urinary catheters are inevitably associated with colonization of the bladder. Attempts to remove such colonization by antibiotics often producing resistant strains. The length of time between catheter changes will depend on the type of catheter used. A variety of fastening devices to the waist or leg are available which can be of great aid in maintaining dignity of the patient.

Suggested reading

Hilton, P. and Stanton, S.L. (1981). Algorithmic method for assessing urinary incontinence. *Brit. Med. J.* **282**: 940–42.

Ouslander, J.G., Uman, H.W., and Uman, G.C. (1986). Development and testing of an incontinence monitoring record, *JAGA* **24**: 83–90.

Teasdale, T.A., Taffet, G.E., Luchi, R.S., and Adam, E. (1988). Urinary incontinence in a community residency elderly population. *JAGA* **36**: 600–606

Williams, M.E., Panill, F.C. (1982). Urinary incontinence in the elderly. *Ann. Int. Med.* **97**: 895–907.

6

Constipation, fecal impaction and fecal incontinence

Bowel problems are extremely important in the geriatric patient population. Constipation is common to all age groups and for many elderly patients needs to be dealt with in the same way as younger patients.

Constipation is said to be present when the individual perceives that the frequency of bowel action is insufficient, or when the stools are hard and difficult to pass. Constipation may be present in an elderly patient and not identified as a problem for a variety of reasons including the inability of the patient to communicate or unawareness due to brain failure.

Complications of constipation are more common in the geriatric population, for example fecal loading, impaction and incontinence. When symptomatic constipation has been present for more than 4 weeks and if available the plain radiograph shows fecal shadowing proximal to the sigmoid; this is referred to as fecal loading. A fecally loaded patient may be found to have hard scybalous stool in the rectum, or firm stool in large amounts in the rectum, and this is referred to as fecal impaction. Fecal incontinence is used to describe the involuntary loss of stool through the anal sphincter in any amount. In other words this would include soiling.

These problems will be better understood as each is discussed and as the pathophysiology is looked at in more detail.

1. Problem: fecal loading and impaction

Predisposing factors

Predisposition to constipation in the elderly is not well understood. In one population study 99 per cent of those questioned had bowel movements between 3 times a day and 3 times a week, and there was no difference between those people over 60 and those under 60. Studies using balloon distension of the rectum have not recorded any age difference and studies of anorectal manometry similarly have failed to show any effect of age. Aging alone cannot therefore be considered to be a predisposing factor for constipation and its complicatons.

Precipitating factors

The precipitating factors can be considered under the headings of general and local causes (Table 6.1). Population studies, although not showing objective evidence of excess constipation in the elderly do however, report a difference in laxative use. Those over 60 being more frequent users with a higher percentage of those over 60 being regular users. Habitual laxative use particularly of the stimulant type may lead to fecal loading, or megacolon. It has been shown that there is degeneration of the myenteric plexuses in mice given purgatives in large doses. The same mechanism seems likely for cathartic colon in man where the patients have been taking the drug for 30 or 40 years. It is important to determine the laxative use of the patient and to recognize that the regular users are predisposed to the bowel problems being discussed.

With advancing age there is an increase in the likelihood of the patient seeing a physician due to the increasing frequency of various diseases. With that comes the increased chance of receiving various drugs. Many drugs have an adverse effect on bowel motility and the most notorious of course are the antidepressants with anticholinergic side effects. Other drugs such as the tranquilizers, sedatives, hypnotics, analgesics and antacids may slow transit times through the bowel or increase the consistency of the stool.

A diet that is low in bulk is another important predisposing factor. Many of the present generation of elderly are used to diets that are low in bulk, using products of highly refined flour. Bowel transit times are prolonged in those patients with lower bulk in their diets. To this may be added reduced overall intake of food and fluid which might further predispose the individual to slow transit times and constipation.

Immobility predisposes to constipation, and for many individuals as their bodies become progressively slower so do their bowels. It is well recognized that propulsive activity only occurs in the physically active patient. Immobility or reduced mobility is a common form of functional impairment in the elderly patient and any pathophysiological process that produces these changes will predispose to constipation and its complications. Bowel transit times have been shown to be prolonged in patients on long-stay wards and is commonly secondary to immobility as well as poor hydration.

One side effect of chronic confusion and memory failure is decreased awareness of some bodily functions. Being unable to remember the time of the last bowel movement or of the last meal could easily have deleterious effects on the function of the bowel. Such individuals are more likely to be constipated and not to be aware of it or bring it to the attention of the family or their physician. Decreased awareness therefore predisposes to constipation which then leads to the complications of fecal loading, impaction and incontinence. Such patients are also likely to receive the types of drug that would reduce gastrointestinal motility which have been discussed.

Table 6.1 Precipitating factors to constipation

General:		
	Immobility/reduced mobility	
	Low fiber diet	
	Poor hydration	
	Poor habit	
	Drugs:	laxative abuse
		iatrogenesis (e.g. anticholinergics)
	Hypothyroidism	
	Hypercalcemia	
	Diabetes mellitus	
	Neurological (paraplegia, Parkinsonism, depression)	
Local:		
	Aganglionosis	
	Anal fissure/hemorrhoids	
	Stricture:	inflammatory bowel disease
		scleroderma
		ischemic colitis
		carcinoma

All of the factors that have been described in the last section may co-exist and the important thing is to remember that the elderly patient, particularly the constipated patient, is 'primed' and needs little more to induce the development of fecal loading or impaction. The physician looking after such patients needs to be aware of this, and to recognize when the problem is present and treat it. Perhaps of greater importance is to introduce preventive treatment in the susceptible patient before the problem develops.

There may be perianal, anal or rectal pathologies that precipitate these problems, and these are referred to as 'local' precipitants. Examples would be anal fissure or thrombosed hemorrhoids. In these situations defecation becomes painful and thus voluntarily inhibited. Other diseases of the bowel, particularly inflammatory bowel disease such as Crohn's disease or ulcerative colitis can lead to constipation in rare instances when the motility of the bowel wall is compromised. One of the most important diagnoses to make in the patient developing constipation for the first time is of course mechanical narrowing or obstruction, due to carcinoma. Narrowing can also result from the scarring of inflammatory bowel disease and diverticular disease.

Subjective

Inquiry about bowel function is an important part of history taking with the geriatric patient. The frequency and nature of bowel movements and any recent change need to be ascertained – from the patient if possible and if not from the care provider. Questions should be asked with regard to the use of purgatives; duration, frequency and type.

Some patients complain of a constant desire to evacuate their bowels, but being unable to do so. Such patients are usually fecally impacted.

Patients may present with the complications of fecal loading but be unaware of the underlying problem. The patient has some of the features of obstruction and presents with vomiting, loss of appetite and dehydration (fecal impaction dehydration syndrome), or with general non-specific decline. These problems may come to light post-operatively and present as described or alternatively because of the precipitation of Urinary problems – specifically the development of incontinence or retention. With impaction there may be features of obstruction with nausea, vomiting, abdominal distension and pain.

Most geriatric patients have one or more of the predisposing conditions for fecal loading or impaction, and these will become clear when the history is taken. Such patients are recognized as being predisposed and preventive measures can be introduced. This is particularly important for the elderly undergoing surgery, and recognition of the potential may well avoid the frequency of post-operative problems.

Objective

Constipation is usually identified as a problem from the history, whereas the complications of impaction or loading are identified from the examination. In the presence of a loaded colon the feces may be palpated through the abdominal wall. A mass in the right lower quadrant is more likely to be due to feces in the cecum when it is mobile and when the shape can be modified (indentable). Often the bowel can be felt throughout its entire length. With severe loading and impaction there may be abdominal distension, visible peristalsis and borborygmi suggesting the presence of obstruction. Adding to the difficulty in some patients there may be significant tenderness to deep palpation. In obese patients the combination of fat, feces and distended, gas-filled bowels may be difficult to distinguish from ascites and there may even be shifting dullness. Some patients have marked dilatation due to gaseous distension of the colon. This is detected by physical examination, the distension is uncomfortable to the patient and is easily seen. The distended abdomen is also tympanitic.

Rectal examination is essential. The perianal region needs to be visually inspected looking for any abnormality. With digital examination note should be made of the tone of the anal sphincter and the ability to voluntarily contract. The contents will be noted. The rectum may be empty, may contain small amounts of stool, may contain scybalous stool or be impacted with a large amount of stool – either soft or hard and rock like. A large amount of stool indicates impaction, when hard it is more difficult to remove. An empty rectum does not rule out constipation or its complications – the colon may be loaded above the rectum.

The patient should be examined carefully for the presence of dehydration or hypothyroidism.

Assessment

From the history and the examination the bowel problem can be quite accurately defined in most patients as constipation, fecal loading or fecal impaction (Fig. 6.1).

There may be a question of whether the patient has an obstructed bowel and this can usually be resolved by examining the abdominal radiograph and looking at the distribution of air. When air and feces extend throughout the large bowel, including the rectum then complete mechanical obstruction is unlikely.

Identification of these problems allows appropriate management of these patients. Problem solution should be taken to the highest level possible so that etiology might be identified. Different diagnostic and therapeutic approaches will be required and will be discussed in subsequent sections.

Plan

Diagnosis

More information than that available from the history and physical examination is usually required to determine the extent of fecal loading.

In the examination note was made of the patient with a very distended abdomen. Plain radiograph is essential in these patients to confirm the diagnosis of fecal loading or impaction. It is also important to identify those patients with Ogilvie's syndrome, with massive distension of the bowel. The distension seen is this syndrome is truly massive.

At the present time other tests are not considered to be part of the normal investigation but are likely to be included in the future. Once the bowel is empty then rectal manometry and electromyography of the anal sphincter may provide useful information to direct therapeutic choices.

Other tests may be indicated if the history or examination point to the presence of a local precipitant. In this case stool for occult blood, barium enema and endoscopy may be indicated. Such tests should not be routine but must be done when there are clinical pointers. For example, marked weight loss and blood loss point to the possibility of cancer and these tests are all indicated. On the other hand, fecal impaction post-operatively in a 90 year-old with a long history of purgative use would not war-

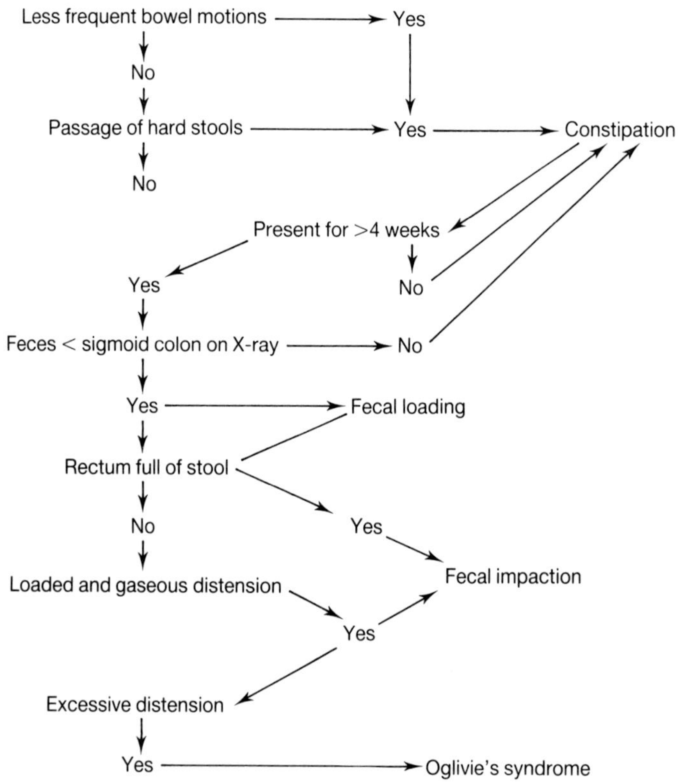

Fig. 6.1 Algorithm for fecal loading and impaction.

rant such a bowel work up and in fact is likely to be detrimental to the well-being of the patient.

Treatment

The treatment of constipation, fecal loading and impaction differs with regard to choice of agents and route of administration. There are certain principles of treatment that can be applied to any of the problems. Complications such as dehydration need to be recognized and corrected. If any general precipitant is identified it should be corrected or treated.

Constipation

Patients identified as being constipated are often used to taking purgatives and there is usually no reason why their favorite agent cannot be continued. There is a wide choice of agents available and there is no logical reason for choosing between the different types in most circumstances. The three major types are lubricant, irritant and bulk.

The lubricant purgatives are widely used and the oldest, namely mineral oil or liquid paraffin, is popular in self-medication. It is not recommended. Stool softeners fall in this category and examples would be dioctyl sodium sulphosuccinate or dioctyl calcium sulphosuccinate. These agents act by lowering surface tension and promoting the penetration of water into the stool. They should not be used with agents containing mineral oil since absorption occurs.

The irritant (stimulant) purgatives contain a variety of ancient agents including cascara and sennokot. These agents act by stimulating the myenteric plexus. Longstanding use results in loss of effectiveness and the development of cathartic colon which has already been mentioned. Another example would be bisacodyl (dulcolax) which is a potent stimulant. Most of these agents can be given either by mouth or in the form of suppository. Perhaps the best place for these agents is in combination usage, which is very effective in geriatric patients – for example with a stool softener, poloxalkol and danthron (Dorbanex),

Docusate sodium with danthron (Doss) Docusate calcium with Danthron (Doxidan)). These agents are cheap, effective and have few side-effects.

The osmotic purgatives, for example magnesium salts, are widely used. These can be used alone as milk of magnesia and efficacy can be increased by increasing the dose. They can be used in combination for example Magnolax and cascara. They act by drawing water into the bowel lumen. Lactulose is a synthetic disaccharide of fructose and lactose that passes to the large intestine undigested. Here it is attacked by bacteria and the products are osmotically active, but also have irritant properties. This agent is effective in geriatric patients. A few patients find the sweet taste unacceptable and cannot tolerate it but for most people this is an effective agent. The usual starting dose is 15 ml once or twice a day and can be increased by 15 ml increments until the desired effect is obtained. It is also available in the form of a gel which is more easily ingested by some people.

Bulk purgatives should be reserved for maintenance therapy or prevention once the constipation is treated. These agents are not useful in the initial management of a fresh problem. In fact their use may aggravate the problem. Once constipation has been relieved and the bowel unloaded then bulk agents can be introduced if dietary manipulation has not been successful. Bulk agents may not be required if the patient can tolerate a high roughage diet with added bran and regular bowel motions are obtained. There are several brands of bulk purgatives available including metamucil, fybyrax and prodiem. The latter is a combination of bulk with the stimulant senna which some patients find particularly effective.

For simple constipation milk of magnesia, a stool softener or softener/stimulant combination is recommended. Purgatives are traditionally given at night for bowel movements the next day but for patients who go to bed very early or who have mobility problems consideration should be given to administering the drug in the morning so that a bowel movement occurs when the patient is up and about later in the day. This reduces the risk of incontinence.

Fecal Loading

The treatment of the loaded patient is more challenging. It needs to be recognized that there is a large quantity of feces to shift and a single large movement is not enough to achieve this. In these patients the rectum may be full or empty. In both situations an oral agent is recommended, and 15 ml of lactulose twice daily has proven satisfactory. If the rectum is full enemas should be started immediately, if empty, enemas can be delayed for one day and then commenced. Simple phosphate enemas are all that is necessary and Fleet enemas should be prescribed on a daily basis. There is no need to go to large volume enemas nor enemas like soapsuds and oil retention. Fleet enemas are continued until the returns are poor. Once the bowel is considered to be empty (this can be confirmed by abdominal radiography) a maintenance regimen is instituted. In patients who have been loaded for some time or who are getting poor results with the previously described regimen, a more aggressive approach is required and alternatives will be discussed in the next section.

Patients with massive distension of the bowel (Ogilvie's syndrome) need to be taken off any medications that may aggravate the condition for example the anticholinergics. Distension is reduced by application of the regimens already described and also the passage of flatus tubes or colonoscopy with suction of as much gas as possible. This manoeuvre may need to be repeated on several occasions and in most instances the bowel will begin to regain tone and function again. It is also possible to use small amounts of cholinergic drugs, bethanechol for example. This can be given orally and a dose of 5 mg should be started, repeated at hourly intervals until the effective dose is determined. The procedure may be stopped by the onset of side effects. The dose is then given 3 or 4 times a day until tone is reestablished. The patients then need to be established on a maintenance regimen which may need to contain a regular dose of a stimulant for some time. It is also important that these patients are never given drugs with anticholinergic side-effects in the future as these may precipitate massive distension again.

Fecal Impaction

The regimen recommended for fecal loading may be also effective in this situation but may need to be combined with manual breakup of the stool mass and often needs to be continued for several weeks. In those patients who are mobile enough to transfer to the toilet or commode an alternative approach is effective. Golytely is a balanced electrolyte solution containing polyethyleneglycol. When used there is no net shift of fluid or electrolytes in or out of the bowel. This agent was originally used for colonoscopic preparation and it is recommended that 3 to 5 litres of the solution is consumed within 1 or 2 hours. In our experience this is a challenge for many elderly patients, and 2 to 3 litres over 3 to 4 hours is effective. This preparation will successfully empty the bowel in 12 to 24 hours and has been shown to be safe and effective in geriatric patients. It is not suitable for the immobile and confused patient. A great advantage of course is that the bowel will be emptied in a short period of time. Golytely can also be given by nasogastric tube at a rate of 250 ml every 10 minutes, to a total of 3 litres. Bowel evacuation can be complete in 3 to 4 hours. This maneuver is possible on an out-patient basis.

Maintenance and prevention

The loaded or impacted bowel tends to be dilated and atonic with gas and feces filled redundant loops. Once the bowel is empty the aim of treatment is to restore normal tone and function. Studies that have been done have not adequately demonstrated that this is always an achievable goal.

The patient with redundant loops, reduced sensation of rectal fullness and incontinence seems to do best with lactulose. It is recognized that this is expensive but we have found patients with very severe problems do well with this preparation only to revert to previous problems on switching to less costly agents. The dosage is adjusted to the patient but is usually 30 ml daily. Patients with less severe problems usually respond to the use of a bulk agent together with an agent to induce daily evacuation – one of the stimulant/softener combinations. Some of these patients can be weaned to bulk plus softener, saving the stimulant for occasional use when a day is missed. Prevention can also be achieved by dietary manipulation, using a high roughage diet and good hydration.

Patient education

Regular evacuation of the bowels, usually daily is an ideal that is worth aiming for. Patients need to understand how to achieve this. Counselling on dietary habits including adequate fluid intake is worthwhile. It is of interest that many elderly are now quite aware of the value of roughage and many make it a regular part of their diet, fewer are aware of the dangers of underhydration.

Excessive purgation should be avoided and this does become a problem in the patient that forgets. Diarrhea induced by overzealous use of cathartics is not unusual and an important clue is that this settles immediately upon hospital admission. Patients or their care providers should be counselled as to the type of purgative that is recommended and when to take.

2. Problem: fecal incontinence

This is a less common problem than incontinence of urine. However incontinence of feces has been reported to occur in as many as 45 per cent of geriatric patients in long-stay wards. For many care providers of demented patients the emergence of fecal incontinence as a problem is the factor that precipitates the demand for institutionalization. Fecal incontinence simply means the involuntary loss of feces from the rectum. This can take the form of passage of very small amounts of feces or soiling, or complete bowel movements at inappropriate times and without control.

It is important to recognize that there are three main types of fecal incontinence. First of all, incontinence may simply be a manifestation or symptom of an underlying bowel problem, the bowel disease itself precipitating the incontinence. Secondly, fecal incontinence may be a complication of fecal loading or impaction. Thirdly, fecal incontinence is a result of neurological disease affecting the defecation process – this might be termed idiopathic.

Predisposing factors

Fecal continence is maintained by a complex series of factors. In simple terms the rectum serves as a distensible reservoir which accommodates fecal material descending from the sigmoid colon. There is a sensory mechanism (S 2–4) which is sensitive to the distension (stretch receptors in the muscles) and indicates when the reservoir is reaching full capacity so that evacuation should occur. The parasympathetic system controls contraction of the sigmoid and rectal musculature and relaxation of the internal sphincter. The sphincter mechanism consists of the internal sphincter and the voluntary muscle controlled external sphincter, contains the rectal contents and prevents premature evacuation or spillage. Studies using the technique of single fiber electromyography have revealed that the motor unit fibre density of the sphincter increases in elderly patients. This indicates that there is underlying muscle atrophy with denervation. The fibers are similar to those found in other muscle groups with aging. These and other studies indicate that neurogenic damage to the anal sphincter reduce the functional reserve of elderly people and predispose to incontinence.

Precipitating factors

These should be considered under the three headings already considered.

1. Constipation, fecal loading and impaction
2. Local causes
   Bowel pathology: diarrhea, diverticular disease, irritable bowel, carcinoma, ischemia
   Destruction of anal sphincter: cancer, neurological disease
3. Idiopathic or neurogenic

Incontinence results when the anal sphincter mechanisms can no longer contain the rectal contents. Obviously there are two main factors that influence the outcome of filling the rectal reservoir. One is the integrity of the sphincter mechanism and we have already seen that aging may result in muscle atrophy. The other is the pressure exerted by the rectal contents. It is easy to understand that the rapid movement of a large volume of liquid stool is more threatening to the integrity of the sphincter than a slow moving, small, semiformed stool. Sudden rectal distension with a large volume of liquid stool can result in incontinence in individuals with strong healthy anal sphincters, and this is not uncommon in younger individuals during outbreaks of infectious diarrhea. This is also true for those with irritable bowel syndrome, or with other pathologies when the propulsive movement forward of liquid or semiformed stool is enough to overcome the sphincter mechanisms. In one study of irritable bowel incontinence was found in a significant number of young individuals.

It is apparent that destruction of the anal sphincter by neoplastic, inflammatory or neurological disease will result in incontinence.

In the preceding section fecal loading and impaction were discussed. Impaction can precipitate fecal incontinence. The impacted stool sitting high in the rectum results in reflex relaxation of the internal sphincter. Liquified stool then travels down into the anal canal and the external sphincter is unable to retain the liquid stool. The incontinence may be in the form of soiling, or the patient reports diarrhea (spurious diarrhea).

Subjective

The importance of a careful history of the problem cannot be overemphasized. The patient complains of the involuntary loss of stool. Questions need to be asked with regards the patient's awareness of rectal distension and call to stool. Also the preceding bowel habit is very important to determine if you are dealing with constipation, impaction and spurious diarrhea. What is the nature of the incontinent stool and what is the frequency of the incontinence? This is obviously important to determine if the incontinence is related to 'stressing' the system with large volumes of loose stool – diarrhea. Inquiry into associated problems is important, the questions are obvious and relate to the other problems already mentioned such as cancer, diverticular disease, irritable bowel syndrome or inflammatory bowel disease for example.

It needs to be recognized that a significant number of patients with this problem do not volunteer the information that it is present. This may be because of associated problems like dementia or because the patient is embarrassed or feels that it is not the sort of problem that a physician can help with. In this case the questions alluded to above need to be asked of the caregiver. This may be useful to explore in the setting of a team conference. For example, in a long-term care team conference a patient was identified as being a problem. The patient had advanced dementia he was fecally incontinent and was smearing feces over everything. It turned out that the stool was loose, pale in color and offensive. It was passed in very large amounts. Incontinence was a problem but it appeared secondary to diarrhea. During further questioning of the team a nurse's aide commented on the fact that the patient consumed vast quantities of milk. The patient had been observed to raid the nourishment cart and to steal from other people's trays. This led to the possibility of lactose intolerance. When the patient's actual consumption was recorded it turned out to be over 3 quarts of milk a day. By diverting the patient and substituting a lactose free beverage the diarrhea ceased and the incontinence was controlled.

Objective

The patient needs to be carefully examined with an emphasis on examining the abdomen and the rectum. Palpation of the abdomen may reveal the presence of a loaded colon or other masses. With the patient lying on the left side the buttocks should be separated and the anus inspected visually. As this is done note should be made of the state of the underwear and the presence of feces on the skin in the perianal and perineal regions. In this way the problem may be identified in those patients not complaining of it.

Digital examination of the rectum should include determination of the contents of the rectum, the size of the rectal cavity, the nature of the rectal wall, whether there are any masses or abnormalities external to the rectum and the tonicity of the anal sphincter.

A plain abdominal radiograph should be obtained to determine whether there is fecal loading or impaction. The value of additional investigations has yet to be established. However, in those patients who are designated idiopathic fecal incontinence, where neurological degeneration is suspected it is likely that anal manometry and rectal pressure studies will become important in the near future.

Assessment

The logical assessment of the patient with fecal incontinence is vital. The algorithm will help in this (Fig. 6.2).

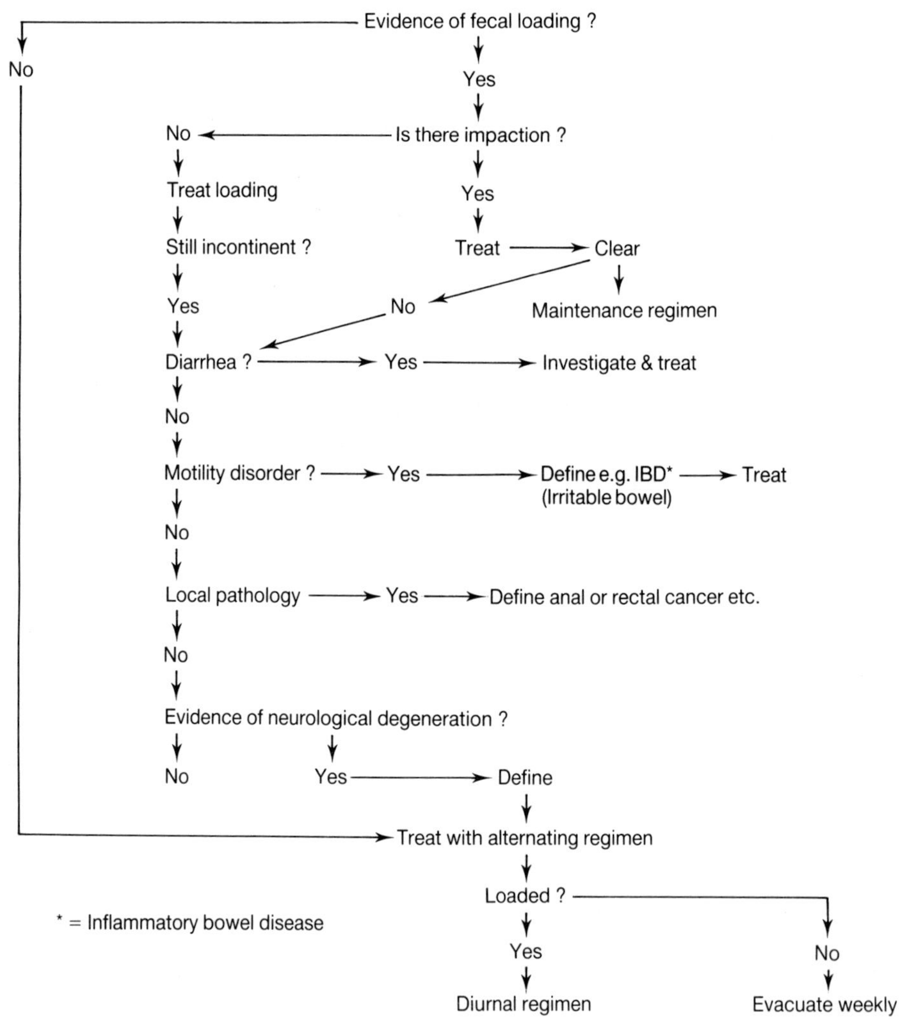

Fig. 6.2 Algorithm for fecal incontinence.

There is no doubt that the idiopathic group will contain patients with incontinence of varying etiologies. It is anticipated that these will be better defined in the future and at that time treatment may be more directed and less empiric. At the present time, however, recognizing these major groupings allows effective treatment in most patients.

Plan

Diagnosis

The steps that need to be taken to determine the type of fecal incontinence that a patient has have already been dealt with. A minimal diagnostic work up includes a plain abdominal radiograph. Patients who are fecally loaded when incontinent and who remain incontinent after the bowel is emptied should have anal manometry if available. In this way a definitive statement can be made about the anal sphincter and our experience in this regard has been positive in helping to design effective treatment. A patient with an inadequate anal sphincter will inevitably become incontinent in the presence of impaction and it therefore becomes important to keep the patient free of any impaction.

If the examination and minimal investigations mentioned so far indicate the possibility of other pathology then the appropriate investigations should be done. These might include barium enema, sigmoidoscopy or colonoscopy, small bowel follow through, and so on.

Treatment

Treatment of the fecal impaction and loading should be as already discussed in the previous section.

Any local cause such as diarrhea, anal carcinoma or inflammatory bowel disease should be treated appropriately. Those with established fecal incontinence labelled as idiopathic or neurological need to be treated empirically. This is also true for some of the patients in the other groups where a cause is identified but nothing can be done about it.

Those patients who are also loaded or impacted clearly have a problem within the colon as well as a problem with the defecation process. For this reason attention must be directed here. It is recommended that the patient who is cleared needs to be placed on a maintenance regimen to ensure that the colon does not once again become loaded. This can be done by the use of a bulk/stimulant combination. A proprietary preparation like Prodiem which is psyllium hydrophilic mucilloid plus senna works well; or any of the bulk agents with milk of magnesia has also been found satisfactory. This combination is given before retiring to bed. The next morning, following breakfast when the gastrocolic reflex is anticipated a suppository (such as bisacodyl) is given to induce a bowel movement. Following rectal evacuation the patient is then given loperamide which is repeated at midday. The cycle is then repeated.

For the patient who is not loaded or for whom the stimulation does not work or the patient with advanced cognitive impairment a longer cycle needs to be used. There are several available. An example would be to use a softener/stimulant preparation in the evening followed by an enema the next morning. The rest of the time between enema administrations the patient is given binding agents such as loperamide. The timing of the cycle depends upon the individual patient and their requirements. Some patients continue to soil or be incontinent. Those with advanced dementia can usually be managed by a combination of diapering and anticipation. There are several different products available to handle this kind of problem and there are none with obvious advantages over the others.

It has been our experience that surgical attempts at correction have not been successful and approaches such as the use of a Thiersch wire are not recommended. There is little experience with other techniques like biofeedback or electrical stimulation in this age group.

Patient education

This depends upon the cognitive abilities of the patient. Obviously those patients who are cognitively intact or who have minimal impairment find this problem most distressing. Patients can be very successfully involved in their management particularly when they have a good understanding of the rationale of the therapeutic interventions. Patients of advanced age, with varying disabilities have been successfully recruited to manage their own problem and to administer their own suppositories for example. We are convinced there is a great deal of unexplored potential with regard to retraining via biofeedback.

Suggested reading

Brocklehurst, J. C. (1972). Bowel management in the neurologically disabled. The problems in

old age. *Proceedings of the Royal Society of Medicine*, **65**: 66–9.
Brocklehurst, J. C. and Khan, Y. (1969). A study of fecal stasis in old age and use of Dorbanex in its prevention. *Geront. Clin.*, **11**: 293–300.
Brocklehurst, J. C., Kirkland, J. L., Martin, J. and Ashford, J. (1983). Constipation in elderly patients: its treatment and prevention by Lactulose, Poloxalkol, Dihydroxyanthroquinolone and phosphate enema. *Gerontology*, **29**: 181–4.
Connell, A. M., Hilton, C., Irvin, G., Lennard Jones, J. E. and Misiewicz, J. J. (1965). Variations in bowel habits in two population samples. *Brit. Med. J.*, **ii**: 1095–99.
Holdstock, D. J. (1970). Propulsion (mass movements) in the human colon and its relationship to meals and somatic activity. *Gut*, **11**: 91.
LoeningBaucke, V. and Anuras, S. (1984). Anorectal manometry in healthy elderly subjects, *J. Amer. Ger. Soc.*, **32**: 636–9.
Percy, J. P., Neill, M. E., Kandiah, T. K., Swash, M. (1982). A neurogenic factor in fecal incontinence in the elderly. *Age and Ageing*. **11**: 175–9.
Ryan, D., Wilson, A., Muir, T. S., Judge, T. G. (1974). The reduction of fecal incontinence by the use of Duphalac in geriatric patients. *Current Med. Res. Opinion.*, **2**: 329–34.

7

Cardiac failure

The term 'cardiac failure' refers to a syndrome in which cardiac dysfunction results in a failure to pump blood at the rate required by metabolizing tissues. It is often, but not always, caused by a primary defect of myocardial contraction and must be distinguished from non-cardiac causes of circulatory failure (e.g. hemorrhagic shock). It is usually, but not always, associated with reduced cardiac output. Some times the myocardium functions relatively normally at rest but the abnormality is uncovered on exercise. Occasionally, the clinical features of cardiac failure are seen in the presence of an increased cardiac output (e.g. anaemia, fever, thyrotoxicosis, Beri Beri, Paget's disease of bone) and in these cases, treatment is largely aimed at these underlying causes.

It is conventional to think of heart failure as either left sided (increased left heart pressures and volumes and later, pulmonary oedema) or right-sided (increased right-sided pressures and volumes associated with peripheral oedema). When both left and right-sided heart failure co-exist, the terms 'biventricular failure' and 'congestive cardiac failure' are often used and this syndrome is the one most frequently encountered when cardiac failure is chronic. The usual sequence of events is the development of chronic left-sided heart failure which then induces right heart failure by increasing pulmonary vascular resistance, reducing renal perfusion and inducing salt and water retention.

Pathophysiology of Heart Failure

Many of the responses to cardiac failure probably evolved to sustain life in the presence of circulatory collapse induced by trauma and hemorrhage. Those same responses may however, be disadvantageous when the myocardium is malfunctioning or when there is obstruction to ventricular outflow.

An increase in *preload* results in lengthening of the sarcomeres in diastole towards an optimum length for contraction and for any given level of cardiac contractility, there is a clear relationship between ventricular end-diastolic volume and stroke work. Preload is determined by venous return which is increased by venoconstriction caused by sympathetic activation. The increase in preload is transmitted to the left heart through the pulmonary circulation and results in an increase in left ventricular end-diastolic pressure and hypertrophy of cardiac myocytes. As this progresses to ventricular dilation a fall in stroke volume occurs due to dilation of the atrio-ventricular valve rings, resulting in functional incompetence.

Reduced cardiac output results in activation of baroreflexes with sympathetic activation and this helps maintain cardiac output (by increasing force of contraction and increasing heart rate) and there are often very large increases in plasma catecholamine concentrations with even modest exertion. With chronic heart failure, cardiac noradrenaline is reduced as is the number of catecholamine receptors, though adrenal-derived catecholamines continue to be secreted. This induces constriction in the resistance vessels and a fall in stroke volume because of increased *afterload*. This sympathetic activation also induces renal arteriolar constriction with activation of the renin-angiotensin-aldosterone system and sodium and water retention. The constriction of renal arterioles reduces perfusion of the kidneys and probably explains the oliguria that is often seen in cardiac failure.

Predisposing Factors to Heart Failure with Aging

It would appear that healthy aging individuals without ischemic heart disease have no significant change in their resting cardiac output. There is, however, evidence of reduced increase in heart rate due to exercise and that maintenance of cardiac output is more dependent upon increased cardiac contraction.

A modest reduction in early diastolic filling rate has been noted with age. This is usually compensated for by more vigorous atrial contraction in the last diastole. The commonly observed increased aortic stiffness and increased systolic pressures tend to increase left ventricular afterload. This produces a tendency towards an increase in left ventricular thickness.

Several animal studies have demonstrated changes in myocardial contractility which serve to favour contractile force at the expense of reduced contractile velocity. Contraction is prolonged in senescent cardiac muscle, probably because of slower release of calcium into the myoplasm during systole. Action potential duration is prolonged. The myosin isoenzymes shift to slower forms and adenosine triphosphatase activity declines.

Asymptomatic and symptomatic ichemic heart disease may result in a reduction in ventricular function without overt cardiac disease. The individual may therefore be at risk of developing overt cardiac failure if 'stressed'. It appears that physiological and occult disease changes predispose the elderly to heart failure in the form of reduced reserve capacity.

Table 7.1 Main causes of heart failure in the elderly

Impediments for forward flow:
Systemic arterial hypertension
Aortic valve stenosis
Obstructive hypertrophic cardiomyopathy
Pulmonary hypertension
Impaired cardiac filing:
Ventricular hypertrophy
Pericardial disease
Restrictive heart disease
Ventricular aneurism
Arrhythmias (atrial fibrillation, supraventricular tachcardia, bradycardia, etc.)
Volume overload:
Valvular regurgitation
Increased intravascular volume
Increased metabolic demands (anemia, thyrotoxicosis, etc.)
Arteriovenous shunts
Myocardial failure
Myocardial ischemia
Cardiomyopathy
Myocarditis
Chronic overload

Precipitating Factors to Heart Failure

Generally the principle causes can be considered under four separate categories: impediments to forward flow; impaired cardiac filling; volume overload and myocardial failure (Table 7.1). Systemic arterial hypertension and coronary heart disease are probably the most commonly encountered precipitants. Infection at any site, but particularly in the lungs, is a common precipitant of cardiac failure in an already compromised myocardium. A variety of medications may precipitate heart failure in a vulnerable individual (Table 7.2).

Table 7.2 Drugs commonly causing or exacerbating heart failure

Beta-adrenergic antagonists
Calcium channel blockers
Some anti-dysrhythmic drugs
Non-steroidal anti-inflammatory drugs
Glucocorticoids

Subjective findings

Cardiac failure is seen commonly in elderly patients and should be considered in the differential diagnosis of those conditions listed in Table 7.3.

In acute heart failure there is a sudden decline in left ventricular function which leads to severe dyspnea. The most common cause is acute myocardial infarction but it also occurs fairly often in the setting of previously stable chronic heart failure. Dyspnea is often the most prominent feature of chronic heart failure and it is worse on exertion and lying flat, possibly because both maneuvers induce a rapid rise in left atrial pressure by increasing both systemic and pulmonary venous return. When there is overt pulmonary oedema, dyspnoea will be present at rest and will usually be associated with cough, hemoptysis and bronchospasm (so-called cardiac asthma). Nocturia is also a feature of cardiac failure and is probably caused by the reduction in sympathetic tone during sleep resulting in improved perfusion of the kidneys.

Table 7.3 Conditions often associated with cardiac failure

Edema
Dyspnoea
Confusional states
Falls
Collapse and syncope
Poor mobility
Fatigue
Malaise
Anorexia/cachexia

Peripheral edema is a characteristic feature of chronic heart failure and there is still controversy about the precise underlying mechanisms. It is most obvious around the ankles of ambulant patients and over the lumbo-sacral region of those who are bed-fast. Ankle swelling is common in old people and is most often attributable to local factors affecting leg veins and lymphatic vessels and sometimes, hypoproteinemia. The presence of edema in heart failure reflects considerable fluid retention and it has been estimated that there must be a net retention of several litres before edema becomes apparent. Venous engorgement may also affect the intestine and liver giving rise to anorexia, nausea, vomiting, malabsorption, constipation and ascites. All these changes lead to the appearances characteristic of quite severe malnutrition and is sometimes termed 'cardiac cachexia'.

The reduced cardiac output is probably responsible for the tiredness and fatigue so commonly described by patients with cardiac failure and is thought to be due to reduced perfusion of skeletal muscle.

Both fatigue and dyspnea limit the ability to undertake exercise and the severity of heart failure is often graded in this way (Table 7.4). Such a classification is of limited value for heart failure in old age since the capacity for exercise may be limited for other reasons.

A careful history may be helpful to establish the underlying cause of chronic heart failure. Angina of effort or previous myocardial infarction provide good evidence that the heart failure is due to coronary artery disease, though the absence of one of these features does not preclude the diagnosis. Angina of effort may occur with normal coronary arteries, particularly in aortic stenosis. A history of rheumatic fever should prompt a careful search for evidence of valvular heart disease. A number of drugs may induce or exacerbate cardiac failure (Table 7.4) and, as always, a thorough review of drug treatment is indicated.

Table 7.4 The New York Heart Association grading of heart failure

Class I	No limitation of physical activity
Class II	Slight limitation of physical activity
Class III	Marked limitation of physical activity
Class IV	Inability to perform any physical activity without discomfort

Objective findings

Physical examination of a patient with heart failure relates both to the assessment of the heart failure and to a search for causative factors. The general appearance in severe cardiac failure reflects sympathetic nervous activity. Signs include sweating, agitation, pallor and cold, clammy skin. Peripheral cyanosis reflects diminished peripheral perfusion and central cyanosis may follow pulmonary edema. Peripheral pitting edema is usually obvious. Liver engorgement and ascites may be present and sometimes jaundice.

The systemic blood pressure may be low, normal or high depending on the degree of left ventricular dysfunction. The fall in right ventricular output and venoconstriction results in an increased systemic venous pressure. This is detected by observing the distended and pulsating superficial jugular veins. If there is tricuspid incompetence, a prominent 'v' wave can be observed in the jugular venous pulsation. Cardiac enlargement is common, particularly in chronic cardiac failure. Localization of the apical impulse may be difficult, usually because of chest wall deformities and lung disease. A forceful apical impulse is indicative of left ventricular hypertrophy, a diffuse impulse suggests ventricular dilation and a tapping impulse may be found with mitral stenosis.

The presence of a third heart sound is good evidence of heart failure but a fourth heart sound should be assigned no special significance. A pansystolic murmur representing mitral or tricuspid incompetence – usually due to dilated valve rings but also to papillary muscle dysfunction and primary valvular disease – may be heard. An ejection murmur occurs in over 50 per cent of old people, even in the apparent absence of heart disease. Clinical examination may not permit it to be distinguished from true aortic stenosis.

Basal lung crackles (sometimes unilateral, most often left-sided) occur in left ventricular failure but also occur in pulmonary fibrosis and bronchiectasis. Bronchial mucosal congestion may cause wheezes and lead to confusion with primary lung diseases with airflow limitation. Pleural effusions (transudates) are common in congestive heart failure and are usually bilateral.

Assessment

Clinical diagnosis of heart failure usually presents few problems, though on occasion it can be very difficult. The aims of the further assessment are fourfold: to confirm the diagnosis, to detect underlying causes, to assess severity and to plan appropriate treatment.

Chest radiography is often considered to be a fairly sensitive investigation. Cardiac dilation leads to an increased cardiothoracic ratio (>50 per cent) but this is difficult to assess in the presence of chest wall abnormalities (so common in old age). Gross cardiac enlargement should alert the physician to the possibility of pericardial effusion. Isolated left atrial enlargement usually indicates mitral stenosis. The plain radiograph may suggest other causes such as aortic dissection, calcification of mitral and/or aortic valves, constrictive pericarditis and left ventricular aneurysm.

Congested lung-fields, indicative of increased pulmonary capillary pressure, a reflection of increased left ventricular filling pressure, may be seen. When pulmonary capillary pressure increases to around 13 mm Hg, basal vessel constriction is prominent and upper lobe vessel diameter equals or exceeds that of lower lobe vessels (reverse of the normal pattern). Interstitial pulmonary oedema is usually seen with pulmonary capillary pressures greater than 20 mm Hg and is seen as Kerley B lines and peri-vascular haze. Frank alveolar oedema and pleural effusions tend to occur with pressures over 25 mm Hg.

The electrocardiogram provides evidence of ventricular dysfunction and possible causes. Left bundle branch block and bifascicular block are strongly indicative of left ventricular dysfunction. Pathological Q waves in an appropriate pattern suggest ischaemic heart disease as the underlying cause of heart failure. Evidence of left ventricular hypertrophy is suggestive of hypertension, aortic stenosis or hypertrophic cardiomyopathy as the underlying cause.

Many would regard echocardiography as a routine investigation in the assessment of heart failure and is widely available. The maximum information is provided by a combination of M mode (most widely available) and Doppler studies. It is possible to derive information about function (e.g. ejection fraction) as well as the pathological anatomy.

Dilated ventricles indicate poor ventricular function and is most often due to ischaemic heart disease. A markedly dilated right ventricle raises the possibility of congestive cardiomyopathy. Regional abnormalities of wall movement and variations in wall thickness are features of ischaemic heart disease. In advanced cases, it may be impossible to distinguish between ischaemic heart disease and congestive cardiomyopathy as causes of heart failure.

Normal left ventricular dimensions suggest that an abnormality in filling is responsible for the heart failure and an increase in wall thickness supports this as an explanation. Marked left ventricular hypertrophy suggests hypertension, aortic stenosis or hypertrophic cardiomyopathy. Another feature of a poorly compliant left ventricle is early closure of the mitral valve due to a rapid rise in ventricular pressure. More detailed information about ventricular function can be gained from Doppler echocardiography. Echocardiography is also useful in the diagnosis and assessment of pericardial disease, valvular heart disease and infective endocarditis.

Radionuclide studies are not widely available for cardiac imaging in non-teaching hospitals. Such techniques permit the making of measurements previously only available by cardiac catheterization. It is possible to image the blood pool and to calculate ejection fraction and responses to drug intervention. Segmental wall movements (e.g. in left ventricular aneurysm) can be detected. Isotope preparations are also available to image areas of ischaemia and infarcts.

Profoundly hypotensive patients may benefit from measuring central venous pressure to exclude hypovolaemia. The placement of a Swan–Ganz catheter can give an indirect measure of left ventricular filling pressure (in the absence of mitral valve disease or ventricular septal defect). Cardiac output can also be determined. Formal cardiac catheter studies are not indicated unless surgery is likely to be a realistic option.

Treatment

Acute Heart Failure

The patient should be sat upright and given oxygen by facemask or nasal specula. Intravenous morphine (5–10 mg depending on body size) over a few minutes is beneficial since it relieves anxiety and reduces sympathetic activation (thus inducing some vasodilation). Morphine is contraindicated in the presence of severe lung disease, in which case intravenous aminophylline (250 mg) may be given slowly. Intravenous loop diuretics (e.g. frusemide, bumetanide) also give rapid relief of dyspnoea, probably also by inducing vasodilation. More recently, sub-lingual and intravenous nitrate preparations and calcium antagonists (principally nifedipine) have been widely used in the treatment of acute heart failure.

Failure to respond rapidly is very serious and demands urgent reevaluation. It may be that the heart failure is a terminal event and symptomatic relief with oxygen and further morphine is the only treatment indicated. If it is judged that further active treatment is needed, the most logical step is to insert a Swan–Ganz catheter and maintain the left atrial pressure at about 18 mm Hg with an infusion of nitroprusside or nitroglycerin. If urine output does not improve, an inotropic agent such as dobutamine (a selective beta-1 adrenoreceptor agonist) may be infused. Aortic balloon pump counter-pulsation should only be seen as a prelude to surgery (e.g. for post-infarct mitral incompetence and ventricular septal defect).

Chronic heart failure

Treatment in chronic heart failure depends on severity. Nevertheless, some general advice is applicable to all patients. Obese patients should lose weight and smokers ought to desist from their habit. Alcohol consumption should be minimized and excessive salt intake should be avoided. Salt-free diets are impractical.

Diuretics are still the mainstay of heart failure therapy and in mild cardiac failure may be the only drug treatment required. They promote salt and water excretion, thus reducing plasma volume and atrial pressures. They do not improve cardiac output and may even reduce it by reducing pre-load. Furthermore, in stimulating the renin-angiotensin system, they may exacerbate the vicious cycle of increasing vascular resistance and falling cardiac output.

Thiazide diuretics (Table 7.5)

For mild heart failure, thiazide diuretics are still the treatment of choice. Thiazides inhibit the reabsorption of sodium in the distal nephron as well as promoting potassium loss. They are of little use in the presence of renal failure with the possible exception of metolazone. The most frequent side-effects of thiazides are listed in Table 7.6. Perhaps the best known side effect of thiazide diuretics is hypokalaemia and this is potentiated by the co-administration of beta-adrenergic antagonists. While hypokalemia is undisputable, it appears to be associated with minimal (if any) change in total body potassium. However, it is the low potassium concentration that is dangerous (Chapter 20) and steps should be taken to prevent it. Adequate supplements (around 100 mmol/day) necessitates approximately 8 Sando K tablets, 12 slow K or 14 Kloref. In the presence of hypomagnesemia, potassium supplements will not achieve a normal plasma potassium concentration unless the hypomagnesemia is corrected. It is usually acceptable to give a potassium sparing agent (amiloride or triamterene), usually as a combined preparation with a thiazide (Moduret, Dyazide). While this combination conserves both potassium and magnesium, it may predispose to hyponatremia and hyperkalemia (Chapter 20) and should not be used in renal failure or when angiotensin converting enzyme inhibitors are used. Hypomagnesemia may occur, and should be suspected when the serum sodium and potassium are normal and the patient has persistent weakness, vertigo or ataxia.

Table 7.5 Some thiazide diuretics used in heart failure treatment

Drug	Maximum dose	Duration of action
Bendrofluazide	10 mg	~12 h
Cyclopenthiazide	0.25 mg	~12 h
Hydrochlorthiazide	100 mg	~12 h
Metolazone	20 mg	18–24 h
Chlorthalidone	50 mg	>24 h

Table 7.6 Common side effects of thiazide diuretics

Hypokalemia
Hyponatremia
Dehydration
Urinary incontinence
Sense of disequilibrium
Lethargy
Impotence
Glucose intolerance
Increased total and LDL cholesterol
Hypomagnesemia

Loop diuretics

If thiazide treatment does not provide adequate control, a loop diuretic (e.g. frusemide, bumetanide) may be substituted. These agents are sulphonamide derivatives and act in the ascending limb of the loop of Henle by inhibiting enzymes necessary to pump chloride across the lining cells. The effect is that chloride, sodium, potassium and hydrogen ions remain in the tubule and are lost in the urine. Clearly, this action may induce hypochloremia, hyponatremia, hypoklaemia and alkalosis. Other side effects are similar to those encountered with thiazides except that they may also be ototoxic. The duration of action is between 4 and 6 hours with an onset within 10 minutes of intravenous administration and one hour of oral administration. Other properties of loop diuretics of value in moderate to severe heart failure are:

1. they are effective (in high doses) when there is co-existent renal failure
2. they reduce pre-load
3. they are more powerful than thiazides.

In moderate cardiac failure, between 40 and 80 mg of frusemide (1–2 mg of bumetanide) is usually adequate therapy. In the presence of renal failure, considerably higher doses will often be needed (up to 2 grams of frusemide per day). In the absence of renal failure, such high dose regimens are rarely used except as a last resort. Nowadays, it is much more acceptable to add an angiotensin converting enzyme inhibitor.

Angiotensin converting enzyme (ACE) inhibitors

These drugs act as mixed arterial and venous vasodilators. They act to inhibit the formation of angiotensin II, a potent vasoconstrictor, potentiator of sympathetic nervous system activity and potential mediator of vasopressin release. Angiotensin II also promotes the synthesis and release of aldosterone which induces salt and water retention and has a direct constrictor effect on vascular smooth muscle. These actions of ACE inhibitors are beneficial in the treatment of heart failure and there is even evidence that these drugs improve survival.

Captopril was the first of this group of drugs to become widely available. Others soon followed: enalapril, quinapril (both pro-drugs) and lisinopril. Captopril has a short duration of action, quinapril is intermediate and enalapril and lisinopril are long. The clearance of all 4 drugs is reduced in old people, largely due to an age-related fall in glomerular filtration rate. Heart failure is also associated with a reduction in clearance of these drugs as well as with a fall in volume of distribution. In such circumstances, the peak dose and the area under the plasma concentration–time curve may be greater than expected.

ACE inhibitors should not be used in the presence of bilateral renal artery stenosis, unilateral renal artery stenosis in a single kidney, immune-mediated renal disease, severe renal impairment, preexisting hypotension and preexisting neutropaenia. They should be used with caution in mild renal impairment and patients with collagen vascular diseases (in whom immune-mediated side-effects are more frequent). The side-effects of ACE inhibitors are summarized in Table 7.7. Cough as a side effect of captopril is important to recognise, and may be a long standing problem. It is extremely rewarding to be able to stop the medication and to stop a very troublesome problem which may be being treated by other medications.

It is our practice to introduce ACE inhibitors when heart failure is not controlled by 40–80 mg of frusemide per day. Captopril should be commenced in a dose of 6.25 mg twice daily and the first dose is best given on retiring to bed since it not infrequently induces moderate to severe hypotension. The dose should be gradually increased, provided blood pressure and renal function are well maintained, to a maximum of 25 mg 2 or 3 times a day.

Table 7.7 Side effects of ACE inhibitors

First dose hypotension
Persistent hypotension
Neutropenia
Proteinuria
Renal failure
Eosinophilia
Angioedema (? commoner with enalapril)
Cough (captopril)

Digoxin

Digoxin is undoubtedly a useful drug for the control of atrial fibrillation. However, considerable controversy persists about its use in heart failure without atrial fibrillation. The debate revolves around whether or not it has any useful inotropic effect in the setting of heart failure. It is our current practice only to use this drug when atrial fibrillation is present or occasionally in the short term treatment of acute cardiac failure.

Despite its bad reputation for producing side effects, digoxin therapy is usually well tolerated by older people and the dose should be titrated by response (usually 125–250 micrograms per day). Measurement of drug concentration in plasma is not particularly useful except in the diagnosis of toxicity. Toxicity is unlikely with a plasma concentration less than 2 nmol/l and almost inevitable when it is greater than 3 nmol/l. The features of digoxin toxicity are well known (Table 7.8). A number of drugs may impair digoxin clearance (quinine, quinidine, captopril, amiodarone, spironolactone, verapamil) and antibiotic treatment may enhance its absorption.

Table 7.8 Features of digoxin toxicity

Anorexia
Nausea
Vomiting
Fatigue
Confusion
Xanthopsia
Cardiac dysrhythmias

Xamoterol

This drug is a partial beta-1 agonist. When endogenous adrenergic activity is low (at rest) it has a moderate inotropic and chronotropic effect but when adrenergic activity is high (exercise) it functions predominantly as an antagonist. Too little information is available to give firm guidelines for its use. It should not be given to patients with a high resting sympathetic drive (moderate to severe heart failure).

Vasodilators

Long-acting nitrates, hydrallazine and alpha-adrenoreceptor antagonists (e.g. prazosin) have all been used successfully in the treatment of chronic heart failure. The major limiting factor for their use is that tolerance often rapidly develops.

Refractory heart failure

Heart failure that does not respond to a combination of loop diuretic and ACE inhibitor should be treated in hospital. Fluid intake needs to be restricted to between 1 and 1.5 l/day. Body weight and urine output need to be measured daily. Loop diuretics can be given intravenously. We rarely give more than 160 mg of frusemide per day by this route and will usually introduce metolazone at this stage. If there is no response in a severely edematous and uraemic patient, an infusion of dopamine (2.5–5 ug/kg/min) can produce dramatic responses. If the patient is hypotensive, dobutamine can be given (15ug/kg/min). There is usually a marked response over 48–72 hours of treatment and the improvement is often sustained over several weeks, after which the treatment can be repeated. Failure to respond to these measures usually indicates very severe heart failure and supportive measures and relief of distress should then become the prime considerations.

Suggested reading

Anon. Digoxin: new answers; new questions [Editorial]. *Lancet, (1989)*. **ii**:79–80.

Applefeld M.M., Newman, K.A., Grove, W.R., Sutton, F.J., Roffman, D.S., Reed, W.P., Linberg, S.E. Intermittent, continuous outpatient dobutamine infusion in the management of congestive heart failure. *Am. J. Cardio.*, **51**:455–8.

Cody, R.J., Torre, S., Clark, M. and Pondolfino, K. (1989). Age-related hemodynamic, renal and hormonal differences among patients with congestive heart failure. *Arch. Int. Med.*, **149**:1023–8.

Firth, J.D., Raine, A.E.G., and Ledingham, J.G.G. (1988) Raised venous pressure: a direct cause of renal sodium retention in oedema? *Lancet*,. **i**:1033–6.

Fleg J.L., Congestive heart failure in the elderly. *J. Ger. Drug Therapy.*, **3**:5–22.

Harris, P. (1988). Role of arterial pressure in the oedema of heart disease. *Lancet.*, **i**:1036–8.

Liang, C-S., Sherman, L.G., Doherty, J.U., Wellington, K., Lee, V.W., Hood, W.B., (1984). Sustained improvement of cardiac function in patients with congestive heart failure after short term infusion of dobutamine. *Circul.*, **69**: 113–19.

8

Hypertension and hypotension

1. Hypertension

In the developed countries, both systolic and diastolic blood pressure (BP) tend to rise, until about the age of 60, beyond that, systolic pressure may continue to rise, whereas the diastolic pressure tends to stabilize or decline. In contrast, in some primitive societies, neither systolic nor diastolic BP increases with age; hypertension is practically non-existent. This has been attributed to the lesser amounts of dietary sodium (< 60 mEq per day) of these populations.

According to the Joint National Committee's 1988 Report on the Detection, Evaluation, and Treatment of High Blood Pressure, systolic pressure elevation is defined as 140 mm Hg or greater and diastolic pressure elevation as 90 mm Hg or greater. Patients whose diastolic pressures are < 90 mm Hg with systolic pressures between 140 and 1 59 mm Hg have borderline systolic hypertension. By definition, isolated systolic hypertension (ISH) is a systolic pressure of 160 mm Hg or greater. When the diastolic pressure is > 89 mm Hg, the condition is called systemic arterial hypertension.

The reported high prevalence of elevated arterial pressures in the USA has led many to believe that a rising arterial pressure associated with aging is normal and innocuous. To the contrary, several multicenter prospective studies have shown that the higher the systolic or diastolic pressure, the greater are the cardiovascular and total morbidity and mortality rates. Moreover, these studies have also shown that an elevated systolic pressure is a better predictor of cardiovascular complications than is an elevated diastolic pressure. An isolated systolic pressure elevation imparts a two to five-fold excess risk of cardiovascular death, a 2.5 times greater risk of stroke, and a 51 per cent, excess overall mortality as compared with age-, race-, and sex-matched normotensive individuals.

In general, hypertension predisposes the affected individual to heart failure, stroke, renal failure, coronary heart disease, and peripheral vascular disease. Antihypertensive therapy reduces the risk of developing many of these catastrophic complications. For example, treatment of hypertension has contributed to a reduction in the incidence of fatal stroke in the USA by 50 per cent, and deaths from myocardial infarction (MI) by 35 per cent. Similar treatment benefits have been reported by the European Working Party on Hypertension in the Elderly, which demonstrated a 60 per cent, reduction in fatal MI.

Pathophysiology of Hypertension in the Elderly

The hemodynamic characteristics of elderly hypertensives are similar to those of younger patients. Thus, arterial pressure is the product of 2 hemodynamic variables: cardiac output (CO) and vascular resistance. The CO, in turn, is the product of 2 variables, heart rate and stroke volume; and the latter may be increased by enhanced myocardial contractility or venous return. Vascular resistance may be increased by adrenergic stimulation, increased renopressor activity, and many circulating hormonal or humoral substances. In considering hypertension in the elderly it is necessary therefore to consider all of these factors.

Atherosclerotic disease, so common in the elderly, reduces large artery distensibility, resulting in elevated systolic pressure as the left ventricle ejects its stroke volume into a more rigid and less compliant aorta. This reduced distensibility of the aorta and other large arteries is a major factor in the pathophysiology of ISH and also impairs left ventricular impedance. Other pathologic conditions that can contribute to systolic hypertension in the elderly are hyperthyroidism, aortic insufficiency, malnutrition (with clinical or subclinical beriberi), diseases with arterio-venous fistulae, and fever.

As the vascular resistance increases, so do systolic and diastolic pressures. The heart adapts to this progressively increasing afterload by a process of concentric hypertrophy. This pressure-overload left ventricular hypertrophy is eventually associated with myocardial ischemia. This process may be aggravated further if exogenous obesity coexists. Obesity is associated with expanded intravascular volume, increased venous return to the heart, and elevated CO. This volume overload provides an eccentric component to the left ventricular hypertrophy, offering an explanation for the facilitated cardiac failure observed in obesity-associated hypertension.

In contrast to the plasma volume expansion that occurs with obesity, intravascular volume contracts as arterial pressure and total peripheral resistance rise in most patients with essential hypertension. In the elderly, however, activity of the renopressor system seems to be reduced, so an attenuated relationship between intravascular volume and the renopressor system results. Plasma renin activity and angiotensin II levels are suppressed in elderly individuals with hypertension. Malignant hypertension therefore in the absence of renal artery stenosis is uncommon in the elderly.

Catecholamine levels, particularly norepinephrine, have been found to be elevated with increased age; and beta-adrenergic receptor responsiveness suggests these receptors are down-regulated. However, beta-adrenergic receptors seem to be unchanged.

Because atherosclerosis is common in the elderly, the presence of an atherosclerotic renal arterial lesion is a major secondary etiologic consideration. Such a lesion may produce an elevated arterial pressure de novo or aggravate prior essential hypertension. Underlying endocrine diseases (e.g., thyroid diseases, hypercalcemic diseases, release of humoral agents from malignant tumors, primary aldosteronism, and pheochromocytoma) also may account for recent-onset hypertension in the elderly.

Elderly patients frequently have multiple medications and these should be carefully considered when identifying the etiology of recent onset, aggravation, or complication of hypertension. For example, use of digitalis and a diuretic may cause hypokalemia-related cardiac dysrhythmias; chronic diarrhea and laxative abuse may also predispose to hypokalemia; corticosteroids may produce a hypokalemic form of hypertension; cyclosporine, tricyclic antidepressants, monoamine oxidase (MAO) inhibitors, and phenyl-Propanolamine or other vasoconstrictors contained in cold preparations may also elevate arterial pressure.

Subjective and Objective Findings

Hypertension, when uncomplicated and not associated with target organ involvement, is usually a silent disease. The medical literature suggest hypertension is associated with headaches, epistaxis, and tinnitus. These complaints are non-specific.

Symptoms and signs occur more often in hypertensive patients with secondary forms of hypertension. Thus, pheochromocytoma may be associated with headache, flushing, BP lability and hypermetabolism. Occlusive renal arterial disease may produce sudden onset or worsening of BP elevation, headaches, and renal arterial bruits that are systolic and (more significantly) diastolic in timing. Patients with renal parenchyma disease may experience recurrent Urinary tract infection and symptoms of frequency, nocturia, impaired urinary concentratability, microscopic or gross hematuria, and anemia (with advanced disease). The co-existence of hypertension and anemia in younger patients indicates renal parenchymal disease (if hemoglobinopathy is excluded); however, in the elderly, it suggests the possibility of co-existent neoplasm.

Patients with thyroid disease show the characteristic symptoms of hyper- or hypothyroidism. Those with primary aldosteronism exhibit muscle weakness, nocturia, isosthenuria, altered carbohydrate metabolism, and hypokalemic alkalosis. Cushing's disease is also suggested by the presence of hypokalemic alkalosis and the typical facies, hirsutism, purplish abdominal striae, buffalo hump, and new appearance of acneiform lesions.

In patients with essential hypertension, the presence of symptoms or signs suggests target organ involvement. With cardiac involvement, the earliest complaints are easy fatigability, palpitations, and atrial or ventricular ectopic cardiac beats. Chest pain in patients without occlusive coronary disease reflects increased myocardial oxygen demand, with persistently elevated arterial pressures and cardiomegaly (left ventricular hypertrophy). More advanced stages of cardiac involvement are marked by symptoms and signs of heart failure: exertional dyspnea, orthopnea, peripheral edema, and increased ventricular irritability. Edema in the absence of cardiac failure suggests a secondary form of hypertension. A third heart sound (ventricular gallop rhythm) may develop, usually in association with a fourth heart sound (atrial gallop), which reflects the reduced distensibility and compliance of the hypertrophying left ventricle. Sudden onset of back pain and hypertension suggest aortic dissection.

The earliest symptom of renal involvement is nocturia, but nocturia is almost universal in the elderly; later symptoms and signs are those of renal impairment: frequency, proteinuria, anemia, and edema.

Sensory or motor deficits signal involvement of the brain; subtle symptoms of TIAs include transient speech impediments, numbness of fingers and extremities, or unusual weakness. Sudden onset of a severe vertical headache and hypertension suggests a subarachnoid hemorrhage.

All patients should be examined for hypertensive retinopathy. This should not be confused with the sclerotic changes of increased arteriolar light-striping, arteriovenous nicking, and tortuosity. Arteriolar (and venular) constriction and the appearance of hemorrhages, exudates, and papilledema suggest advancing and more severe degrees of hypertensive vascular disease. The physician should listen for renal, carotid, aortic, brachial, and femoral arterial bruits. For example, the presence of a carotid bruit with symptoms of transient ischemic attach suggests embolic phenomena from that vessel.

Assessment

Laboratory studies in patients with hypertension should include: a blood count (with hemoglobin, hematocrit and white blood cell); an electrocardiogram (to identify early evidence of left ventricular hypertrophy, left atrial abnormality, and dysrhythmias); selected blood chemistries such as fasting blood glucose and serum levels of creatinine, uric acid, potassium, and lipids (including high- and low-density cholesterol fractions); and a urinalysis. Hyperuricemia may indicate that the patient is taking a diuretic; has the inborn potential for gout; or, in the untreated hypertensive patient, that renal blood flow is reduced.

The chest x-ray is less sensitive than the ECG for detecting cardiac enlargement. ECG evidence of left atrial enlargement provides an early clue to left ventricular hypertrophy, before it can be detected by the usual criteria of increased voltage, delayed intrinsic deflection of the QRS complex, or left ventricular hypertrophy and strain pattern. The enlarged left atrium does not indicate atrial disease per se. Rather, it indicates reduced left ventricular distensibility associated with development of hypertrophy of the left ventricle.

Even more sensitive than the ECG is the echocardiogram, which can clearly demonstrate ventricular hypertrophy in patients whose ECG shows left atrial abnormality only. Moreover, before systolic functional changes occur as a result of left ventricular hypertrophy, diastolic functional changes are revealed by echocardiographic or radionuclide studies showing a reduced left atrial filling rate. Echocardiographic evidence of left ventricular hypertrophy usually precedes early evidence of renal functional impairment, which includes slightly reduced renal blood flow in proportion to the height of serum uric acid concentration. Later evidence of renal impairment includes rising serum creatinine or blood urea nitrogen concentrations, as well as reduced creatinine clearance (glomerular filtration rate) and urine concentratability.

Hypercalcemic states are frequently associated with hypertension, and when they are present, the clinician should think first of hyperparathyroidism in younger persons but metastatic bone disease in older patients. Because hypercalcemia is frequently associated with diuretic therapy, this possibility should be carefully explored in the history taking.

Proteinuria occurs infrequently in patients with uncomplicated essential hypertension. When daily urinary protein excretion exceeds 400 mg, nephrosclerosis (associated with essential hypertension or aging) is not likely to be the cause; the entire differential diagnosis of renal parenchymal disease should be considered. A fresh urine sample with an alkaline pH suggests hypokalemia or primary aldosteronism.

Plan

Diagnosis

The diagnosis of hypertension depends on demonstration of elevated arterial pressure. The elevated pressure should be documented on at least three separate occasions, with at least two separate BP measurements taken on each occasion.

Proper technique in BP measurement is especially important in the elderly patient. BP should be measured in both arms during the initial examination and periodically thereafter. Frequently, occlusive atherosclerotic disease of the subclavian or brachial arteries reduces systolic pressure in one arm, as evidenced by an abrupt, unexplainable decline.

Measurements should be obtained in supine or sitting and standing positions, because postural (orthostatic) hypotension is common in elderly patients, particularly after meals. If pressures are persistently and strikingly elevated but cardiac size is normal according to chest X-ray and ECG criteria, the physician should suspect 'pseudohypertension.' This finding occurs when the sphygmomanometer cuff is unable to compress a sclerotic brachial artery. To verify the phenomenon, a direct arterial pressure measurement may be needed. Once actual hypertension is diagnosed, the physician must determine whether the condition is of primary or secondary origin.

Treatment

Non-pharmacological treatment includes maintaining an ideal weight, moderating alcohol intake, controlling dietary sodium (100 mEq/day), and avoiding smoking. Studies show that smokers who take certain antihypertensive drugs, such as propranolol, have more complications of hypertension than smokers who receive other treatment, such as thiazide diuretics. These therapeutic measures may not control arterial pressure completely, but they may be adequate to control pressure in some patients or reduce the number and dosages of antihypertensive drugs in others.

Isolated systolic hypertension (ISH)

The efficacy of reducing systolic arterial pressure in patients with ISH has not yet been adequately demonstrated in clinical studies. However, it appears that ISH patients are at greater risk than non-hypertensive individuals and the elevated pressure and larger heart of the elderly ISH patient increases myocardial oxygen demand. The feasibility study for a large multicenter study of systolic hypertension in the elderly (SHEP) strongly suggests that elevated systolic pressure can be controlled by diuretics (e.g., hydrochlorothiazide, starting with 25 mg and increasing, if necessary, to 50 mg). Alternatively, beta-adrenergic receptor blocking agents or Ca entry antagonists may be effective. If one of these agents alone is unable to control the elevated pressure, a second drug may be added (e.g., a diuretic and a beta-blocker).

Mild hypertension

Patients whose diastolic pressure falls between 90 and 104 mm Hg, and whose pressures are not controlled by non-pharmacologic means, may respond to a diuretic, beta-adrenergic receptor blocker, an angiotensin converting enzyme (ACE) inhibitor, or a Ca entry antagonist in submaximal doses. The European Working party on hypertension in the elderly study demonstrated a clear advantage to treatment of mild asymptomatic hypertension for individuals of both sexes, between the ages of 60 and 79 years with a K sparing, thiazide diuretic combination. If the initial dose fails to control pressure, the dose may be increased. This concept is consistent with the currently advocated 'individualized stepped care' approach to treatment.

A second agent may be added to low-dose drug administration to prevent development of side effects from full doses of the first agent. Thus, adding a beta-blocker to hydrochlorothiazide 25 mg daily may prevent hypokalemia and hyperuricemia. In general, elderly patients respond to diuretics. Ca entry antagonists are also effective with these patients, as well as with blacks and with patients who have not responded to lower doses of beta-blocking drugs prescribed for concomitant angina pectoris.

More severe stages of hypertension

In patients with moderate or severe hypertension, any of the first-step agents may be prescribed. If this does not control BP adequately, however, a second or third agent may be necessary. These can be added sequentially, using lower doses first, then increasing doses or adding different agents.

It has to be appreciated that side-effects of medication can be common in the elderly and this may modify treatment goals. If the patient is already using digitalis, a diuretic should be prescribed with care. Serum potassium levels should be closely followed to obviate cardiac dysrhythmias associated with hypokalemia. Impotence may result in male patients treated with diuretics, adrenergic inhibitors, and beta-blockers; the ACE inhibitors and Ca entry antagonists have been reported to produce fewer side-effects. Although elderly hypertensive patients have no more side-effects from prolonged treatment than younger patients, they are more likely to have postural (orthostatic) hypotension from agents that inhibit adrenergic function. Also, agents with central actions may be more likely to cause depression, forgetfulness, vivid dreams or hallucinations, and sleep problems. Patients with chronic obstructive lung disease, asthma, or heart block (greater than Ist degree) should not be treated with beta-blocking drugs; Ca entry antagonists may be more appropriate. Patients with low heart rates may be good candidates for Ca entry antagonists that do not markedly reduce heart rate.

2. Orthostatic hypotension

Many healthy elderly people have wide variations in postural BP. Orthostatic hypotension is defined as a reduction of at least 20 mm in systolic BP upon standing upright. Orthostatic hypotension is a common clinical manifestation of impaired BP homeostasis, occurring in 20 to 30 per cent of non-institutionalized elderly persons. A strong relationship exists between postural BP change and basal supine BP; when basal supine BP is highest, the decline in postural BP is greatest.

Pathophysiology of hypotension in the elderly

Many physiologic changes that occur with aging affect blood pressure control. Baroreflex mechanisms regulate systemic BP by resisting transient decreases and damping transient increases in arterial pressure. With age, baroreflex response to changes in blood pressure progressively declines. This attenuation of baroreflex response may be caused partly by arterial stiffening that results in a damping of baroreceptor stretch and relaxation during changes in arterial pressure. Reduced adrenergic responsiveness by the aged heart may also result in diminished baroreflex-mediated cardioacceleration during hypotensive stimuli. These changes in baroreflex response become clinically significant when common hypotensive stresses, such as posture change, can no longer be offset by compensatory homeostatic mechanisms.

A progressive decline in cerebral blood flow occurs with advancing age and is enhanced by risk factors for cerebrovascular disease (e.g., hypertension, heart disease, diabetes mellitus, and hyperlipidemia). Thus, since elderly patients with such risk factors have reduced cerebral flow, relatively small reductions in BP may produce cerebral ischemia. Current data suggest that autoregulation of cerebral blood flow is generally maintained with age, except in certain individuals who have symptomatic orthostatic hypotension. Chronic hypertension raises the threshold for cerebral autoregulation and acute reductions in BP might not be tolerated well by hypertensive elderly patients.

Subjective and Objective Findings

Orthostatic hypotension in the elderly has 2 distinct clinical presentations: (1) physiologic, attributable to normal aging, and (2) pathologic, attributable to disease.

Physiologic orthostatic hypotension in healthy elderly persons varies dramatically from day to day, is related to BP elevation and associated with the exaggerated plasma norepinephrine response to postural change. Although generally asymptomatic, transient orthostatic hypotension may become clinically significant when associated with other hypotensive stresses; for example, volume depletion, ingestion of hypotensive drugs, or performance of Valsalva's maneuver during voiding. Prolonged bed rest may further compromise physiologic mechanisms, resulting in severe postural hypotension. Postural systolic BP reductions greater than 20 mm Hg have been shown to be significant risk factors for syncope and falls in elderly patients.

Pathologic orthostatic hypotension is usually symptomatic and is associated with postural dizziness, syncope, and symptoms of autonomic dysfunction; for example, a fixed heart rate, constipation, inability to sweat, heat intolerance, impotence, and fatigue. In young patients, the absence of cardioacceleration upon standing is considered a distinguishing feature of autonomic dysfunction (rather than hypovolemia) as the cause of orthostatic hypotension. However, since the response is often impaired in normal elderly persons, it is not useful in the diagnosis of pathologic orthostatic hypotension in the geriatric population. Pathologic orthostatic hypotension may be secondary to any of numerous diseases or to drugs commonly taken by elderly patients (Table 8.1).

Table 8.1 Causes of orthostatic hypotension

Idiopathic orthostatic hypotension
Central nervous system disorders
Shy–Drager syndrome
Brainstem lesions
Parkinson's disease
Myelopathy
Multiple cerebral infarcts
Peripheral and autonomic neuropathies
Diabetes mellitus
Amyloidosis
Tabes dorsalis
Paraneoplastic syndromes
Alcoholic and nutritional diseases
Drugs
Phenothiazines and other neuroleptics
Monoamine oxidase inhibitors
Tricyclic antidepressants
Antihypertensives
Levodopa
Vasodilators
Beta-blockers
Ca channel blockers

Idiopathic orthostatic hypotension is characterized by lower basal plasma norepinephrine levels in the supine position, no increase in norepinephrine level upon standing, a lower threshold for the pressor response to infused norepinephrine, and a greater pressor response to tyramine, despite release of less norepinephrine at the sympathetic nerve ending. These findings suggest that norepinephrine is depleted from sympathetic nerve endings, resulting in postsynaptic denervation supersensitivity.

Patients with the Shy–Drager syndrome have normal levels of circulating norepinephrine and a normal response to infused norepinephrine and tyramine, but they also have no increase in plasma norepinephrine levels upon standing. This syndrome is associated with the degeneration of neurons in several areas of the central nervous system, including the corticobulbar, corticospinal, extrapyramidal, and cerebellar systems of the brain, as well as intermediolateral columns of the spinal cord. Thus the Shy–Drager syndrome is a central disorder of sympathetic BP control, usually associated with extrapyramidal and cerebellar symptoms.

Disorders of the peripheral autonomic nervous system are other major causes of pathologic orthostatic hypotension. This includes insulin-dependent diabetes mellitus, in which severe peripheral neuropathy and other end-organ damage is evident. Much less common causes are conditions such as amyloidosis, vitamin deficiencies, and the neuropathies associated with malignancies, particularly cancers of the lung and the pancreas.

Probably the most common cause of orthostatic hypotension is the use of medications, such as antihypertensive drugs, phenothiazines, tricyclic antidepressants, and antianxiety agents. Orthostatic hypotension may occur even from doses within the therapeutic range, which poses a dilemma, in that a positive therapeutic effect is achieved at the expense of this adverse effect.

Plan

Diagnosis

The proper management of orthostatic hypotension begins with a clear demonstration of a clinically significant symptomatic reduction in BP upon standing. The BP and pulse rate should be measured after the patient has been recumbent for at least 5 minutes and again at 1 and 3 minutes after the patient has been standing quietly. These measurements should be obtained on several occasions to confirm that the reduction of BP is consistent. The goal of therapy should be reduction or elimination of symptoms, which often can be achieved without complete correction of orthostatic hypotension.

Treatment

Initial therapeutic considerations include correction of hypovolemia and evaluation of all medications the patient is taking in order to identify a possible offending agent. The patient with chronic orthostatic hypotension should be instructed to rise slowly from bed or chair after a long period of lying or sitting. Dorsiflexing the feet before standing often promotes venous return to the heart, accelerates the pulse, and increases BP. Initiating a high salt intake program may produce modest weight gain but also will reduce symptoms of orthostatic hypotension in many individuals. Elastic stockings that cover the thigh as well as the calf may also be effective. Elevating the head of the bed 5 to 20 degrees prevents the nocturnal diuresis and supine hypertension caused by nocturnal shifts of interstitial fluid from the legs to the rest of the circulation.

If the patient remains symptomatic despite these measures, medications may be necessary. Various drug regimens have been attempted, but most of them either have been ineffective or require further study. One agent that is often helpful is fludrocortisone acetate. This mineralocorticoid, given in daily doses of 0.1 to 1.0 mg orally until mild peripheral edema develops, produces an increase in extracellular fluid and plasma volume, and sensitizes blood vessels to the vasoconstrictive effect of norepinephrine. These physiologic changes appear to offset the homeostatic defect that occurs on arising in most persons with mild or moderately severe orthostatic hypotension. Except for the occasional development of supine hypertension or heart failure, complications of treatment are rare. Hypokalemia with large doses of mineralocorticoids is usually not a problem.

Other drugs currently under study in the management of pathologic orthostatic hypotension include NSAIDs, such as indomethacin, the central alpha 2-antagonist yohimbine, the alpha 2-agonist clonidine, and beta-blockers that block beta 2-vasodilator receptors or have intrinsic sympathomimetic activity such as pindolol.

3. Post-prandial hypotension

Post-prandial hypotension is another recently recognized clinical abnormality of BP homeostasis in the elderly. Studies of clinically stable, unmedicated elderly patients, both institutionalized and non-institutionalized, show significant reduction in BP after morning and noon meals, which does not occur in younger persons or in the absence of a meal in the elderly. About one third of healthy elderly have a postprandial BP decline of at least 20 mm Hg within 1 hour of eating a meal. This decline can be even greater when hypotensive medications are given before a meal. The incidence of post-prandial hypotension is greatest in hypertensive elderly persons and in patients who have post-prandial syncope or autonomic dysfunction. This phenomenon is probably a common cause of syncope and falls in the elderly.

The mechanism of postprandial hypotension is unknown but is thought to be related to impaired baroreflex compensation for splanchnic blood pooling during digestion. The BP should be evaluated before and after meals in geriatric patients who experience post-prandial dizziness, falls, syncope, or other cerebral or cardiac ischemic symptoms.

In the absence of clinical trials to evaluate treatment of postprandial hypotension, management relies on common sense. Symptomatic patients should avoid taking hypotensive medications before meals and should lie down after eating. Reduction in dosage of hypotensive medications and ingestion of small, frequent meals may also be helpful. Recent studies of patients with autonomic insufficiency suggest that indomethacin, caffeine with or without subcutaneous dihydroergotamine, or parenteral somatostatin given by experimental protocol before a meal may ameliorate postprandial hypotension. Caffeine (with dihydroergotamine) should be given only in the morning so the caffeine effect wears off by evening, allowing sleep and preventing tolerance to the drug. Other agents given a half-hour or so before the meal last for only a few hours.

Suggested reading

Black D.M., Brand, R.J., Greenlick, M. et al. (1987). Compliance to treatment for hypertension in the elderly patients: the SHEP pilot study. *J. Gerontol.* **432**: 552–7.

Hagberg J.M., Montain, S.J., Martin, W.H. III and Ehsani, A.A. (1989). Effect of exercise training in 60 to 69 year old persons with essential hypertension. *Amer. J. Cardiol.*, **64**: 348–53.

Lipsitz, L.A., Pluchino, F.C., Wei, J.Y., Minaker, K.L., and Rowe, J.R. (1986). Cardiovascular and norepinephrine responses after meal consumption in elderly (older than 75 Years) persons with postprandial hypotension and syncope. *Amer. J. Cardiol.*, **58**: 810–15.

Lye, M., Vargas, E., Faragher, E.B., Davies, I., and Goddard, C. (1990). Haemodynamic and neurohumoral responses in elderly patients with postural hypotension. *Eur. J. Clin. Invest.*, **20**: 90–96.

Materson, B.J., Cushman, W.C., Goldstein, G. et al. (1990). Treatment of hypertension in the elderly: results of a Department of Veterans affairs cooperative study, parts I and II. *Hypertension*, **15**: 348–69.

Siegel, D., Kuller, L., Lazarus, N.B. et al. (1987). Predictors of cardiovascular events and mortality in the systolic hypertension in the Elderly Program Pilot Project. *Amer. J. Epidemiol.*, **126**:385–99.

Staessen J., Bulpitt, C., Clement, D. et al. (1989). Relation between mortality and treated blood pressure in elderly patients with hypertension:

Report of the European Working Party on High Blood Pressure in the Elderly. *Br. Med. J.* **298**: 1552–56.

Wilking, S.V.B., Belanger, A., Kannel, W.B., D'Agostino, R.B., Steel, K. (1988). Determinants of isolated systolic hypertension. *J. Amer. Med. Assoc.*, **260**: 3451–5.

Woo, J., Woo, K.S., Kin, T., Vallance, Owen, J. (1987). A single blind, randomized, cross-over study of angiotensin converting enzyme inhibitor and triamterene and hydrochlorothiazide in the treatment of mild to moderate hypertension in the elderly. *Arch. Int. Med.*, **147**: 1386–9.

9

Pyrexia, heat stroke and hypothermia

1. Pathophysiology of body temperature control

Normal humans can maintain the core body temperature constant to within a degree. The normal range of core temperature is usually taken to be between 36.5 and 37.5 degrees Celsius. It tends to be lower in the mornings and higher with exercise. Peripheral or skin temperature may vary a great deal. Core body temperature is sensed by peripheral skin receptors which are sensitive to either heat or cold; and temperature sensitive receptors in deeper areas of the body which monitor blood temperature. There are also temperature sensitive neurones, within the preoptic area of the anterior hypothalamus. These neurones form the thermostat for core body temperature and are 'set' to a central reference temperature. The hypothalamus also integrates the information from the peripheral and deep receptors elsewhere in the body. As the temperature rises the inhibitory activity from the anterior hypothalamus increases, conversely it diminishes as the temperature drops. Body temperature is therefore controlled by altering heat loss and heat production.

The receptors in the anterior hypothalamus in response to a temperature drop release the posterior hypothalamus resulting in adrenergic vasoconstriction. Heat loss mainly occurs through the skin and can be reduced by vasoconstriction. There is also an accompanying piloerection which is of little importance in humans. Reduction of heat loss is accompanied by increased generation of heat through release of the shivering center from inhibition. The resulting increase in muscle tone and muscle metabolism, and onset of shivering results in a rise in heat production. With increased production of epinephrine and norepinephrine there is uncoupling of phosphorylative oxidation, leading to increased oxidation of foodstuffs. Thyroxine production will also be increased which would lead to increased cellular metabolism and increased heat.

Conversely, when the temperature rises heat loss is promoted. This is done by vasodilatation and increasing loss through the skin. Sweating is increased to increase loss by evaporation. Heat production is held constant.

2. Age changes in body temperature control.

The elderly are less able to detect ambient temperature differences, in fact about one-quarter of the elderly population show very poor temperature discrimination. The ambient temperature of the private dwellings of the elderly have been shown to be lower than other groups but there may be many factors that influence this, including economic ones.

Apart from the detection of ambient temperature, and the decreased ability to 'fine tune' the environment, there is also deterioration in the mechanisms that control body temperature (Table 9.1). In one study of normal people living at home about a half of them had abnormal peripheral blood flow in response to moderate cooling and warming. Shivering in response to cooling only occurred in 12 per cent. Elderly individuals may require a greater fall in body temperature to initiate shivering. It would appear that there is a proportion of the elderly population that have impairment of temperature regulation and that the proportion increases with advancing age. This impairment is not restricted to temperature regulation but is manifest in other areas of the autonomic nervous system, and correlates with the presence of postural hypotension.

Apart from normal aging, there are changes related to disease that impair thermoregulatory mechanisms – these would include stroke, head injury, spinal cord injury and Wernicke's encephalopathy. Myoedema may lower body temperature. Some drugs inhibit the ability to control body temperature, for example by inhibiting shivering. Examples would be the major tranquilizers like chlorpromazine, or barbiturates or antidepressants (Table 9.1).

Table 9.1 Impaired thermoregulation

1. Normative aging:
   - Detection of change
   - Control ambient temperature
2. Disease:
   - Impaired thermoregulatory reflexes
     - stroke
     - head injury
     - Wernicke's encephalopathy
     - extensive skin lesions
     - steatorrhoea
     - spinal cord lesion
   - Metabolic effects
     - hypothyroidism
     - malnutrition
     - immobility
     - diabetic coma
   - Drugs
     - tranquilizers (chlorpromazine)
     - barbiturates
     - antidepressants
     - alcohol

3. Pyrexia

Impaired febrile response in old age

It has been accepted for a long time that in old age infections can occur without the development of fever. Indeed Hippocrates noted this in his 'Aphorisms'. But how frequently does this occur, and is the absence of fever more common with advancing age? These are important questions and it is not clear that the answers are forthcoming.

The majority of elderly people develop fever in response to infection, but some do not. In one study of patients with pneumococcal bacteraemia it was clear that the maximum temperature attained during infection was lower in those over the age of 65, when compared with younger groups. The number of elderly patients that do not become pyrexial in the presence of a definite infection ranges between 5 and 65 per cent from different series. When temperature is recorded by the rectal route, and every 4 hours, the number without fever in the presence of definite pneumonia is between 12 and 15 per cent.

For accurate recording of core body temperature, the rectal route is preferred. Oral temperature is inaccurate in the elderly for various reasons. The majority of elderly patients manifest a normal febrile response and cannot be distinguished on this basis from younger age groups. It is not clear if the proportion with an afebrile response increases with age.

The reasons for the lack of fever in some infected individuals are not understood. It has been seen in the previous section (Table 9.1) that many factors contribute to impaired temperature regulation. The same factors are relevant here, so that disease, drugs or a low environmental temperature could result in a failure to develop fever.

The autonomic nervous system has been shown to deteriorate with age which has a variety of effects. These changes are thought to account for the altered sensitivity to visceral pain, the development of postural hypotension, the impaired thermoregulation and the altered presentation of disease. Undoubtedly these changes could lead to an impaired febrile response, there being an inability to restrict heat loss or to generate more heat. The humoral mediator of the pyrexial response, endogenous pyrogen or interleukin 1, IL-1, has also been looked at in old age. It has been postulated that impaired production by circulating monocytes, and altered sensitivity of the hypothalamus, with advancing age might account for the impaired febrile response. Studies that have been done have shown no consistent aging effect in humans.

Failure to mount a febrile response may be of clinical significance by masking the clinical picture and causing a potential delay in diagnosis. There is no apparent difference in morbidity or mortality, and the group that are febrile have no special features that allow their separation or identification.

It is common clinical practice to reduce the temperature of the febrile patient. This is done by a combination of physical and pharmacological methods, such as acetaminophen or aspirin to reduce the temperature or use of a fan over ice. Such measures are appropriate and may well make the patient feel better. However, there is no good evidence that this approach is beneficial to the patient. Morbidity and mortality do not appear to be affected. When the fever is very high as in heat stroke there may be permanent brain damage and it is essential to reduce the temperature.

It is possible that fever is beneficial. Immune responses may be enhanced by a rise in temperature. Survival is enhanced in the neonate by a higher ambient temperature, and premature infants are more likely to die if in incubators with lower temperatures. There is no comparable data for the elderly, and the usual clinical practice is to reduce fever and provide symptomatic relief.

Detection of fever in old age

In order to detect fever, body temperature must be accurately recorded. There is some evidence that this becomes more difficult with advancing age. The temperature of the mouth does not accurately reflect core body temperature. It is difficult to ensure adequate closure, particularly in those patients with raised respiratory rates. It has been shown that the accuracy of oral temperatures can be improved by using electronic recording methods. However this is not generally available, whereas rectal thermometers are. It should be noted that rectal temperature in the elderly is usually higher than oral by 0.3 to 1.2°C, therefore even with a core temperature of 38.5°C the oral temperature may be 'normal'.

Central body temperature is reflected by the temperature of the esophagus, the external auditory meatus or the urine. None of these can be recorded easily. The best site for recording is the rectum, this most accurately reflects the core body temperature.

Our recommendation is to record rectal temperatures, and if searching for fever these should be taken every 4–6 hours.

Heat stroke

Predisposing factors

The normative age changes which lead to deterioration of the thermoregulatory mechanisms obviously predispose the elderly to the problems of heat stroke or hypothermia. Age itself would appear to be a predisposing factor to heat stroke, the mean age of those dying from heat illness has been shown to be in the early 70s. Like many other situation there is loss of reserve with aging and the older adult is less able to withstand the stress of a hot climate. In the same way elderly individuals are less able to acclimatize to a hot climate.

Disease may also predispose an elderly patient to heat stroke if the disease is impairing the thermoregulatory reflexes. For example patients with hypothalamic lesions or damage to the spinal cord. Some patients with extensive skin lesions can be considered to be poikilothermic. Hyperpyrexia may also occur following exposure to certain drugs. This would appear to be rare.

The elderly who are most likely to die from heat stroke are those who are suffering from ischemic heart disease or cerebrovascular disease.

Precipitants

The most common precipitant is a high environmental temperature. The clinical entity of heat stroke in the elderly usually occurs when there is a heat wave, a period of time when the ambient temperature is particularly high. The crisis occurring when there is a power failure or a mechanical breakdown of air conditioning.

The frail elderly who are residing in areas poorly equipped to cope with heat waves, are particularly vulnerable. It has been reported that up to 4 per cent of nursing home residents may die during a heat wave. Drugs, including anesthetic agents, can rarely precipitate heat illness.

Subjective

The patient suffering from heat illness is unable to give a history. The ambient temperature will be high. The most likely story is that the patient will have experienced a significant decline in function becoming increasingly lethargic.

Initially patients will sweat in response to the rise in temperature, although in some elderly patients the temperature rise required to produce sweating is higher than in younger age groups. Intense sweating is usually followed by a period of anidrosis. Patients may complain of headache and dizziness. They are likely to develop restlessness and confusion and then go on to develop signs of more profound disturbance.

Objective

The body temperature is elevated, and in one study the mean core body temperature was 41.3°C. The patient is often hyper- ventilating, which in turn may produce a fall in pCO2 and increase in fluid loss. Many patients will show an elevation in blood pressure with a high cardiac index. Others show a drop in blood pressure with a low cardiac index.

Patients are usually dehydrated and develop profound metabolic disturbance leading to shock. Patients may develop cardiac dysrhythmia, gastrointestinal bleeding, purpura and pneumonia. They will develop increasing impairment of consciousness with impending coma.

Plan

Diagnosis

Awareness of prevailing environmental conditions alerts the physician to the possibility of this problem. Diagnosis is reached by recognition of the constellation of signs mentioned above and the finding of a raised body temperature.

Blood should be taken for routine biochemical screen as well as complete blood count. An electrocardiogram should be obtained.

Management

Therapy is aimed at reducing the temperature by cooling and correcting any fluid and metabolic abnormalities. Speed is essential to avoid permanent brain damage. The body is cooled by using ice water and evaporation. With return of temperature to normal the patients should be carefully watched for infection and treated if detected.

Hypothermia

In order to define the problem of hypothermia an accurate body temperature needs to be recorded. If this problem is suspected a special low reading thermometer should be used. Hypothermia is recognized when the body temperature (rectal) is below 35°C.

Predisposing factors

Hypothermia can occur at any age. It results from exposure of the body to low environmental temperature and conditions that promote cooling – for example immersion in cold water. The ability to withstand low environmental temperatures decreases with advancing age. Thus old individuals may develop hypothermia in environments that do not appear to be hostile.

The age changes within the host that have been described, result in impaired thermoregulatory reflexes. In extreme old age there is weight loss (see Chapter 16) which results in loss of insulation, and a decreased ability to retain body heat. Diseases as well as aging predispose to poor temperature control (Table 9.1).

Another important predisposing factor is a hostile environment. In some societies there is an increasing likelihood of poverty with advancing age. Such individuals may not keep their environment warm.

Precipitants

Sudden exposure to extremely cold temperature will precipitate hypothermia if the exposure is of sufficient duration. Anything that promotes cooling will also increase the risk of hypothermia, for instance immersion in water. It has been seen in hospital environments, for example in an intensive care unit when a shocked patient is rapidly transfused with cool solutions and exposed to air conditioning.

Drugs, particularly alcohol may play an important role. For example in the case of an inebriated individual who falls asleep in a snow bank.

An elderly person who falls in a relatively hospitable environment but lays immobile on a cold floor for a long period may develop hypothermia. In the cold Canadian climate hypothermia remains rare except in relation to alcohol intoxication. Most dwellings are centrally heated, and other complications of falls are more common.

Subjective

In the early stages the patient may experience feeling cold, but as the problem progresses and there is increasing disturbance of normal neurological function the patient becomes unable to give a history. The patient becomes apathetic, listless, confused and develops hallucinations and paranoid ideation.

Objective

The patient is obviously cold and feels cold to the touch. The temperature (rectal) needs to be recorded with a low reading thermometer. The skin is usually pale. The finding of a body temperature below 35°C allows the diagnosis to be made.

The patient may be in coma, or if not at that stage may show ataxia, prolonged reflexes, slurred speech, confusion, meningism or muscle rigidity. The pulse slows with associated heart block and various arrhythmias. All patients show a degree of heart block, the Q-T interval is usually prolonged with inversion of the T wave and the development of a J wave. The respiration becomes slow and shallow, often with periods of apnoea. Various organs may be damaged by the low temperature, it is important to remember that there may be features of acute pancreatitis.

Signs of life may be so difficult to record that a premature 'diagnosis of death' may be made.

Plan

Diagnosis

The diagnosis is established by the recording of a low body temperature. A number of initial screening tests need to be done because of the various complications that can occur. This would include a complete blood count, a standard biochemical screen, serum amylase and serum thyroxine. An ECG is indicated and patients with moderate to severe hypothermia need cardiac monitoring.

Management

The most important aspect of treatment is rewarming. Patients with mild hypothermia (32–35°C) need slow and gentle rewarming. The patient should be placed in a warm environment and wrapped in blankets (space blankets) and rewarmed at a rate of 0.5°C per hour. Patients with severe hypothermia need rapid core rewarming. This requires admission to an intensive care unit and the use of one of several different techniques to rewarm – for example peritoneal dialysis with warm fluids (38–43°C) or extracorporeal rewarming of blood.

Patients should be cardiac monitored and corrective action taken for any arrythmia. The airway will need to be protected and some patients may require endotracheal intubation. Fluid balance must be carefully controlled and when fluids are replaced the solutions should be warmed.

Antibiotics (ampicillin) and hydrocortisone are recommended for patients with severe hypothermia.

This problem, when severe, carries a significant mortality of between 30 and 70 per cent. Most patients with mild hypothermia (>32°C) recover. Intensive treatment does save some elderly patients with severe hypothermia, but it remains difficult to say which approach is most beneficial.

Perhaps the most important aspect is prevention. It is of interest that in Canada hypothermia is rare compared to the United Kingdom. The cold Canadian winter demands central heating, better insulation with double glazing of the windows. Thus the elderly person who falls on their way to the bathroom usually falls in a warm environment. Those that fall outside rapidly succumb to sub-zero temperatures or suffer form other problems such as frost-bite. Hypothermia is seen in the alcoholic or the individual who falls whilst inebriated. Indeed one clinical pointer to this is observing the loss of digits or partial amputation of feet as a result of a fall in a snow bank. These individuals, whilst old, are usually the young old or even late middle-aged.

References

Barley, S. L. and Evans, E. J. (1970). Hypothermia in the elderly. *Lancet*, **i**: 1003–4.

Berman, P. and Fox, R. A. (1985). Fever in the elderly. *Age and Ageing*, **14**: 327–32.

Buetow, K. C. and Klein, S. W. (1964). Effect of maintenance of 'normal' skin temperature on survival of infants of low birth weight. *Pediatrics*, **34**: 163–70.

Collins, K. J. (1986). Low indoor temperatures and morbidity in the elderly. *Age and Ageing*, **15**: 212–20.

Collins, K. J., Dore, C., Exton Smith, A. N., MacDonald, C. and Woodward, P. M. (1977) Accidental hypothermia and impaired temperature homeostasis in the elderly. *Brit. Med. J.*, **i**: 353–56.

Collins, K. J., Exton Smith, A. N. and Dore, C. (1981) Urban hypothermia, preferred temperature and chemical perception in old age. *Brit. Med. J.*, **i**: 282;175–7.

Finkelstein, M. S., Petkun, W. M., Freedman, M. L. and Antopol, S. C. (1983) Pneumococcal bacteraemia in adults. *J. Amer. Ger. Soc.*, **31**: 19–27.

Fox, R. H., Woodward, P. M., Exton Smith, A. N., Green, M. F. and Donnison, D. V. (1973). Body temperature in the elderly: a national

study of physiological, social and environmental conditions. *Brit. Med. J.*, **i**: 200–206.
Macpherson, R. K., Offner, F. (1971). The febrile response in the aged. *Med. J. Aust.*, **i**: 292–5.
McAlpine, C. H., Martin, B. J., Lennox, I. M. and Roberts, M. A. (1986) Pyrexia in Infection in the elderly. *Age and Ageing*, **15**: 230–4.
Rudd, A. G., Bannerjee, D. K. (1989). Interleukin 1 production by human monocytes in ageing and disease. *Age and Ageing*, **18**: 43–6.

10

Disturbance of consciousness

Most of the causes of loss of consciousness are not peculiar to the elderly, although some are more common than others. Those individuals with transient loss of consciousness may be able to give a reliable history but failing that a careful history should be sought from witnesses, usually the care providers. This must be followed by a complete physical examination which will usually clarify the situation. In this section we will restrict ourselves to the assessment of syncope, seizure and coma.

The term syncope needs to be understood and implies a transient loss of consciousness due to failure of adequate blood supply. Syncope may arise from a fall in cardiac output, a fall in peripheral resistance or a local abnormality of the blood vessels supplying the brain. There are various types of syncope linked to different physiological situations such as cardiac, vasovagal, cough, micturition, defecation and carotid sinus.

Cardiac syncope is not uncommonly due to cardiac rhythm disturbances. In vasovagal attacks an excessive vagal tone results in bradycardia associated with peripheral vasodilatation in muscles. Carotid sinus hypersensitivity can give rise to syncope by extreme sinus bradycardia or asystole or to acute peripheral vasodilatation. Cough syncope results from a combination of diminished venous return, raised intrathoracic pressure and baroreceptor reflexes stimulated from pressure transients from repeated coughing. Micturition and defecation syncope have been ascribed to a failure of venous return especially when straining. In both of these situations circulatory changes similar to a Valsalva maneuver have been noted.

1. Subjective

In the event that the patient can give a history, details of the feelings and experiences of the patient should be sought. Syncope is characteristically associated with a feeling of dizziness, visual disturbance, nausea and hyperventilation immediately prior to the loss of consciousness. Recovery occurs within a few minutes, particularly in the recumbent position. There may be a history of anxiety, pain, emotional stress or of standing for long periods. Alternatively, there may be a history of recent medical procedures such as venepuncture, rectal examination or esophageal dilatation. These situations will be obvious to the physician and it should be noted that such syncopal episodes are not common in the elderly. There are certain medications that may increase the likelihood of vasovagal episodes, such as phenothiazines, tricyclic antidepressants and antihypertensive agents (Table 10.1).

Cardiac syncope is often due to cardiac rhythm disturbances. The patient is likely to experience symptoms of palpitations and may have a past history of cardiac disease and previous rhythm disturbances. These changes may be associated with typical anginal chest pain. If the patient is taking drugs such as quinidine, disopyramide or lithium then cardiac arrhythmia needs to be considered (Table 10.1).

Cough syncope should be obvious from the history of repeated coughing spells and the association of the fainting spell with these. There is usually

Table 10.1 Drugs and transient loss of consciousness

	Drugs
Vasovagal (syncope)	Phenothiazines, tricyclic antidepressents, antihypertensives
Cardiac syncope	Quinidine, disopyramide, lithium
Carotid sinus hypersensitivity	Beta-blockers, digitalis, alpha methyl dopa
Postural hypotension	L-dopa, bromocryptine, diuretics, antihypertensives, anticholinergics alcohol, glyceryl trimitrate

nothing in the history that will indicate the likelihood of carotid sinus hypersensitivity, although some drugs may be associated (Table 10.1).

If the syncopal episode occurs when the person first stands, for example when first rising from bed in the morning or on getting up from a chair after sitting for some time then postural (orthostatic) hypotension should be considered. In these individuals there may be a history of diabetes or Parkinson's disease and the patient is usually on a number of medications (Table 10.1).

A seizure should be readily distinguishable from syncope. The patient is unlikely to be able to give a clear history immediately afterwards. The loss of consciousness is sudden and usually not related to posture. An aura is possible but rare. During the episode the patient is likely to be rigid and there may be clonic movements as well as incontinence of urine or more rarely feces. Following the seizure there may be a period of drowsiness or disturbed behavior. The patient with a transient ischemic attack has a short lived disturbance of consciousness with focal neurological features (Chapter 15).

In the patient who has become unconscious information should be sought on any associated conditions or any drugs that are taken. When unconsciousness is maintained most information of clinical importance is obtained from the examination but the history must not be overlooked and any significant other should be carefully questioned. A medication history is particularly relevant including agents not normally taken by the patient but available to them.

2. Objective

In any individual with persisting disruption of their level of consciousness it is important to establish a baseline and to monitor it subsequently for change. The Glasgow coma scale which was developed to help with the management of head injuries, is useful (Table 10.2). This scale includes a rating of motor functioning, verbal responses and eye opening to painful or verbal stimuli. Patients with aphasia may score low, but it remains particularly useful for repeated assessments over time. The observation of movement, positioning and tone of the limbs may be helpful in the evaluation of the comatosed patient. As indicated in the Coma scale the presence of motor responses can be tested for using painful stimuli.

Table 10.2 Glasgow coma scale

Test	Score	Response
Eye opening	1	no response to pain
	2	open eyes to pain
		open eyes to herbal stimulus
	4	eyes open spontaneously
Best motor response	1	none
	2	extension to pain
	3	flexion to pain – abnormal
	4	flexion to pain – normal
	5	localizes painful stimulus
	6	normal
Best verbal response	1	none
	2	incomprehensible
	3	inappropriate
	4	confused
	5	fully alert and orientated

Examination of the respiratory pattern is helpful in localizing the level of the lesion, and in indicating the presence of raised intracranial pressure and coning. A prolongation of apnea following periods of hyperventilation is characteristic of bilateral hemispheric damage. Cheyne–Stokes respiration may occur with hemispheric damage but is more typical of damage to pathways running between the cerebral hemispheres and the pons. Hyperventilation is suggestive of midbrain damage. Ataxic breathing, with completely irregular patterns of inspiration, both in depth and frequency, suggests medulla damage and heralds complete respiratory collapse.

The pupils and eye movements are likewise of value in diagnosis and prognosis. Pupillary changes are a very late feature of metabolic coma with a few notable exceptions. Barbiturates and phenothiazines are important causes of non-reactive pupils. Hypothermia and acute anoxia may also produce non-reactive pupils. Body temperature needs to be accurately measured. A deepening level of coma with pupillary changes of dilatation or fixed constriction or apneic episodes, implies raised intracranial pressure with coning.

Deviation of the eyes to one side or the other suggests a lesion of the same cerebral hemisphere or pontine tegmentum. With hemispheric lesions the eyes look towards the lesion and can be brought back by caloric testing or the oculocephalic maneuver. Transient deviation to the side away from the lesion may occur with frontal or occipital lobe seizures. A predominantly unilateral lesion of the pontine tegmentum causes a lateral gaze palsy towards the side of the lesion, which is not affected by the caloric or oculocephalic maneuver. Fixed deviation of the eyes below the horizontal meridian signifies brain stem dysfunction, which is usually due to a structural lesion but may be caused by hepatic encephalopathy. Forced downward deviation of the eyes during caloric testing often occurs in coma induced by drugs. Sustained upward gaze palsy may be seen with anoxic encephalopathy.

Neck stiffness may suggest the presence of meningeal irritation. In the presence of an atypical history for a haemorrhagic stroke or a subarachnoid haemorrhage the possibility of cerebral infarction must be considered.

Focal neurological signs are unusual with metabolic encephalopathy but can occur, for example hemiplegia with hypoglycaemia. Decorticate and decerebrate rigidity may also be seen. In patients with light coma the limbs will fall slowly when released, in contrast the affected limbs will drop like a dead weight in stroke.

Cardiac, hypovolaemic and endotoxic causes should be sought in both transient and persisting disruptions of consciousness. Aortic stenosis, aortic valve incompetence, left atrial myxoma or ball valve thrombus of the mitral valve may present with syncope. Apart from the diagnosis of valvular lesions the peripheral pulses need to be checked including a search for bruits and aneurysms. If postural hypotension is suspected the patient needs to have their blood pressure taken after lying for at least 20 minutes, and then repeated on standing. A drop of at least 20 mm Hg which is present after 2 minutes indicates significant postural hypotension. An elevated blood pressure is a common accompaniment of stroke and should not be taken as evidence of pathological hypertension. The blood pressure should not be reduced in the acute situation. Atrial fibrillation is the commonest arrhythmia found in association with stroke, finding it does not indicate that embolus is the cause of the stroke.

There may be other features on general examination which help to explain the cause of a metabolic encephalopathy such as the features of chronic liver disease or a bounding pulse in hypercapnia.

Assessment

Most causes of transient or persistent loss of consciousness can be discerned following a careful history, examination and basic haematological and biochemical screen. If the patient is unconscious the conscious level should be determined and probable causes investigated. There are many metabolic conditions that can be associated with disturbance of consciousness and disorders of anemia, hyponatremia, uremia, dehydration, liver dysfunction, hypocalcemia, hypercalcemia, hyperglycemia and hypoglycemia should be readily detected (Table 10.3). A very high erythrocyte sedimentation rate (ESR) raises the question of vasculitis. At this point the correct route of investigation should be clear. A sepsis screen should be seriously considered including a lumbar puncture. If hypoxia or hypercapnia are suspected then an arterial sample should be obtained for blood gases. If the coma is thought to be linked to a toxin, a toxins or poisons screen should be done.

An electroencephalogram (EEG) may help in diagnosis since diffuse, symmetrical slow wave activity is found in metabolic encephalopathy, but there are other causes and it remains a test of limited value in this context. Computerized axial tomography (CAT) is obligatory if tumour, subdural haematoma or abscess is seriously considered. If the CAT scan makes the diagnosis of space occupying lesion unlikely then a lumbar puncture should be carried out if sepsis or subarachnoid hemorrhage is considered.

Table 10.3 Principal metabolic conditions associated with change in state of consciousness

Anoxia	
anoxic anoxia:	Pulmonary insufficiency
stagnant anoxia:	Cardiac disease
	Hyperviscosity states
anemic anoxia	
postanoxic	
Chronic renal failure	
uremic encephalopathy	
dialysis encephalopathy	
Pancreatic disorders	
hypoglycemia	
pancreatic encephalopathy	
Hepatic disorders	
portosystemic encephalopathy	
Electrolyte abnormalities	
hyponatremia	
hypernatremia	
Vitamin deficiency states	
thiamin	
B12	
folate	
niacin	
Endocrine disorders	
hypothyroidism	
thyrotoxicosis	
parathyroid abnormalities	
adrenal disease	
panhypopituitarism	

Plans

Management

Treatment is directed towards reversing or modifying precipitating factors, preventing immediate complications such as aspiration, tissue injury, hypothermia and dehydration, and later complications like immobility, deconditioning, impaired balance and dependency in self-care.

The general approach is similar to that for the stroke patient (Chapter 15) and an adequate airway should be ensured, ventilation should be adequate, cardiac output and peripheral circulation should be optimized. It is advisable to ensure an intravenous access site, unless the patient is clearly in extremis and there is no hope of recovery. If the fluid status needs to be closely monitored then a catheter should be inserted into the bladder and output carefully documented. The results of the various tests should give specific guidance to immediate actions and it will be obvious which tests are necessary to repeat to monitor the patient appropriately.

11

Stroke

Stroke is a clinical syndrome which has been defined by the World Health Organization (WHO) as 'rapidly developing signs of focal (or global) disturbance of cerebral function, lasting more than 24 hours or leading to death, with no apparent cause other than a vascular origin'. Put more simply, it is a sudden onset of neurological deficit caused by focal ischemia or hemorrhage. Embolism, thrombosis and hemorrhage account for the majority of cases. Sometimes the stroke is transient, with complete resolution of symptoms and signs within a short time period. When this resolution is complete within 24 hours, we speak of a transient ischemic attack (TIA). When recovery is complete within a few days, but more than 24 hours, the term reversible ischemic neurological deficit (RIND) is sometimes used.

1. Definition

Transient Ischemic Attack (TIA)

The occurrence of TIAs suggest the affected individual is at high risk of developing a full stroke. It is estimated that between 15 to 25 per cent will so progress. In addition there is an increased occurrence of serious heart disease. It is believed that particularly ominous TIAs are those affecting the anterior circulation, and where there are multiple episodes in a short period of time. The causes of TIA are listed in Table 11.1.

Table 11.1 Causes of TIAs

Microembolization from carotid or vertebrobasilar atheroma
Embolization from valvular vegetations, mitral stenosis or myocardial infarction
Hypertension or hypotension
Cardiac arrhythmias
Hyperviscosity syndromes
Polycythemia or anemia
Degenerative cervical arthropathy
Intracranial space occupying lesions

Stroke

It is generally felt that there is a stroke incidence rate of 150–250 per 100,000 of the population per year in Western countries. There is an age-related variation in the incidence. The incidence rate rises from 60–180/100,000/year at age 45–54 through 600–1200/100,000/year for ages 65–74 up to 4000/100,000/year at age 85+.

The incidence of the various pathological types of stroke are less certain. The diagnosis of intracranial hemorrhage is uncertain unless a CAT scanner is used within the first 72 hours. The Oxfordshire Community Stroke Project (1983) found a 13 per cent incidence of hemorrhage. Distinction between embolic and thrombotic strokes are difficult, about 30 per cent of strokes are embolic.

2. Predisposing factors

It is generally agreed that there is an association between the risk of cerebrovascular disease (stroke or TIA) and the level of blood pressure. Information from the Framingham Study suggests that the risk of stroke was related to their level of blood pressure at entry, especially their systolic reading. It is suggested though that high blood pressures, first detected in senescence, may have less relevance to the risk of stroke.

Diabetes mellitus has been shown in several studies to increase the risk of stroke by between two and four times. The relationship between stroke and rheumatic heart disease is well attested. The Framingham Study showed that 75 per cent of stroke victims had some evidence of heart disease. Left ventricular hypertrophy on electrocardiography or chest radiograph, coronary heart disease, heart failure or atrial fibrillation all contributed to the risk of stroke independent of hypertension. Probably the association is partly explained by stroke and cardiovascular disease being separate manifestations of atherosclerosis.

It is hardly surprising that patients with evidence of cerebrovascular disease have an increased risk of stroke. Studies suggest that 18 to 26 per cent of patients suffering an acute stroke have a past history of strokes, and probably a further 10 per cent have a history of TIAs.

The Framingham Study has found an inverse relationship between obesity and stroke risk in the elderly (i.e. fat people are less likely to suffer a stroke), possibly due to the inverse risk associated with a raised low-density lipoprotein (LDL) level.

The risk associated with an asymptomatic carotid bruit remains to be defined, but such patients do not appear to be any more likely to suffer ipsilateral strokes.

It is generally agreed that a pathologically high hematocrit, as in polycythemia ruba vera, increases the likelihood of arterial thrombosis. Prospective studies from Framingham have shown a relationship between the level of hemoglobin and the risk of stroke even at 'normal' levels. Hyperviscosity syndromes as may be seen in myeloma and Waldenstrom's macroglobulinemia can present with the stroke syndrome.

Other factors such as smoking, elevated serum cholesterol and alcohol consumption have not been shown to increase the likelihood of stroke in individuals over the age of 55 years.

There appears to be a definite association between the season and the rate of stroke. Usually there is a higher rate in the cold months, although there may be two separate peaks, one in early spring (March/April) and one in late autumn (October/November).

3. Precipitating factors

Events such as myocardial infarct, arrhythmias, hemorrhage, pulmonary infarct, and so on, which reduce cerebral perfusion pressures may precipitate a stroke, particularly in a predisposed individual. Subjects with long-standing hypertension tend to have higher, upper and lower limits for autoregulation of cerebral blood flow and so are very vulnerable to hypotensive events.

Embolization is more likely at certain times. It has been suggested that the risk of embolization is greatest at the onset of atrial fibrillation. Other cardiac sources of embolization include myocardial infarcts, bacterial endocarditis and atrial myxoma.

Clotting disorders may rarely present with hemorrhagic strokes. The commoner types of clotting disorders are those seen from the use of anticoagulants or in association with leukemias and marrow aplasias.

4. Subjective

Stroke is essentially a clinical diagnosis made on the basis of the history and examination. The salient feature is the sudden onset of a disturbance of neurological function.

Sudden is a relative term but probably 95 per cent are completed within 24 hours and most within 5 minutes and 5 hours. There are a wide number of possible permutations and combinations of symptoms and signs of strokes. Some of the more common clinical features are listed in Table 11.2.

About 30 per cent of patients present with alteration of level of consciousness as their major clinical feature, and a further 10 per cent will be drowsy in addition to their other symptoms. Confusion is particularly common in the elderly, and needs to be looked at closely to avoid missing dysphasia. The differential diagnosis of disturbance of levels of consciousness and confusion is large and discussed in depth in other chapters.

Table 11.2 Clinial feature of stroke

Disturbance of	Frequency (%)
Level of consciousness	30–40
'Confusion'	45
Visuospatial neglect	?
Dysarthria	30
Dysphasia	30
Motor weakness	50–80
Dysphagia	30
Cortical sensory function	25
Visual fields	7
Seizure	6–9

Paralysis (hemiplegia) or weakness (hemiparesis) of one side of the body are fairly obvious symptoms of a stroke, but are seen in only about 50 to 80 per cent of cases. The patient may be aware of a hemiparesis as an inability to stand or tendency to fall. Involvement of the upper limb may be complained of as clumsiness, with spilling of food and fluids.

Disturbances of sensory function are often not mentioned by the subject specifically, although there may be referral to 'numbness' or altered perception. Milder degrees may present as walking into objects, falls or apparent incoordination. In its more severe degrees there may be failure of recognition of limbs and complaints of 'molestations' by foreign limbs.

Complaints of difficulty in swallowing and slurring of speech are common in the first few days after a stroke. Difficulties with speech can be particularly distressing and may result in frustration and aggressive behavior. They are discussed more fully in another chapter.

Strokes may present as an epileptic seizure. This can present diagnostic problems with the Todds paresis, seen sometimes after a seizure. Occasionally a stroke may present for the first time with status epilepticus but before accepting this, other metabolic factors such as hypoglycemia and hypocalcemia must be excluded.

There are a number of other conditions which should be distinguished from the stroke syndrome (Table 11.3). Infective diseases are important to consider because of the high morbidity and mortality associated with them. A complaint of headache and pain on flexing the neck should raise the possibility of meningitis. A cerebral abscess may present as a stroke syndrome but the history is usually that of progressive symptoms of more than 24 hours duration.

Table 11.3 Differential diagnosis of stroke

Subdural hematoma
Extradural hematoma
Epilepsy
Meningitis
Cerebral abscess
Cerebral neoplasm
Hypoglycemia
Hyperglycemia
Hypothyroidism
Hypothermia
Renal failure
Hepatic failure
Vasculitis

A history of treated diabetes mellitus must lead to the suspicion of hypoglycemia. Hyperglycemia with its disturbed level of consciousness, and sometimes focal neurological signs should also be considered.

A history of head trauma should raise the possibility of an extradural or subdural hematoma. A subdural hematoma is usually insidious in its onset, and a progressive, fluctuant history is unusual for a stroke. In an extradural hematoma the onset of neurological symptoms is usually clearly associated, to within a few hours of a head injury.

Cerebral tumours are usually insidious in their onset but can sometimes present rapidly, especially following hemorrhage into the tumour. A progressive history of headache may be suggestive. Another diagnosis to consider with a history of headache, especially temporal, is cranial arteritis.

The symptoms and signs reported in a TIA depend on the vascular territory affected. It is convention to divide them into anterior territory and posterior territory strokes. Transient monocular visual impairment (amaurosis fugax) due to a retinal embolus is one presentation of an anterior territory TIA. When the embolus is largely comprised of platelets, resolution is very rapid. It may or may not be associated with contralateral arm and/or leg weakness. Isolated complaints of hemiparesis or cortical sensory disturbance may be seen. Transient dysphasias may occur.

A TIA in the posterior territory (vertebrobasiliar distribution) manifests itself principally by brainstem dysfunction. Typical features include diplopia, ataxia, dysarthria, dysphagia and drop attacks. Hemiparesis and hemisensory loss may be seen. Transient global amnesia is occasionally associated with evidence of vertebrobasiliar insufficiency.

5. Objective

The examination and assessment of the stroke patient can be divided into attempts to identify potentially remedial conditions and those to clarify the disabilities present.

The examination of the patient with TIA is essentially the same as that of the completed stroke. The main considerations are the complete remission within 24 hours and the careful search for etiological factors.

Degenerative cervical disc changes and osteoarthrosis of the cervical diathrodial joints may increase the likelihood of vertebral artery compression. Severely affected individuals may develop transient neurological deficits, especially nystagmus and dysarthria on rotation and extension of the neck.

The cardiovascular system should be carefully examined for potential sources of embolization and arrhythmias. Carotid bruits should be looked for. Valvular lesions should be sought. Features of endocarditis may be present but care must be exercised in the interpretation of sphincter hemorrhages in the nail beds. These are common in old people, especially in the presence of mobility disorders. Most disorders associated with cerebral vasculitis will usually present with additional signs in other systems.

Many patients with stroke, and conditions which must be considered in its differential diagnosis, present with an alteration of level of consciousness, which may hinder accurate assessment. It is important that some form of accepted rating of conscious level be used, if accurate longitudinal review of the patient is to be possible. One useful scale is that for measuring coma from Glasgow, originally developed for the assessment of head injuries. It should be appreciated that in the presence of aphasia the patient may score artificially low, but it is still useful as a longitudinal tool.

The value of assessment of the respiratory pattern, pupil status and eye movements in the diagnostic and prognostic assessment of the patient is discussed elsewhere (see 'The unconscious patient' in Chapter 10).

Neck stiffness may suggest the presence of meningeal irritation. In the presence of an atypical history for a hemorrhagic stroke or a subarachnoid hemorrhage the possibility of cerebral infection must be considered.

The observation of movement, positioning and tone of the limbs may be helpful in the evaluation of the comatosed patient. The presence of motor responses in the lightly comatosed patient can be tested for with painful stimuli. A hemiparesis is unusual with metabolic encephalopathies other than hypoglycemia but patterns such as decorticate and decerebrate rigidity may be seen. In light coma, the limbs when released tend to fall slowly to the resting position, whereas in a stroke they will fall like a 'dead weight'. Asymmetrical motor findings are against the diagnosis of a metabolic encephalopathy.

Measurement of the blood pressure and pulse characteristics are important. Hypotension if rectified may produce reversal of neurological deficit. In patients with TIAs postural hypotension should be checked. Cardiac, hypovolemic and endotoxic causes should be sought. An elevation of blood pressure is a common accompaniment of a stroke and should not be taken as evidence for pathological hypertension. Reduction of blood pressure should not be attempted in the acute situation. A full volume pulse is characteristic of metabolic encephalopathies such as hypercapnea. An irregular pulse may be of clinical significance as an etiological factor in embolization or in reducing cerebral perfusion. Atrial fibrillation is the commonest arrhythmia seen in stroke patients.

Identification of the particular arterial territory and type of stroke, is often attempted on clinical findings. A number of syndromes have been described, linking together particular patterns of symptoms and signs. A knowledge of the arterial anatomy and various stroke syndromes is of some value in assisting stroke diagnosis, in that atypical cases, which are not readily explained will be noted and investigated further. As far as patients are concerned, however, the more relevant factor is the functional effect of their stroke.

The examination of the patient should also include careful assessment of function.

It is the contention of the authors, that each patient needs a detailed assessment, directed toward delineating deficits and putting them into perspective, with the patient's functional needs. We feel it important to stress the functional assessment of the stroke patient. The detection of sensory deficits are more than just academic exercises, their presence may explain difficulties with rehabilitation of elderly patients, and allow measures to overcome them, to be initiated. A suggested outline to the approach is indicated in Table 11.4.

As indicated above a reduced attention level is often seen after a stroke and may add to the patients frustrations. An allowance for impaired level of consciousness and reduced attention level must be made for in any assessments of communication, intellectual function, motor function and sensory deficit.

Normal communication is a complex function with many components and contributory factors. Its assessment is described in more detail in another chapter. Obvious things such as hearing defects must be excluded before raising the possibilities of dysphasia.

In the conscious patient, it is important that the presence of swallowing difficulties be looked for, by

Table 11.4 Functional assessment of stroke

1 Conscious level
2 State of hydration and nutrition
3 Hearing and visual acuity
4 Language
5 Muscle power and tone assessment
6 *Presence of perceptual problems:*
  (a) Somatic:
    • neglect
    • extinction
    • two point discrimination
    • proprioception
    • agnosias
  (b) Visual:
    • neglect
    • field defect
    • cortical blindness
    • agnosias
  (c) Auditory:
    • neglect
    • agnosia
7 *Presence of problems of integration:*
  (a) Apraxias – General:
    • ideomotor
    • ideational
  (b) Constructional Apraxias (specific)
    • dressing
    • gait
    • speech
  (c) ADL assessment

observing the patient taking a glass of water and then solids. Many of these patients will also have a coexisting dysarthria.

One of the commonest used measures of voluntary power is that devised by the Medical Research Council (UK). The scale (Table 11.5) has the drawback of lacking sensitivity at the upper range.

Tone is the term used to describe the resistance felt when the limb is passively moved by an external examiner. Problems arise in the assessment of tone in a patient partly because of effects of anxiety, comprehension, temperature and the patient's posture. Spasticity refers to the increased excitability of motor neurones in the spinal core, manifested clinically as an increased resistance to passive stretching of a muscle and by an increased amplitude of the stretch reflex. We prefer not to apply it to the abnormal postures and movements adopted at joints, arising from the unbalanced and uncontrolled forces of several muscle groups.

Table 11.5 MRC muscle power grading

Grade	Strength
0	No movement or contraction
1	A palpable contraction but no movement seen
2	Movement at the appropriate joint with gravity eliminated
3	Able to move the joint against gravity
4	Able to move the joint against resistance but less than normal
5	Normal power

Probably the main value of tone and spasticity measurement is in the assessment of the stability at a joint. In some circumstances increased tone may be beneficial, as in the early stages of recovery of the lower limb, by enabling a standing posture to be attained, but in later stages may be detrimental by encouraging an abnormal gait, predisposing to falls.

Cortical perceptional loss may be defined as impairment of recognition or appreciation of sensory stimuli, in the presence of an intact sensory input system. There are problems creased in the assessment of perception by the lack of uniformity in the classifications and the actual measures used. One possible classification based on the sensory system involved and the nature of the defect is shown in Table 11.6.

Table 11.6 Classification of perceptual disorders

Visual	Unilateral neglect
	Agnosia
	Cortical blindness
Somatic	Unilateral/bilateral neglect in body awareness
	Agnosia
Auditory	Agnosia

Visual neglect means that a patient consistently ignores one half of his visual field, and may result in complaints of knocking furniture, eating only part of a meal, and so on. Traditionally it is tested for by asking the patient to fill in the numbers on a clock face. Alternatively a patient may be asked to copy a simple shape such as a house or cross. Another approach to the demonstration of visual neglect, favoured by psychologists, are cancellation tasks. The test usually takes the form of the patient being asked to search through a series of letters or numbers and asked to strike out certain items.

Damage to the posterior areas of either hemisphere can lead to visual neglect, but is usually more common and more severe in lesions of the right hemisphere. In one study of 400 patients, 15 per cent had visual neglect and it occurred ten times more commonly in those with right cortical damage.

Visual neglect is not uncommonly seen in association with other perceptual problems of somatic and auditory types resulting in the unilateral neglect syndromes.

Visual object agnosias are the commonest form of visual agnosias seen. The patient will be unable to recognize a familiar object and therefore unable to name it or indicate its use. Sometimes the use of another sensory modality, such as handling the object, will result in sudden recognition of the object. In the presence of language disorders a visual agnosia may be difficult to demonstrate.

There are problems with reproducibility of two point discrimination because of the considerable explanation, concentration and time needed to do it properly. Commonly used tests of proprioception are the thumb finding test or using the good arm to mimic the position of the affected limb. The thumb finding test is one of the few clinical tests which have some predictive value of outcome. Although vibration testing is relatively easy to perform its value remains to be established.

Somatic attentional disorders may be unilateral or bilateral. If the disturbance is mild it may take the form of simple indifference to the limb, but when marked the patient may deny any problem with an otherwise useless limb. The patient may deny the affected limb as their own and even suggest it belongs to the assessor. Sometimes a touch on the affected limb is localized to the correct spot but on the opposite limb.

The main specific somatic agnosia is astereognosis: the inability to recognize an object or shape by touch. Other agnosias of body somatic perception include problems in ability to localize and name parts of the patient's body.

The main auditory perceptual disorder forms part of dysphasia and is discussed in a separate chapter. Auditory agnosia is where the patient is unable to recognize the significance of a sound, for example, telephone ringing. It is very uncommon.

Apraxia refers to the inability to carry out a voluntary, learnt movement in an alert and orientated patient, in the absence of motor or sensory dysfunction. The problem is one of a failure of integration of available sensory information with intact motor control systems, resulting in defective motor output. They may be divided into general apraxias and the specific apraxias.

The general apraxias include the motor (ideomotor) and the ideational apraxias. In motor apraxia a patient may successfully perform a particular movement automatically but be unable to repeat it on demand. They may not surprisingly be associated with aphasia. Ideational apraxia is characterized by the failure to hold on to the ideas necessary to carry out an action. This disorder is particularly associated with bilateral parietal damage.

The specific apraxias include apraxias of construction, speech, dressing and gait. Constructional apraxias involve a disturbance of the organization of individual spatial elements into a complete whole. This may be readily demonstrated by asking the patient to reproduce patterns using coloured blocks. Constructional apraxias are often involved with right hemisphere damage. Apraxias of gait are said to be associated with frontal lobe damage. It takes the form of a difficulty of initiation and maintenance of a normal walking pattern.

The significance of the previous deficits will be measured by their effects on the ability of the patient to function within their environment. A variety of activities of daily living (ADL) scales have been developed and are discussed in Chapter 1.

6. Plan

Diagnostic

The investigations which are indicated in a patient with stroke are outlined in Table 11.7. Some such as the hemoglobin, blood sugar, urea and electrolytes require to be done urgently, since they may indicate abnormalities which require immediate treatment.

Others such as the chest radiography or electrocardiagram (ECG) can often wait a few

Table 11.7 Investigation of stroke

Hemoglobin Urea and Electrolytes Blood sugar	Urgent
White cell count and differential Erythrocyte sedimentation rate (ESR) Liver function test Cardiac enzymes Chest radiograph Electrocardiogram (ECG)	Routine
Skull radiography Echoencephalogram Electroencephalogram (EEG) CAT scan Isotope scan	Occasionally indicated
Arteriography	Rarely indicated
PET scan NMR scan (MRI)	Research tools

hours unless particular clinical factors alter the situation.

The skull radiography will be indicated in any possible case of head trauma, and in the presence of pineal calcification may show midline shift. Areas of abnormal calcification or rarefaction may be seen. Echoencephalopathy can also be of assistance as a non-invasive investigation of midline shift within the first 24 hours.

A lumbar puncture is associated with some risk and should only be undertaken if specific indications are present. It is advisable, if the facility is available, that computerized axial tomography (CAT) be performed first, so that any large hemorrhage or space-occupying lesion can be excluded.

A CAT scan is not indicated in the routine evaluation of a stroke, although many would consider it standard. The Oxfordshire Community Stroke Project demonstrated that a careful history and examination was very accurate in the diagnosis of stroke. Less than 1 per cent of subjects had undiagnosed, potentially treatable causes of the stroke syndrome, found by CAT scan. The availability of CAT scanning has not improved diagnostic accuracy. It should be reserved for atypical presentations where other pathology, such as tumour, are considered or where it is important to identify cerebral hemorrhage.

In a number of situations isotope scans are the only detailed, non-invasive investigation available. They are generally less sensitive than the CAT Scan but will occasionally detect lesions missed by CAT scan. The tend to be unreliable at distinguishing tumour and stroke.

Other procedures such as positron emission tomography (PET) scans and nuclear magnetic resonance (NMR) scans are proving of use as research tools. They have not as yet been shown to have any beneficial effect upon patient management.

Arteriography is now rarely indicated. Its main role is to delineate areas of arterial damage where surgery is a realistic prospect. In clinical practice it will normally be used to investigate the carotid arteries. Occasionally it may be of value in the clarification of a subdural hematoma.

Table 11.8 Common problems after a stroke

General:	Bronchopneumonia
	Bedsores
	Constipation
	Deep vein thrombosis
	Pulmonary embolus
Local:	Shoulder pain/limitation
	Contractures
	Falls and fractures
Cerebral:	Epilepsy
	Thalamic pain
	Associated movements
Long term:	Further stroke
	Multi-infarct dementia
	Myocardial infarction

Management

The available evidence suggests that young people with stroke seem to have a milder degree of disability, when measuring activities of daily living, at two weeks following the stroke. Probably the maximum ability reached decreases with advancing age, so that in the under 65 year old age group, as many as two-thirds will reach a mild degree of deficit compared to less than 50 per cent of those in the 65–74 age group, and only about one-third of those in the over 75 age group. These observations are sometimes used to back up the feeling that elderly stroke victims are a very difficult group to rehabilitate. However, they have a very high mortality rate, when only about a third of those in the over 75 year old age group being alive at three months following the stroke, compared to three quarters of those in the under 65 group. If therefore the survivors of stroke at one year are assessed, then a different pattern emerges, in that there tends to be no difference in the amount of recovery which is achieved, all age groups seeming to do equally well, or for that matter, equally badly. This needs to be taken into consideration in designing rehabilitation programs for an elderly stroke. Time factors are especially crucial.

Another problem of rehabilitating the elderly individual with a stroke, is that they tend to have more than one problem present at a time. Conditions such as unsteadiness and falls continue to increase markedly with advancing age. We therefore find that about 60 per cent of elderly patients already had balance problems prior to the onset of their stroke.

Most recovery of physical function will occur in the first six months after a stroke. Sensory function tends to be disturbed in about half of patients but especially in those with a right hemisphere lesion. About 70–80 per cent of people who survive will be able to walk within six months of their stroke. About 75 per cent have some impaired arm function initially and in about one-third there will be very little functional recovery in the arm by six months.

In general terms the prognosis for functional recovery is dependent upon the initial degree of loss of function. Some important prognostic factors have been demonstrated:

1. *Level of consciousness*. The early mortality is much higher in patient who present with reduced levels of consciousness. They as a group are also more likely to be hospitalized and less likely to be independent six months after their stroke.
2. *Poor performance on cognitive testing*. A number of studies have shown a poor functional outcome, in subjects who score badly at tests of intellectual function, such as WAIS. Part of this may be explained by perceptual disturbances showing up as poor performance in some of the subsets, such as block design and object assembly tests.
3. *Proprioceptive loss and/or spatial neglect*. These are more common in right hemisphere damage. Approximately 50 per cent show evidence of resolution within a three month periods. Those arising from cerebral hemorrhage tend to have a better prognosis.
4. *Poor arm function*. Two major studies have confirmed the importance of this variable in predicting ultimate ADL scores.
5. *Poor sitting balance*. Postural control is an important predictive parameter of outcome.
6. *Hemianopia or other visual field loss*. The presence of a visual field defect in older patients has been found to increase the mortality at 15 months by a factor of over 4. There was also a poor prognosis for ADL achievement in the presence of visual field defect. The median time for resolution of visual field has been reported as 32 weeks.
7. *Urinary incontinence*.

It would appear then that the presence of perceptual problems may be at least as important as power loss in determining outcome. This is hardly surprising, since in the presence of visual and tactile neglect, difficulties may arise in the eliciting of full patient cooperation in the rehabilitation program. Agnosias and apraxias may create difficulty to the carers in rehabilitation problems the patient is experiencing.

The first essential of treatment is correction of any underlying conditions, which may be contributing to the clinical picture. This will involve ensuring adequate cerebral perfusion with appropriately oxygenated blood and normoglycemia.

Some agents such as dexamethasone, dextran and glycerol have been advocated to reduce the size of the stroke but conclusive proof of their value remains to be demonstrated. Glycerol may reduce mortality in the early weeks but leave a very disabled patient. Claims have been made for naftidrofuryl to reduce the length of hospitalization with stroke but they require confirmation.

A problem of whether to anticoagulate embolic stroke is sometimes raised, there is still no evidence that immediate anticoagulation is beneficial.

Surgical evacuation of an intracerebral hematoma has not been shown to alter outcome with the possible exception of cerebellar hemorrhage. This type of stroke is however, uncommon and comprises less than 10 per cent of all hemorrhages. Procedures for the restoration of the blood supply to the brain, either through carotid endartectomy or by anastomosing the superficial temporal artery to the middle cerebral artery, are still under evaluation. The present evidence suggests however, they will not have a major role because much of the damage of the stroke occurs very quickly and the mortality of carotid endartectomy can be extremely high.

The next stage of treatment to be considered is that of general symptomatic care. The common problems seen in the first few days of a stroke are summarized in Table 11.7. Approximately 30 per cent of patients will be comatosed and will need all of the care normally given to the unconscious patient (see Chapter 10). This will include protection of the airway, maintenance of fluids and nutrition, frequent turning to prevent bedsores and care of joints and limbs with good positioning.

It should be appreciated that problems with fluids and nutrition are not restricted to the unconscious patient. Approximately 10 per cent of conscious patients have marked difficulty with swallowing. Intravenous fluids may be necessary, although in most cases they can manage small sips of water. Milk products increase mucous production and should be avoided. Patients may have significantly more problems with liquids than semi-solids and 'jelled' materials, and in this case adequate fluid intake can be maintained with a minced and semi-solid diet. As swallowing improves liquid can be better tolerated and the total amount increased. Dietary advice should be sought during this period to ensure adequate calorie, protein, vitamin and mineral intake. In a few cases where the dysphagia is prolonged a fine-bore nasogastric tube may be required. However conscious patients with swallowing problems should have a careful swallowing assessment by occupational therapy (OT) or speech therapy. Permanent feeding tubes via a gastrostomy should be done rarely, and only when swallowing is unlikely to return.

Excretion may raise considerable problems. Many patients are incontinent of urine for several days because of a number of factors including reduced level of consciousness, impaired communication, immobility, and reduced awareness of bladder filling. It is probably reasonable to use a drainage device where the patient is unconscious but otherwise they should be avoided. They will in fact often delay rehabilitation by producing prolonged incontinence secondary to urethritis, infection and loss of bladder tone. Regular toileting using a commode is often sufficient to control the situation and the act of transferring to the commode several times a day becomes part of the rehabilitation program.

Problems with apparently confused behavior are quite common. Often the situation can be helped by the appreciation of the contribution of communication and perceptual problems to such behavior. Emotional distress and frustration can manifest in apparent aggressive behaviour. In addition other factors such as infection or poor hydration may be present. The use of sedatives or isolation should be avoided.

The rehabilitation of stroke patients starts immediately following the onset of the stroke itself. It is the responsibility of all carers and should not be considered to reside solely with physiotherapists or occupational therapists. The acts of dressing, transferring, toileting, feeding, and so on. throughout the whole 24 hours should be treated as sessions of rehabilitation. It is essential that the level of assistance in each task be appropriate and consistent for the patients functional capacity.

There is some evidence to suggest that therapy may be of value in speeding resolution of perceptual problems. Measurable improvements in visual fields occur with stimulation of the impaired area, after as little as 6 hours of training. Block design training may also improve visual perceptual defects. Interestingly the improvement carried over onto several other unrelated functions, possibly by allowing them to overcome other perceptual problems by improved visual scanning. There is a need for further investigation of these interesting experiences.

It would seem reasonable that certain simple measures be followed when treating patients with perceptual problems. The initial procedure is to anticipate their presence, especially in lesions of the right hemisphere, and accurately demonstrate them. All carers should be made aware of their presence. Allowance for them should be made in the positioning of food, fluid and personal belongings. During contacts with the patient the neglected side should be maximally stimulated by whatever measures are available. Reassurance and encouragement of the patient who is coping with a series of frustrating problems is essential.

The major function of rehabilitation in the early stages will be to prevent complications arising and therefore allow optimal conditions for natural recovery. There are three conditions which must be prevented in the early stages. The first is the development of abnormal tonal patterns; the second is the painful hemiplegic shoulder and the third pressure sores. All of these can be controlled by the correct positioning of the patient, whether lying in bed or sitting.

The dominant tonal patterns following a stroke usually results in depression of the shoulder, internal rotation of the arm, flexion of the elbow and the wrists and abduction of the fingers. With the hip the problem is one of extension of the leg. The positioning used will be an attempt to reverse these and place the limb in a more neutral and comfortable position. When the patient is lying on his back, it is essential to keep him well supported with the shoulder brought forward, the arm extended and slight flexion of the knee. When lying on the non-affected side, the same type of position is maintained using pillows to support the arm and leg. It may be necessary to support the back also to prevent the patient rolling over. Another less satisfactory position is for the patient to lie on his affected side. Here there is great danger of the shoulder being trapped, causing further tension. Maintaining the arm in the appropriate positioning throughout the day can be extremely difficult and some help can be gained by use of inflatable splints.

Protection of the shoulder joint is critical in the long term management of the stroke patient. The humerus is very loosely supported within the glenoid fossa, a firmer attachment would be difficult since the shoulder needs to move through very wide angles. There is therefore a danger to subluxation of the shoulder when the tone is decreased, or it being tied down by the increased tone around the scapula. This is particularly true of the patient with unilateral tactile neglect since they usually have flaccid limbs allowing subluxation of the shoulder.

Attempts to splint the arm using a triangular bandage has problems, first it maintains the arm in the dominant pattern which is undesirable; secondly it inhibits normal activity of the arm; thirdly it disturbs the body image. In addition, it does not prevent subluxation of the shoulder, since, inevitably, the arm will sag. A more satisfactory technique of supporting the shoulder is the figure of eight splint, as this allows good movement of the arm while providing some support to the humerus within the axilla.

It is also essential that the shoulder capsule is not over stretched. This is particularly relevant in patients with spasticity, since the arm can only be elevated about 120 degrees before the scapula itself has to turn to allow further elevation to 180 degrees. For this reason, the overhead pulley has a great tendency to disrupt the shoulder joint and produce further pain.

Similarly, patients should not be helped out of a chair under the armpits. A more satisfactory position is to stand in front of the patient supporting the knees with those of the attendant; and supporting at shoulder level rather than lifting at the shoulder. The patient then is encouraged to bring their weight forward and to stand up.

Part of this will require position sense training, however, many patients find it difficult to bend forward particularly patients with left hemiplegia. Many of these patients will benefit from having either a bed or a stool placed in front of the chair to carry out these activities. This will be one of the first steps to train the patient in the balance techniques for standing.

Whilst sitting at a table it is important that the patient is kept in a good upright position with the knees kept at right angles. They can also use this position to maintain a good body image by correctly placing the hands on the table. They can also use the table as a method of extending the fingers to release spasticity. Normally it is advisable to encourage bilateral hand techniques, of which there are many available, whilst sitting at the table.

Once good sitting balance has been achieved, then the patient can progress on to a standing balance. This must be achieved before the patient starts to walk. There are many simple techniques, one is to get the patient to start with a good stable base by standing at a table. They can then move further off the centre of gravity by carrying out activities at the table. Games can be used to encourage changes in position including elevation of the arm.

Many therapists prefer to encourage walking without the use of any aids at all. This is certainly feasible in many young individuals, though in the elderly, who often had walking aids prior to the stroke, this is unrealistic. The main purpose is to maintain the pelvis on a horizontal plane, encouraging lifting of the knee. This can also be used even in the presence of foot drop. A variety of aids are used in the rehabilitation of strokes, especially in the elderly. It is important that they be appropriate.

The quad cane (stick) has the advantage of being relatively easy to use early on and allowing some degree of mobility, with beneficial effects on patient morale. It does, however, encourage the patient to lean to the non-affected side, with the weight being transmitted between the good leg and the cane. This results in hitching up of the affected side and produces an abnormal walking gait. The other disadvantages of quad canes is that they do have a tendency to catch on furniture and may cause a fall.

The use of a cane (walking stick) has similar disadvantages although some therapists advise the use of a tall walking stick, since this prevents weight bearing whilst allowing it to be used for balancing. This has, in fact, progressed to a further stage of using a long cane or shepherd's crook in an attempt to avoid weight bearing and produce better positions of the arms. In many elderly patients the use of a pulpit frame or gutter frame (elbow walker) has the advantage of encouraging the weight to fall between the two feet, whilst giving a greater stability of 4 point support. The disadvantage of this is that it tends to encourage flexion at the hips.

Many patients may then progress on to a walker with or without wheels. The advantage of the triangular folding frame, is that it takes up less room, and therefore is more maneuverable around furniture, and is capable of being easily folded to fit in a car.

Calipers have been in use for many years for the treatment of footdrop. They are however, somewhat heavy on a rather weak leg, unattractive and require special adaptation to shoes. For these reasons, several other forms of footdrop splint have come into use. The polypropylene ankle splint has the advantage of being light, unobtrusive and can fit into almost any shoe. Its disadvantage is that it can cause discomfort, especially on the sole of the foot and needs to be carefully measured. An alternative approach is the clasp brace which clips on to the back of the shoe. This is more unsightly but is light and does not require new shoes to be specially adapted. A final type is a very light spring loaded sole which fits under the normal shoe. The disadvantage of this is that any spring loading of the foot encourages further spasm within the calf muscles and therefore increases tone, producing further foot drop.

As mentioned before time factors are particularly relevant to the management of the elderly stroke. An early assessment needs to be made of the environment they will be discharged to and potential helpers need interviewing. The sizes of doorways, presence of stairs, amount and type of furniture will affect the ability of the patient to live an independent existence and the aids they might use. Helpers should be involved in the rehabilitation of the patient. It is important to ensure that the level of help will be appropriate after discharge, if a 'caring' helper is not to inadvertantly undo the benefits of a rehabilitation program. After discharge useful improvement and maintenance of function are often achieved by the use of community physiotherapists or day hospital facilities.

Management of TIAs is directed at any precipitating factors to reduce the chances of progress to completed stroke. This includes treating underlying hemodynamic factors and other conditions such as vasculitis, hyperviscosity syndromes, and so on. The management of cases felt to be due to carotid or vertebrobasilar microemboli is less clear. The main arguments are between surgery and medical therapy.

Carotid endartectomy has not been demonstrated to have any advantage over conservative treatment and indeed may have a higher mortality, but definitive trials are still ongoing.

Anticoagulation may reduce the risk of stroke for the first few months after the initial TIA. There is of cause a real risk of cerebral hemorrhage especially in the elderly. It is contraindicated in the presence of hypertension, previous history of cerebral hemorrhage or likely poor compliance. A CAT scan should be performed before commencing therapy.

A variety of antiplatelet drugs, including aspirin and dipyridamole, have been used, based on the observation that the core of an arterial thrombus is a mass of platelets surrounded by leukocytes and fibrin. The Canadian Cooperative Study Group (1979) showed a modest benefit in stroke reduction with aspirin use, for men under the age of 55 but not in women or older men. Any benefit of antiplatelet treatment in the elderly patient with TIAs remain to be demonstrated.

Suggested reading

Adams, G. F. (1974). *Cerebrovascular Disability and the Aging Brain.* Churchill Livingstone, Edinburgh.

Aho, K., Harmsen, P., Hatano, S., Marquardsen, J., Smirnov, V. E. and Strasser, T. (1980). Cerebrovascular disease in the community: results of a WHO collaborative study. *Bull. WHO,* **58**: 113–30.

Caplan, L. R., Hier, D. B. and C'Cruz, I. (1983). Cerebral embolism in the Michael Reese stroke registry. *Stroke,* **14**: 530–6.

Cerebral Embolism Study Group (1983). Immediate anticoagulation of embolic stroke: a randomized trial. *Stroke,* **14**: 668–76.

Demeurisse, G., Demol, O. and Robaye, E. (1980). Motor evaluation in vascular hemiplegia. *Eur. Neurol.,* **19**: 382–9.

Fuller, J. H., Shipley, M. J., Rose, G., Jarrett, R. J. and Keen, H. (1983). Mortality from coronary heart disease in relation to degree off glycemia: the Whitehall study. *BMJ,* **287**: 867–70.

Haberman, S., Capildeo, R. and Rose, F. C. (1981). The seasonal variation in mortality from cerebrovascular disease. *J. Neurol. Sci.* **52**: 23–36.

Hecaen, H. (1962). Clinical symptomatology in right and left hemisphere lesions. In: Mountcastle, V. B. (ed.) *Interhemisphere Relations and Cerebral Dominance,* Johns Hopkins University Press, Baltimore, MD.

Hellma, K. M. and Watson, R. T. (1977). Mechanisms underlying the unilateral neglect syndrome. In: Weinstein, E. A. and Friedland, R. P. (eds) *Advances in Neurology,* vol. 18, Raven Press, New York, pp. 93–106.

Imms, F. J. and Edholm, O. G. (1981). Studies of gait and mobility in the elderly. *Age and Aging,* **10**: 147–56.

Kannel, W. B. and Wolf, P. A. (1983). Epidemiology of cerebrovascular disease. In: Russel, R. W. (ed.) *Vascular Disease of the Cerebrovascular System.* Churchill Livingstone, Edinburgh, pp. 1–24.

Norris, J. W. and Hachinski, V. C. (1982). Misdiagnosis of stroke. *Lancet,* **i**: 328–31.

Oxfordshire Community Stroke Project (1983). Incidence of stroke in Oxfordshire: first year's experience of a community stroke register. *BMJ* **287**: 713–16.

Prescott, R. J., Garraway, W. M. and Akhtar,

A. J. (1982). Predicting functional outcome following acute stroke using a standard clinical examination. *Stroke*, **13**: 641–7.

Teasdale, G., Murray, G., Parker, L. and Jennet, B. (1979). Adding up the Glascow Coma Scale. *Acta Neurochir.*, Suppl. **28**: 13–16.

Walker, A. E., Robins, M. and Weinfeld, F. D. (1981). Clinical findings. In: Weinfeld, F. D. (ed.) The National Society of Stroke. *Stroke*, **12**: Suppl. 1, 13–44.

Wolf, P. A., Kannel, W. B., McGee, D. L., Meeks, S. L., Bharucha, N. E. and McNamara, P. M. (1983). Duration of atrial fibrillation and imminence of stroke: the Framingham Study. *Stroke*, **14**: 664–7.

Yatsu, F. M. and Hart, R. G. (1983). Asymptomatic carotid bruit and stenosis: a reappraisal. *Stroke*, **14**: 301–4.

Young, G. C., Collins, D. and Hren, M. (1983). Effect of pairing scanning training with block design training in the remediation of perceptual problems in left hemiplegia. *J. Clin. Neuropsychol.*, **5**: 201–12.

Zihi, J. and Von Cranon, D. (1979). Restitution of visual function in patients with cortical blindness. *J. Neurol. Neurosurg. Psychiat.*, **42**: 312–22.

12

Disorders of speech and language

Disorders of speech and language should become apparent during the initial contact with the patient. Those of us who have frequent contact with elderly people will immediately recognize the characteristic speech of ill-fitting dentures and of the absence of dentures. Familiarity with these problems may save needless examinations. When a disorder of speech or language is detected it is as well to examine it immediately rather than leaving it and adding to a more formal neurological examination later.

The production of speech requires the complex integration of those muscles which produce an adequate air stream, the muscles of the larynx which modify the air stream and produce changes in the pitch, and the muscles of the soft palate, tongue, cheeks and lips which are responsible for the accurate articulation of speech. Each of these events may be modified by anatomical abnormalities which are congenital or acquired secondary to aging or disease.

Dysphonia refers to a problem with the production of sound from the larynx. Dysarthria refers to problems of articulation and pronunciation. The words can be found by the patient who knows how to express himself but the speech is unclear. Dysphasia or aphasia refers to the problems of communication which involve language. The patient may have difficulty in understanding, conceptualizing and creating speech. Sounds can be produced and there is no problem with articulation.

1. Subjective

The patient may or may not be able to express themselves with regard to their problem of communication. The important features of the history pertain to the nature of the problem as described by the patient or significant other. The timing of onset should be determined, as to whether rapid and of short duration or whether the onset is insidious and has been gradually worsening.

In order to understand the nature of the problem and to determine likely etiology the associated symptoms and signs are of great importance. The patient with dysphasia secondary to stroke is likely to have associated hemiparesis. The patient with dysarthria secondary to myasthenia is likely to have symptoms of weakness and rapidly progressive fatigue, and so on. The Parkinsonian patient with dysphonia and dysarthria is likely to have the associated symptoms of Parkinson's disease.

2. Objective

Examination commences as soon as the patient begins to communicate, and it is important for the physician to determine the nature of the speech problem at the outset – dysphonia, dysarthria or aphasia. Simple observation can give much information and when conversing with the patient the examiner focusses on the various aspects of speech production.

It is good to have a regular system of examining patients with speech problems. A simple schedule we have found useful is:

1. Encourage spontaneous speech by engaging conversation and noting the articulation, the sound production, the use of filler words, the presence of paraphasias and the overall content.
2. Proceeding to a simple screen for the presence of understanding or comprehension by using one,

two and three stage commands and carefully avoiding the use of inadvertant body cues.

3. The patient is then given a short piece of prose to read and then understanding is determined.
4. The ability to name is then tested which should include objects as well as body parts.
   Repetition should be tested and the patient asked to repeat simple phrases.

Abnormal airflow tends to give rise to the production of speech in short phrases with breaths in between. This can be due to disorders of thoracic musculature and its innervation; to weakness of laryngeal adductors (often accompanied by abductor weakness and audible inspiration); or to airflow obstruction which may be anatomical or due to sustained contraction of laryngeal adductors. The patient needs to be carefully examined during two or three cycles of slow, deep ventilation. The voice also assumes a strained quality in pseudobulbar palsy or in dystonic disorders. Phonation during inspiration is characteristic of deafness since childhood. Tremor of the voice may occur in timing with tremors elsewhere.

A nasal quality to the voice with inability to produce consonants is seen in bulbar palsy and other lesions affecting the lower cranial nerves. This is due to weakness of the soft palate and there is incomplete separation of the oropharynx from the nasopharynx. When the nasal quality increases as speech progresses myasthenia gravis should be considered and appropriate examination made. Adenoidal speech occurs when the nasopharynx is blocked such as due to an anatomical abnormality from a neoplasm.

Lesions of the tongue will lead to problems in the production of consonants (t,d,l, and s). Facial palsy produces dysarthria and difficulties with bilabial consonants (p and b). In the presence of cerebellar disease the rhythm of speech is abnormal with inappropriate stresses. This is referred to as scanning or prosodic speech.

In Parkinson's disease the voice is reduced in volume and often somewhat monotonous. Speech is often slow with episodes of phonatory festination and a slowness or inability to finish off the consonants.

Spastic dysarthria is most often found in pseudobulbar palsy. Speech tends to be monotonous, low pitched and strained. There is frequently a problem with production (dysphonia) as well as with articulation, particularly with those consonants and vowels dependent upon tongue movements.

In flaccid dysarthria air frequently escapes into the nasopharynx producing a nasal quality to the voice. Articulation is abnormal, particularly for vowels and consonants due to tongue movements.

Examination may reveal that the patient has no problem with any of these areas and that the problem rests with the generation or understanding of language. Once the problem is recognized as a dysphasia it needs to be identified as fluent or non-fluent. The patient should be asked to name simple objects. If fluent the patient will readily produce an incorrect name – the wrong one or a neologism. In response to commands there may be inappropriate responses with all types of paraphrases and neologisms or 'word salad' – a surfeit of words with a deficiency of meaning. Repetition is abnormal. These patients have great difficulty in understanding and may have a right homonymous visual field defect. Before testing reading abilities it is important to ensure that there are no visual difficulties and that the patient has learned to read in the past.

Fluent dysphasia, associated with buccofacial and upper limb dyspraxias is due to a lesion in the posterior Sylvian fissure. This is also known as conduction dysphasia.

Fluent dysphasia may be difficult to distinguish from dementia, for example when there is an empty, circumlocutory style of speech without hemiparesis, and is seen in posterior parieto-temporo-occipital lesions. The dysphasia is fluent but there is impaired understanding and repetition is well preserved. This is known as transitory sensory dysphasia.

The patient with aphasia may be mute and attempt to communicate with grunts and gestures. Lesser degrees of non-fluent dysphasia are characterized by agrammatic speech without filler words. Repetition is abnormal. There may be phonemic, semantic or neologistic substitution. In phonemic substitution one correct phoneme is substituted for another for example 'poor' for 'door'. The problem may be predominantly with expression, alternatively it may be with understanding or more commonly a mixture of the two. Dysphasia of this type is frequently associated with limb dyspraxias, right hemiplegia, hemisensory loss or homonymous field defects. Speech is usually represented in the dominant hemisphere and it should be determined if the patient is right or left handed. When there are extensive neurological deficits the dysphasia is more likely to be more profound.

Apraxia is the inability to perform complex motor acts which cannot be explained on the basis of weakness alone and may be performed automatically. In these patients there is difficulty in initiating speech and there may be stuttering or short explosive outbursts. Automatic movements are usually well preserved such as eating and drinking, the patient may be able to recite nursery rhymes. The patient is likely to be unable to lick his lips or to blow out a candle on command. Written language may be well preserved. Patient's with dyspraxia may have difficulty in naming and therefore questions should be constructed that will allow 'yes/no' answers.

Assessment

At the completion of the examination the physician will have determined the nature of the communication problem and whether it is dysphasia, dyspraxia, dysphonia or dysarthria. The extent of associated problems will be apparent which will have a bearing on the direction of further investigations. In interpreting the findings it has already been mentioned that knowledge of whether the patient is right or left handed is important. The patient's native language as well as educational attainments should also be known. The likely causes of dysphonia and dysarthria have already been discussed. Dysphasia is most frequently found as a result of cerebrovascular disease. Dysphasia and language dysfunction also occurs as a result of dementia. Much more rarely aphasia develops due to what appears to be a primary neurodegenerative disorder in the absence of dementia.

Plan

Diagnosis

Most patients with speech disorders should be seen by a health professional skilled in the assessment of communication problems – a speech pathologist or a therapist. This is of great help in the diagnosis of the problem and identification at the pathophysiological level. Other investigations may be indicated such as neuropsychological assess-

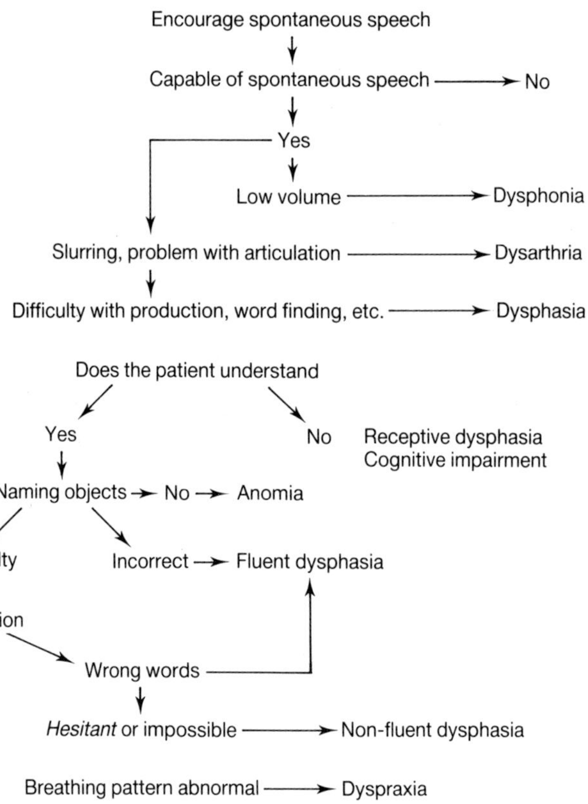

Fig. 12.1 An approach to understanding speech and language dysfunction.

ment. CAT scanning may be indicated, as well as nuclear magnetic resonance (if available) in some of the more difficult problems. The type of investigation should be directed by the associated findings.

Treatment

The speech pathologist may recognize that treatment and further training is likely to be of benefit to the patient and will commence such therapy. Often the patient can be taught exercises that the other health professionals and family can continue throughout the period of time when there is no formal treatment. Involvement of family and other care providers can help a great deal in motivation. When treatment options are limited and improvement unlikely the speech pathologist can help to set up a system of communication that is then followed consistently by other members of the team and the family. If this is done it may help in preventing reactive depression and also help in avoiding significant behavioral problems which often come with frustration.

Suggested reading

Cummings, J. L., Darkins, A., Mendez, M., Hill, M. A. and Benson, D. F. (1988). Alzheimer's disease and Parkinson's disease: comparison of speech and language alterations. *Neurol.*, **38**: 680–84.

Emery, O. B. and Breslau, L. D. (1989). Language deficits in depression; comparison with SDAT and normal aging. *J. Gerontol.* **44**: M85–92.

Faber-Langendoen, K., Morris, J. C., Knesevich, J. W., LaBarge, E., Miller, J. P. and Berg, L. (1988). Aphasia in Senile Dementia of the Alzheimer type. *Ann. Neurol.*, **23**: 365–70.

Kirshner, H. S., Tanridag, O., Thurman, L. and Whetsell, W. O. Jr (1987). Progressive aphasia without dementia; two cases with focal spongiform degeneration.

Knepper, L. E., Biller, J., Tranel, D., Adams, H. P. Jr, Marsh, E. E. III (1989). Etiology of stroke in patients with Wernicke's aphasia. *Stroke*, **20**: 1730–32.

13

Movement problems: gait and involuntary movement

Disorders of movement are extremely common in the geriatric population and present great challenges in diagnosis and management. Frequently the problems can be identified, recorded and no further action taken since they are of no concern to the patient and do not significantly interfere with function. In others, however, the disorder of movement results in an impairment of function and warrants further investigation and treatment. This is particularly true of impaired mobility when the problem has been developing over a period of time, but almost imperceptibly to the patient. The problem which becomes apparent to the physician has not been recognized by the patient.

In this chapter the problems with movement, walking and dressing for example, and movement disorders, such as tremor and dystonia, will be discussed. It is important to understand the usual problems of aging which are poorly described in most texts and to understand that these can be intermixed with the identifiable pathological problems which are dealt with in most neurological texts.

1. Age changes

The most obvious change in walking that occurs with aging is the decline in walking speed and these changes have been discussed (Chapter 3). There is an associated decline in balance and increase in sway (Chapter 4). There are no abnormal movements that can be considered a normal part of aging.

However, with advancing age there are an increasing number of individuals who develop tremor of the hands, head or face which are of no pathological significance. Senile or essential tremor occurs in the limbs and are constant repetitive movements, often made worse by movement or by maintaining a posture. Similar movements are seen in the face, particularly the jaw and lips. Another very common problem is titubation of the head when the head shakes from side to side or back and forth. These can be very disturbing to those observing, such as family members but are often scarcely noted by the person themselves.

2. Specific pathologies

The slow protective gait of the elderly should be easily recognized and has been discussed. There are many other lesions that will give an abnormal gait which can be recognized clinically (Table 13.1).

3. Subjective

Patients with movement disorders, either spontaneous movements or difficulty with moving, are likely to complain of problems in looking after themselves, in ambulating and often in maintaining balance. These individuals frequently have a typical geriatric presentation with loss of mobility and falling. Presentation to the physician is often by a third party – the spouse, family member or care provider brings it to the attention of the physician.

The abnormal movements may make fine movements extremely difficult to control and the patient will have difficulty in dressing or in feeding themselves for example. These complaints are prominent in patients with Parkinson's Disease, and associated problems include deterioration in writing

Table 13.1 Common causes of movement disorders in the elderly

- Parkinson's disease
- Parkinsonism
  - Post-viral encephalitis
  - Drugs
  - Toxins (Carbon monoxide, MPTP, Manganese)
  - Trauma
  - Degenerative
    - Progressive supranuclear palsy
    - Shy–Drager Syndrome
    - Olivo–Ponto–Cerebellar Atrophy
    - Striatonigral degeneration
  - Trauma
  - Multi-infarcts
  - Anoxia
- Tremor
  - Essential
  - Cerebellar
  - Hyperthyroidism
  - Metabolic
- Chorea
  - Iatrogenic (phenothiazines, anticonvulsants, L-dopa, lithium)
  - Huntington's disease
  - Senile
  - Alzheimer's disease
- Dystonia
  - Iatrogenic (Neuroleptics, L-dopa, Anticonvulsants, Metoclopromide)
  - Viral encephalitis
  - Tumours
- Tardive dyskinesias
- Myoclonus
  - Physiological
  - Dementia (Alzheimer's, Jacob–Creutzfeldt disease)
  - Metabolic (hepatic and renal failure, hyponatremia, hypoglycaemia)
  - Toxic
  - Basal ganglion degeneration
  - Viral encephalopathy
  - Post-hypoxic encephalopathy
  - Post-traumatic

skills. The patient may complain of decreasing ability to speak or sing, with a loss of volume.

The slowness in ambulation is usually noticed, with complaints of increased stiffness of the joints, sometimes with aches and pains interpreted by the patient as arthritis. The difficulty in initiating movements may be a prominent complaint, as well as the difficulty in stopping – for example a patient who is walking down an incline complains that they are walking faster and will be unable to stop. Eventually they will fall or collide with something, frequently injuring themselves. Occasionally patients find novel ways of coping with this problem, such as progressing down a street by moving from one lamp post to the next, – grabbing each one as they approach it.

The involuntary movements of Parkinson's disease may be a problem for the patient, typically such movements decrease during voluntary movement and disappear during sleep. On the other hand, the patient with increasing essential or senile tremor will note that it gets worse when they are trying to do something – for example when drinking from a cup. The interference with voluntary movements is what brings the problem to the patient's, and in turn the physician's, attention.

The involuntary movements of tardive dyskinesia usually follow on from treatment with major tranquilizers. Like all patients with involuntary movements these may at first be unnoticed by the patient and cause little or no complaint. They are frequently distressing to family members who seek medical attention on the patient's behalf. However as the problem increases the patient is more likely to complain. The abnormal movements and the continued activity that comes with akathisia can be very tiring for the elderly patient. Some patient's will lose weight as a result of the continued activity. Other's will complain of continued aches and pains, for example neck pain, due to the abnormal activity.

There may be associated problems of mood or cognition. Patients with increasing difficulty in moving and coping, and those distressed by the movements may develop a depression and become quite withdrawn. This needs to be distinguished from the patient who is much more withdrawn because of an inability to cope with everyday problems due to impaired cognition. Those patients with marked slowing of gait, frequently associated with falls, often have brain failure and it is the cognitive impairment that leads to the problems and the crises that bring them to the attention of physicians.

4. Objective

Examination begins from the moment that the patient is first seen and can be observed. The patient's gait and their ability to negotiate doorways can be noted. Whilst the patient is still dressed and wearing usual footwear there should be a more formal assessment of gait. The 'get up and go' test is an appropriate test of mobility and balance. The patient is asked to sit in a conventional straight-backed chair, to stand up, walk a short distance (3 metres), turn around, return and sit down again. The physician or nurse should be very close, ready to assist and prevent accidents. The overall effort is assessed and scored from one to five, one being normal and five the most impaired (Table 13.2). The time taken for the 3-metre course from beginning to end should also be recorded.

Table 13.2 The 'get up and go' test

Grade	Description
1	Normal, without assistance and no risk of falling
2	Very slightly abnormal, pushing up from chair with hands. Slight slowing
3	Mildly abnormal, pushes up, pauses after standing, feet widely spaced, gait perceptibly slow
4	Abnormal, as for three, patient staggers, examiner feels uncomfortable and is prepared to help (standby)
5	Severely abnormal, patient unable to rise and walk on own, requires hands on assistance

Source: Modification of the test as published by Mathias, *et al.* (1986)

The different types of gait can be observed during this procedure. During this test the overall posture should be noted. Many elderly patients adopt a flexed posture, most obvious in patients with Parkinson's disease. This has to be distinguished from the flexion of skeletal deformity when there is kyphosis secondary to vertebral collapse in osteoporosis or the rigid flexed spine of ankylosing spondylitis. An actor's characterization of an older person will frequently include the flexed posture, with bowed head and slightly shuffling gait. In mild degree these might be considered to be a normal feature of aging. In Parkinson's disease these will be more obvious.

In Parkinson's disease the patient attempting to walk may hesitate initially, and then set off with shuffling gait, with small steps (*marche a petit pas*), with little arm swing, the arms being held in flexed position by the side with the hands shaking rhythmically due to the tremor. The walking speed may increase with the patient taking rapid, festinating paces. During the walk the patient may stop and be unable to move. In order to start moving the patient leans forward at an angle and then takes a step in order to catch up with their center of gravity. The facial features may be relatively blank and immobile with a stare. On standing, the degree of sway should be noted, and the ability to correct if displaced should be observed. Patients with Parkinson's disease have great difficulty in correcting and may fall if the balance is suddenly disturbed. Eye movements may be abnormal with difficulty in convergence, weakness of upward gaze and fast saccades instead of slow smooth movement when following an object. The tremor is typically 'pill rolling', usually both sides although it may be unilateral. It may also be present in the lower limbs. Muscle tone is increased, and is typical cogwheel rigidity. This may be brought out by reinforcement maneuvers. The patient is likely to have difficulty with fine movements, such as unbuttoning. The ability to write should be checked and there should be a permanent record of the handwriting. The characteristic triad of Parkinson's disease is comprised of the rigidity, the tremor and the bradykinesia or poverty of movement.

Spastic gait, related to hemiplegia, is common and has been described (Chapter 11). When there is bilateral spasticity both legs will be in extension, with bilateral equinus position of the feet. There is usually an accentuated adduction giving a typical scissor gait, which may be so marked that the person literally trips over their feet every time they attempt to walk. This problem can be seen in association with, for example, cervical myelopathy.

Ataxia results in an abnormal gait due to uncoordination of the legs, disequilibrium with pitching and reeling, and disturbance of postural and walking reflexes. This gait tends to be wide based, slower, coarser jerky movements with a lot of swaying. The patient looks unsafe.

When there is loss of dorsiflexion of the foot the patient lifts the leg high and the foot slaps down when it is lowered to the ground. This is known as a steppage gait.

Apraxic gait needs to be recognized. This represents an inability to use or coordinate the motor function despite the absence of any obvious motor or sensory damage. Minor abnormalities can be brought out by giving commands which the patient cannot follow, although at other times normal movement that is involuntary, can be seen. The patient will have profound difficulty with simple actions like kicking a ball. These patients walk slowly and haltingly, and their feet seem to be stuck to the floor. Walking will cease when an obstacle is approached and the patients will have great difficulty in initiating or stopping movements. This problem is due to bilateral frontal lobe dysfunction. Examination of the patient in bare feet will show the toes curled over as if the foot is gripping the floor and some neurologists have interpreted this as an exaggerated plantar grasp rather than a true apraxia.

Patients with severe osteoarthritis of the hips may present with a waddling gait, which bears resemblance to the gait that is seen with severe proximal muscle weakness – with each step the patient rolls and throws the hips up and forward.

The patient may also exhibit involuntary movements which are likely to indicate the nature of the underlying neurological disease. The tremor that is seen in many elderly patients, referred to as senile or essential tremor may be difficult to distinguish from the tremor of Parkinson's disease. Senile tremor may be found at rest, it is more rapid than Parkinson's and not 'pill rolling'. It may be present at rest and gets worse with movement.

Other movements tend to be less regular such as chorea, and patients with Huntington's chorea may present to the geriatrician. These movements are sudden involuntary, jerking movements involving muscles and groups of muscles. Athetoid movements which may be difficult to distinguish are more writhing in nature. Hemiballismus may complicate stroke and is characterized by coarse, flinging movements of one arm. Much more common than any of these are the movements that are seen with tardive dyskinesia. In this condition all parts of the body may be affected and it is characterized by irregular, involuntary, non-purposive movements. Constant chewing, tongue protrusion, lip smacking or grimacing are characteristic. There may be dystonic features where the patient adopts exaggerated postures. Many of these patients have associated akathisia and have great difficulty in sitting still and are constantly on the move.

In the patient with a slow protective gait the neurological examination may yield further useful information. The patients should be examined for primitive reflexes (Chapter 3). The tone may be found to be increased and the patient appear to be quite rigid. This is often paratonic rigidity (gegenhalten) in which the patient has great difficulty in relaxing. As passive movement is checked the patient continues the movement after the examiner has stopped. Limbs may be sustained in posture instead of returning to a relaxed position of rest. This type of rigidity is common and often misleading and mistaken for the rigidity of Parkinson's disease or even spasticity. When examining one limb, and gegenhalten is suspected, the patient should be asked to move the opposite limb. The tone should decrease if gegenhalten is present – extrapyramidal (cogwheel) rigidity will increase.

5. Assessment

In the situations described here problem formulation is achieved by the careful history taking, observation and examination. In most situations the problems will have been clarified from an obvious dysfunction to a pathophysiologic level. There is usually little need for further investigation. Complete assessment should include objective data on level of function. We have found it extremely useful to record on video the state of the patient when first seen, this allows later comparison to determine the effectiveness of treatment and is of great value as a teaching tool.

Idiopathic gait disorder of the elderly (IGDE) is a diagnosis of exclusion. Once the examination is complete the only positive findings will be the slowing of the gait and the impairment of balance. There may be some non-specific neurological findings that are common in the elderly such as failure of upward gaze, absent ankle jerks, loss of vibration sense in the ankles or positive glabellar tap and palmo-mental reflex, but these are of no pathological significance and are no commoner in those patients with IGDE compared with others who walk at a normal speed and who fall less frequently.

The patient with impaired gait due to cerebral atrophy (brain failure) will have associated cognitive impairment, and a variety of extrapyramidal signs. Bradykinesia and rigidity are the usual findings and may lead the clinician to make a false diagnosis of Parkinson's disease. The classical tremor is usually absent although there may be a senile tremor which adds to the confusion (of the physician not the patient). This is an important condition to distinguish from Parkinson's disease since treatment with anti-Parkinsonian medications invariably makes the patient much worse – specifically with their mental state.

The clinical triad of bradykinesia, rigidity and tremor allow the diagnosis of Parkinson's disease to be made.

The nature of abnormal movements which are observed allow problem formulation at a pathophysiological level and in some situations ascent to an etiological diagnosis.

6. Plans

Diagnosis

Apart from the routine investigations which will have been done on these patients, there is usually little need for any further tests. Parkinson's disease remains a clinical diagnosis and computerized axial tomography (CAT scan), for example, adds little. In the patients with abnormal gait, cognitive assessment may need to be completed and will provide useful information. In these patients further imaging of the brain may be of value, for example CAT scan or nuclear magnetic resonance in the diagnosis of multi-infarct state or Binswanger's disease. All patients presenting with disorder of gait and cognitive impairment of short duration should have a CAT scan to determine if normal pressure hydrocephalus is the cause and whether surgical intervention is possible. Further tests for toxic levels of heavy metals may be indicated in some situations when manganese or mercury poisoning are considered a possibility.

Treatment

Physical therapy plays a prominent role in the management of all disorders of movement. When the gait has deteriorated to the extent that it is unsafe the aim of treatment is improve safety as far as possible.

With the idiopathic gait disorder of the elderly, the impaired gait secondary to brain failure and dyspraxic gait, any deconditioning that is present is addressed with an exercise program. Walking is practised and the patient is helped to be as safe as possible. This may mean prescribing a walking aid. For example, those with IGDE are frequently helped a great deal by the use of a cane (stick), in fact many will have discovered this for themselves. The therapist will need to check that this is the correct length for the patient (with the patient standing and the arm hanging by the side the wrist flexion creases should be level with the top of the cane). Patients with associated cognitive decline may find walking aids too difficult and are safer without anything. Those with a dyspraxic gait may be helped by a walker (Zimmer frame) particularly with wheels so that the patient can push it along. The physiotherapy that is appropriate varies from simple conditioning to more complex gait training with progress from parallel bars to independent gait.

The approach by the physiotherapist has to be adjusted to the patient, to their cognitive functioning and ability to remember as well as their degree of dyspraxia. The patient with cognitive impairment needs frequent repetition and simple direction. With dyspraxia automatic movement is encouraged and techniques such as movement to music, dancing, or marching should be tried.

Physiotherapy is extremely important in the patient with Parkinson's disease and much can be done even for the patient with advanced disease. Both patient and care provider can be taught techniques to minimize as far as possible the disability. Occupational therapy is important in training in transfers and in activities of daily living and to determine if the patient will be helped by the use of various aids. For those with severe limitation of walking, wheelchair prescription is important. At first the wheelchair being used for distance outings and later when the gait has deteriorated even further for everyday use.

With the patient with abnormal movements physical techniques are of little value although in some instances tremor can be reduced by the judicious use of weighted cuffs. In this situation various appliances can be adapted to be more spill proof – for example, cups and dishes which adhere to the table.

Pharmacological treatment is not appropriate for IGDE, the impaired gait of brain failure or dyspraxic gait.

Parkinson's Disease

The patient with Parkinson's disease can almost always benefit from pharmacological intervention. In the elderly , particularly with any degree of cognitive impairment, treatment should always begin with small doses with slow increases. The most valuable drug remains L-dopa. This drug in combination with decarboxylase inhibitors should be started in most patients at a dose of 100/125 mg 3 times daily. In the very old and frail, half this dose would be preferable, increasing every 3 days. Many patients can be maintained on 100/25, 3 times a day. In some patients the dosing has to be increased in frequency, usually 5 times a day will be adequate. The most common complications which limit treatment are nausea and vomiting, hallucinations and mental disturbances and orthostatic hypotension.

Anticholinergics, such as trihexyphenidyl, benztropine and orphenadrine, have a very limited role in the elderly because of their marked propensity to produce hallucinations with even a very small dose. Their main use is in the control of tremor.

Bromocryptine has a limited place in the management of the frail elderly and even with very small doses there is a high incidence of side-effects – particularly hypotension and hallucinations. We have managed to use this drug in only a few patients starting with a small dose of 2.5 mg once daily and increasing by 2.5 mg every 3 days until the desired improvement is obtained or the side-effects become unacceptable.

Deprenyl has a limited role and there is limited experience with this drug so far. It is started in a dose of 5-10 mg daily at the beginning of treatment. It may delay the need for L-dopa therapy and prolong the beneficial effects of L-dopa. Like all anti-parkinsonian medications side-effects such as mental disturbances are common in the elderly. In late cases of treated Parkinson's disease, where multiple small doses of L-dopa therapy is necessary to avoid 'on-off' phenomena deprenyl has a role. Often the number of doses of L-dopa can be reduced with a smoothing-out of pharmacological action.

Senile Tremor

Many patients may have found that their tremor improves with alcohol – in fact this helps in establishing the diagnosis. There are a variety of drugs which help when senile or essential tremor is disturbing the patient. Beta-blockers are probably the best drugs to try initially – propranol in a dose of 10 mg 3 times a day should be started and gradually increased (every 3 to 4 days) until control is achieved or side effects limit further increase. Metoprolol may be a better choice and should be started at a dose of 50 mg twice daily. If control is not achieved with 200 mg twice daily and there are no significant side effects then primidone should be added at a dose of 62.5 mg twice daily with incremental increases every 4 days to a maximum of 250 mg 3 times daily. Most patients will be controlled on this regimen. Clonazepam may be of value in some patients and is an important alternative.

Tardive Dyskinesia

This has proven to be a difficult problem to manage in many patients. This is usually secondary to tranquillizer usage and the likely offending drug should be reduced and discontinued to determine the effects. If a tranquilizer is required then the one with the least potential to produce this unwanted side-effect is said to be thioridazine. Many drugs have been tried with little benefit including clonazepam and reserpine. In our hands the most effective therapy is tetrabenazine. This drug should be commenced in doses of 12.5 twice daily, increasing to 3 times daily after a week. Some people are helped by this dose, others will need to be increased up to 75 mg 3 times a day. The effects are dramatic in most patients and the drug will need to be continued.

References

Bendall, M. J., Bassey, E. J. and Pearson, M. B. (1989) Factors affecting walking speed of elderly people. *Age and Ageing*, **18**: 327–32.

Himann, J. E., Cunningham, D. A., Rechnitzer, P. A. and Patterson, D. H. (1988). Age-related changes in speed of walking. *Med. Sci. Sports Exerc.* **20**: 161–6.

Imms, F. J. and Edholm, O. G. (1981). Studies of gait and mobility in the elderly. *Age and Ageing*, **10**: 147–56.

Kotsoris, H., Barclay, L. L., Kheyfets, S., Hulyalkar, A. and Dougherty, J. (1987). Urinary and gait disturbances as markers for early multi-infarct dementia. *Stroke*, **18**: 138–41.

Mathias, S., Nayak, U. S. L. and Isaacs, B. (1986). Balance in the elderly patient: the 'get up and go' test. *Arch. Phys. Med. Rehabil.*, **67**: 387–9.

14

Visual loss

The elderly individual suffering from visual loss is put at risk of falls, has impaired ability to maintain self independence and is at risk of misinterpreting visual stimuli thereby exacerbating confusion. The clinician's aim should be to identify treatable conditions, optimise visual function and, if necessary, modify the environment to compensate for the visual impairment of the patient.

Predisposing factors

There is evidence, that there are age related changes in vision; with deterioration in brightness vision, acuity, colour vision and depth of perception. Changes in accommodation arise from loss of elasticity of the lens, with resultant reduced ability to alter the focal length. The resting diameter of the aged iris is less, tending therefore to admit less light. There would also seem to be impairment in central vision processing. Other changes predispose to pathological processes of the eye, such as reduced depth of the anterior chamber increasing the likelihood of developing glaucoma.

Precipitating factors

The majority of cases of recent visual loss have as their basis lesions within the orbit; macular degeneration, cataracts and glaucoma account for 83 per cent of non-reflective visual loss. They would have to be excluded before considering lesions of the optic nerve and cerebral pathways (Table 14.1). Extraorbital causes are less common and can be detected by associated symptoms and signs.

Table 14.1 Causes of visual loss

Intra-orbital	Vascular	Extra-orbital	Metabolic	Others
Errors of refraction	Arteritis	Neurological Tumour	Diabetes mellitus	Pagets disease
Glaucoma	Retinal artery occlusion	Neuro-syphilis	Vitamin A deficiency	Sarcoid
Cataract	Retinal vein occlusion	Encephalitis	Vitamin B12 deficiency	Toxic
Retinal detachment	Cerebro-vascular accident	Meningitis		
Macular degeneration	Hypertension	Trauma		
Optic neuritis	Arrhythmias	Migraine		
Papilledema	Aneurysm	Epilepsy		
Optic atrophy	Polycythemia			
Vitreous hemorrhage				

An accurate history and examination can often identify these causes of visual impairment without resorting to elaborate tests. In an individual with visual impairment there are often several co-existing factors contributing to the impairment. Each requires identification and treatment on its own merit.

Subjective

The rate of onset of visual impairment can be helpful in determining its cause (Table 14.2). An insidious onset of visual impairment is a feature of cataracts, chronic glaucoma, senile macular degeneration and diabetic retinopathy. Increasing myopia is not uncommon with cataracts. Diplopia may be seen. Senile macular degeneration affects central vision so complaints of difficulties with reading or sewing are common. Chronic glaucoma initially affects peripheral vision and involves central vision only at a very late stage.

Table 14.2 Rate of onset of common causes of visual loss

Rapid onset	Gradual onset
Retinal detachment	Cataract
Acute glaucoma	Chronic glaucoma
Vascular occlusion	Macular degeneration
Ischemic optic neuropathy	Diabetic retinopathy

A history of diabetes mellitus should be sought since 40 per cent of people with diabetic retinopathy, significantly interfering with their vision, are over 70 years of age. They are also prone to cataract formation, macular edema, retinal degeneration and vitreous hemorrhage.

A complaint of blurred vision, associated with halos around bright lights, especially in the evenings, may suggest acute (narrow angle) glaucoma. Less commonly this may be seen also with cataracts produced by light deflection from the lens opacity. Distorted vision is a feature of stigmatism.

Acute glaucoma may present with sudden loss of vision usually associated with pain in or around the eye. This may follow the use of mydriatrics for the purpose of fundoscopic examination. The pain may involve the whole area innervated by the fifth cranial nerve.

An abrupt, painless loss of vision may suggest arterial or venous occlusion. Sometimes in retinal artery occlusion, the loss of vision is produced by amaurosis fugax or perceptions of cloudiness and colours. Occasionally temporal arteritis may give rise to retinal artery occlusion, so a history of headache and/or temporal tenderness should be sought. In retinal vein occlusion vision is usually not completely lost.

A retinal detachment may be suspected by a story of floaters followed by awareness of a shadow over part of the visual field. If the detachment involves the macular area there may be profound loss of visual acuity.

The rate of onset of visual loss and its association with pain is of some diagnostic value and will help define extraorbital causes. A history of preceding temporal headache and tenderness, or limb girdle stiffening with pain, suggests the possibility of arteritis. Acute optic neuritis is associated with rapid loss of vision and pain in the region of the affected eye, which is aggravated by eye movement. Raised intracranial pressure may present with headache, particularly on coughing or straining, and may be associated with amaurosis fugax on those occasions.

The patient's attitude to the loss of vision may suggest certain conditions. Cortical blindness, for instance, is often strongly denied by the patient (Anton's syndrome). The eyes appear superficially normal with preservation of pupillary reactions. The condition may remain static, or gradually recover to one of a number of less intense stages, involving a progressive lightening of greyness and hazy images.

Objective

Examination of the eyelids may reveal the presence of ectropion or entropion, which can produce corneal irritation and ultimately opacification.

A semi-dilated pupil with ciliary injection should suggest the possibility of narrow angle glaucoma. Usually one eye is more affected than the other. An increase in ocular tone may be difficult to assess by simple palpation and tonometry should be performed in any suspect case. In advanced cases, fundoscopy shows the characteristic cupped appearance of the optic disc.

The presence of a bilateral central scotoma with a loss of colour discrimination in a heavy smoker, alcoholic or debilitated patient may suggest a toxic amblyopia.

Refractive errors can be simply tested for by using the pinhole test. A pure refractive area would be corrected by viewing an object through a pinhole. Cataracts are readily detected on routine fundoscopy. It should be appreciated that they may obscure other significant causes of visual impairment and can predispose to glaucoma.

The features of diabetic retinopathy may be found, and their presence should always be an indication for further referral.

In retinal artery occlusion the direct light pupillary reaction is lost, although the consensual reflex is preserved. Arteries distal to the occlusion may not be visualized or may be identified as pale lines. The retina often appears pale. In the region of the macular a cherry red spot may be seen.

Light perception and perception of movement is often maintained in retinal vein occlusion. The retina is hemorrhagic with congested veins, edema and transudates.

Edema of the macular and hyaline bodies associated with pigmentation changes should suggest the presence of senile macular degeneration. A loss of central vision may be found on perimetry. It may be seen in association with cataracts. It should not be considered a contraindication to cataracterectomy as a useful degree of peripheral vision can be restored.

An appreciation of the normal visual pathways is essential in the localization of lesions. Any visual field defect should be carefully documented and confirmed by perimetry.

The appearance of the optic disc may be helpful. Swelling of the disc is a feature of papilledema, venous occlusion and optic neuritis. In the case of papilledema the extent of visual loss is usually mild relative to the degree of changes in the disc. The extent of venous engorgement and hemorrhages from venous occlusion usually allows for ready diagnosis.

A pale, sharply demarcated disc suggests the presence of optic atrophy which can be from a variety of causes (Table 14.3). A unilateral case of optic atrophy should suggest the possibility of either a compressive or vascular lesion.

The presence of a 'Pagetic' skull may be relevant. Narrowing of the optic foramen can interfere with venous return resulting in papilledema and secondary optic atrophy. Retinal artery occlusions, retinal hemorrhage, chorioretinitis and macular degeneration have been described in Paget's disease affecting the skull.

Table 14.3 Causes of optic atrophy

Chronic papilledema
Retinal lesion – chorioretinitis, intra-ocular hemorrhage, etc.
Arterial occlusion
Optic neuritis
Optic nerve compression
Division of optic nerve
Lesion of optic tract

Assessment

Routine investigations may point to the likely etiology of problems for example by the finding of high blood sugar (diabetes) or a high erythrouyte sedimentation rate (ESR) (temporal arteritis). A normal ESR does not exclude the possibility of temporal arteritis, but if the diagnosis is considered probable on clinical grounds then a temporal artery biopsy should be done. Treatment should not await the result, in fact steroid therapy (40–60 mg/day) may be given on a diagnostic trial.

The purpose of the algorithm, Fig. 14.1, is to identify potentially reversible or treatable lesions. In this population of patients there are often more than one contributory cause of visual loss.

Plan

Diagnosis

Many of the intra- and extraocular causes of visual impairment can be identified from the initial assessment, with limited investigations. Further investigation is dependent upon the findings and may include angiography and computerized axial tomography.

Careful perimetry can be of use in the localization of compressive lesions.

Treatment

The presence of problems such as confusion should not be used as a contraindication for treatment of visual disturbance, as distorted visual information may well be exacerbating the confusion.

The indications for the removal of cataract will depend upon the individual's particular visual requirements and the method chosen. Removal via

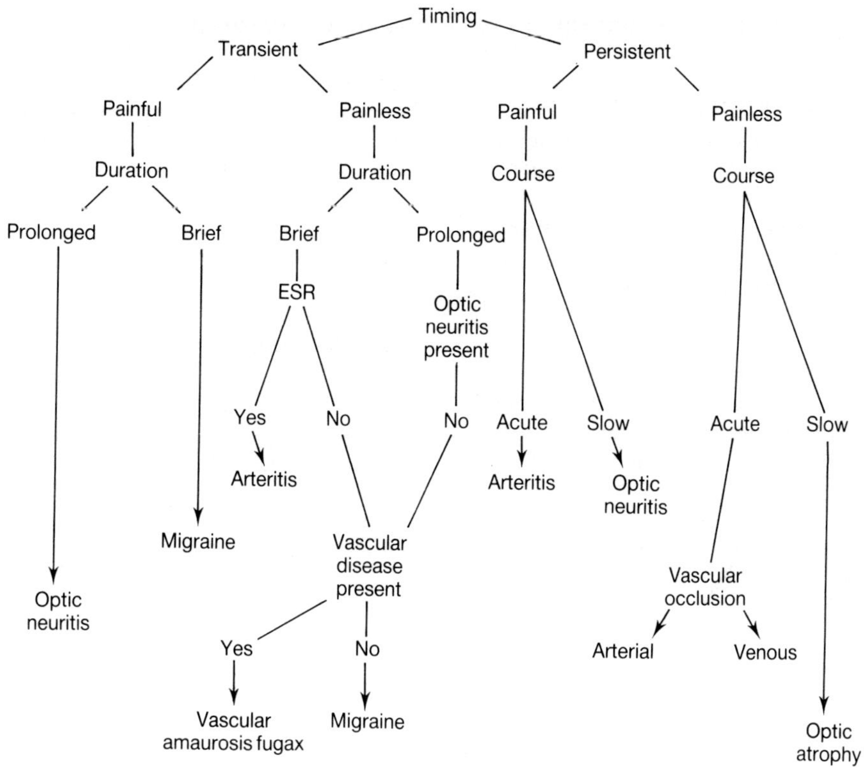

Fig. 14.1 Monocular blindness.

the intracapsular method will produce distortion, alteration in magnification and some restriction of visual fields. It therefore tends to be deferred, until poor vision is clearly adversely modifying lifestyle. The extracapsular type of removal of the lens coupled with the use of acrylic intraocular lenses can restore almost normal optics. This method is therefore being increasingly used, particularly at the early stages of visual impairment.

The only effective therapy for macular degeneration is destruction of sub-retinal neovascular formations using the argon laser, and treatment of areas of pigment epithelial detachment with the krypton or argon laser, to limit their spread. Unfortunately the treatment of neovascularization is limited to those formations not close to the fovea, or between the fovea and the optic disc.

Immediate skilled ophthalmic treatment of acute glaucoma is necessary if permanent visual damage is to be avoided. The pressure can usually be reduced by the use of osmotic agents orally (glycerol) or intravenously (mannitol), or acetazolamide to reduce aqueous secretion and miotics. Most eyes can be rendered safe by the relatively easy procedure of peripheral iridectomy. The control of chronic glaucoma is usually achieved by the use of miotic drugs and in some cases by oral acetazolamide. Timolol can be used topically thereby avoiding the visual effects of miotics.

The management of retinal detachment will depend upon its stage. If a retinal hole is found which is likely to lead to detachment, then the promotion of inflammatory adhesions between the choroid and retina by light coagulation, or the external application of a cryoprobe, is indicated. If detachment has occurred then the choroid and retina need first to be brought into apposition.

Unfortunately, by the time it presents, retinal artery occlusion will usually result in a substantial, permanent loss of vision. Sometimes vasodilators, eye massage or paracentesis of the anterior chamber are used in recent occlusions in an attempt to improve blood flow. In the case of amaurosis fugax, a search should be made for a source of embolization. Low dose aspirin is sometimes prescribed.

Retinal vein occlusion needs reassessment, usually at three months after onset. If little or no recovery has occurred by that time the prognosis is poor. Areas of non-perfusion, which may be demonstrated by fluorescein angiography, may result in new vessel formation with later, fibrosis and traction. In the region of the macular they may further impair vision. In such circumstances their treatment by photocoagulation needs to be considered.

With ectropion the eyelashes may cause chronic corneal irritation, infection or ulceration which requires prompt treatment if scarring is to be prevented. Temporary measures using adhesive tape to prevent the inversion of the lid are useful. Surgical correction is easy and can be done in an out-patient setting under local anesthetic.

Suggested reading

Applegate, W. B., Miller, S. T., Elam, J. T., Freeman, J. M., Wood, T. O. and Gettlefinger, T. C. (1987). Impact of cataract surgery with lens implantation on vision and physical function in elderly patients. *J. Amer. Med. Assoc.*, **257**: 1064–6.

Gardiner, P. A. (1978). Glaucoma. *Brit. Med. J.*, **ii**: 1689.

Gardiner, P. A. (1979). Visual difficulty in old age. *Brit. Med. J.*, **i**: 105–6.

Gordon, D. M. (1974). Eye problems of the aged. In: Chuin, A. B. (ed.) *Working with Older People, Vol. IV: Clinical Aspects of Ageing*. US Department of Health, Education and Welfare, Washington, DC.

Marmor, M. (1977). The eye and vision in the elderly. *Geriatrics*, **32**: 63–7.

15

Deafness

Deterioration in hearing is a common problem amongst the elderly population, and this has been shown in many surveys. The number of elderly people that acknowledge that they have a problem and actively seek assistance is less. Studies of populations in the industrialized West have revealed a pattern of gradual hearing loss with advancing age. The loss begins with the higher frequencies of sound. Pure tone audiometry has revealed a prevalence in population studies varying from 12 to about 40 per cent, with higher rates in certain situations such as mental institutions. Pure tone audiometry detects hearing impairment which does not always result in any significant degree of disability. Hearing disability occurs when there is change in hearing function that causes problems with the perception of speech and environmental sounds, and the individual has a hearing handicap when this interferes with the ability to perform activities of daily living. Self-assessment techniques have been used to determine the degree of disability and handicap and should be considered part of a complete assessment.

1. Predisposing and precipitating factors to hearing changes with age

Hearing loss can be explained by a mixture of aging changes and the increasing incidence of disease. The age change appears to be secondary to the environmental assaults that occur throughout life, it is not a primary aging change that is universal to the species.

The changes that occur with age are predominantly sensorineural. There is progressive degeneration of the structures of the cochlea, with changes in the epithelial and sensory cells. Losses can be shown in both the afferent and efferent nerve fibres. The changes are most prominent in the basal turn of the cochlea and are not found in children but become more prominent beyond the age of 60. There are more central changes, and lesions within the cortex have been identified. The blood supply to the inner ear may also deteriorate with atrophy of the striae vascularis. There are changes within the middle ear with thickening of the tympanic membrane and loss of elasticity. These changes are hastened by environmental factors and exposure to noise will make things worse. Disease states will also exacerbate those changes and include previous middle ear disease and vascular disease.

2. Subjective

Some patients will complain that they have difficulty in hearing, and that the problem is with higher frequencies, the female voice rather than the male voice. Such impairment is likely to start in middle age usually becoming noticeable in the sixth decade. The nature of the impairment is unlikely to be truly reflected by pure tone audiometry findings. The majority of patients have particular difficulty with speech discrimination. So that hearing is reasonably good when there are no interferring noises, the patient being unable to keep track of conversation when there are other noises such as music or other people speaking close by.

In some people hearing loss may be associated with tinnitus – an internal noise generated within the hearing system. This can be a very distressing symptom, much more so than deafness itself. The nature of the noise varies but is often described as 'swishing' or 'ringing'. This needs to be distinguished from abnormal noises like voices or music, which are not tinnitus.

Hypersensitivity to sound is another associated feature with the elderly deaf. Loud speaking or amplification is unpleasant and usually intolerable to such patients.

Questions should be asked about the patient's appreciation of the sound in both ears, and whether it is the same or asymmetrical. Unilateral losses often have a different etiology to bilateral symmetrical losses. The onset of the impairment also needs to be determined, specifically whether it is of sudden onset or more gradual.

3. Objective

Auditory acuity can be tested by a number of relatively simple maneuvers such as rubbing the fingers together beside the ear, speaking in a whisper or using a tuning fork (256 Hz). Although these may not need to be done if the patient is obviously deaf and has difficulty in answering questions. Both ears should be tested. Once established that there is a problem then the ears should be carefully examined otoscopically. If there is wax occluding the ears this will need to be removed. The state of the tympanic membrane should be determined.

Weber's and Rinne's tests remain of value in a limited number of elderly patients with hearing problems. In the presence of unilateral nerve deafness, a vibrating tuning fork placed on the centre of the forehead will be heard in the normal ear (Weber's test). With middle ear disease the fork may be heard better on the affected side. With Rinne's test bone conduction is compared with air conduction. The vibrating fork is placed on the mastoid process and when the sound disappears is placed next to the auricle. It will be heard vibrating in this position with a normal ear and mild nerve deafness. In the presence of middle-ear disease it is louder on the mastoid bone and not heard when moved.

Examination should include an assessment of the patient's perception of the hearing loss. This can be very difficult to achieve in cognitively impaired patients as many disregard any degree of hearing loss and ignore the issue. The patient should be asked questions about the impact on every day function (Table 15.1). For the majority of patients with significant hearing loss there needs to be referral for more detailed audiological assessment. This should define whether a patient has a significant problem with hearing and also whether it is likely to be correctable or helped by amplification.

Table 15.1 Self-perceived hearing loss

Yes (4) Sometimes (2) No (0)

1. Does a hearing problem cause you to feel embarrassed when meeting new people?
2. Does a hearing problem cause you to feel frustrated when when talking to members of your family?
3. Do you have difficulty hearing when someone speaks in a whisper?
4. Do you feel handicapped by a hearing problem?
5. Does a hearing problem cause you difficulty when friends, relatives or neighbours are visiting?
6. Does a hearing problem cause you to attend religious services less often than you would like?
7. Does a hearing problem cause you to have arguments with family members?
8. Does a hearing problem cause you difficulty when listening to TV or radio?
9. Do you feel that any difficulty with your hearing limits or hampers your personal or social life?
10. Does a hearing problem cause you difficulty when in a restaurant with relatives or friends?
11. Can you hear the phone bell?
12. Can you hear over the telephone?
13. Can you hear the door bell?

Interpretation
Score 0–8 no self-perceived handicap
Score 10–22 mild to moderate handicap
Score 24 or more, significant handicap

Assessment

The vast majority of elderly patients with deafness give a history of gradual onset. When the audiological testing reveals high tone hearing loss in the patient with very gradual onset of deafness from middle age onwards the most likely diagnosis is presbycusis.

Deafness may be due to vascular damage. This may be insidious, deafness coming on in middle age and progressing – essentially identical to presbycusis with sensorineural deterioration. When deafness is sudden and unilateral it may be due to cerebral infarction secondary to embolism or hemorrhage in the territory of the artery of the internal auditory meatus. Rarer causes would include viral infections like zoster, neoplasms like acoustic neuroma or trauma or drug ototoxicity.

Plan

Diagnosis

The identification of deafness as a problem is not difficult. More precise definition comes from the audiological assessment and the results of consultation with an otorhinolaryngologist. The investigations that may be required are beyond the scope of this book.

Treatment

Deafness that is considered to be presbyacusis, or that is shown to be sensorineural with no clear etiology may be helped by amplification. It is recognized that many elderly patients have such a problem and have never sought help, or alternatively have chosen to ignore recommendations that have been made. Deafness makes interview and examination very problematical and it is advised that all those dealing with the elderly have an amplification device available. For example a simple binaural amplification system that resembles a 'Walkman' can be obtained easily at a modest cost. This may make communication possible.

The most acceptable means of amplification for most people is a hearing aid. There are various types which will need to be prescribed and fitted by experts. Once in use there is much that can be done by way of training and rehabilitation that will help the patient. Small cosmetically attractive aids may be extremely difficult for some elderly patients to manipulate. Amplification produced by electronic aids may be unacceptable to the patient as the sound produced is too harsh and cannot be tolerated. When this is the case other approaches need to be considered such as learning to lip read. This may be very difficult in some of the elderly because of vision problems. Some people benefit from the use of light-flashing door bells and telephones and built-in amplifiers on telephones and television sets.

Other problems are very difficult to treat such as hyperacusis, for which avoidance seems to be the only solution. Tinnitus is also very difficult problem to help, although some people benefit from the use of a tinnitus masker. This is a piece of equipment like a hearing aid which produces another sound that drowns out the tinnitus.

Physicians and other health professionals can do a lot to improve communication with the elderly deaf. Speaking should be done with a clear moderately loud voice, and shouting should be avoided. The speaker should sit squarely facing the patient in good light and there should be no distractions, audible or visible. Speech should be slightly slower than normal, pronounced in the local accent if possible, leaving longer intervals than normal between sentences. It is interesting how family members will act as a 'translator' or 'mediator' for the physician and can get through to a patient when the professional has failed miserably.

Suggested reading

Bess, F. H., Lichtenstein, M. J., Logan, S. A., Burger, M. C. (1989). Comparing criteria of hearing impairment in the elderly: a functional approach. *J. Speech Hear. Res.*, **32**: 795–802.

Fisch, L. (1985). 'Special senses – the aging auditory system. In: J. C. Brocklehurst (ed). *Textbook of Geriatrics and Gerontology*. Churchill Livingstone, pp. 484–99.

Mulrow, C. D., Aguilar, C., Endicott, J. E., Velez, R., Tuley, M. R., Charlip, W. S. and Hill, J. A. (1990) Association between hearing impairment and the quality of life of elderly individuals. *J. Amer. Ger. Soc.*, **38**: 45–50.

Uhlmann, R. F., Teri, L., Rees, T. S., Mozlowski, K. J. and Larson, E. B. (1989). Impact of mild to moderate hearing loss on mental status testing: comparability of standard and written mini-mental state examinations. *J. Amer. Ger. Soc.*, **37**: 223–8.

16

Weight loss, malnutrition, swallowing problems, anorexia, nausea and vomiting

Introduction

Weight loss, malnutrition, anorexia and nausea are relatively common problems with elderly patients. This is to be expected, since with advancing age the likelihood of serious disease and death increases.

Weight loss may be objectively recorded with precise evidence of the amount that has been lost, or may be perceived but without objective evidence. The patient or family noting that clothes no longer fit, or that progressively smaller clothes have been bought. As the problem of weight loss is pursued it may become apparent by close observation that the patient has a reduced intake of food and that this is due to difficulty in swallowing. It has been suggested that 25 to 50 per cent of patients in an acute care facility for 2 weeks or longer suffer protein calorie malnutrition. The frail old individual is particularly vulnerable in both the hospital and home situation. In one study of a psychogeriatric institutional patients' energy and/or protein malnutrition was present in 30 per cent and obesity in 4 per cent. Micronutrient problems were also common. The prevalence of clinical vitamin deficiencies is probably less than 1 per cent of all elderly in the community, but on biochemical measures the subclinical prevalence is several times this.

Dysphagia is defined as difficulty with swallowing, it is a symptom that is only associated with the act of swallowing. Pain upon swallowing is referred to as odynophagia and is a separate symptom which will be considered here. When there is difficulty the food may stick and then be regurgitated.

Anorexia means the loss of desire for food or loss of appetite. This may be a difficult symptom to define and we need to consider the reasons why patients are not eating, or indeed whether they do in fact have a reduced intake. Anorexia is one of the reasons why there may be weight loss and reduced food intake.

Nausea and vomiting may occur independently of each other, but are usually associated. The presence of nausea limits the appetite, and is usually associated with weight loss if of any significant duration. Nausea means that the individual has the feeling of the imminent desire to vomit. Vomiting is the forceful oral expulsion of gastric contents.

1. Predisposing factors with aging

Weight Loss

Weight loss is commonly associated with aging and may not be indicative of any underlying pathology. Steady weight gain in the adult, after the second or third decade, appears to be a feature of normative aging in 'developed' or industrial societies. Studies that have been done measuring the amount of adipose tissue or skin fold thickness, have shown a steady climb until old age (after 60) and then a decrease. The lean body mass appears to decline steadily from about the third decade throughout adult life. This has been shown in primitive communities as well as in 'Western Man'.

In other words some weight loss might be considered to be a common feature of aging. The loss of lean body mass appears to accelerate in extreme old age – over the age of 75 to 80. It should however, be appreciated that at least some of the lean body mass loss seen with aging may be dietary and lifestyle related. Even at the extremes of age relative modest increases in dietary protein intake and increase in exercise result in improvements in lean body mass.

This age change (weight loss) makes it difficult to be precise about what is normal and what is pathological. It is important to understand what the patient means by weight loss, the gradual change that occurs with normal aging is a different kind of problem that will not be dealt with in this chapter.

Pathological weight loss can be considered to be that which occurred over the preceding six months or at most two years. The amount of weight lost that is significant is difficult to define but should be more than a few pounds, and is likely to be at least 10 pounds. A variety of factors predispose the elderly to pathological weight loss. Access to nutrients may be difficult because of problems of finance, isolation from help, and limited choice because of geographic restrictions. Ingestion may be adversely affected by problems of dentition, and disruption of swallowing mechanisms.

The villi of the small intestine tend to be broader and flatter with advancing age. For the most part this does not have a deleterious effect, but the absorption of monosaccharides appears to be less efficient in the geriatric population. The absorption of calcium, iron and some vitamins show some decline with age. These changes do not lead to overt disease or to clinical problems, however they demonstrate that there may well be decline in functional reserve. Digestion may be affected by interactions with medications, previous stomach and small intestine surgery, and malabsorption syndromes.

Appetite and anorexia

Appetite is controlled by centres in the hypothalamus, there is little information available on normal age changes of these centres. Clinical experience suggests that in the presence of dementia there is damage to these centres, and loss of appetite with profound weight loss is usual in patients with severe dementia. Appetite may also change with the decreased olfactory and taste senses of aging. Physical activity also decreases for many elderly individuals and with this comes a reduced intake of food.

Weight loss occurring in the presence of a normal appetite is unusual in all age groups and even less common in old age. In all age groups patients with malabsorption may lose weight with a prodigious appetite. For those patients who reach old age with malabsorption the weight loss in recent times may be small. The patient is likely to have been undernourished for some time. Other conditions in younger age groups in which one sees weight loss with a good appetite, are modified by old age. For example in thyrotoxicosis there is often an associated loss of appetite in the elderly patient.

Swallowing

The successful ingestion of food is complex and consists of many steps (Fig. 16.1). Food is first of all prepared and rendered suitable for eating or drinking. Once prepared the food needs to be transferred from receptacle to mouth. Further preparation occurs within the mouth where under normal circumstances it is chewed and lubricated prior to the act of deglutition. The process may be impaired at any stage, and with aging often is. Impairment at one stage may also affect other stages.

With aging there may be difficulty with obtaining and preparing food due to problems of cognition and mobility. These have been discussed elsewhere. From the standpoint of swallowing, food should be of such a consistency that it is appropriate to swallow. Large chunks or particularly dry food may initiate problems. If the patient cannot prepare food

- Preparation
  - shopping
  - organization
  - cooking
- Transfer
  - motor dysfunction
- Mastication
  - no teeth
  - painful mouth
  - neurological problems
- Lubrication
  - dry mouth
- Deglutition
  - swallowing dysfunction

Fig. 16.1 Diagram of the stages of food ingestion.

because of visual impairment or loss of motor skills these problems might arise. It is well recognized that with advancing age there is loss of motor skills and of manual dexterity.

Loss of teeth is increasingly common with advancing age. It is also apparent that many older individuals do not wear complete sets of dentures and that many are ill-fitting. For this reason there is often impaired mastication in elderly patients. Saliva production drops with advancing age and there is an increasing incidence of xerostomia. Thus there is an increased chance of food being poorly prepared for deglutition, arriving dry and with a larger than optimal particle size.

Age changes occur in the esophagus, indeed these changes have been described as presbyesophagus. In apparently healthy individuals there is a reduction in frequency and amplitude of peristaltic waves (primary and secondary). At the same time it has been noted that there is impairment of relaxation of the lower esophageal sphincter – the sphincter normally relaxes with almost every peristaltic wave. In older individuals this may decrease to approximately 40 per cent of the time. At the same time as this occurs there is an increase in frequency and amplitude of tertiary waves. The aged esophagus is less efficient at swallowing, demonstrates less reserve and is clearly predisposed to develop further problems.

Nausea and vomiting

There is no information available on the effects of aging on the predisposition to vomit. Nausea and vomiting do not appear to be of any greater or lesser severity in the elderly patient. Having said that it is important to remember that the old patient who is vomiting has less reserve than the younger patient, and the effects of dehydration are seen much sooner.

2. Precipitating factors

When an individual is taking in fewer calories than they are expending there is loss of weight, and we have seen that in old age this usually means a reduction in oral intake. There are many reasons for this (Table 16.1). Many cases of Alzheimer's disease present to the clinician with weight loss secondary to reduced intake (poor attention span to complete meal) and increased activity (wandering) with higher metabolic rate.

Table 16.1 Cause of loss of weight

Reduced food intake
1. Loss of appetite
   - constipation
   - systemic problem (serious)
     infection
     cancer
     inflammatory non-infective
   - GI problem
     early satiety
     stomach cancer
     peptic ulcer
   - Drugs – local or systemic effects
2. Psychiatric problem
3. Fear of symptoms (sitophobia)
   - GI problem – IBD
4. Problem with ingestion
   - Dysphagia (see Table 16.2)
   - Aspiration
   - Small stomach – surgery, scarring or malignancy
5. Lack of awareness (cognitive decline)

Problem with digestion
Malabsorption

Excess loss or catabolism
1. Inflammatory bowel disease
2. Thyrotoxicosis, diabetes, tuberculosis

The aged individual with presbyesophagus is clearly predisposed to swallowing difficulties. There is usually a single major problem that gives rises to a swallowing problem, but as discussed above, the problem often relates to factors outside the pharynx, larynx and oesophagus. Any age change or disease process that leads to difficulty in preparation of food, or in transfer to the mouth may precipitate a swallowing problem (Table 16.2). This may be acute as when large chunks of meat or bread are eaten, which stick at the lower esophageal sphincter. This leads to mechanical obstruction to swallowing.

Mastication may be inadequate or impossible due to disease of teeth or loss of the muscles of mastication. Damage to the fifth or seventh cranial nerves will lead to problems. For example when there is upper motor neurone damage to the seventh with drooping of the corner of the mouth, there is often associated difficulty with retaining food in position to chew. Lubrication may become impaired due to aging, a gradual change. More acute problems may result from radiation therapy for example.

Infection in the mouth may also cause sudden inability to ingest food. For example with oral candidiasis, aphthous ulceration or herpetic stomatitis.

Table 16.2 Causes of swallowing problems

Preparation and transfer	Mastication	Deglutition	Esophagus
Visual loss	Tooth loss	Motor neurone	Web
Impaired motor skills	Oral pathology	Myasthenia gravis	Motility problem
Cognitive loss	Radiation candidiasis	Cerebrovascular disease	Achalasia stricture
Mechanical obstruction to chunks	Aphthous ulceration	Syringomyelia	Carcinoma
		Multiple sclerosis	Infection
		Trauma	
		Infection	

Tongue movement is important in preparation for swallowing as well as the act of deglutition. Damage to the muscle or twelfth nerve will result in difficulty with these stages of swallowing.

The act of deglutition may be impaired as a result of neuromuscular dysfunction due to various disease states at a variety of different anatomical sites. The muscles of deglutition are supplied by the ninth, tenth and eleventh nerves. Bulbar palsy occurs when the nuclei or the cranial nerves themselves are damaged. Damage to the nuclei occurs as a result of motor neurone disease, tumours or syringomyelia. The nerves themselves may be damaged by trauma, infection or tumour. Pseudobulbar palsy occurs when the innervation of the nuclei from the motor cortex is damaged. The most common cause of this in this age group is of course cerebrovascular disease, but it may also occur with motor neurone disease, multiple sclerosis and Parkinson's disease.

Dysphagia may also occur with myasthenia gravis, and this problem may dominate the clinical picture.

The bolus of food may be transferred to the upper pharynx without any problem, but there is a problem with the act of swallowing beyond this point. The cricopharyngeus is in a constant state of tonus during its resting stage. During normal deglutition this muscle relaxes, and then increases in tone behind the bolus. Damage to the tenth cranial nerve, or its nucleus within the brain stem may result in a hypertonic state of the cricopharyngeus. Thus food arriving meets an obstruction and is then likely to be aspirated or be regurgitated. There may be pooling of fluid in the pyriform fossae. Food may also be retained within Zenker's diverticulum which forms as a result of the obstruction.

Rarely in advanced iron deficiency states there may be a cricopharyngeal web. Within the body of the esophagus there may be motility problems, achalasia, stricture resulting from inflammatory disease or radiation damage,carcinoma or infection (candidiasis).

Nausea and vomiting may result from a wide variety of diseases. It is useful to consider systemic causes, and local disease states (Table 16.3). Certain problems are much more common in old age, specifically adverse drug reactions, gastrointestinal infections and severe constipation.

Table 16.3 Causes of nausea and vomiting in old age

Systemic response
1. Metabolic problem (renal failure, diabetes, heart failure)
2. Infections (viral or bacterial illness)
3. Drug toxicity (e.g. digoxin, opiates, alcohol)
4. Other toxicity (radiation)
5. Psychosomatic

Local causes
1. Upper gastrointestinal
   - peptic ulceration
   - gastritis
   - outlet obstruction
   - pancreatitis
2. Lower gastrointestinal
   - constipation
   - inflammatory bowel disease
3. Distant site
   - raised intracranial pressure

3. Subjective

The patient is asked if they have lost any weight if they have not already volunteered this. The patient should be asked what they consider to be a normal weight, the frequency of weighing themselves and the timing of the last weight. Change in clothes size or belt notch may be a useful indicator.

A full dietary history should be obtained. It may be necessary for the dietician to obtain this information by speaking with a care provider. Care providers usually have an accurate picture of the daily intake of the patient.

If it is decided that weight loss is significant, then the history should be directed to determine the likely factors that might be contributing. Is there loss of appetite, or a true lack of desire for food? Because loss of appetite is such a non-specific symptom and can result from a variety of causes questions might be asked to see if there are problems in any system. There are some patients who appear to have a loss of weight secondary to loss of appetite and no physical problem. It needs to be remembered that psychiatric problems suppressing appetite can also surface in old age. There are patients who have a syndrome that is very close to anorexia nervosa, and this will be discussed again later.

Is intake inadequate for needs? This might be the case where there are problems with attention span such as in the demented, mobile wanderer?

Is there a failure to eat because of fear of the symptoms that might result? The patient will volunteer that they would like to eat but that a certain discomfort is stopping them. The patient should be asked if they are tempted by food and if they would like to eat. The patient with genuine loss of appetite will state quite clearly that they have no desire for food and that they could not care less if they ate.

Is there difficulty with eating, with chewing the food and with swallowing? Does posture make a difference? Does the patient choke when eating and is this with solids or liquids or both?

The patient who states that they cannot 'get their food down' or cannot swallow needs to be closely questioned to find exactly where the problem is. In the early stages of swallowing there are characteristic symptoms. Patients complain of food 'going down the wrong way', which leads to choking, coughing and gagging when eating. This is often worse for liquids. When there is neurological damage to the soft palate, liquid may be regurgitated through the nose. Material may collect within diverticula (Zenker's) and cause greater obstruction until emptied, usually by regurgitation.

Mechanical obstruction due to extrinsic compression, or due to encroachment of the lumen by cancer, post-inflammatory scarring or foreign body results in dysphagia with the sensation that food is sticking. The patient can usually point to the level at which the food sticks – for example the patient with a web will point high, the patient with a stricture between the middle and lower third will point to the appropriate level. This may be accompanied by pain. The pain is due to esophageal spasm and is usually located anteriorly in the center of the chest or to the left of the sternum. The pain may feel gripping in character and is often difficult to distinguish from the pain of myocardial ischemia. The pain and the sensation of sticking may be relieved by dislodging the food. The patient may do this by trying to wash the food down with water or by inducing vomiting. Passage of the food or regurgitation will result in relief. When the esophagus is narrowed the patient will experience dysphagia for solid material rather than fluids, and at first for food that is ingested in large chunks. When the narrowing is progressive, as with an encroaching carcinoma, the dysphagia gets progressively worse. At first, difficulty is experienced with large chunks of meat or bread, later becoming difficult for even minced foods. The patient with a post-inflammatory stricture will often give a history of preceding heartburn and other symptoms of reflux.

Motility problems, particularly the tertiary spasm in presbyesophagus, are characterized by their intermittent nature (Table 16.4). Although the overall symptomatology may become gradually worse, more frequently, the dysphagia is inconsistent. The patient characteristically experiences difficulty with either solids or liquids, which comes on at any time during a meal. Once relieved the patient may be able to continue eating. The dysphagia may be precipitated by hot or cold liquids. These symptoms are often accompanied by odynophagia, as already described.

Is the patient cognitively intact and aware that they have a problem? This should become clear early in the interview, but not always so.

Weight loss may be secondary to the other symptoms of nausea and vomiting, and questions should always be asked of this. Furthermore, if the patient does not have weight loss and yet is complaining of long-standing and significant nausea, then it is difficult to place much emphasis on the problem. When

Table 16.4 Differentiation of esophageal motility problems

Characteristic	Motility presbyesophagus	Narrowed lumen cancer/stricture
Timing	Intermittent	Constant
Progress	Increased frequency	First for solids then liquids
Temperature of foods	Made worse by very hot/cold	No effect
Weight loss	Yes	Extreme

complaining of nausea there should be inquiry into any associated symptoms. A careful drug history is required, and if the patient is on a number of drugs the timing of these in relationship to any meal.

There is a need to distinguish between saliva, water-brash, retching, regurgitation and vomiting. Vomiting is itself of two main types. Regular vomiting which has a variety of causes; and projectile vomiting which implies outlet obstruction. Questions might be asked to determine the timing of vomiting in relation to meals and whether it is true vomiting or simply regurgitation. Are there associated problems of pain or diarrhoea? Are any associated symptoms relieved by the vomiting?

Weight loss occurring in the presence of apparent normal intake and activity should always raises suspicions of some underlying problem such as malabsorption, neoplasm, and hyperthyroidism. If so is the patient constipated? If the answer is yes, the normal bowel habit and any recent changes need to be determined.

4. Objective

In those patients who have weight loss identified as a problem from the history, there is usually objective evidence of this. Findings on examination may also reveal for the first time that this as a problem (Fig. 16.2). It is important to look for objective evidence in the form of actual weight measurements. Estimates of height are often used in calculating several indices of nutritional statuses. The presence of kypho-scoliosis or flexion deformities of the legs make difficult such measurements. The height is often expressed as a ratio of weight. Skin fold measurements made at multiple sites are useful in estimating subcutaneous tissue proportions. In a clinical setting, the recording of serial weights is often the most practical method of assessing significant fluctuations in nutritional status.

The clinical evaluation of nutritional status requires careful examination of the mouth, skin, hairs, eyes, nails, lower extremities and various organs. Angular stomatitis and glossitis may be seen in a variety of vitamin deficiencies, including niacin, riboflavin, or pyridoxine deficiency. A rolled appearance of the tongue with papillary atrophy associated with niacin deficiency and a magenta color reflects riboflavin deficiency. It should be appreciated however that poor hygiene, peridontal disease, systemic antibiotics, and uremia may cause glossitis and discoloration of the tongue. Soft and spongy bleeding gums are indicative of ascorbic acid deficiency, but will only be seen in gross cases.

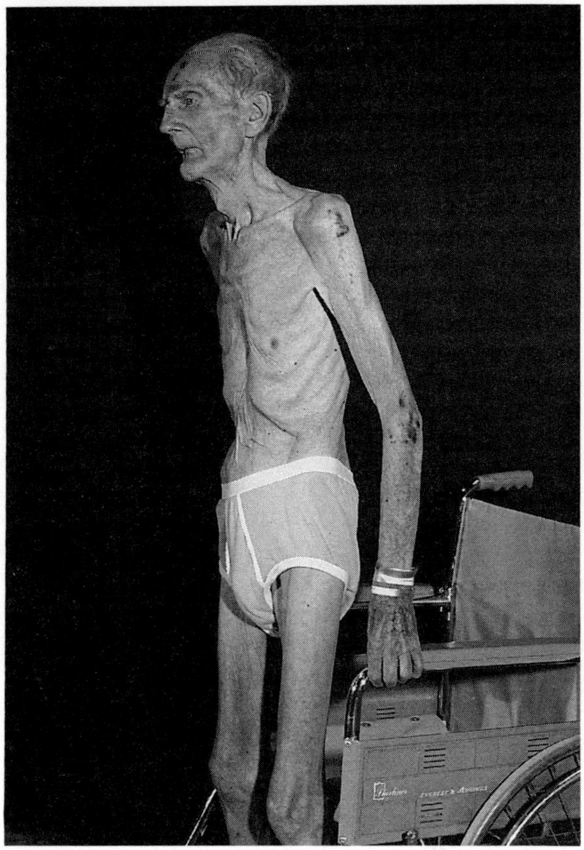

Fig. 16.2 A patient with multiple problems and severe weight loss.

Dryness, thickening, and a paleness of the conjunctivae are seen in severe vitamin A deficiency. Pale mucous membranes and koilonychia of the nails are suggestive of inadequate iron.

The skin may reveal useful information concerning malnutrition. Skin lesions are seen in exposed parts of the body with niacin deficiency. Corkscrew coiling of body hair, thorax and abdomen may be seen in early scurvy.

Edema of the extremities may be associated with hypoalbuminemia or anemia. Peripheral neuropathies may be seen especially with deficiencies of water-soluble vitamins.

Physical examination is not particularly accurate in assessing the degree or severity of weight loss. With normal aging there is loss of lean body mass, specifically of muscle. The finding of limited musculature with redundant skin folds may not be pathological in an extremely old individual.

Obviously if weight loss is identified as a problem the physical examination should be complete looking for any physical sign that might provide an explanation. Patients with significant swallowing problems usually experience weight loss which will be detected on examination.

Much information may be gathered by observing the patient whilst eating. This is particularly important in the patient with deglutition problems. The speech therapist may during a bedside assessment detect evidence of problems with naso-pharyngo-laryngeal mechanisms.

A careful examination of their mouth looking at the teeth, natural or artificial, as well as the tongue, the palate and the pharynx should be conducted. The gag reflex should be tested as part of the neurological examination of the ninth to twelfth cranial nerves. Apart from the gag reflex the sensation of the pharynx and posterior third of the tongue need to be tested. The movements of the palate during phonation and the movements of the tongue should be checked.

When dysphagia is suspected as part of a generalized neurological disorder then other signs of that disorder should be looked for during the complete neurological examination.

When nausea and vomiting are problems the examiner needs to pay special attention to the nervous system to be certain that there are no signs of raised intracranial pressure. The abdominal exam must be complete, looking for any evidence of gastrointestinal pathology. This includes a rectal examination, particular attention is paid to the presence of stool and its characteristics. Fecal impaction may present with anorexia and intermittent vomiting.

5. Assessment

When investigating a non-specific problem like weight loss or loss of appetite, it is never clear exactly where the investigation will lead. Investigation should always follow the direction

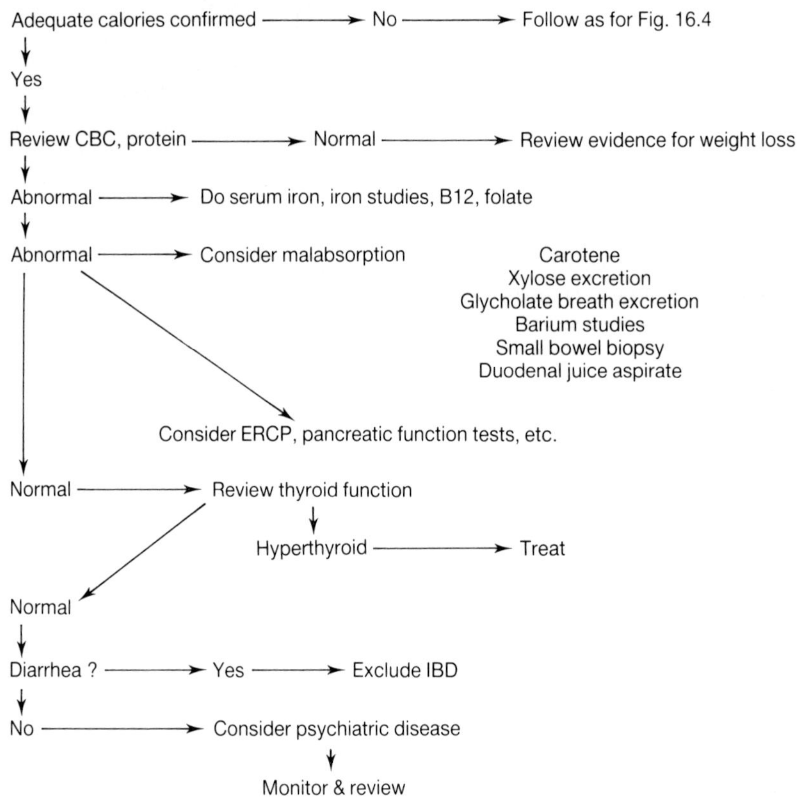

Fig. 16.3 Weight loss with adequate calorie intake.

indicated by the findings. In the absence of any pointers the approach should be conservative and investigations delayed until objective evidence of weight loss is obtained. If this is available then minimum investigations would include the standard geriatric screen (Chapter 1), examination of stools for occult blood and visualization of the upper gastrointestinal tract. This would also be true for the investigation of nausea and vomiting. Investigation of these patients will depend upon the symptoms and signs and should follow a logical path (Fig. 16.4).

In the patient with weight loss dietary consultation is useful. There are a number of methods for collection of objective data on food intake. The 24-hour recall provides a retrospective record of the amount of food consumed in the previous 24 hours. Its simplicity and rapid means of obtaining information makes it attractive. Unfortunately, it tends to yield unreliable data in the elderly. Information may be improved by prospective recording for a longer period of perhaps three days. This can give an indication of a dietary pattern but often information about quantities of

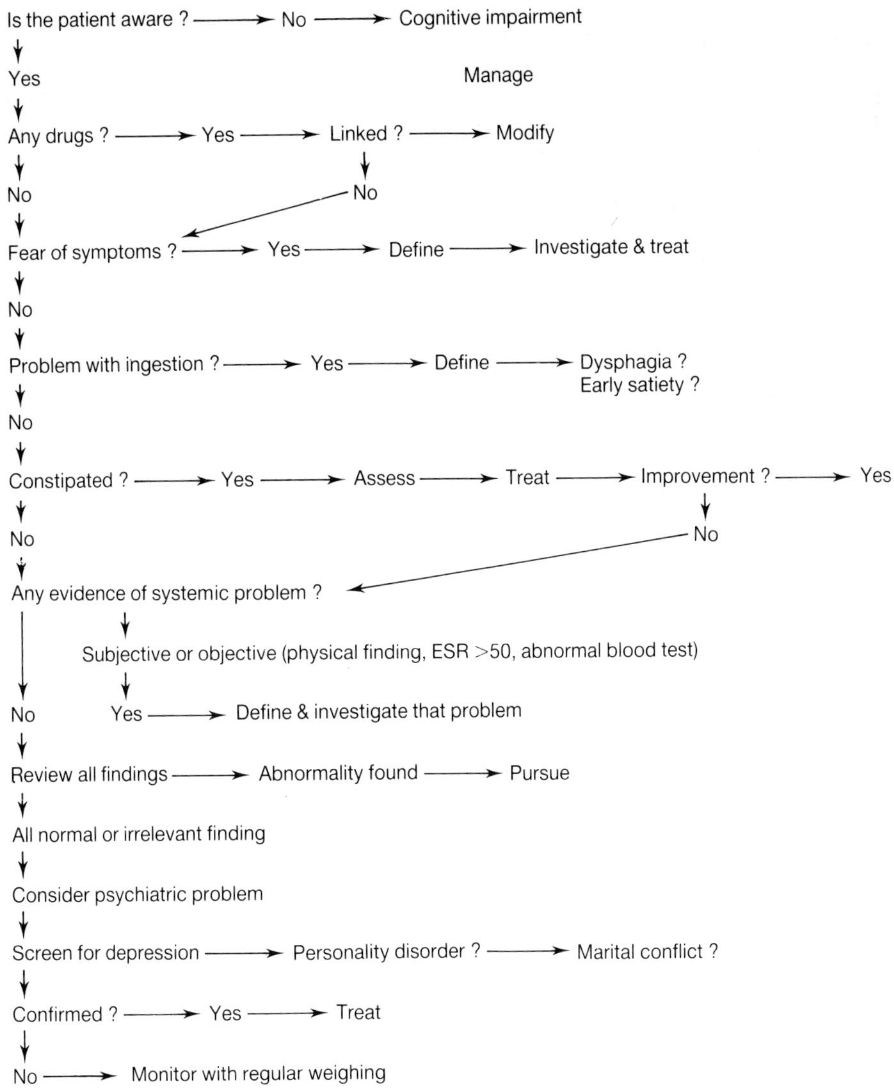

Fig. 16.4 Weight loss due to reduced intake.

individual food products and method of cooking is lacking, thereby limiting the data use. If the dietary consultation reveals that the patient has an adequate intake of food, but has still lost weight then investigations will be directed at determining if there is malabsorption (Fig. 16.3).

Initial laboratory evaluation should include hemoglobin, hematocrit, white cell count, differential, total proteins and albumin. A suspicion of nutritional problems should indicate further evaluations, including a serum iron, transferrin, red blood cell folate, serum B12, phosphorous, alkaline phosphatase, urea, creatinine, and lipids. Trace proteins, such as the retinal binding protein, are thought to be better indicators of protein status than the serum albumin and total protein. Assays, if available, of specific micronutrients can be considered. It should be appreciated that factors other than malnutrition may affect the measurement. Serum ascorbic levels, for example, tend to reflect recent dietary intakes and not the body's reservoir. Plasma zinc is a measure of body zinc and a small shift from intracellular fluids may markedly increase the plasma concentration. Thus, changes in plasma zinc are seen with infection, trauma, myocardial infarction, and low dose estrogen treatment. Any abnormality could point to the possibility of malabsorption. In this case further investigations might include serum carotene, xylose tolerance test, radio-labeled glychocholate breath test, barium studies, small bowel biopsy and duodenal juice aspirate. Xylose tolerance test is problematic because of difficulties in collection and because of associated renal failure. If this proves to be a dead end then there are few other things that would give weight loss.

In patients with dysphagia, visualization of the upper gastrointestinal tract during swallowing is an essential investigation and this is best done radiologically with barium. The swallow is recorded on videotape. With this technique all stages of swallowing can be visualized including deglutition. If there is narrowing of the lumen this can be well visualized with radiographs. The appearance of the narrowing will usually allow identification of a stricture, carcinoma or achalasia for example. Plain chest radiographs are required before embarking upon barium studies. If there is extrinsic compression of the esophagus other views might be necessary.

Esophageal endoscopy will also be indicated with biopsy of any lesion. Those patients who appear to have a motility disorder or achalasia should have esophageal manometry which will reveal the presence of tertiary waves, the nature of the peristaltic waves and the pressure of the lower esophageal sphincter and its ability to relax (Fig. 16.5).

When there is nasal regurgitation or aspiration the barium swallow needs to be performed with caution. Such patients should have inspection of the pharynx and larynx by an otolaryngologist.

There are patients who have dysphagia and who have a clearly defined cause, for example a stroke. In such patients there are practical considerations of feeding and the risk of aspiration. It is important to carry out a detailed swallowing assessment. A tray is prepared for a meal on which there are foods of differing texture, consistency and particle size. The patient is then assessed for their ability to swallow the different items. This may be performed by various health professionals such as speech pathology, occupational therapy or nursing. The information obtained may well confirm the swallowing problem but will also allow an appropriate treatment protocol to be developed.

6. Plan

Diagnosis

A common occurrence in geriatric practice is for a care provider to raise concerns with regard to weight loss in the patient who is cognitively impaired. Weight loss is common, if not usual, in the patient with dementia. Rejection of food occurs in the patient with advanced dementia and contributes to the final demise. It is also common in earlier stages when patients are living at home, fending for themselves and of course forgetting to prepare or forgetting how to prepare food. Also with reduced attention span, food may be left unattended, to be burnt or to become cold and so 'less tasty'. These people tend to 'snack' and often on items that do not provide a well-balanced diet. Such patients have difficulty in explaining their concerns or their symptoms to the physician. Weight loss is accepted as a consequence of the cognitive decline if there are no other pointers that there is a problem – for example no observed difficulty with swallowing, no pain, a normal ESR and normal screening blood tests.

A major problem with elderly patients is multiple drug use. Many, if not most, drugs can affect the gastrointestinal tract. Nausea is a common side-effect found. The more medications that a patient

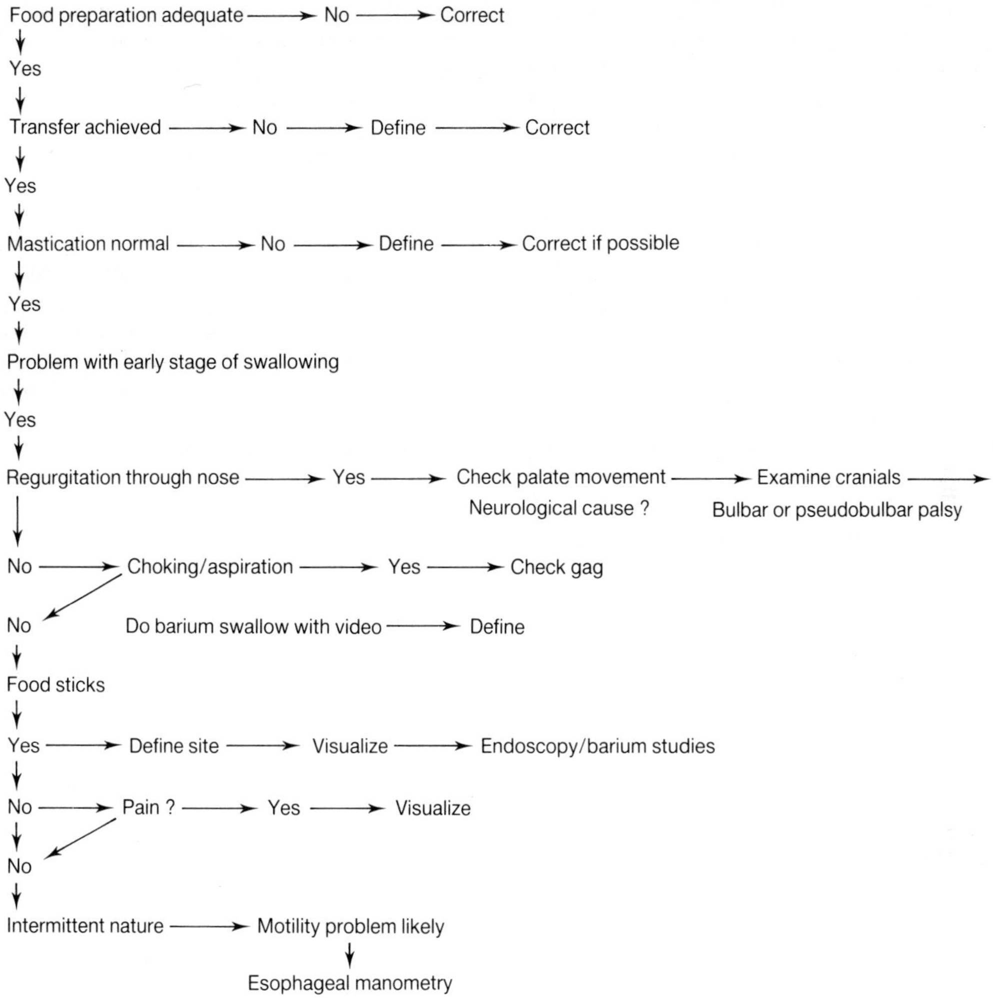

Fig. 16.5 Decision analysis in swallowing problems.

takes the more likely that there is to be a side-effect. The physician should be aware of the medications that are being consumed, and the possible effects on appetite.

Even after a careful and logical approach to the assessment and investigation has been followed one may be left with a patient who has an unexplained problem. It should be remembered that weight loss can be caused by depression which may be difficult to diagnose. Chronic alcohol abuse should also be considered. There are patients who have objective evidence of weight loss or of being undernourished and some of the features of anorexia nervosa. There is no single clear-cut syndrome but some patients appear to have anxiety, situational depression, a personality problem and often marital conflict. Such patients are likely to have had many exhaustive investigations and once identified should have no further investigations. These patients are difficult to manage but may improve gradually with psychotherapy.

Some patients with chronic nausea may be left with no adequate explanation for the problem. Symptomatic treatment is the only option.

Treatment

Treatment can be considered in two ways, first of all that which is specific to the problem and will depend upon the etiology. Different treatment options are discussed in the different chapters. Secondly, treatment may be symptomatic. It is difficult to improve appetite unless the etiology is defined. Indeed in many instances treatment appears to be designed to allay the fears of the relatives and care providers rather than the patient. If loss of appetite appears to be an inevitable result of a systemic problem little can be done apart from making sure that food is palatable and suited to the patient's preferences. Appetite stimulants are of little value, although aperitifs and tonics may be tried.

The individual with dementia and weight loss due to poor attention span can be helped by the provision of frequent nutritious cold snacks. Explanation and reassurance will help allay the care provider's fears. Those patients who are demented and refuse to eat may be helped by the use of a major tranquilizer such as chlorpromazine or thioridazine. A small dose may result in the early return of a good appetite. It is particularly useful in those patients who become agitated and paranoid, it is of no value in the most advanced cases. In advanced dementia where the care provider has been spending a long time in assistance with feeding, the patient may begin to spit out food, or to hold it in their mouth without swallowing (Hamster syndrome) or simply to keep the mouth tightly clenched. In patients with the 'Hamster syndrome' it is important to check the mouth carefully after any meal or administration of any drugs. When food or medicine is retained in the mouth there is a higher risk of aspiration or asphyxiation. This behaviour in severe dementia often results in profound weight loss. Such changes mark the terminal phase of dementia and should be accepted as such. There is no evidence that such patients are hungry, indeed evidence points to the contrary. A recent study indicates that survival is not enhanced by the use of artificial means of nutrition. Such patients should continue to be cared for with good nursing care, mouth toilet should be maintained but no extraordinary measures to provide nutrition should be employed. Feeding tubes by mouth or via gastrostomy are not indicated and should not be employed.

Treatment of swallowing problems should be both definitive and symptomatic. Definitive treatment will depend upon the problem that is identified. Such treatments are dealt with in other textbooks and will not be covered in great detail here.

Patients with motility problems are difficult to manage. Antacid therapy may be helpful if the patient notes that heartburn precipitates spasm. Metoclopramide may sometimes be of value although there is a 25 per cent incidence of central nervous system side effects, cisapride is a much better choice. Domperidone does not appear to be of great value in this problem. Occasionally mechanical dilatation reduces the stricture and temporarily helps the problem.

It may be necessary to provide extra nutrition to the patient who has lost a great deal of weight. It is preferable to use regular oral feeding with food supplements. A swallowing assessment may be invaluable in this regard.

The recovering stroke patient can often take purěed foods or minced items. They may well have difficulty with liquids or large particle items. Thus liquid is given in the form of gels often with good effect. It is also useful to stimulate the swallowing mechanism with temperature differences, to start the meal with a popsicle for example. Patients should also be sitting vertically out of bed. In order to avoid mucus build-up patients are also encouraged to avoid milk and milk products. In this way many patients, with impaired gag reflexes, can be retrained and recovery promoted. This should not be done with a nasogastric feeding tube in place and it is important to have suction readily available during the early phases. When the input remains limited the food that is taken can be enriched to boost calorie and nutrient intake.

An important principle is that nutritional deficiency is rarely an emergency situation. It is possible to allow some time to pass before beginning replacement. In patients with stroke or other neurological problems swallowing may be impaired. After a few days (maintaining hydration via a peripheral route) nasogastric intubation may be necessary. The tube can subsequently be removed when the patient recovers or if no neurological recovery occurs and the patient persists in coma or vegetative state. Those patients with no return of ability to swallow who are conscious and wish it may benefit from a feeding gastrostomy. Gastrostomy should be delayed until this time and not performed early in the management of these patients. Because various technical means of supplying nutrition are available there is a tendency to use them frequently. Careful thought should go into evaluating the burdens as well as the benefits from the various methods. It needs to be emphasized that the natural oral route is always preferred and that there is always time to follow the patient to determine what will happen (Table 16.5).

If the cause of nausea or vomiting can be found

then it should be treated. Symptomatic treatment can be effective and simple treatment with a drug like dimenhydrinate is usually effective. For more severe cases domperidone is an effective drug. Starting dose should be 10 mg prior to each meal up to 4 times a day. This dose can safely be increased if necessary up to 160 mg daily. It is preferred to metoclopramide which has up to 25 per cent incidence of central nervous system side-effects in this age group. Any other antiemetic may be used but care should be taken with potential side-effects. For the patient unable to swallow medications, suppositories provide a satisfactory alternative.

Patient education

Those patients with weight loss and poor appetite as a result of a significant illness such as cancer or dementia, are likely to persist with a limited intake unless the underlying problem is addressed. When the patient is receiving palliative care the patient is allowed to control what and how much they eat. Mouth toilet can be maintained but there should be little concern with the intake and its adequacy. Because food plays such an important role in our lives in a social and ceremonial way, it is very hard emotionally for patients, but more so for families and care providers to accept limited intake. When death appears to be both imminent and inevitable then concerns of comfort should supersede those of adequate nutrition.

In those patients who have poor understanding of nutritional necessities then education is called for, and significant care providers should receive the instruction too.

The nutritional state can be monitored by weight measurement and by performing calorie counts and measuring input. During the periods of retraining those with neurological problems, patients need to be closely monitored to make sure that not only is there adequate intake but that there are no complications developing. Great patience and perseverance are required to attain success, and attempts to get patients to swallow again should not be abandoned too early. Patients and their care providers need to be educated with regard to the techniques to enhance swallowing.

When the oral route of feeding appears to be impossible because of the nature of the problem the alternatives need to be explained to the patient, with a full discussion of the potential benefits as well as the burdens. In a situation where there is potential for recovery, or for continued deterioration it should be explained that treatments once started can be stopped. For example nasogastric intubation may be necessary in the stroke victim

Table 16.5 Nutrition and hydration

Route	Advantages	Problems
Oral	Natural Patient acceptance	Aspiration Poor if appetite poor
Nasogastric intubation	Simple Temporary Effective	Discomfort GI irritation Ulceration, bleeding Aspiration
Gastrostomy	Efficient 'Technical'	Permanent Burden on patient Distances care giver Stoma sepsis
Peripheral	Maintain hydration	Nutrition limited Vein Sepsis, phlebitis
Central line	Efficient Effective	Expensive Sepsis, trauma Fluid overload Confusion
Hypodermoclysis	Effective Easy, inexpensive Well tolerated	No nutrition Slow

unable to swallow but when there is no recovery of consciousness it is ethically acceptable to stop that form of treatment. Gastrostomy is of a more permanent nature, but may still be reversed if the patient so chooses or if recovery occurs.

In the very old there may be a combination of many problems although one appears to dominate the clinical picture. It is important to council with the patient to determine that definitive treatment is desired and that it is likely to help. For example a patient may have a cricopharyngeal problem but will also be suffering from depression and is not eager to eat because of the environment. The patient may be residing in a nursing home for example and he finds the other residents unacceptable and the food unappetizing. One has to correct as much as is possible and leave the decision with regard to treatment to the patient. In this milieu the results are not always as satisfactory as one would anticipate.

Suggested reading

Castell, D. O. (1976). Achalasia and diffuse esophageal spasm. *Arch. Int. Med.*, **136**: 571–9.

Khan, T. A., Shragge, B. W., Crispin, J. S., Lind, J. F. (1977) Oesophageal motility in the elderly. *Amer. J. Diges. Dis.*, **22**: 1049–54.

Mills, C. P. (1973). Dysphagia in pharyngeal paralysis treated by cricopharyngeal sphincterotomy. *Lancet*, **i**: 455–7.

Singh, S., Mulley, G. P. and Losowsky, M. S. (1988). Why are Alzheimer's patients thin? *Age and Ageing* **17**: 21–8.

Soergel, K. H., Zboralske, F. F. and Amberg, J. R. (1964). Presbyesophagus: oesophageal motility in nonagenarians. *J. Clin. Invest.*, **43**: 1472–9.

Zboralske, F. F., Amberg, J. R., Soergel, K. H. (1964). Presbyesophagus, Cineradiographic manifestations. *Radiology*, **82**: 463–7.

17

Abdominal pain and diarrhea

In the setting of geriatric practice pain remains a frequent and important problem. It continues to be important as a harbinger of serious morbidity. It needs to be remembered however that one of the characteristics of aging is a changing threshold for pain. This is by no means uniform, but it does appear that in many people with advancing age there is less appreciation of visceral pain.

Attenuation of symptoms or reduced acuity of pain has been recorded for some time in the case of the acute abdomen; and potentially serious problems may remain masked. The patient presents late with more serious disease. Some patients of course are unable to relate their experience of pain because of communication difficulties or cognitive decline and one has to interpret their actions and perhaps surmise that they do indeed suffer pain. There is no doubt that in this setting treating some agitated, confused patients for pain may result in dramatic improvement in the patients mental state.

Abdominal pain may be associated with other symptoms or signs such as jaundice, urinary retention or hematuria. In these cases, the problem is approached from the standpoint of jaundice or hematuria, not the pain. In this chapter, abdominal pain alone or with diarrhea is discussed. Diarrhea is also identified as a problem for diagnosis.

The term diarrhea means, for some, a change in stool consistency and the passage of loose or soft stools. For others it means an increase in frequency of stool passage, the normal range being from one bowel movement every three days to three a day. For an individual having one bowel movement every three days, an increase to one daily of looser consistency would constitute diarrhea. It is therefore important to recognize that this is an individual definition, and in labelling a bowel function as diarrhea there needs to be a clear understanding of what has been normal before.

For these reasons it is difficult to generalize about the problem of diarrhea, and problem definition should be precise from the history and examination of stool.

1. Age related predisposing factors

With advancing age there may be changes in the ability to perceive pain related to the pathophysiological changes within the nervous system. The threshold for visceral pain, induced by balloon distension of the esophagus, has been shown to change with advancing age such that a greater degree of distension is required before it is perceived. This means that in some patients pain is a less prominent feature and in some may be absent, in situations where in younger patients one would anticipate significant and serious pain.

The effect of age, for the most part, is to reduce the appreciation of pain. Those individuals that survive into old age with chronic pain problems may find their symptoms deteriorating, due to compounding psychological problems. It is held by some that depression increases in frequency with advancing age, and it is well recognized that the psychological state of the patient has a profound effect on the patient's ability to tolerate pain.

The effect of cognitive decline has been mentioned. Note should be taken of another significant problem that occurs in patients with dementia. Some patients in the earlier stages of decline become unduly preoccupied with bodily problems, constantly mentioning a symptom such as abdominal pain which results in excessive investigation and therapy. But this is a situation that requires all the skills of a good clinician to sort out and it would be foolhardy to ignore such complaints.

There is an increasing likelihood of impaired defence of the gastrointestinal tract with advancing age (Table 17.1). Infectious diarrhea occurs as a result of contaminated material ingested orally. Defence is less efficient. One of the age changes that is important is impaired acid production in the stomach (achlorhydria). Achlorhydria has been detected in up to one-third of those over the age of 60. It is recognized that there is a steady decline in maximum acid production with advancing age. The incidence of chronic atrophic gastritis increases with age. These two observations may well be linked so that the achlorhydria is in fact secondary to the atrophic gastritis. An association between campylobacter pylori infection and advancing age has been shown, and the atrophic gastritis is thought to result from this.

Table 17.1 Predisposing changes in the elderly

1. *Increased susceptibility to infection*
   - reduced acid production
   - increased exposure
   - reduced motility (drugs)
2. *Reduced absorption*
   - shortening and broadening of villi
   - impaired monosaccharide absorption
   - impaired mineral and vitamin absorption

Any agent that reduces acid production may predispose the patient to enteric infection, indeed this has been shown in some outbreaks. Many elderly patients are prescribed agents like cimetidine or ranitidine which would add to the problem of reduced acid production.

There is no evidence that the mucus of the gastrointestinal tract changes with age. Secretory immunoglobulins do not appear to change with age.

Bowel motility is an important part of the normal defence mechanism. Thus infectious organisms in small amounts may be swept through the bowel and eliminated. Many drugs that the elderly take alter bowel motility which predisposes to them to enteric infection as well as constipation and its complications.

2. Precipitating factors

Abdominal pain can be brought on by many different pathologies, and it would be difficult to provide a fully comprehensive list. In order to facilitate hypothesis generation it is useful to consider the site of origin of the pain and the likely pathology (Table 17.2).

Table 17.2 Abdominal pain

1. *Originating outside the abdomen*
   - A. Spine: vertebral collapse, osteoarthritis
   - B. Other parts of skeleton: e.g. pelvic fracture
   - C. Neurogenic: zoster, causalgia, spinal stenosis
   - D. Muscle
   - E. Chest: myocardial infarction, pneumonia
2. *Originating within the abdomen*
   - A. Peritoneum: perforated viscus - bacterial or chemical
   - B. Obstruction of hollow viscus
     - intestine (including constipation)
     - biliary
     - urinary
   - C. Pathology of organ: peptic ulcer, cholecystitis, pancreatitis
   - D. Vascular: ischemia
3. *Systemic causes:* toxins, metabolic – uremia, diabetes
4. *Unknown or functional*

Abdominal pain can arise outside the abdominal cavity and a common site of origin in geriatric practice is the spine. Degenerative osteoarthritis is a frequent cause of pain. Osteoporosis is common, and collapsed vertebrae may precipitate pain. This is usually easy to diagnose and can be localized to the back. Trauma may also cause fracture in other parts of the skeleton and pelvic fractures can be an important cause of abdominal pain.

The pain associated with Herpes Zoster may be difficult to diagnose and easily confused with other causes when it precedes the vesicular rash. Pain may also result from systemic disease and is occasionally seen with no other identifiable pathology in diabetes or uremia.

Within the abdomen there are many problems that give rise to pain. The parietal peritoneum is sensitive to nociceptive stimuli, the two most important being bacterial or chemical contamination. The latter occurs when there is perforation of a viscus, for example a perforated peptic ulcer or acute pancreatitis. Bacterial contamination can occur with perforation, for example of a colonic diverticulum, or from an inflamed appendix. Occasionally spontaneous infection can occur.

Any of the hollow organs within the abdomen can become obstructed and the pain that results from that usually takes on a typical cramp-like or colicky characteristic. There are often symptoms associated with this which will depend upon the organ that is obstructed. The intestine can be obstructed at any level with resulting pain. A common cause of abdominal pain is 'incomplete' obstruction of the large intestine, the pain associated with functional bowel syndrome, diverticular disease or constipation and fecal impaction.

Inflammation or tumour of the various organs can give rise to pain. The pain is usually produced by the stretching of the capsule from the tumour or from the edema associated with inflammation. For example hepatitis, peptic ulceration, cholecystitis and pancreatitis.

Diarrhea can be precipitated by a variety of different factors (Table 17.3). When the diarrhea is of acute onset and characterised by the passage of large volumes of watery stool then it is most likely due to an infectious agent. The etiological agents in the elderly are similar to other age groups. There are now a number of reports of outbreaks of infective diarrhea in different settings, such as inpatient geriatric units, day hospitals or day care centers. There is no doubt that the elderly that gather in such settings are at greater risk for exposure to these various organisms. The pain associated with this diarrhea is usually cramp like, and may be severe.

Table 17.3 Precipitants of diarrhea

1. *Acute*
   - drugs (purgatives)
   - antibiotics
   - enteric pathogens
   - malabsorption
   - inflammatory bowel disease
   - constipation – overflow or spurious
   - ischemia
2. *Chronic*
   Irritable bowel (diverticulosis), as for acute

The most common bacterial infections are shigella, salmonella, campylobacter and clostridium difficile. In each case the diarrhea is likely to have an explosive onset and be characterized by the passage of large amounts of watery, bloody stool together with severe cramping abdominal pain. The exception is Clostridium difficile infection which may commence as a result of antibiotic administration. This may have a more insidious onset, and patients often have a longer history of diarrhea of up to 48 days, often without any pain.

There are a number of viral infections that may cause diarrhea, and many examples of presumptive viral diarrhea. The two most common agents being rotavirus and the Norwalk agent. These agents cause acute diarrhea in elderly patients. The features differ from younger age groups in that the disease often lasts a little longer.

Diarrhea with less explosive onset may result from a variety of causes within the small or large bowel. Inflammatory bowel disease may present for the first time in old age, indeed ulcerative colitis has a second peak in the fifth or sixth decade. With Crohn's disease, the repeated cramping abdominal pain may be the most important feature. Carcinoma of the large bowel with progressive narrowing of the lumen may allow only a liquid stool passage and produce spurious diarrhea.

Vascular disease is increasingly common with advancing age. Vascular occlusion to some of the vessels of the large bowel may result in an ischemic colitis with sudden onset of bloody diarrhea and abdominal pain.

Malabsorption is an important cause of diarrhea and should always be considered. For example lactase deficiency may result in lactose intolerance and diarrhea. These patients usually have a long history of bloating, excessive flatulence and cramping abdominal pain. Most of the recognized causes of diarrhea can occur in the elderly but become increasingly uncommon with advancing age, usually presenting in younger age groups.

It is important to remember that a loose, watery stool does not necessarily equate with diarrhea. Spurious diarrhea is one of the more common problems that one deals with in geriatric practice. The patient is in fact fecally loaded and impacted and passes liquefied stool. Patients who abuse purgatives often have diarrhea and this is one of the most important precipitants of fecal incontinence in the elderly.

3. Subjective

The most important feature in the history of abdominal pain is to determine the location, character, duration and associated features. Pain is a subjective experience, the character only being known to the patient. It is important to try to get some understanding as to the severity of the pain, recognizing that this may be very difficult. The patient should be asked for information with regard to the quality of the pain and its characteristics. Careful note should be made of the patient's choice of words and whether the pain is sharp and stabbing or perhaps colicky and cramp like, or crushing.

The localization will help determine the likely offending organ if it is an intra-abdominal source.. For example, pain in the epigastrium is likely to have arisen from the stomach, esophagus or associated fore gut structures such as the biliary tract. Colonic pain is most likely located below the umbilicus.

The mode of onset and the duration of the pain often provide valuable diagnostic clues (Table 17.4). Associated features are also of importance, for example the pain of ischemic colitis is usually of abrupt onset, situated in the lower abdomen and cramping. There may be rectal bleeding in association with this pain as well as vomiting, diarrhea and fever. The patient will usually have features of arteriosclerosis elsewhere. Consideration should be given to those things that might aggravate the pain such as respiratory movement or ingestion of food. Such findings would point to diaphragmatic involvement or location within the upper gastrointestinal tract respectively.

Table 17.4 Characteristics of pain

Location
Quality
Severity
Mode of onset
Duration
Aggravating factors
Relieving factors
Associated features

A common problem in this age group is diverticular disease. There are two types of pain which are important to distinguish. First of all the chronic intermittent pain which is associated with the functional bowel problem linked with diverticulosis. This can occur in any part of the abdomen. It is characteristically cramp-like, aggravated by stress and sometimes by eating, relieved by the passage of flatus or a bowel movement, and usually associated with alternating or changing bowel habit. The other type of pain is that associated with diverticulitis. This pain is localized to the quadrant of the abdomen containing the involved bowel, usually the left lower quadrant. The pain may be accompanied by fever and chills, and a change in bowel habit.

A history of diarrhea may direct the inquiry along a different path. The normal bowel habit of the patient should be inquired after, as well as the use of purgatives and other drugs. Obviously the duration of the change in bowel habit and the exact nature of the change should be known. How many bowel motions a day, the consistency of the stool and whether there is blood, mucus or undigested food particles present. If the patient is passing small amounts of stool, but has a constant or frequent desire to empty the bowel then it is likely to be of large bowel origin. On the other hand, large stool diarrhea is likely to be of small bowel origin.

Associated symptoms should be asked about, specifically abdominal pain, vomiting, rigors, and so on. It is important to know of potential exposure to infectious agents such as a recent trip abroad; or whether there is a high risk situation, for example the patient attends a day care centre and several others are affected in the same way. Severe, cramping abdominal pain with profuse watery diarrhea points to an enteric infection.

Fecal incontinence is a common presentation of diarrhea. When a patient complains of fecal incontinence, questions should be asked about the nature of the stool, appearance and odour, the frequency of the episodes of incontinence and the degree of urgency. The patient who has a sense of urgency, who is repeatedly incontinent of watery or bulky offensive stools obviously has diarrhea. The problem would be defined as such, and resolution of the diarrhea is likely to resolve the secondary problem of incontinence.

4. Objective

The objective findings from examination or laboratory data are dependent upon the nature of the underlying problem. The history provides the most important information with regard to the likely cause of abdominal pain, and if this pain is acute, whether it is life-threatening and so demanding emergency therapy (Table 17.5).

It is important to record temperature accurately. Pyrexia points to infection, peritonitis or abscess for example. Some patients develop a subnormal

Table 17.5 Features of acute abdomen

1. *General*
   - fever (subnormal temperature)
   - tachycardia
   - hypotension
2. *Local*
   - tenderness
   - rebound tenderness (peritonism)
   - bowel sounds (absent or increased)

temperature in response to infection, particularly gram negative bacilli. A proportion of patients will not become pyrexial with infection.

Other features on examination which point to the acuity of the problem are the increase in pulse rate and features of shock with hypotension.

The finding of tenderness is important but often unrewarding. False positives and negatives occur in this age group. Tenderness indicates that there is a problem but often no more than this. If there is rebound then this is more supportive of the presence of peritoneal inflammation.

Auscultation is important, listening for bruits as well as bowel sounds. Bruits are frequently found and may not be associated with the problem presenting, but may be an important clue raising the possibility of vascular disease and possible ischemic pain. In the presence of peritonitis the bowel should be quiet, and the failure to hear bowel sounds is an important observation. In the restless delirious patient, the only clue to an intra-abdominal catastrophe such as a ruptured aneurysm or perforated viscus, may be a silent abdomen. In the presence of intestinal obstruction bowel sounds may be increased.

An examination is not complete without a rectal examination with a statement on the anus, rectum, rectal contents and adnexae. In the female there should be a pelvic examination. Inspection of the perianal area is important not only with regard to understanding the nature of the problem but also in managing complications such as skin breakdown. Inflammatory bowel disease can present for the first time in this age group and the presence of anal fistulae, or perianal abscesses and granulomata, may be important findings supporting a diagnosis of Crohn's disease.

Rectal examination will usually reveal if there is fecal impaction and thus spurious diarrhea, although it should be remembered that up to thirty per cent of patients with fecal loading have high impaction beyond the reach of the examining finger.

Needless to say the examination of patients should be complete and important clues may be picked up from evidence of disease elsewhere. It should be appreciated however that many geriatric patients have multiple problems which may not be etiological in the pain or diarrhea. One should therefore be cautious of trying to attribute all symptoms and signs to one pathology.

In considering the common problems in this age group the skeleton should be carefully assessed, particularly when there is any trauma or accidental fall. The skin needs to be inspected looking for any rash with a dermatomal distribution. Evidence of systemic disease such as uremia, sepsis, and so on should be sought.

When a patient has diarrhea of acute onset it is important to determine the well being of the patient, dehydration occurs very rapidly in the very old. With dehydration comes a number of other types of functional impairment particularly reduced mobility and confusion.

5. Assessment

The geriatric investigational screen will provide useful information. An elevated white blood cell count or shift to the left supporting the diagnosis of infection. A raised sedimentation rate and anemia pointing to infection, inflammation or malignancy. The liver function tests may reveal a liver problem, but it should be remembered that several conditions within the abdomen can give rise to non-specifically abnormal enzyme values. Urinalysis will indicate if there is the likelihood of an urinary tract infection, or red cells will point to a calculus.

Additional blood tests may be required, for example serum amylase if acute pancreatitis is suspected. A plain abdominal radiograph is important for most patients with abdominal pain. The film may reveal evidence of obstruction, fecal impaction with pseudo-obstruction or perforation with free air within the peritoneal cavity. Other findings may be important like the presence of pancreatic calcification, or biliary or urinary calculi.

Other investigations will be indicated depending upon the symptoms for example ultrasonography. This might be indicated if aortic aneurysm is suspected, or biliary obstruction.

In the assessment of diarrhea, the search for an etiological agent, should follow a logical course (Fig. 17.1). In patients with acute diarrhea, where the features point to an infectious etiology it is essential to collect specimens to search for the etiological agent, although defining the nature of the agent is unlikely to alter treatment. The importance of this often rests with limiting any potential outbreak particularly in the setting of in-patient geriatric units or day care facilities. It is important to define the infectious agent when this is part of a wider outbreak and to identify the source.

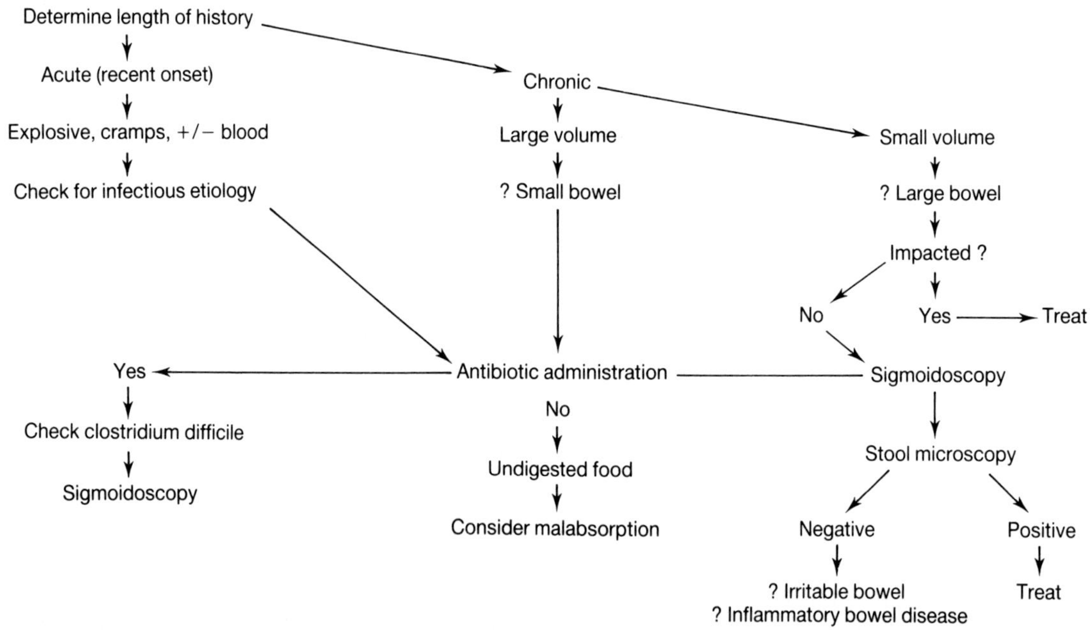

Fig. 17.1 Diarrhea – an approach to diagnosis.

When the diarrhea follows antibiotic administration, and the problem has become less acute, investigation should include sigmoidoscopic examination of the rectum and lower sigmoid colon. The examiner looking at the state of the bowel wall and for the presence of membrane overlying inflamed mucosa (pseudomembranous colitis). Stool should be sent for examination for clostridium difficile and the toxin.

Individuals with a history of passing small amounts of liquid stool frequently and often incontinently, should be checked for impaction. A plain abdominal radiograph is indicated.

Patients with more chronic diarrhea may need various investigations which will depend upon the associated clinical picture. The most important part of the investigation is to chart the bowel movements. Each bowel movement is recorded, and note is made of the appearance. Often this simple investigation enables better problem definition. It is remarkable that many patients improve by being brought into hospital and observed. It is likely that such patients are in fact laxative abusers – a common problem in the elderly population.

If the stools are bulky and malabsorption is considered a possibility, then investigation should be directed towards this end. If the diarrhea is persistent, stool culture, plain abdominal radiograph and sigmoidoscopy have been done and are unrewarding, then investigation should proceed with radiographic visualization of the large bowel by barium enema. Barium studies of the small bowel might be indicated. Inflammatory bowel disease (IBD) may present for the first time in the very old and other investigations might include colonoscopy and biopsy. Obviously the results of some blood tests, specifically sedimentation rate and a low hemoglobin, might point to the importance of looking for such problems as IBD.

6. Plan

Diagnosis

The accurate diagnosis of the cause of abdominal pain and/or diarrhea in all age-groups is strongly dependent upon a careful history and examination. It has to be appreciated that the non-specific presentation of confusion, falls, immobility and social crisis may attenuate the accuracy of the history and the examination. Their recent presence, however, may also be a clue to the presence of serious pathology and give more relevance to vague complaints of pain which are poorly localized.

Some patients survive into old age with long-standing abdominal pain. Many of these patients will have lost their gall bladders, uterus and appendix and may have had a variety of other forms of investigation and surgery. Such patients are difficult to manage and are usually left undiagnosed. There is a group of patients who have pain of unknown origin or functional pain, but this remains a designation that is applied after exclusion of other causes.

Treatment

Therapy will be dependent upon the diagnosis, and achieving a diagnosis is of paramount importance. Symptomatic therapy may be required in some patients, and this will depend upon the pathophysiological changes that are taking place. When straightforward pain relief is required the principles of treatment are the same as in younger age groups. It should be noted that certain analgesics are less effective, particularly pethidine or demerol because of its protein binding characteristics. Adequate pain relief is important, and it is of interest that confused patients may improve significantly with regard to their confusion as the pain is relieved.

There is an increasing incidence of gall bladder stones with advancing age, so that their presence does not necessarily imply a relationship with the pain. In those patients with pain that is difficult to diagnose, no therapy should be undertaken lightly. Cholecystectomy should not be performed for the patient over the age of 75 with gall stones unless there is good evidence that they are truly symptomatic.

The patient with recurrent or chronic pain in whom a diagnosis cannot be reached should be assessed psychiatrically.

Diarrhea might result in dehydration and electrolyte imbalance. Severe diarrhea results in hypovolemia, with depletion of sodium and potassium and often an acidosis. Intravenous replacement appropriate to the deficits becomes more likely with advancing age and the increasing loss of reserve. When fluid loss is less severe replacement should be oral, preferably with lactose free, glucose containing drinks which are palatable to the patient.

For the most part infectious diarrhea is best left untreated and allowed to run its course. However when it is severe, associated with incontinence or skin breakdown the physician should treat symptomatically – recognizing that this might prolong the period of infectivity. A number of agents can be used to 'bind up' the bowels, the preferred choice is loperamide – 4 mg as an initial dose with 2 mg following each bowel movement. It is not unusual to find patients who are on purgatives with diarrhea. The medications of patient with diarrhea should be carefully checked and any purgatives discontinued.

It is rarely necessary to treat most forms of infectious diarrhea with antibiotics. There is no treatment for the viral types, which are self-limiting anyway. Shigella, salmonella and Campylobacter will only need treatment when there are significant systemic symptoms. In the case of Clostridium difficile when symptoms are moderate to severe the patients should receive vancomycin in the dosage of 0.5 to 2 gm daily. Any other antibiotics should be stopped. Alternatives include metronidazole and cholestyramine.

The treatment of the fecally impacted patient has been discussed in Chapter 6.

There are no special considerations for the management of inflammatory bowel disease in this age group, and the usual treatment modalities should be employed. If corticosteroids are required then an adequate dose should be used with a reduction and discontinuation as soon as the clinical condition permits. In elderly patients with problems such as osteoporosis the potential for side-effects is much higher than in younger age groups.

Irritable bowel syndrome, the functional abnormality associated with diverticulosis, is a relatively common problem and although constipation is more common, diarrhea is also seen. The main approach to therapy is the use of bulk – either by increasing dietary roughage or if flatus is a problem by the use of agents such as metamucil. Milk and milk products should also be withdrawn from the diet. When the diarrhea is associated with distension and passage of excessive amounts of flatus an agent such as simethicone in sustained release form is often of considerable benefit. Antispasmodics should not be used, particularly those combinations which contain agents like phenobarbitone. Other agents, which change bowel motility, may be tried and have been deemed to be of benefit – for example trimebutine maleate (200 mg 3 times a day for 4 to 6 weeks).

Monitoring and patient education

The course of the diarrhea and the response can easily be monitored by the maintenance of an elimination record. The oral intake needs to be watched closely, it is advisable for patients to be placed on a lactose free diet for any acute diarrhea which results in damage to the intestinal mucosa.

Purgative abuse when discovered needs to corrected. The patient may need bowel reeducation and the development of a regimen which ensures regular bowel evacuation without the potential of overuse of purgatives.

The patient with acute pain and systemic manifestations will be monitored in the same way as any other acutely ill patient. Definitive treatment of the underlying problem is essential in optimizing the patient's physiological status. The patient who is less emergent needs to be monitored with regard to the relief of the pain. Patient's may need help in modifying their diet or activities when any of the aggravating factors can be determined.

Suggested reading

Andrews, B. J., Haneman, B. and Arnold, B. (1967). Atrophic gastritis in the aged.

Baron, J. H. (1963). Studies of basal and peak acid output with an augmented histamine test. *Gut* **4**: 136–44.

Barston, G. R. and Moore-Smith, B. (1970). Occult surgical emergencies in the Elderly. *Brit. J. Clin. Prac.*, **24**: 239–43.

Bullamore, J. R., Gallagher, J. C., Wilkinson, R. Nordin, B. E. C. and Marshall, D. H. (1970). Effect of age on calcium absorption. *Lancet* **ii**: 535–7.

Horan, M. A., Gulati, R. S., Fox, R. A., Glew, E., Ganguli, L. and Kaeney, M. (1984). Outbreak of Shigella sonnei dysentery on a geriatric assessment ward. *J. Hos. Infec.*, **5**: 210–12.

Montgomery, R. D., Haeney, M. R., Ross, I. N., et al. (1978). The aging gut: a study of intestinal absorption in relation to nutrition in the elderly. *Quart. J. Med.*, **186**: 197–211.

Roberts, S. H., James, O. and Jarvis, E. H. (1977) Bacterial overgrowth syndrome without blind loop. A cause for malnutrition in the elderly. *Lancet*, **2**: 1193–5.

Webster, S. G., Leeming, J. T. (1975) Assessment of small bowel function in the elderly using a modified xylose tolerance test. *Gut*, **16**: 109–13.

18

Pruritus and common skin conditions

1. Age-related changes in the skin

The major morphological changes of the skin with age include wrinkling, laxity, uneven pigmentation, and a variety of proliferative lesions. One of the most consistent histological changes seen is flattening of the dermo-epidermal junction with reductions in the numbers of interdigitating papillae and rete pegs, resulting in a smaller contiguous surface between the two compartments. The average epidermal thickness is relatively constant in the sun-protected skin with advancing age.

A decrease of 10 to 20 per cent of the skin's enzymatically active melanocyte population each decade reduces the protective barrier against irradiation. The number of melanocytic naevi progressively decrease with age from a peak of 15 to 40 in the third and fourth decade to an average of 4 to a person after the age of 50. A reduction in the number of morphologically identifiable epidermal Langhans's cells of the order of 40 per cent occurs by late adulthood.

Loss of dermal thickness approaches 20 per cent in elderly individuals and may account for the paper-thin quality of the skin. The remaining dermis is relatively acellular and avascular. There is a reduction in mast cells of approximately 50 per cent. The striking age-associated loss of vascular bed is believed to underline many of the physiological changes in old skin as well as the gradual atrophy and fibrosis of hair follicles, eccrine, apocrine and sebaceous glands.

Loss of the melanocytes is believed to occur more rapidly in hair than in skin and probably explains the greyness of the hair with age. Advancing age is also accompanied by a gradual decrease in the number of hair follicles and remaining hair follicles may be smaller in diameter and grow more slowly.

The number of eccrine sweat glands decrease in average number during adulthood in most sites and accumulate lipofuscin. Sebaceous gland size and numbers do not decline with age, although there is evidence of decreased function. The functional consequences of these age-associated changes in skin function are summarized in Table 18.1.

2. Pruritus

Pruritus is one of the commonest presenting symptoms in dermatology and includes both local and

Table 18.1 Age-associated changes in skin function

Functional loss	Probable consequence
Barrier function	Increased entry of allergens/irritant
Cell replacement	Decreased epidermal turnover rate, slow wound healing
Dermoepidermal adhesion	Tendency to torn skin, abrasions and blisters
Immune responsiveness	Reduced skin hypersensitivity reactions
Injury response	Reduced wound healing
Sensory perception	Increased frequency of injury
Sweat production	Impaired thermoregulation

generalized itching with or without accompanying eruption. A wide range of conditions may be associated with pruritus in the elderly. They can be broadly divided into four main categories:

1. Xeroses and asteatotic eczema. These are frequently seen in the elderly, particularly in relation to the use of alkaline soaps, low humidity, rough clothing, poor nutrition and alcohol excess. The dry skin, most commonly seen over the lower legs may fissure, appear shiny and crack, with subsequent inflammatory change. On inspection the skin looks pale and dry with attached irregular small scales.
2. Infections and infestations. This includes conditions such as scabies, fungal and yeast infections.
3. Hypersensitivity reactions, particularly in relation to drug reactions.
4. Generalized causes of pruritus such as malignancy (especially haematopoietic), uremia, cholestatic liver disease, iron deficiency anemia, diabetes, thyroid disease and psychiatric disorders.

The approach to the patient with pruritus follows several directions:

1. Identification of probable precipitating factors, such as anemia, renal disease, liver disease, diabetes, and so on.
2. A search for evidence of infection or infestation requiring appropriate treatment.
3. The use of general prophylaxis methods such as good hygiene; restricting the use of alkaline soaps and amount of bathing; and the use of emollients.
4. In the case of marked inflammation, short-term topical cortico-steroids may be considered and should be combined with appropriate emollients.
5. Pruritus, if severe, may require symptomatic treatment with antihistamine agents, ideally non-sedating types.
6. Where hypersensitivity is believed to be a factor, removal of the offending agent.

3. Fungal infections

There are several important conditions to consider in the differential diagnosis of a superficial fungal infection which includes a non-infective eruption such as intertrigo, eczema, psoriasis, erythema multiforme or other superficial infections such as erythrasma, and candidiasis. The non-infective conditions may become secondarily infected as well. Simple friction intertrigo is usually readily discernible from candida lesions in that it produces less pruritus and is poorly demarcated without satellite lesions. Distinction of ringworm, erythrasma and seborrhoeic dermatitis is usually possible. If corticosteroids are considered for use it is desirable to take scrapings. If available a Wood's ultraviolet light readily distinguishes between the three conditions.

Erythrasma is a low-grade superficial bacterial infection caused by Corynebacterium minutissimum. The disorder affects the flexures predominantly, causing slightly pink, scaly patches. It generally involves much larger areas than fungal infections and seborrhoeic dermatitis. A Wood's ultraviolet lamp shone on the affected area reveals a characteristic coral pink fluorescence. The condition is responsive to the same topical agents as ringworm.

The commonest type of skin candida involvement in the elderly is flexural intertrigo. The obese are particular at risk in the inframammary region, axillae and groin areas. The affected area usually has a glazed, red appearance which is sharply demarcated with satellite papules and pustules. Simple 'friction' induced intertrigo is usually less symptomatic, lacks pustules and is less well demarcated.

A different profile of ringworm infections are seen in the elderly compared to other age groups. Tinea corporis (body ringworm) consists of well-defined, red scaly patches with a tendency to central clearing. If corticosteroids are used in their treatment the micro-organism may proliferate and give rise to tinea incognito with involvement of unusually large areas of skin, often with a bizarre appearance. Most cases of rashes in the groin in elderly men referred to as tinea cruris are in fact due to seborrhoeic dermatitis. The two conditions can usually be readily distinguished by the fact that seborrhoeic dermatitis is symmetrical and has a diffuse, irregular border. It is, however, wise to take scrapings from any groin eruption if corticosteroid use is considered to avoid 'tinea incognito'. Persistent infection of toe nail plates by ringworm infection (tinea unguium) is common in the elderly male population. The involved nail is usually thickened, opaque and discolored yellow or brown, and irregular. It may be readily confused with other conditions such as psoriasis or simple dystrophic changes. The diagnosis can be confirmed by microscopic examination of toe nail clippings after they have been softened in 20 per cent potassium hydroxide. Other types of ringworm infection in the elderly are much less common than in other age groups.

The three commonest dermatophyte skin conditions are tinea corporis, tinea cruris and tinea unguium. For localised areas of skin infection, topical treatment is adequate. The various imidazole preparations are effective with very few side-effects. Topical treatment should be used at least daily for three weeks. When infection is extensive and the nails are involved, systemic treatment may be required. Griseofulvin (250 mg 6-hourly for 4 to 6 weeks) is usually adequate for skin infection. Ketoconazole has a broader anti-fungal activity than griseofulvin but can cause hepatotoxicity and should be reserved for serious infections.

Most of the agents used for ringworm are also effective against candidiasis but nystatin, 5-fluorocytosine and amphotericin B can be considered in certain situations. Nystatin solutions are particularly helpful for mucosal candidiasis. More general treatment will consist of good skin hygiene and keeping the affected areas dry and free from moisture.

4. Neoplastic conditions

Neoplasia associated with age is particularly common in the skin. Most adults have one or more benign proliferative growths present. Skin tags are common in the lateral neck and areas of friction, especially in obese individuals. Seborrhoeic keratoses (raised, slightly scaly, light brown plaques) are most often found in the face and trunk. Cherry angiomas (bright red papules) are seen commonly on the trunk.

Actinic keratoses are exceedingly common, especially in fair-skinned elderly individuals. They are best recognized by their sandpaper-like texture and are usually red-brown and slightly scaly. They often go through a period of near total regression after several months of sun avoidance.

All cutaneous malignancies can be attributed to the effects of chronic sun damage rather than aging per se. The three main conditions seen are basal cell carcinoma, squamous cell carcinomas and melanoma. The basal cell carcinoma is the commonest and early lesions are asymptomatic. Firm pearly papules are seen with more than 90 per cent occurring on exposed areas of the face and neck. They typically enlarge slowly and lesions of less than half a centimetre may have been present for several years. The large rodent ulcer is less common today with greater physician awareness but can still be identified by its firm, opalescent, pearly, rolled border.

The squamous cell carcinoma may occur at sites of chronic ulceration or other skin damage. Its firm red papules are relatively circumscribed.

The malignant melanoma is much less common than the above. Of concern are signs of enlarging size, indistinct borders, varying colour, surrounding inflammation, ulceration and easy bleeding.

5. Pressure ulcers

Pressure ulcers are unfortunately one of the most common health risks of the immobilized elderly. They are otherwise referred to as decubitus (from the latin 'to lie down') ulcers or bed sores. It should be appreciated that they may occur at any site and from any posture, not just lying in bed. A pressure ulcer is an area of soft tissue breakdown usually over a bony prominence. They are therefore most often seen over the sacral prominence in the supine position, the greater trochanter when lying on one's side, and the tuberosities of the ischium in the sitting position. Other sites where they may be seen are the posterior aspects of the heels, ankles, and knees, the iliac crests, the elbows, ribs, and occasionally the ears and scalp.

Pressure is the primary pathophysiological mechanism in the formation of these ulcers. Prolonged pressure unrelieved by change in position leads to ischemia, anoxia and cell death followed by necrosis. In order for ischemia to occur, the pressure must exceed the capillary pressure in the skin of approximately 35 mm Hg. Microscopic changes in the tissue can be seen in pressures as low as 60 mm Hg. Time is an additive factor in that ulcers can develop after 12 hours at 100 mm Hg but after only 2 hours at 500 mm Hg. In the sitting position, one half of the body's weight is supported on only 8 per cent of the sitting surface. Pressures in excess of 300 mm Hg are commonly seen beneath the ischial tuberosities. It is therefore inevitable that sitting or lying immobile for periods of time (as little as 2 hours) will result in tissue ischemia and necrosis. The same process can occur relatively quickly by the shearing effect where skin and subcutaneous tissues are pulled taut and overstretched. This tissue disruption greatly accelerating the tissue necrosis in vulnerable areas.

A number of other factors which interfere with tissue perfusion, integrity and healing may aggravate the effects of pressure and shearing forces making pressure ulcers more likely. They include reduced sensation, protein-calorie malnutrition, avitaminosis and various trace element deficiencies, anemia, hypoproteinemia, peripheral vascular disease, diabetes mellitus, maceration of the skin, infection, fecal incontinence and poor hygiene. Incontinence of urine is often quoted as a predisposing factor but objective evidence for this is lacking. Aging changes of the skin with reduced subcutaneous tissues will predispose to pressure effects. Obesity although increasing subcutaneous padding, creates the problem of enhancing immobility and making regular position changes difficult in an immobilized patient.

The management of pressure ulcers necessarily involves their anticipation, prevention or minimization. There are a number of scales which have been developed to help in identifying the high-risk patient. They generally include factors such as general health, mental status, activity, mobility in bed, and incontinence. Some also make allowance for nutritional status. The use of such a scale could focus special preventative approaches. Such measures would include at least 2-hourly turning, protective padding over bony prominences, use of special mattresses or flotation pads to reduce pressure at sites by distributing pressures more evenly. It is also necessary to optimize the patient's condition by correcting nutritional deficiencies, anemia, and dehydration; treating underlying infections; and dealing adequately with incontinence.

An essential part of the approach would be regular review of skin status. Any area of skin redness which does not fade promptly should be considered at imminent risk of developing a pressure ulcer. An area of skin which does not blanche on pressure already has its integrity compromised. Evidence of compromised areas means immediate pressure removal must occur. Local treatment including good hygiene, lubricating with oils, and massage are thought to be beneficial in this situation. If a pressure ulcers occurs it should be classified according to one of the accepted methods. One example is the following:

Stage 1: Blanching hyperemia. Reactive hyperaemia causes a distinct erythema after pressure is released but blanching will occur with light pressure indicating the microcirculation is intact.

Stage 2: Non-blanching hyperemia. Microcirculatory disruption is present, with inflammation and edema of tissues. Superficial damage may present as swelling, induration, blistering or epidermal ulceration which might expose the dermis. Pain will be present if sensory pathways are intact.

Stage 3: Ulceration progresses through the dermis to the junction with the subcutaneous tissue. The ulcer edges are distinct but surrounded by erythema and induration.

Stage 4: Ulceration extends into the subcutaneous fat. Fat necrosis occurs, the underlying muscle is swollen and inflamed.

Stage 5: The necrosis extends through to the deep fascia with muscle destruction. Bursae, joints and bone becomes exposed and involved.

The management of pressure ulcers necessarily involves the application of several principles:

1. Accurate determination of extent. Often the extent of tissue damage is much greater than initial impressions suggest. The area of tissue damage should be considered to extend to the margins of non-blanching. Ulceration may be present with undermining of superficial tissues so sinuses and fistulas are not uncommon.
2. Factors predisposing to poor skin integrity and healing need resolution.
3. Pressure has to be removed from all affected areas if further extension is not to occur.
4. Any infection has to be eradicated by removal of necrotic tissue, use of local bacteriostatic/bactericidal agents and systemic antibiotics where indicated.
5. Necrotic tissue will delay healing, and promote infection so its removal must occur though debridement. Debridement may be surgical, chemical or enzymatic. In large pressure ulcers the different methods of debridement may be combined. The use of impermeable hydrocolloids such as Duoderm or Comfeel Ulcus aids in debridement by maintaining a moist environment and softening the necrotic plates. This may avoid sharp debridement and simplify other debridement procedures. It should be noted that the impermeable (occlusive) hydrocolloids should not be used on an infected ulcer.
6. Encouragement of healing. The optimal conditions for wound healing are a moist, nutrient-rich environment. Heat loss should be avoided as leucocyte activity is very temperature sensitive. Lengthy frequent wound changes are

to be avoided to prevent heat loss and dehydration. Hyperosmolar conditions although inhibiting bacterial growth also interfere with phagocytosis so may affect debris removal. Oxygenation is important for healing so wound coverings should be oxygen permeable. Movement of wound margins are undesirable and will seriously disrupt epithelialization.

Dressings play a major role in modifying the wound environment. Generally, with a small sore the priorities will be towards preventing infection, so covering with an oxygen permeable dressing such as Op-Site will prevent dehydration and contamination. A deeper ulcer may necessitate necrotic tissue removal and infection treatment. Debriding is often necessary and thereafter the wound should be kept clean and infection-free until closure occurs. Packing may be necessary to prevent premature closure of the 'neck' of the wound. It should be realized that packing exerts its effect by inhibiting healing so care is necessary if negative effects on wound closure are not to be seen. Wound drainage is commonly necessary with 'deep ulcers' and has to be balanced against the risks of dehydration and wound margin disruption by frequent dressing changes. Traditional gauze dressings have the problem of requiring frequent changes with adherence to the wound. Non-adherent dressings offer only marginal advantages. A variety of agents have been developed for use in deep ulcers aiming at addressing some of these problems and include substances such as Op-Site, Debrisan, Varidase, Synthaderm, Silastic form, Mesalt.

The authors suggest that these guidelines be followed:

1. For shallow pressure ulcer a semi-permeable dressing is preferable, providing infection is not present and Op-Site is a suitable product to consider.
2. For a necrotic ulcer debridement is necessary and surgical measures are quicker.
3. For the infected wound removal of bacteria and excess exudate is desirable. Osmotic wound-cleansing agents and wound irrigation can help achieve this. Dressings which minimize interference with the wound are desirable but take second place to the needs of debridement and infection clearance (see treatment of leg ulcer).
4. A variety of adjuvant treatments to promote wound healing have been suggested including hyperbaric oxygen, infrared, ultraviolet, and ultrasound. Their use might be considered in certain cases.

6. Local Wound Care

Care of pressure ulcers and leg ulcers are in terms of cleaning wound, removing necrotic tissue, eradication of infection and dressing.

The choice of dressing to be used in ulcer management is dictated by:

1. the site of the wound,
2. whether the wound is infected, and
3. consideration for the underlying condition.

For infected or discharging, moist wounds a combination of Mesalt and ETE has proven to be effective.

Mesalt is a 100 per cent cotton gauze treatment pad with a high content of crystalline sodium chloride (15 per cent by weight) which is hypertonic. It effectively promotes the drainage and healing of discharging wounds in the inflammatory stage by creating a hypertonic environment which helps remove exudate, bacteria and necrotic material from the site through a 'wicking' effect.

To increase this 'wicking' effect, ETE is added on top of the Mesalt with the 'matted' side down. The ETE is a pad made up of rayon fibers to which a highly absorbent rayon wadding is stitched in a checkered pattern. Wound secretions are absorbed by the rayon fibres which swell to give a cushion-like effect. The stitching also limits the spread of wound secretion beyond the margins of the wound so that the surrounding delicate skin is not irritated.

The Mesalt should be applied to the draining wound once or twice a day as indicated by wound assessment. The wound should be irrigated with normal saline to remove any debrided tissue or secretions. The Mesalt can be applied directly on the wound or loosely patted into an ulcer cavity. The ETE is added on top and the combination is fixed to the wound with appropriate adhesive or bound with a gauze 'cling' dressing.

The appearance of a green discoloration in the dressing may indicate a pseudomonas infection, but with the Mesalt/ETE combination, it is a common finding unrelated to pseudomonas infection. If the dressing is adherent to the wound, soaking with normal saline will expedite removal.

Some patients report painful stinging at the site of the dressing, particularly at night. This can be managed either by mild analgesics or by applying the dressing only during the day. The Mesalt/ETE combination is not effective in dry, mummified ulcers, such as those associated with arterial insufficiency, because of ischemia.

When the inflammatory phase is over and there is no evidence of infection, and granulation is proceeding to epithelialization, a hydrocolloid dressing can be used.

Other aspects of ulcer management such as the use of skin grafting at the appropriate time need to be considered. Any attempts to heal an ulcer using only a dressing rather than basic education of the patient, and the application of the other physical and supportive measures, is likely to be ineffective.

7. Leg ulcer

There are a large number of conditions which play an aetiology in leg ulcers (Table 18.2). By far, the most common cause of peripheral ulcers of the lower extremity is venous stasis and it is estimated that venous stasis is responsible for 70 to 90 per cent of peripheral ulcers, particularly in the older age group. Varicose veins develop as a result of incompetence of the venous valvular system, and incompetent communicating veins between the deep and superficial venous system. Deep venous thrombosis may be a preceding event to venous stasis. In the pathophysiology, edema is a result and clinically there is tissue induration with prominent veins and stasis dermatitis with or without cellulitis. It is the increased venous pressure that causes the edema in combination with the incompetent venous system.

Stasis dermatitis develops showing the classical signs of edema, erythema, and crusting which then becomes indurated and secondarily infected. This leads to cellulitis and an eventual loss of the continuity of the skin and the clinically recognizable ulcer. Tissue 'staining' is a sign of chronic venous stasis, and is the result of extravasation of blood (bruising) and hemosiderin deposition in the skin. It is this hemosiderin that gives the brown to black skin discoloration (or 'staining').

Venous stasis ulcers are large, shallow moist lesions with a base of granulation tissue. They occur about the malleoli in areas of brawny hemosiderin deposition. Stasis ulcers are associated with dull aching pain in dependency that is relieved by elevation.

Arterial ulcers are commonly located in the distal circulation usually toes and feet. The lesions are painful, again often relieved by dependency. They occur in areas of mottled, rubrous skin. The ulcers show little granulation tissue and little bleeding occurs with debridement.

Table 18.2 Causes of leg ulcers

Metabolic ulcers include those related to:
- diabetes mellitus
- necrobiosis lipoidica diabeticorum
- porphyria cutanea tarda

Haematologic causes include:
- thalassaemia
- polycythemia rubra vera
- leukaemia
- dysproteinemia (multiple myeloma; Waldenström's macroglobulinemia)

The *tumors* that cause skin ulcers include:
- basal cell carcinoma
- squamous cell carcinoma
- malignant melanoma
- Kaposi sarcoma

Secondary tumors that cause cutaneous ulcers are:
- metastatic carcinoma
- lymphoma

Infection causes include both primary and secondary infections. These include:

bacterial	*fungal*	*viral*
staph	coccidioidomycosis	herpes
strep	blastomycosis	AIDS
syphilis	sporotrichosis	
mycetoma	cryptococcosis	

Vasculitic causes include:
- necrotizing vasculitis
- periarteritis nodosa
- systemic lupus erythematosus
- cryoglobulinemia
- rheumatoid vasculitis
- AIDS (associated with a leukocytoclastic vasculitis)

Vascular causes include:
- venous stasis and arterial insufficiency and the rarer conditions of
  - Raynaud's Syndrome
  - Livedo Reticularis
  - Hypertension
  - Arteriosclerosis Obliterans
  - Thromboangiitis Obliterans

Neurotrophic ulcers occur in areas of pressure, friction or chronic trauma such as the metatarsal heads. The ulcers are deep, punctate, and surrounded by callous formation. Patients with these lesions commonly have suffered from conditions such as diabetes mellitus complicated by peripheral neuropathy. They will often bleed profusely when debrided.

Management

A similar approach to factors such as blood supply, infection, concomitant disease, and so on have to be taken as with pressure ulcers. There are however, some general points relevant to venous and arterial ulcers worth stressing.

Venous ulcers

- leg elevation and bed rest
- compression bandaging
- support hose
- pressure relief
- exercise

The exercise should be supervised by a physiotherapist initially and the referral to the physiotherapist should specifically indicate exercise for relief of venous stasis.
Supportive measures include:

- weight reduction
- optimal skin hygiene, and
- vein stripping or vein sclerosis

Arterial Ulcers

Physical methods for arterial ulcers include:

- controlled and supervised warming
- bed rest
- leg placement at a dependent level (that is, not elevated)

Supportive measures for the arterial ulcer include:

- analgesics
- consideration for bypass surgery

A number of 'vasodilator' agents have at different times be advocated for the use in healing of arterial leg ulcers. They have not however, generally been very useful. Pentoxifylline is a hemorrheologic agent which is claimed to improve red cell deform ability and alter blood viscosity. Pentoxifylline is currently approved for treatment of intermittent claudication and treatment of superficial ulcers on the dorsum of the feet, toes and ankles, as an adjunct therapy. It is important to note that early consultation with a vascular surgeon is desirable at the first clinical sign of impaired arterial circulation.

19

Abnormalities of the complete blood count

The complete blood count (CBC) consists of measurement of hemoglobin concentrations and the indices, the white blood cell count (WBC) and differential, and the erythrocyte sedimentation rate (ESR). Only those aspects which are of most importance in the frail elderly will be discussed here.

The finding of a reduced hemoglobin indicates anemia. There is no change in the normal range of hemoglobin concentration or of number of erythrocytes with advancing age. The accepted lower limit of normal in men is 13 g per dl for hemoglobin and 12 g per dl for women.

The normal range for the white blood cell count is up to 11000 per cu. mm, so that values at this level or above are considered abnormal. It is well recognized that in the elderly patient the total WBC may not be raised or if elevated may not be as high as in younger individuals. In our experience the blood film will almost invariably be abnormal, showing a shift to the left with the presence of immature neutrophils with toxic granulation, in the circulation.

The normal range for the ESR in the elderly is wider than in younger age groups. However, in one study of 258 non-hospitalized elderly subjects the conclusion reached was that ESR determination was of limited value with a normal range of from 3 to 65 mm/hr. In contrast another study found a similar range for the ESR but showed that after post-mortem study a raised ESR in an elderly patient always indicated underlying pathology.

How high should the ESR be to invite further investigation? It needs to be high and the best available evidence indicates that a value of 50 mm/hr or above should be investigated. It is important to emphasize that we are not simply investigating a high ESR. This is a high ESR in the setting of presentation of the elderly patient to a physician. In this setting there is good evidence that investigation of elderly patients is worthwhile and that a raised sedimentation rate is a good indicator that further diagnostic evaluation is required.

1. Anemia

Predisposing factors with aging

Normal healthy old people are not anemic and although mortality due to anemia increases with age, information on the incidence of anemia with advancing age is conflicting. Studies have been done which show a gradual decline in hemoglobin with age, but that the level remains within the normal range. The bone marrow is endowed with its full complement of stem cells at birth, usually in adequate numbers for life. There is no doubt that throughout life these cells are subject to radiation damage and to other effects that reduces their ability to self repair and possibly their ability to differentiate and proliferate. It appears logical to conclude that these changes will lead to a loss of reserve and less resilience within the bone marrow. In other words anemia is more likely to develop with deficiency states. Patients that are seen by departments of geriatric medicine have a high incidence of anemia ranging from 6 to 50 per cent.

In the surveys that have been done the most common form of anemia due to nutritional deficiency is iron. Approximately one-third of all anemias are macrocytic with folate and B12 deficiency being the most common causes. Other deficiencies also occur. Increasing disability may predispose the elderly to anemia. With declining mobility and declining cognitive function there may be deficient intake of various nutrients. With advancing age there is decline in gastric acidity with a resulting reduction in iron absorption.

Precipitants

Anemia will result from impaired production or from destruction or loss of erythrocytes. It is important to understand that there are many things that will produce anemia and the classification into the 3 types according to cell size helps in reducing the number of possible variables (Fig. 19.1).

Normocytic Anemia

The bulk of patients with normocytic anemia are normochromic and the condition is secondary to impaired production. There are many problems that give rise to this which would include infection, malignancy, collagen vascular disease, rheumatoid arthritis, temporal arteritis or polymyalgia rheumatica, renal failure, hypothyroidism, hypoadrenalism or nutritional deficiency, like scurvy (Table 19.1). It is important to recognize that aplastic anemia falls in this category and that usually no precipitants can be identified. This may, however, be associated with leukemia or other myeloproliferative disorder.

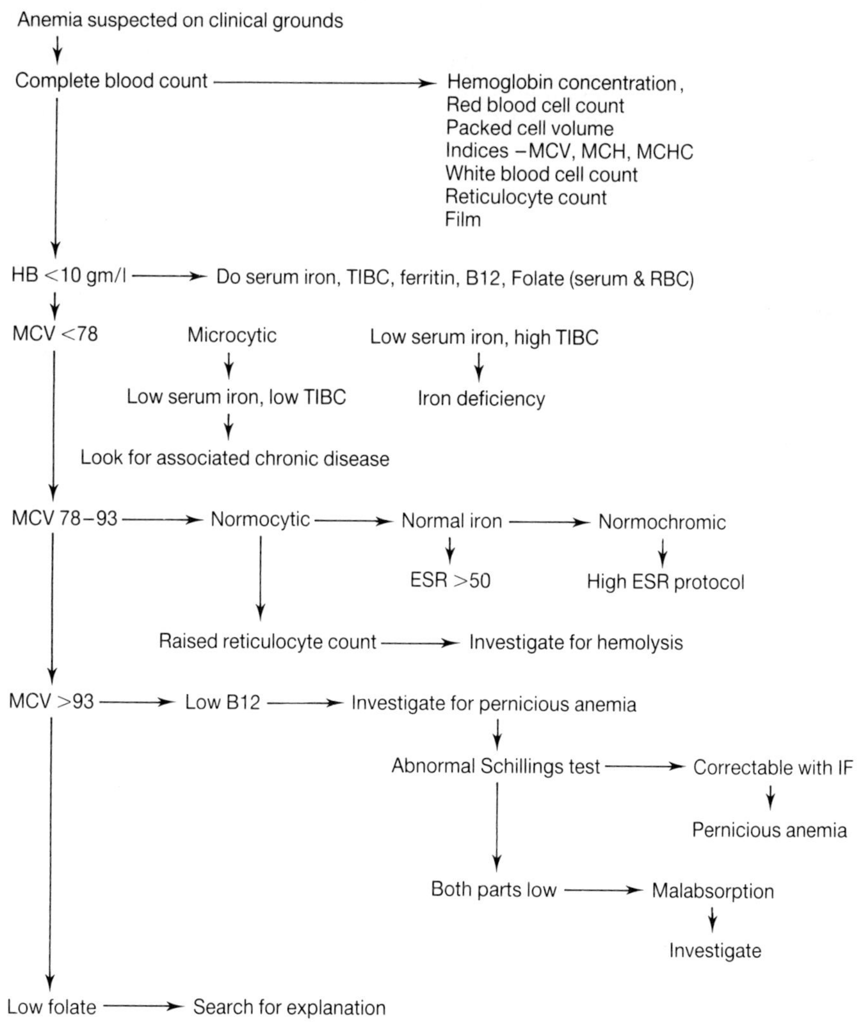

Fig. 19.1 The classification of anemia.

Occasionally it is found associated with mild hypochromia related to recent blood loss, or early and excessive destruction of erythrocytes secondary to drugs or toxins – hemolytic anemia. Autoimmune hemolytic anemia may also be of this type. Since there is increased production of erythrocytes in this situation the red cells may be abnormal and macrocytic.

Macrocytic Anemia

Most of these are megaloblastic and the most common are related to vitamin B12 or folic acid deficiency. These may be related to inadequate intake or inadequate absorption.

Normoblastic macrocytic anemia is not uncommon in the elderly. It may be related to alcohol. There are many diseases that may precipitate this including hypothyroidism, scurvy, leukemia, aplastic anemia, hemolytic anemia, lead poisoning, malaria, protein malnutrition and liver disease.

Microcytic Anemia

The most important precipitant of this type of anemia is iron deficiency. This may be related to blood loss or to inadequate intake, nutritional deficiency. There are patients with this type of anemia who have normal iron levels, some of these are related to pyridoxine deficiency.

Subjective

The symptoms of anemia can be considered first of all as those related to the anemic state, and secondly those related to the specific type of anemia (Table 19.1).

General symptoms

The symptoms of anemia are related to the reduced ability of the blood to carry oxygen. At any age the symptoms of tiredness, lethargy, lack of energy or general feeling of being unwell develop slowly and are difficult to recognize by the patient. Such complaints may be quite long-standing before medical advice is sought. This is of particular importance in old age and the lethargy of anemia may be difficult to distinguish from the symptoms of other chronic diseases.

Aging is often associated with a reduction in functional reserves in several systems, anemia may therefore result in decompensation in one or more systems. The most frequent complaints relate to shortness of breath and the development of symptoms of cardiac decompensation such as ankle edema and orthopnea. Symptoms of myocardial ischemia may appear in those with underlying ischemic heart disease. Cerebral symptoms may dominate the clinical picture and these would include confusion, apathy, depression, hallucinations or dizziness.

Patients with anemia may well have a geriatric presentation. Anemia is a common precipitant of the major functional problems of old age, namely confusion, reduced mobility, falling and incontinence of urine.

Specific symptoms

a) Normocytic Anemia

This type of anemia is also known as symptomatic anemia and it is important to look for symptoms of any of the other conditions that would give rise to this problem. In other words questions should

Table 19.1 Symptoms of anemia

General	Normocytic	Macrocytic	Microcytic
Tiredness	Associated	Burning	Sore tongue
Lack of energy	Chronic disease	Sore tongue	Dysphagia
Feel unwell	e.g. rheumatoid		Blood loss
Functional impairment	arthritis, polymyalgia rheumatica etc.	Confusion	Dyspepsia
Confusion		immobility	
Immobility		falling	Hematuria
Falling	Various	incontinence	
Incontinence	Chronic		
Dyspnea	Diseases	Paresthesiae	
Angina			
Orthopnea			
Ankle edema			

be asked which might support the diagnosis of problems such as temporal arteritis, polymyalgia rheumatica, infection, neoplasm, connective tissue disease, renal failure, scurvy, hypothyroidism, hypoadrenalism or hypopituitarism. The other normocytic anemias resulting from decreased marrow production for example are not associated with any specific symptoms that would point to this as the likely problem.

b) Macrocytic Anemia

The most common types of macrocytic anemia are megaloblastic and due to deficiencies of vitamin B12 or folic acid. Burning or soreness of the tongue can occur in either deficiency state and is also found in iron deficiency.

B12 deficiency is associated with symptoms related to the neuropathology. Confusion and other mental symptoms are common. There may be paresthesiae of the extremities. Other sensory changes may occur, particularly ataxia related to posterior column loss. Due to the combination of sensory and motor deficits, patients may well complain of difficulty with walking and an increased frequency of falling.

There are many causes of folate deficiency (Table 19.2). Folate deficiency may be associated with alcoholism and there may be features of this problem. There should be no symptoms referable to neurological disease, and if found in the presence of megaloblastic anemia would point to B12 deficiency. However the alcoholic with folate deficiency may well have an alcoholic peripheral neuropathy which would make diagnosis more challenging. Folate deficiency may be related to malabsorption or inadequate dietary intake. In these cases features of these particular problems should be identified, diarrhea for example. A careful dietary history should be obtained from these patients to determine if one is dealing with a case of 'tea and toast' syndrome. It is important to ask about the presence of any skin problems since dermatitis herpetiformis is associated with malabsorption. A careful drug history should also be obtained since trimethoprim or anticonvulsants for example may be associated with folate deficiency.

Table 19.2 Causes of folate deficiency

Reduced intake
- poor diet
- malabsorption (dermatitis herpetiformis)
- alcoholism

Antagonists (drugs)
- anticonvulsants, diphenylhydantoin, primidone, barbiturates
- cytotoxic, methotrexate, aminopterin

Increased utilization
- hemolytic anemia
- neoplasia

Increased loss
- exfoliative dermatitis
- psoriasis

c) Microcytic Anemia

Microcytic anemia implies red cells with inadequate hemoglobinization. The most important cause being iron deficiency. This type of anemia is rarely so advanced that specific symptoms are seen, however patients may complain of dysphagia which is due to the development of a post-cricoid web after 10 to 15 years of severe iron deficiency (Plummer Vinson or Smith Kelly Patterson syndrome).

Apart from this problem due to the iron deficiency there may be symptoms related to the precipitating factor(s). Questions must be asked to determine if there has been any obvious blood loss from any site, the most important being, of course, the gastrointestinal tract. Occult blood loss is also important and therefore inquiry should be made to see if there is anything that might contribute to this. In this regard the most important thing is the taking of any of the non-steroidal anti-inflammatory drugs. These have been shown to be linked to 'silent' peptic ulceration. A full drug history, a dietary history and whether there has been previous gastric surgery are all important considerations.

Objective

General features

Pallor can be detected on examination, although it may be difficult in the very old. The buccal and lingual mucosae and the nail beds should be inspected. There may be findings on examination of the consequences of anemia such as heart failure, or dyspnea with minimal exertion or postural hypotension.

Specific anemias

a) Normocytic Anemia

The important findings on examination are related to the associated conditions. There are no signs that are peculiar to this type of anemia. In most circumstances this type of anemia is normochromic, although if there is associated recent blood loss it may be hypochromic. Other tests may be helpful in indicating the likely reason for the anemia, the most important being the ESR and the biochemical screen including urea, creatinine and electrolytes.

b) Macrocytic Anemia

The majority of these anemias are megaloblastic. There may be features on examination that point to the probability that one is dealing with a megaloblastic anemia. In B12 deficiency there is often an associated glossitis and the tongue appears smooth, shiny and atrophic on examination. Neurological examination may reveal the findings of subacute combined degeneration of the spinal cord. There may be a sensory level, or a peripheral neuropathy. Motor deficits may be a combination of upper and lower motor neurone damage. B12 deficiency may occur as a result of malabsorption so that there may be features of deficiency of other essential nutrients.

Folate deficiency is not associated with neurological damage although there may be features of alcoholism on examination. These patients may have a peripheral neuropathy or spinocerebellar degeneration for example.

c) Microcytic Anemia

Findings on examination that point to iron deficiency are only found in advanced cases. Koilonychia is rarely seen, although the nails may be brittle and ridged. Finding a post cricoid web as a cause for dysphagia is also rare. There may be important findings on examination that reveal the site of blood loss, for example a rectal carcinoma.

Assessment

On receipt of the initial blood tests anemia may be diagnosed and also the type of anemia should be apparent. However because of overlap and the presence of mixed pictures most patients should have measurement of serum iron, iron binding capacity, ferritin, serum B12 and folate. Most patients with a hemoglobin below 9 gm and without a clearly identified type of anemia from the blood tests should have an examination of the bone marrow. Iliac crest is the preferred site and bone marrow should be both aspirated and biopsied. The specimen should always be stained for iron. Further testing will be directed by the nature of the results.

Plan

Diagnosis

The further investigation of anemia will depend upon the CBC, iron studies, B12, folate, and bone marrow results.

a) Normocytic Anemia

The film and mean corpuscular hemoglobin concentration will reveal whether it is a normochromic anemia. The results of other investigations may indicate the presence of chronic renal or hepatic disease and offer a reasonable explanation for the anemia.

The association of a very high ESR and a normochromic, normocytic anemia suggests several important diagnostic options including arteritis, collagen vascular diseases, tuberculosis, and underlying malignancy.

An important diagnosis to consider is temporal arteritis or polymyalgia rheumatica. Both conditions are readily treatable and if ignored the consequences in terms of loss of vision can be catastrophic. Biopsy confirmation of temporal arteritis is desirable as one is subjecting the patient to months or years of treatment which has potentially lethal side-effects. Unless however, typical symptoms of headache, fatigue, tenderness are present the yield from blind biopsy is negligible. Treatment should not be delayed until biopsy is arranged and if vision is threatened should start as soon as a clinical diagnosis is made. If temporal arteritis is diagnosed then the patient should be treated with steroids – 40–60 mg prednisone a day. If the diagnosis is correct there will be amelioration of symptoms within days and the ESR should drop to at least half its former level within 7 to 10 days. The patient who complains of fatigue and aches and pains and stiffness in the muscles, particularly in the proximal muscles of the upper limbs with a high ESR may have polymyalgia rheumatica and should be treated as such. In the absence of a clear history then clinical judgment needs to be invoked and a decision as to the likelihood of a diagnosis of polymyalgia rheumatic. If a decision is made to treat then the patient should be given a dose of approximately 15 mg prednisone a day. If the diagnosis is correct the patient's symptoms should improve rapidly and the ESR drop by 50 per cent in the first week. In the difficult patient this can be used as a diagnostic test.

Dermatomyositis or polymyositis might be considered if muscle tenderness is a feature. A simple punch biopsy is a relatively innocuous procedure and may help establish a diagnosis. In patients that we have seen where this test has proved diagnostic, appropriate treatment of the patient with high dose steroids has resulted in dramatic improvement.

Collagen vascular diseases may be possible and furthers test to consider include serum complement levels, antinuclear antibodies and rheumatoid factor. Positive tests would need to be acted upon in the appropriate manner.

Other conditions to consider would be myeloma, malignancy and tuberculosis. Usually plasma protein electrophoresis will clarify the situation with regards to myeloma and indicate the need for bone marrow aspiration and biopsy. Tuberculosis has an increasing incidence in the elderly, both from new infection and reactivation of a latent focus. The chest radiograph should be carefully examined and a skin tuberculin test performed.

A search for occult malignancy can be very exhaustive and in the frail elderly patient this needs to be tempered. If there are no clinical pointers, then the stool should be examined for occult blood. If positive then a full investigation of the gastrointestinal tract needs to be considered. A bone scan should be done and if positive this may modify the need for further investigation with the diagnosis of metastatic malignancy. Another investigation that should be considered in a search for occult neoplasm is an abdominal ultrasound looking at the areas where cancer can be silent, particularly the pancreas.

b) Macrocytic Anemia

The film should indicate whether the anemia is megaloblastic. If the serum B12 comes back below the normal range there are three major possibilities – pernicious anemia, malabsorption or 'idiopathic'. If the serum folate is also low malabsorption might be more likely, the red cell folate should also be measured if one suspects deficiency.

The definitive test to diagnose pernicious anemia is the Schilling's test. The patient is given a loading dose of vitamin B12, and then an oral dose of radiolabelled B12. The excretion of the latter is measured in the urine over a 24-hour period. If below the normal range the test should be repeated with intrinsic factor and if this now corrects the previous reduced absorption then pernicious anemia is confirmed. If the absorption is still impaired, then malabsorption is the problem. The difficulty in geriatric practice is the accuracy of the collection of urine over a 24-hour period. It may not be possible to confirm a diagnosis of pernicious anemia and one may be left with the only option of treating. Other tests which might help but are not diagnostic, include serum antibodies to gastric parietal cell or to intrinsic factor. Measuring B12 metabolites in the serum can be diagnostic, but this is not widely available at present.

If malabsorption is suspected then this will need to be investigated, by visualization or biopsy of the gastrointestinal tract and other tests of absorption.

c) Microcytic Anemia

In iron deficient hypochromia the serum iron will be reduced and the serum total iron binding capacity will be raised above the normal upper limit. Serum ferritin reflects the amount of storage iron and should be reduced. In acute inflammatory states however, the ferritin behaves as an acute phase reactant and may be raised well above the normal range.

If iron deficiency is found from the above tests then it is important to determine if there is blood loss. At least three stools should be collected and tested for occult blood. If these are positive or there are features from the history or examination that point to a gastrointestinal site of blood loss then further examination is indicated, with upper and lower intestinal endoscopy and radiology.

Urine should be examined on more than one occasion for the presence of blood. Hemoptysis is a rare cause of iron deficiency anemia and in most circumstances there would be indication from the history. Chest radiograph will also have been done as part of the initial investigations. Finding any lesion will point to the type of additional investigation that will be required. In those patients who have iron deficiency but no evidence of blood loss a decision must be made as to the most appropriate management. The very old and the functionally impaired can be made worse by unnecessary investigation, and in many instances it is appropriate to simply observe the patient, rechecking the hemoglobin at intervals to see if there is further lowering of the value.

Iron absorption may be impaired in the elderly due to reduced acid production in the stomach, or as a result of a previous gastrectomy. Intake of iron in the diet may be deficient and inadequate intake can be a legitimate cause of iron deficiency anemia in the elderly. When this diagnosis is reached patients should be carefully monitored to be certain that this is the case. For some patients the blood film is not characteristic or there may be a mixed picture, with some hypochromic cells. Such patients should have a bone marrow examination. It is only with a bone marrow that sideroblastic anemia can be diagnosed, in this condition intense erythroblastic hyperplasia is seen with many ring erythroblasts.

Treatment

Treatment should be both symptomatic and specific. Symptomatic treatment should only be given when the necessary investigations have been obtained. The patient with angina or a history of ischemic heart disease or cardiac failure is clearly at increased risk of further problems. The patient who has significant functional impairment as a result of anemia should also have the anemia treated to enable rehabilitation to be commenced sooner and more effectively. These patients categories should be transfused at least two units of packed cells. This should be done slowly and often with the concomitant administration of an appropriate diuretic like frusemide intravenously.

The deficiency anemias need to be treated with appropriate replacement. If pernicious anemia is diagnosed then vitamin B12 will need to be given for life. The initial dosage is 1000 ug on alternate days for 4 doses. If there are neurological signs then this frequency is continued for a month and then the same dose given weekly for six months. Without neurological problems or at the end of this time the frequency of injection should be reduced to monthly. Patients with macrocytic anemia who have low serum B12 values and in whom further investigation is impossible should be treated by monthly injections of B12 for the rest of their life. It has been found that in elderly individuals a low B12 in the absence of hematological or neurological effects may arise because of impaired binding by the carrier protein, cyanocobalamin. The low B12 in this situation is not of pathological significance. In these patients even after several doses of B12, the serum level will not rise to within the normal range.

When there is folate deficiency any identifiable cause should be treated. Folate should be replaced by giving 5 mg three times a day until corrected, and then maintained at 5 mg daily. Patients who receive folate should have had B12 deficiency excluded.

Patients with iron deficiency anemia should have any identifiable problem corrected or any gastrointestinal irritant removed. Iron needs to be given until the hemoglobin is once again normal and then continued for about three months afterwards. Since absorption is often a problem in the elderly vitamin C can be given at the same time as the iron. Those patients who fail to respond may do so through failure to take the tablets, failure to absorb the iron or a failure of the bone marrow to respond. In the latter case this may be because of associated chronic disease, and the diagnosis needs to be carefully checked. If there is failure to absorb then iron can be administered parenterally and a good way of doing this is by total dose infusion. It is possible to do this in a day hospital setting for example.

Other deficiency anemias such as that found in scurvy should be treated by appropriate replacement.

Sideroblastic anemia is often unresponsive to therapy but pyridoxine and folate should be given. A limited number of patients will respond to other agents such as Danazol, a pituitary gonadotropin inhibitor. This should be given for at least 6 weeks at an initial dosage of 50 mg 3 times a day.

Patients with impaired production of red blood cells – aplastic anemia, myelodysplastic state or pure red cell aplasia usually need to be treated symptomatically. Other forms of treatment have been tried – including anabolic steroids or cyclosporine. Such patients need specialist hematological investigation and management.

Patient education

When a cause of anemia is defined successful treatment is often dependent upon the compliance of the patient to a therapeutic regimen which includes replacement of those factors that are deficient. This may require considerable patient education. In the patients treated symptomatically by repeated transfusions, education is required with regard to the recognition of significant symptomatology. Any agents that have been identified etiologically need to be avoided in the future. There may need to be dietary counselling.

Elevated white blood cell count

The most likely causes of an elevated white blood cell count (WBC) are infection, inflammation, and leukemia. A peripheral film will usually clarify if there are abnormal cells or an excess of lymphocytes which would allow a diagnosis of leukemia. An elevated WBC in association with a high ESR and pyrexia identifies the problem as possible infection.

Such a problem definition may come about as a result of presentation with falls, immobility, confusion or incontinence. If the possibility of infection is being considered in an elderly patient because of functional decline then a careful 'Infection Screen' is recommended. It needs to be remembered that infection is one of the two most common causes of functional decline in the elderly, the other being adverse reaction to medications.

Subjective

The geriatric presentation has been discussed in previous chapters. In the setting of the hospital the functional decline may be manifest as a change in behavior, an unwillingness to cooperate with rehabilitation for example. The changes may be slight at first and come on gradually, so that the patient may neither complain nor bring anything to the attention of the physician. It may well be a care provider who expresses concern and alerts the physician who instigates an infection screen. There are features in the history that might indicate the presence of infection, for example the development of chills, rigors or night sweats. In illnesses like influenza the patient may have systemic complaints like the presence of muscle aches and pains or headaches. Careful questioning may also reveal the presence of symptoms referable to an infection in certain systems.

Objective

There are certain findings which increase the likelihood that infection is the problem that needs to be investigated.

The most important is pyrexia. The control of body temperature has been discussed in a previous chapter (Chapter 11). It is essential that rectal temperature monitoring be undertaken before the absence of pyrexia can be confirmed. A subnormal temperature may also be found in certain types of infection and may be a clinical pointer. Some patients develop herpes labialis during the presence of infection although it should be remembered that the type of infection is usually respiratory. There may be more specific findings in the different systems which raise the problem definition above that of possible infection (e.g. chest infection or urinary tract infection).

Assessment

The erythrocyte sedimentation rate will also be raised, usually to values greater than 45 mm/hr. There are other tests which indicate an acute phase reaction, such as transferrin or C-reactive protein. When these are elevated the possibility of infection needs to be considered. The liver switches from albumin to globulin synthesis in the face of infection and so an unexplained fall in albumin, in the absence of a protein-losing state, should be treated with suspicion.

Plan

Diagnosis: screening for infection

It is most important to be certain that all relevant questions pertaining to symptoms of the various types of infection have been asked. Care providers and family members should always be questioned for any additional information. Diagnosis should pursue a logical path, with use of invasive tests only when clearly indicated (Fig. 19.2).

Tuberculosis should always be considered in the history to determine if the patient or family members have had it diagnosed and if adequately treated.

If the patient identified as possible infection is within a supervised setting then body temperature should be recorded regularly – for instance at 6-hourly intervals. The temperature recording should be as accurate as possible and the rectal route is preferred. It is our experience that when pyrexia is searched for in this way it is usually found, and this is important in substantiating the diagnosis of infection.

The patient should be reexamined with great care and if negative should be reexamined on a regular basis (daily). On examination attention should be paid to the lymph nodes, the skin, joints and fundi. The respiratory rate should be checked and the chest carefully reexamined. It is recognized that crepitations at the base of the lungs is a common finding in elderly patients but asymmetrical findings are more likely to indicate serious underlying pathology. The abdomen is

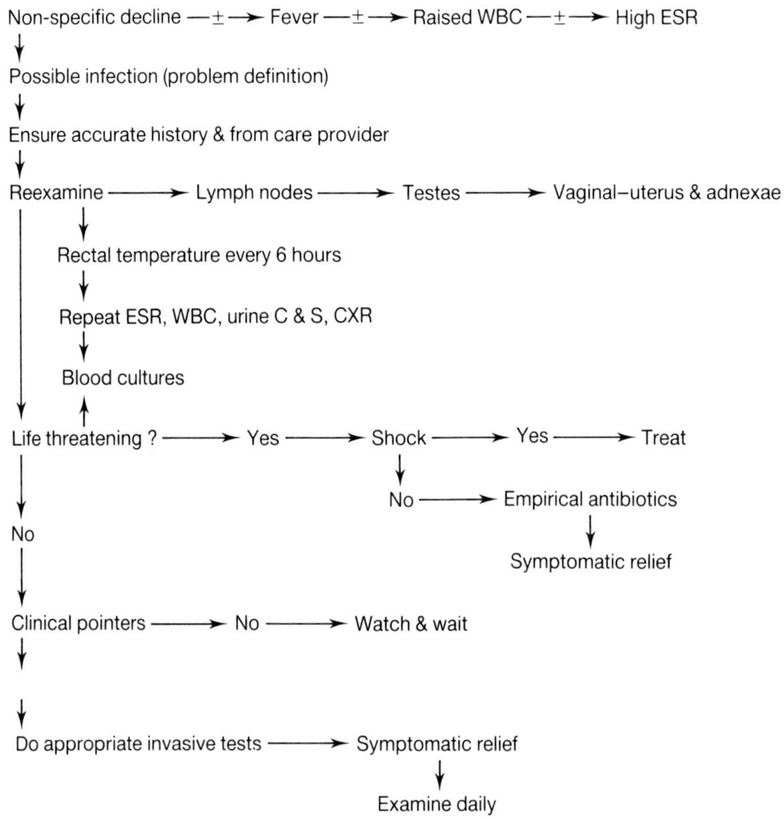

Fig. 19.2 Infection screen.

examined looking for organomegaly. The bowel sounds are listened for and the finding of a silent abdomen raises the possibility of a perforated viscus with intraperitoneal infection. In the male the testes and related organs need to be carefully palpated – epididymoorchitis is not an uncommon finding, the patient may be afebrile without any localizing symptoms. This is of particular importance in the patient who has had urinary tract infection recently treated, or who has undergone any form of genitourinary instrumentation. In the female the genital area also needs very careful examination, with per vaginal examination of the pelvic organs. Intrauterine infection may easily be missed.

In discussing fever of unknown origin it has been recommended that the nail beds should be carefully examined on a regular basis. In the elderly the finding of splinter hemorrhages is of no pathological significance, appearing to result from minimal trauma of any kind.

The ESR will have been done, indeed a high ESR is one of the findings that will have identified the problem as possible infection. The ESR should be repeated. There appears to be no value in performing other tests looking at non-specific markers of infection for example the C reactive protein. Further specimens of urine should be obtained for replicate cultures and for microscopy and analysis. The chest radiograph should be carefully reexamined, and if of poor quality repeated.

All patients should have blood cultures done, a minimum of 3 is recommended. One might expect a yield of approximately 10 per cent positive cultures.

Tuberculin skin testing (5 T.U.) should be done, a strongly positive result indicating the need for further testing. This would include early morning urines for acid fast bacilli, gastric aspirations and possible bone marrow examination.

Further invasive testing is only recommended if any of the above bear fruit. If there are findings consistent with infections in various sites then a variety of tests might be done including barium studies of the gastrointestinal tract, intravenous pyelography, ultrasonography of gall bladder, bone marrow or liver biopsy.

If the patient does not appear to be in a life threatening situation then investigations can wait and empirical treatment avoided. The patient is closely followed. In the long term care setting many febrile patients with possible infection can be followed for a few days and the fever settles, the patient improves returning to normal function without further treatment or investigation.

Treatment

The purpose of further investigation is to identify the site of infection and if possible the etiological agent. If this is achieved, therapy can be directed by the results. If diagnosis does not go any further and the problem remains identified as possible infection then there are two important considerations with regard to treatment – symptomatic relief and empirical therapy.

a) Symptomatic Relief

The patients may feel unwell. Often no specific treatment is required. The patient is allowed to rest, hydration and nutrition is maintained. The finding of a high body temperature appears to produce a reflex response in health professionals and a strong desire to bring it down to normal. There is some evidence that pyrexia is beneficial to the host so there is no urgency to treat. However patient's with extreme pyrexia are often delirious and may need treatment. Administration of acetaminophen orally is usually sufficient. Other approaches to treatment consist of simple physical measures to maintain the comfort of the patient.

b) Empirical Therapy

The patient may be quite ill with fever and general debility or may in fact be in septic shock. When this occurs the diagnostic approach outlined above is followed immediately and then the patient is treated. Shock is treated by intravenous fluid infusion and careful monitoring. Antibiotics are administered. Such patients will require intravenous antibiotics. A suitable empirical choice would be the combination of intravenous ampicillin and an aminoglycoside. These would be changed if cultures yielded positive results with differing sensitivities or if the patient fails to respond. Ampicillin should be given in the dose of 500 mg every 6 hours. After a loading dose of aminoglycoside further dosage schedule will depend upon the renal function and should be carefully monitored by blood levels.

Patient education

Patients and their families may need reassurance particularly when the problem is not further defined. In this situation keeping the patient and family fully informed helps to assuage anxiety. When an expectant approach is adopted all have to be content to wait and see. It is reassuring that in many instances the patients get better and the reason for the deterioration and the fever is never forthcoming. It is our experience that when surveillance is good, detection rate of infection increases, morbidity and mortality drop. It is important to note that if the empirical use of antibiotics is kept to a minimum it is of benefit to the patient and to the institution. Patients can be reassured by this knowledge.

Raised ESR

A raised ESR, with no other abnormality is unusual, although irritatingly common in the cognitively impaired elderly. The ESR should be over 50 mm/hr before investigation is undertaken. When the presentation warrants further investigation, then a logical pathway must be pursued (Fig. 19.3).

This approach will help identify the most important and frequent diseases associated with a high sedimentation rate. The high ESR is a good indicator in this population that a patient is in need of further diagnostic evaluation. If at the end of the investigations that have been recommended nothing has shown up then the patient's should be followed. If anything changes with the passage of time it may become obvious that more specific testing is warranted. Alternatively the correct decision may well be to accept that the ESR is high but of no apparent clinical significance.

With this approach the patient is not left in limbo and the physician is able to make a clear statement with regard to the patient. In our experience in the majority of patients with a geriatric presentation and a high sedimentation rate an explanation is forthcoming and the patient benefits.

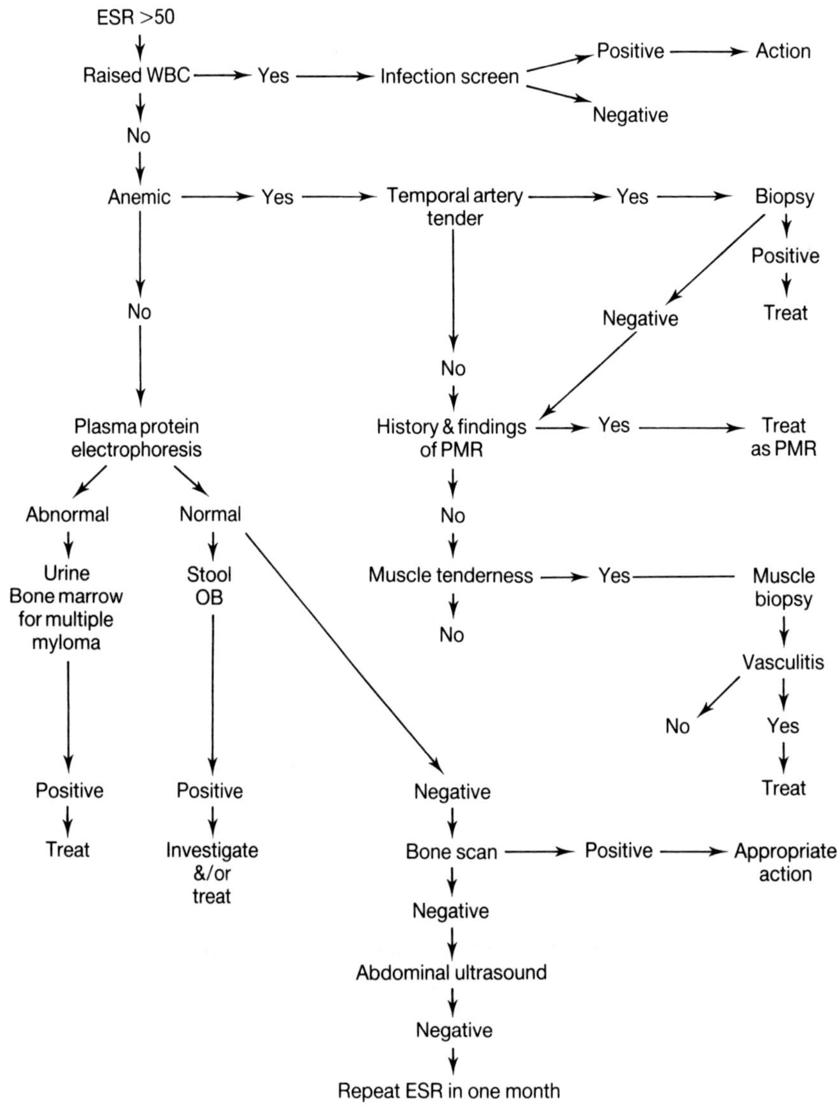

Fig. 19.3 Flow chart for high ESR (erythrocyte sedimentation rate).

Suggested reading

Andrews, J., Fairley, A. and Barker, R. (1976). Total dose infusion of iron dextran in the elderly. *Scot. Med. J.*, **12**: 208–15.

Berman, P., Hogan, D. B. and Fox, R. A. (1987). The atypical presentation of infection. *Age and Ageing*, **16**: 201–207.

Cartwright, G. E., Lee, G. R. (1971). The anemia of chronic disorders. *Brit. J. Haematol.*, **21**: 147–52.

Crawford, J., Eye-Boland, M. K. and Cohen, H. (1987). Clinical utility of erythrocyte sedimentation rate and plasma protein analysis in the Elderly. *Amer. J. Med.*, **82**: 239–46.

Denham, M. J. and Chanarin, I. (1985). *Blood Disorders in the Elderly*. Churchill Livingstone, London.

Downton, J. H., Andrews, K. and Puxty, J. A. H. (1987). Silent pyrexia in the elderly. *Age and Ageing*, **16**: 41–44.

Finkelstein, M. S., Petkun, W. M., Freedman, M.

L. and Antopol, S. C. (1983). Pneumococcal bacteremia in adults. *J. Amer. Ger. Soc.*, **31**: 19–27.

Gibson, I. J. M. (1972). The Value of erythrocyte sedimentation rate in the Aged. *Gerontol. Clinica*, **14**: 185.

Horan, M. A., Puxty, J. A. H. and Fox, R. A. (1983). Gynecologic sepsis as a cause of covert infection in old age. *J. Amer. Ger. Soc.*, **31**: 213–215.

Lipschitz, D. A., Mitchell, C. O. and Thompson, C. (1981). The anemia of senescence. *Amer. J. Hematol.*, **11**: 47–54.

MacLennan, W. J., Andrews, G. R., MacLeod, C. and Caird, F. I. (1973). Anemia in the elderly. *Quart. J. Med.*, **42**: 1–13.

Marrie, T., Haldane, E. V., Faulkner, R. S., Durant, H. and Kwan, C. (1985). Community acquired pneumonia requiring hospitalisation. Is it different in the elderly? *J. Amer. Ger. Soc.*, **33**: 671–80.

Puxty, J. A. H. and Andrews, K. (1986). The role of chest radiography in the evaluation of the geriatric giants. *Age and Ageing*, **15**: 174–6.

Sharland, D. E. (1980). Erythrocyte sedimentation rate: the normal range in the elderly. *J. Amer. Ger. Soc.*, **28**: 346–8.

Tinetti, M. E., Schmidt, A. and Baum, J. (1986). Use of the erythrocyte sedimentation rate in chronically ill, elderly patients with a decline in health status. *Amer. J. Med.*, **80**: 844–8.

Williamson, J. (1979). Adverse reaction to prescribed drugs in the Elderly. In: Crooks J., Stevenson, I. H. (eds) *Drugs and the Elderly*. Macmillan, London, pp. 239–46.

Young, J. and Mulley, G. (1987). Splinter hemorrhages in the elderly. *Age and Ageing*, **16**: 101–104.

20

Abnormalities of water, sodium and potassium

Fluid and electrolyte disturbances are common findings in the ill elderly. Both fluid overload and plasma volume depletion are commonly associated with changes in serum sodium concentration which in turn is often linked to changes in serum potassium. In this chapter we will review the age-related pathophysiological changes which impact on them, the consequences of these changes and suggest plans for assessment and management strategies.

1. Age related changes

Sodium, Potassium and Osmolarity

The maintenance of plasma sodium concentration, plasma potassium concentration and osmolarity within very strict limits is essential to the *milieu interieur* and normal bodily function. Aging alone is not associated with any change in the normal range for plasma sodium (135–48 mmol/l), plasma potassium (3.6–5.2 mmol/l) or plasma osmolarity (285–99 mosm/kg). Nevertheless, elderly people appear to be peculiarly vulnerable to the development of disorders of fluid and electrolyte balance when subjected to stresses (e.g. infection, cardiac failure, unusual water or electrolyte loads, drugs). This is probably due to a combination of rather subtle changes that are present to a greater or lesser extent in most elderly people.

In old age, the renal response to reduced sodium intake may be considerably slowed. Even with a minimal sodium intake, it can take several days to reduce renal sodium excretion and, since sodium and water are lost together, predisposes to volume depletion. Two factors appear to be involved. First of all, loss of nephrons places an increased osmotic load on those that remain, resulting in a mild osmotic diuresis. Secondly, basal and stimulated levels of renin and aldosterone are considerably reduced in many elderly people, predisposing them not only to sodium loss but also to retention of potassium.

In addition to a problem in sodium conservation, there are problems in dealing with an excess sodium load. This is largely attributable to a fall in glomerular filtration rate (which also impairs the ability to excrete a potassium load). Such sodium loads may derive from injudicious fluid therapy, unusually high dietary intake of sodium or the administration of sodium-rich radiographic contrast media (as may be used for intravenous urography). Even modest extra-cellular fluid volume expansion can induce overt cardiac failure, especially when there is some underlying myocardial dysfunction.

The sensitivity of the anti-diuretic hormone (ADH) response to an osmotic load is increased (leading to a tendency to hypo-natremia), while the sensitivity of the response to volume depletion is reduced (leading to a tendency to hypovolemia). The maximum concentrating capacity of the kidneys is reduced to about 850 mosm/kg (about 70 per cent of that observed in younger people), and this is probably due to an age-related decline in sensitivity to ADH. Little is known about the influence of age on the production of atrial natriuretic peptide (ANP), which has a potent diuretic action causing increases in the excretion of sodium, water, calcium and magnesium. The ANP concentration appears to be elevated in heart failure, and the magnitude of this increase seems to be greater in old people than younger ones.

Aging is associated with a fall in whole body potassium which in some people is greater than can be explained by the age-related decline in lean body mass. The aged kidneys can conserve potassium as well as young ones but there is an obligatory potassium loss in urine which may lead to whole body potassium depletion when potassium intake is low.

Aging is associated with a mild hyporeninemic hypoaldosteronism and it has been suggested that the abnormality lies at the level of the juxta-glomerular apparatus. This predisposes to retention of potassium and an impaired ability to excrete a potassium load. Hyporeninemic hypoaldosteronism is also seen with several renal interstitial diseases, particularly hypertension, diabetic nephropathy and obstructive uropathy. It may also be induced, or at least exacerbated by drugs, particularly angiotensin converting enzyme inhibitors (e.g. captopril, enalapril), non-steroidal anti-inflammatory agents and heparin.

The glomerular filtration rate is diminished in many elderly people but rarely gives rise to hyperkalemia until it is below 20 ml/min. Hyperkalemia may occur with a higher glomerular filtration rate if there is an abnormally high potassium load, if potassium-sparing diuretics are used, or if one of the conditions mentioned above which predisposes to hyperkalemia is present.

Urea and Creatinine

Population studies show that aging is associated with an increase in plasma concentrations of both urea and creatinine. The increases are only modest and a reference range of 3.9–9.9 mmol/l for urea and 52–159 umol/l for creatine may be used.

Urea is a product of protein metabolism. Amino acids may be de-aminated to form ammonia which is converted to urea in the liver. Urea production is largely determined by the dietary intake of protein except in severe liver disease. Creatinine derives from muscle and dietary intake of meat contributes little. Creatinine production reflects lean body mass and may be low in the frail elderly even in the presence of moderately impaired renal function.

Urea excretion occurs in the kidneys and depends on renal blood flow, glomerular filtration rate and the rate of urine flow. Urea is reabsorbed and the rate of this varies inversely with the rate of urine flow. Creatinine is not significantly reabsorbed but is secreted in the renal tubules which explains why creatinine clearance tends to overestimate the glomerular filtration rate.

2. Hyponatremia

Definition and Pathophysiology

Hyponatremia is the commonest electrolyte disturbance to be encountered in geriatric practice. It is said to be present when the plasma sodium concentration is less than 135 mmol/l, but rarely causes symptoms until the plasma sodium concentration is below 125 mmol/l. It may occur with normal, increased or decreased total body sodium. Symptoms and signs tend to be severe in elderly people, though the rate at which the sodium concentration falls is the major determinant of severity. Acute decreases in plasma sodium concentration are generally associated with the most severe clinical manifestations and greater mortality. Such acute decreases are frequently encountered post-operatively, especially when 5 per cent dextrose or dextrose-saline have been given to excess or when the bladder has been irrigated with water during trans-urethral resection of the prostate gland. In contrast, chronic hyponatremia may be almost entirely asymptomatic.

The evaluation of hyponatremia will depend entirely on the urgency of the clinical setting and some diagnostic maneuvers may have to take second place to therapy until the patient's condition improves. It is important to seek the features of volume depletion (see later) as well as sending a sample of urine for estimation of sodium concentration and osmolarity. Specific gravity can be measured at the bedside (using a hygrometer or reagent strips) and, in the absence of glucose, protein or mannitol, correlates well with osmolarity (Table 20.1).

Table 20.1 Correlation of specific gravity with osmolarity

Specific gravity	Osmolarity (mosm/kg)
1.010	350
1.020	700
1.030	1050
1.040	1400

Subjective Findings

The symptoms and signs of hyponatremia are largely those of raised intra-cranial pressure and reflect the excess of intra-cellular water. They depend upon both the severity and the rate at which the hyponatremia develops. Anorexia, nausea and lethargy are often early features, but these may be masked by various neuro-psychiatric complaints such as disorientation (delirium), psychotic manifestations and seizures.

The remainder of the subjective assessment is directed towards elucidating possible causes of the hyponatremia. Specific enquiry should be made about vomiting and/or diarrhea and a thorough drug history should be taken paying particular attention to those drugs listed in Table 20.2. The opportunity should be taken to review any fluid balance charts that may be available, noting not only the volume but also the nature of the fluids ingested. This is particularly important for post-operative patients. A similar situation to that occurring post-operatively may develop less acutely in patients who maintain an adequate fluid intake but fail to take in adequate amounts of solutes in the form of food. This may be a particular problem in the long-term care setting.

Table 20.2 Drugs associated with hyponatraemia

Non-steroidal anti-inflammatory drugs*
Tricyclic antidepressants*
Monoamine oxidase inhibitors*
Carbamazepine*
Phenothiazines*
Sulphonylureas*
Thiazide diuretics
Combination diuretics (e.g. thiazide and amiloride)

Note: * = associated with the syndrome of inappropriate antidiuresis

It is important to elicit any history of renal or adrenal disease or treatment with glucocorticoids that may have been withdrawn. A history of cardiac, pulmonary or liver disease will also be valuable in the subsequent assessment. A history of head injury is relevant.

Objective Findings

Confusion, hallucinations, delusions and seizures should not be difficult to elicit. Other neurological findings associated with hyponatremia include diminished deep tendon reflexes with slow relaxation times, muscle twitching, pseudo-bulbar palsy, hemiparesis and a depressed conscious level. These signs are useful in the assessment of the severity of the problem and the urgency of therapy.

The most useful signs to aid diagnosis are those used to assess the state of hydration ('volume status') of the individual. Signs of volume depletion include tachycardia, postural hypotension, recumbent hypotension and an abnormally low central venous pressure. Volume depletion with hyponatremia implies a greater fall in total body sodium than in total body water.

Hyponatremia with fluid overload is always associated with edema. Important conditions in this category are congestive heart failure, nephrotic syndrome and liver cirrhosis. One important warning is that edema does not always indicate a generalized volume expansion and may simply arise from local mechanical factors or represent the 'sick cell syndrome'. In the presence of edema, it is still important to search for features of any disease or patho-physiological process known to induce hyponatremia. One important example is the patient with ankle swelling from mechanical causes who is given a thiazide diuretic which depletes plasma volume and induces hyponatremia while the peripheral oedema may still persist. The edema of the 'sick cell syndrome' is non-pitting and results from a change in cell membrane permeability with movements of sodium and water into cells while potassium moves out. The syndrome is usually seen in very ill patients who are hypoxic and in those suffering circulatory shock.

The abnormal pigmentation of Addison's disease and haemochromatosis will lead to a further search for these conditions. Finally, the abdomen should be examined for tenderness or abnormal distension arising from paralytic ileus or pancreatitis, two important conditions associated with fluid and electrolyte losses into a 'third space'.

Plan – Diagnosis and Treatment

Hyponatremia of acute onset is usually found in the first 24 hours following surgery and tends to arise for one of two reasons. The commoner of the two is the administration of 5 per cent dextrose or dextrose-saline intravenously as post-operative fluid replacement. The less common cause is irrigation of the bladder with distilled water after prostatectomy. Quite often, the plasma sodium is below 125 mmol/l and may exist with normal or somewhat expanded plasma volume. It is usual for plasma ADH levels to be elevated following anaesthesia and surgery and in some patients may remain elevated for 4–5 days. In this setting, the administration of hypotonic fluids leads to water retention and hyponatremia. Most elderly people do not need 5 per cent dextrose in the first 24 hours after surgery and for uncomplicated cases, two litres of normal (0.9 per cent) saline will suffice.

The mortality of acute, severe hyponatremia is high and the need for treatment is urgent. Unfortunately, there is no agreement about the optimal rate at which the correction of the hyponatremia should take place. We suggest that one should aim to restore plasma sodium to at least 125 mmol/l within 8 hours and to within the normal range in 24–48 hours. This is usually achieved by the administration of 2.7 per cent sodium chloride (450 mmol/l). More concentrated solutions can be very dangerous and we do not recommend their use. The number of millimoles of sodium to give may be calculated as follows:

First 8 hrs (mmol) = 60 per cent × wt (kg) × (125 – Na concentration)

Next 16 hrs (mmol) = 60 per cent × wt (kg) × (135 – Na concentration)

It is essential to examine the patient frequently to ensure unwanted volume expansion does not occur and if there is any doubt, a central venous line should be inserted and the pressure maintained between 8 and 10 cm of water. If volume expansion starts to become a problem, frusemide should be administered. Some authors recommend that initial treatment should be by replacing frusemide-induced salt losses with a hypertonic solution (e.g. 2.7 per cent sodium chloride).

Subacute and chronic hyponatremia can be conveniently classified on the basis of the measured plasma osmolarity. Hyponatremia with normal osmolarity (pseudo-hyponatremia) is of little consequence and any treatment given is that of the underlying disease. Hyponatremia associated with a raised osmolarity is usually caused by hyperglycemia. The management of this condition is discussed in Chapter 24. Hyponatremia with a low plasma osmolarity is also called hypotonic hyponatremia and forms the subject of the remainder of this discussion.

Hypotonic hyponatremia can be further categorized on the basis of the patient's volume status. Clinical examination is usually quite adequate for this purpose but occasionally, central venous pressure must be measured.

The commonest form of hypotonic hyponatremia is that induced by thiazide diuretics, especially in combination with the potassium-sparing diuretic, amiloride. Similar synergy may exist with triamterene and spironolactone, two other potassium-sparing diuretics. Hyponatremia seldom occurs as a result of frusemide administration since this drug actually induces some resistance to ADH at the level of the kidney. For mild cases of thiazide-induced hyponatremia, withdrawal of the drug is usually the only treatment needed. More severe cases require 0.9 per cent sodium chloride intravenously but more concentrated solutions are hardly ever needed.

Other causes of hypotonic hyponatremia with volume depletion are summarized in Table 20.3. They may be separated into 'renal' and 'non-renal' on the basis of the urine sodium concentration. Urine sodium concentrations over 20 mmol/l suggest renal sodium wasting. The term 'salt-losing' nephritis refers to a group of disorders characterized by renal salt-wasting and tubulo-interstitial disease. Other evidence of tubular dysfunction is almost always present. Salt wasting is also a feature of progressive chronic renal failure and may occur when an obstructive uropathy is relieved and is due to a mixture of tubular dysfunction and the osmotic diuresis due to urea. Metabolic alkalosis and renal tubular acidosis will both be discussed later.

If the urine sodium concentration is less than 20 mmol/l, extra-renal salt and water losses are likely. Important causes are listed in Table 20.3. The treatment of hypotonic hyponatremia with volume depletion, whether it is renal or extra-renal in origin, is 0.9 per cent sodium chloride intravenously plus treatment aimed at the underlying disorder.

With elderly patients, there may be some difficulty in distinguishing hypotonic hyponatremia

Table 20.3 Assessment of hypotonic hyponatraemia with hypovolemia

Urine sodium >20 mmol/l
Diuretics
Metabolic alkalosis
Renal tubular acidosis
Osmotically active substances (glucose, urea, mannitol)
Adrenal insufficiency
Urine sodium <20 mmol/l
Gastrointestinal fluid loss
'Third spaces'
burns
pancreatitis
peritonitis
ileus
muscle trauma
Severe skin diseases
Treatment: isotonic saline

with mild volume depletion from the syndrome of inappropriate antidiuresis (SIA). Table 20.4 lists the features of SIA. A similar syndrome may accompany myxedema which responds to treatment with thyroxine. The SIA may arise from almost any intra-cranial disorder, either acute or chronic (Table 20.5). It may also arise in association with respiratory diseases, particularly severe infections, small cell carcinoma of the bronchus and respiratory failure. Plasma uric acid is usually diminished in SIA but tends to be elevated in the presence of hypovolemia. In more severe volume depletion, pre-renal uremia will be present which will exclude SIA.

Treatment of SIA is aimed at the underlying disorder, including the withdrawal of offending drugs (Table 20.2). If specific treatment is thought necessary, fluid restriction to 500–1000 ml/day is usually effective. If this fails, judicious treatment with frusemide should be added since it reduces renal sensitivity to ADH. Thiazides should not be used as they will make the problem worse. Dimethylchlortetracycline should be avoided since it may cause a deterioration in renal function and lithium carbonate might be considered as a possible alternative, but in this case, careful monitoring of plasma lithium levels will be needed.

Hypotonic hyponatremia with volume expansion (oedema states) usually carries a poor prognosis and is difficult to treat. Diuretics, together with salt and water restriction, are the mainstay of treatment in most of these disorders. It has been suggested that hyponatremia in congestive heart failure is associated with a high plasma renin concentration. In this event, treatment with angiotensin-converting enzyme inhibitors (e.g. captopril and enalapril) would seem logical.

Management of the 'sick cell syndrome' comprises treatment with insulin (with potassium unless plasma potassium is high). High doses of synthetic glucocorticoids are usually given and plasma expanders may be needed to correct the hypovolemia and salt-poor albumin is to be preferred for this purpose.

Table 20.4 Features of the syndrome of inappropriate antidiuresis

Hypotonic hyponatremia
Absence of hypovolemia
Absence of edema
Inappropriate antidiuresis
Urine sodium >20 mmol/l

Table 20.5 Assessment of hypotonic hyponatremia with no change in volume status

Urine sodium >20 mmol/l
Syndrome of inappropriate antidiuresis
• brain lesions (e.g. injury, infection, neoplasm)
• lung lesions (e.g. infection, neoplasm)
• drugs (Table 20.1)
• cryptogenic
Renal failure (inadequate solute intake)
Hypothyroidism
Urine sodium <20 mmol/l
Potassium depletion
Water intoxication
Treatment: water restriction

3. Hypernatremia

Definition and Pathophysiology

Hypernatremia is always associated with dehydration and is usually diagnosed when the plasma sodium concentration equals or exceeds 150 mmol/l. It is a rare but dangerous electrolyte disorder and is encountered more often in elderly people than in young ones. Its presence implies a preferential loss of water over sodium (eg in respiratory infections) or inadequate water intake due to impaired thirst or lack of availability of water (Table 20.6).

Table 20.6 Approach to hypernatremia with volume depletion

Urine sodium >20 mmol/l
Osmotic diuresis (glucose, urea, mannitol)
Urine sodium <20 mmol/l
Excessive sweating
Diarrhea

Several features of the elderly may predispose to this electrolyte abnormality. Diseases and disorders leading to a loss of hypotonic fluids are common. There is also an age-associated deficit in renal concentrating capacity and the central thirst mechanism may not function normally. The dependent elderly may have very restricted access to 'free water' (in the form of drinks) and hyperosmolar oral or nasogastric feeds may not be adequately supervised.

There are several causes of an osmotic diuresis but only two are encountered with any regularity. Hyperglycemia (with uncontrolled diabetes mellitus) and urea following the relief of obstructive uropathy. A slightly raised or even normal plasma sodium in the context of severe hyperglycemia is quite inappropriate (since the egress of water from cells should lower the plasma sodium) and indicates a significant water deficit. Osmotic diuretics occupy the place of electrolyte solutes in urine and in this way, water is lost in excess over sodium.

Subjective

The symptoms of hypernatremia are attributable to cellular dehydration in the brain and include headache, lethargy, restlessness, irritability and seizures (either focal or generalized). All these features are rather non-specific.

Aspects of the past medical history that may be of use in the later assessment are the presence of chronic renal failure, the presence of malignant disease (metastases are the commonest cause of diabetes insipidus in the elderly), the presence of diabetes mellitus and perhaps other electrolyte disorders (especially hypokalemia and hypercalcemia). The fluid balance chart should be reviewed and an effort made to determine whether the patient has been taking hyperosmolar feeds without additional water. It is also important to note the setting and whether proper prophylaxis is likely to have been given to the disabled or unconscious patient.

Objective

Hyper-reflexia, muscle twitching, seizures and depressed conscious level are all features of hypernatremia but are unhelpful when trying to determine the cause. Perhaps the most important part of the examination is an assessment of 'volume status' which is discussed under 'hyponatremia'. Since significant hypernatremia carries such a poor prognosis, the slightest doubt should prompt the setting up of a central venous line.

Plan – Diagnosis and Treatment

The commonest form of hypernatremia seen in geriatric practice is 'euvolemic'. The patient is often in some continuing care establishment and not adequately supervised to ensure an adequate 'free water' intake. It is most likely to develop in hot weather or in the presence of fever (in which case, a search for the site of infection is mandatory). It is also seen when hyper-osmolar diet supplements are given without adequate access to water. Treatment is with 5 per cent dextrose. The water deficit may be calculated in litres as follows:

$$\left[\frac{\textit{measured Na}}{140} \times 60\%\ \text{weight (kg)}\right] - \left[60\%\ \text{weight (kg)}\right]$$

There is little agreement about the optimum rate to administer the fluid. In general, one should aim to correct the disorder over two to three days.

Euvolemic hypernatremia also occurs in diabetes insipidus. The central form of this disorder is most likely due to a metastasis or a vascular lesion in elderly people. Nephrogenic diabetes insipidus is most likely to complicate other electrolyte disorders (hypokalemia and hypercalcemia) or treatment with lithium. Treatment is as outlined above with correction of any *underlying* electrolyte disorder or withdrawal of offending drugs. The central form will require further investigation together with replacement treatment in the form of a pitressin spray.

Hypovolemic hypernatremia usually follows fluid losses from the gut, either as a result of infection or vigorous purgation. Infective causes may be associated with fever and sweating which may further contribute to the losses of salt and water and water replacement may be inadequate. If signs of hypovolemia are present, intravenous therapy is indicated. Initially, haemo-dynamics should be restored by the infusion of 0.9 per cent sodium chloride followed by 5 per cent dextrose or 0.45 per cent sodium chloride.

The volume expansion associated with the hypernatremia of Cushing's syndrome or Conn's syndrome is always mild and diuretic treatment with water replacement is usually adequate. The volume expansion which follows excessive infusion of sodium bicarbonate during cardio-pulmonary resuscitation may be very severe. In this case, diuretics with fluid replacement may not be adequate and then, peritoneal dialysis should be performed.

4. Hypokalemia

Definition and Pathophysiology

Hypokalemia may be defined as a plasma potassium concentration below 3.5 mmol/l. It is often an incidental finding but may be suspected by the presence of U waves and flattened T waves in the electrocardiogram. In practice, there is little to be gained by investigating and initiating treatment when the plasma potassium concentration is above 3.0 mmol/l and some authors suggest that concentrations above 2.5 mmol/l do not merit investigation unless the patient is taking digoxin or has some other problem where whole body potassium depletion is likely such as vomiting and/or diarrhea.

A low plasma potassium concentration does not always reflect whole body potassium depletion but may arise from movement of potassium into the intra-cellular compartment (remember over 90 per cent of whole body potassium is inside cells). Such re-distribution probably explains the variation seen in plasma potassium concentration over a 24-hour period. It is also worth noting that considerable potassium depletion may be present with a normal plasma potassium concentration and this is particularly likely to be observed with a metabolic acidosis (e.g. diabetic keto-acidosis, uraemia) and in congestive heart failure.

There is considerable renal capacity to regulate potassium losses over quite a wide range. Nearly all filtered potassium is reabsorbed prior to the proximal part of the distal convoluted tubule and most of the potassium that appears in urine is actively secreted in the distal convoluted tubule and possibly in the collecting ducts. Aldosterone acts mainly at the level of the distal convoluted tubule and stimulates potassium losses as well as sodium retention. These two effects are, at least in part, independent of one another. The rate of fluid and sodium delivery in the glomerular filtrate are also major regulators of potassium losses.

Several problems influence the interpretation of plasma potassium results, particularly the circumstances of sampling and how the sample is subsequently handled. A tourniquet kept in place too long can cause potassium leakage from arm muscles and haemolysis may occur with 'difficult' venepunctures. Unless the plasma is separated quite soon, there is a steady loss of potassium from red cells, regardless of the temperature at which the sample is kept and is not prevented by keeping the sample at 4°C.

Changes in acid-base balance affect plasma potassium concentration and these are dealt with later in this chapter. Alkalosis (respiratory or metabolic) results in potassium movement into cells and renal potassium wasting in an attempt by the kidneys to conserve hydrogen ions. Likewise, hypokalemia exacerbates alkalosis because the availability of potassium ions for exchange with hydrogen ions is reduced.

Subjective Findings

Hypokalemia may be seen as an isolated finding or in the setting of an ongoing medical problem which predisposes to potassium re-distribution or depletion. Hypokalemia is usually asymptomatic unless moderately severe and concentrations below 2.5 mmol/l are almost always associated with symptoms. The dominant symptoms are neuromuscular and muscle weakness is the best known of these. It may be so severe that the presentation masquerades as a quadriparesis. Tetany is very rarely encountered and may in fact be due to an associated magnesium deficiency. Muscle cramps and constipation are also common and paralytic ileus may be seen, particularly after surgery. Hypokalemia may induce some autonomic impairment and cause symptomatic postural hypotension, particularly in the elderly. Elderly patients are also more likely to manifest neuro-psychiatric symptoms such as apathy, fatigue, anorexia and occasionally, thirst.

It is essential to review medication. Diuretics are the most important drugs in this regard but treatment with carbenoxolone, de-glycyrrhizinated liquorice, carbonic anhydrase inhibitors and laxatives may all induce potassium losses. Treatment with vitamin B_{12}, β_2 agonists and insulin may lower the plasma potassium concentration because of re-distribution. Rarely, treatment with lithium salts, penicillin and gentamicin may be associated with hypokalemia.

Other aspects of the clinical setting may reveal the cause of hypokalemia. A dietary history is important but may be very unreliable. It is therefore important to seek some external corroboration since a sizeable minority of older people appear quite content to live on 'tea and toast'. Edematous states with secondary aldosteronism (liver cirrhosis, nephrotic syndrome, congestive heart failure and cor pulmonale) are often associated with potassium wasting. Diabetic ketoacidosis, naso-gastric suction and initial vitamin B_{12} treatment in pernicious anemia will be obvious and hypokalemia should be actively sought under such circumstances.

Objective Findings

The general appearance of the patient may suggest severe nutritional deprivation but a more detailed assessment will be needed to reveal less overt cases. A flaccid quadriparesis will be obvious but more subtle degrees of muscle weakness require very careful examination for their detection. Signs of cardiac failure, nephrotic syndrome, liver cirrhosis and cor pulmonale are important for the further assessment of the condition. Fecal loading should be sought and the presence of 'melanosis coli' on proctoscopy suggests prolonged laxative abuse.

Plan

Diagnosis

Potassium re-distribution may lead to very severe and symptomatic hypokalemia. These conditions are listed in Table 20.7 and will often be obvious from the clinical setting. In the situations listed in this table, it is essential to be aware that hypokalemia may ensue and many would give prophylaxis in the form of potassium supplements (see below).

Table 20.7 Hypokalemia with re-distribution of potassium

Hyperaldosteronism
Catecholamines
β_2-agonist drugs
Insulin
Vitamin B_{12} therapy
Alkalosis

In the absence of re-distribution of potassium, hypokalemia is most likely to arise from treatment with diuretics (especially in edema states with secondary aldosteronism), or from overt gastrointestinal disorders such as vomiting, diarrhea and laxative abuse. If one of these disorders is clearly present, it can reasonably be considered to be the explanation for the hypokalemia. Hypokalemia associated with diuretic treatment is just as likely to occur when potassium supplements or potassium-sparing agents are given as when they are omitted. Vomiting is associated with secondary aldosteronism and alkalosis, both of which contribute more to the hypokalemia than do direct potassium losses in the vomit.

If the cause of the hypokalemia remains elusive, the above disorders are not ruled out since laxative and diuretic abuse can be very difficult to detect. The diagnostic procedure at this stage (Fig. 20.1) depends on an assessment of urinary potassium and acid-base status. With urine potassium losses over 20 mmol/l, it is safe to assume that the hypokalemia is caused by renal potassium wasting. Its association with an alkalosis implies diuretic treatment, vomiting with bicarbo-naturia or a mineralocorticoid effect (most often, secondary aldosteronism). Acidosis is most likely due to

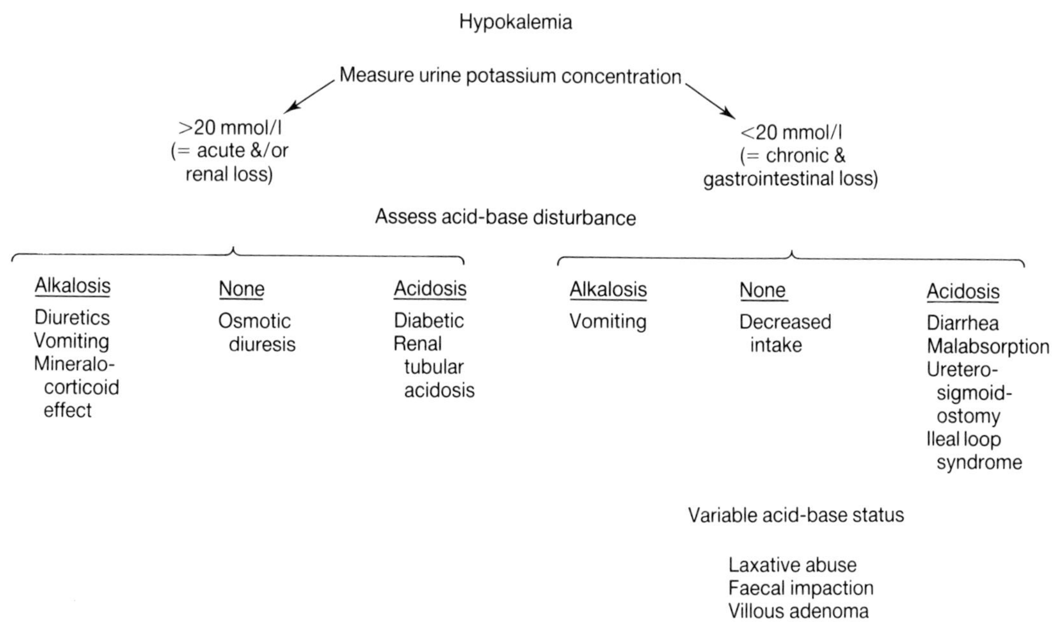

Fig. 20.1 Diagnostic approach to hypokalemia.

uncontrolled diabetes mellitus or an acquired form of renal tubular acidosis. Renal tubular acidosis refers to a group of disorders of the kidneys, either intrinsic or extrinsic, in which the ability to secrete hydrogen ions is impaired (leading to a metabolic acidosis) but glomerular function is more or less normal. The most likely causes of renal tubular acidosis in old age are conditions associated with high globulin concentrations (chronic active hepatitis, primary biliary cirrhosis, cryoglobulinemia) or abnormalities of immunoglobulins (myeloma, light chain disease, amyloid disease). In the absence of acid-base disturbance, an osmotic diuresis is the most likely cause. This may arise from the administration of osmotic diuretics such as mannitol or the presence of endogenous osmotically active substances such as glucose or ketones and urea (following nutritional deprivation).

Low urine potassium concentration ($\leqslant$ 10 mmol/l) associated with an alkalosis is most likely caused by vomiting, usually without bicarbonaturia, but may occur with laxative abuse, fecal loading and villous adenoma. These latter 3 disorders may also be associated with acidosis or there may be no detectable acid-base disturbance. Acidosis is more typical of ureterosigmoidostomy, ileal loop syndrome and diarrheal illnesses (including malabsorption).

Treatment

Treatment (when necessary) can usually be effected by the oral route. In most cases, potassium chloride as a syrup is effective. In the presence of alkalosis, potassium citrate and potassium gluconate simply add to the bicarbonate load and potentiate potassium losses. In the presence of acidosis, potassium citrate or potassium gluconate should be given. Commercial effervescent potassium preparations such as Kloref and Sando–K contain a mixture of potassium salts including chloride and bicarbonate. In the presence of alkalosis, these preparations may not be as effective as anticipated.

For most purposes, 40–50 mmol/day of potassium is an adequate oral treatment. This is the equivalent of about 3 grams of potassium chloride per day in divided doses. Intravenous therapy is very rarely needed for the correction of hypokalemia and is usually given in the form of a potassium chloride addition to some other intravenous fluid. Concentrations of potassium chloride greater than 40 mmol/l should not be used, no more than 20 mmol should be infused over one hour and no more than 150 mmol should be given in a single day. Furthermore, frequent plasma potassium estimations are needed when a potassium salt is infused intravenously.

5. Hyperkalemia

Definition and Pathophysiology

Hyperkalemia is said to be present when the plasma potassium concentration is greater than 5.2 mmol/l. It is best detected in plasma rather than serum since platelets and leukocytes release potassium during blood coagulation. Factitious hyperkalemia may also arise from keeping a tourniquet in place for too long or when red cells are disrupted during or after blood sampling.

Like hypokalemia, hyperkalemia can arise from redistribution of potassium and is particularly associated with either a metabolic or respiratory acidosis since hydrogen ions move into cells and potassium ions move out *pari passu*. However, it is not a uniform feature of acidosis and does not occur when the hydrogen ion plus anion (e.g. lactate) move into cells. Redistribution may also be induced by drugs, particularly beta-blockers and insulin.

As mentioned earlier the elderly are predisposed to potassium retention by their relatively low renin and aldosterone levels. Drugs such as the non-steroidal anti-inflammatory agents by inhibiting production of prostaglandins (PGE2 and PGI2) further aggravate the situation so hyperkalemia may result.

Subjective findings

Hyperkalemia is usually asymptomatic until plasma potassium rises above 6.5 mmol/l. Symptoms are non-specific. Early on, hyperkalemia causes partial depolarization at muscle membranes which is associated with neuro-muscular excitability. Eventually, sodium permeability decreases which makes the muscle cells less able to generate action potentials and weakness and eventually paralysis ensue.

Hyperkalemia may be first suggested by changes in the electrocardiogram. These comprise tall, peaked T waves in the precordial leads followed by a decreased R wave amplitude, widened QRS complex, prolonged P–R interval and reduced amplitude P waves. Eventually the QRS complex seems to blend into the T wave to give a sine wave type of pattern. Serious ventricular dysrhythmias may occur at any stage of this progression. If the electrocardiogram shows none of these changes, the plasma potassium concentration should be measured again, taking great care to ensure the sample is optimal for potassium estimation. A normal ECG is not grounds for complacency about treating hyperkalemia as serious dysrhythmias may occur rapidly without pre-warning.

The clinical setting will usually give important clues regarding the cause of hyperkalemia. Fluid charts should be examined to assess whether the patient has been subjected to abnormally high potassium loads, especially intravenously. The prescription chart should be reviewed paying special attention to potassium-sparing diuretics, non-steroidal anti-inflammatory drugs, angiotensin-converting enzyme inhibitors, heparin (even low-dose sub-cutaneous therapy), beta-blockers and insulin. Other biochemical results should be reviewed in a search for uraemia and acidosis.

Objective findings

As with hypokalemia, paralysis associated with hyperkalemia should be obvious but more subtle degrees need more careful assessment. This is probably not worthwhile since the need for treatment is urgent. It is worthwhile looking for the abnormal pigmentation of Addison's disease (though this disease is rare in geriatric practice).

Plan – diagnosis and treatment

Having established that the hyperkalemia is not an artefact of sampling, it is important to establish whether or not there is co-existing acidosis or renal failure since both may require specific therapy. Where possible, offending drugs should be withdrawn.

If the plasma potassium concentration is less than 6.5 mmol/l and the electrocardiogram is normal or only peaked T waves are present, no further treatment other than restricting potassium intake may be required, though polystyrene sulphonate resins may be given orally or *per rectum*. Calcium resonium should be avoided in hyperparathyroidism, myeloma or metastatic carcinoma and resonium A should be avoided in cardiac failure and with severe renal impairment. The appropriate dose is 15 grams 3–4 times daily in water or as an enema (30 grams in methylcellulose solution to be retained for 9 hours). Rectal ulceration may complicate the treatment when given as enemas.

If the plasma potassium concentration is greater than 7.0 mmol/l, more urgent treatment is needed and an electrocardiographic monitor is required. The most rapidly acting treatment is intravenous calcium gluconate (10–20 ml of 10 per cent solution over 5 minutes) to antagonize the peripheral neuromuscular and myocardial effects of hyperkalemia (effective within minutes but the effect lasts only 30–40 minutes). Cellular uptake of potassium can be stimulated by glucose and insulin or by sodium bicarbonate infusion. A 10 per cent glucose infusion (500 ml over an hour is a suitable dose) together with soluble insulin, 5 units intravenously every 15 minutes. The use of sodium bicarbonate is limited by the amount of sodium that can be tolerated. If these treatments are not succeeding or if fluid overload is worsening, dialysis should be considered.

These urgent measures are temporary in their effect and, if the cause cannot be removed, an attempt must be made to remove potassium from the body by using a low potassium diet and polystyrene sulphonate resins. If there is an associated acidosis, sodium bicarbonate or calcium carbonate may be given to buffer hydrogen ions extracelluarly and prevent them moving into cells with consequent egress of potassium. In the presence of hypoaldosteronism, fludrocortisone may be given but its use is limited by sodium retention.

6. Plasma urea and creatinine; renal failure.

Causes of a low plasma urea concentration are listed in Table 20.8.

Table 20.8 Causes of low plasma urea concentration

Severe liver disease
Protein malnutrition
Hemodilution
Overhydration
Nephrotic syndrome

Elevations in urea concentration (Table 20.9) occur following a heavy protein meal or after a gastro-intestinal bleed. In the absence of renal dysfunction, levels rarely exceed 20 mmol/l under these circumstances and the creatinine concentration is usually normal or only slightly raised. A combined increase in the concentrations of urea and creatinine reflect reduced renal blood flow (dehydration, shock and cardiac failure), intrinsic renal disease or obstruction of urinary outflow Table 20.9).

Table 20.9 Raised urea and creatinine (renal failure)

1. Pre Renal
   - dehydration
   - shock
   - haemorrhage
   - volume depletion
2. Renal
   - nephrotoxic medications
   - end stage nephrosclerosis (hypertension)
   - end stage chronic infection
   - glomerular nephritis
   - diabetes, etc.
3. Post Renal
   - outlet obstruction: prostate calculus

Subjective

The symptoms of renal failure will depend upon the nature of the precipitant and the acuity. Acute renal failure is seen more frequently in the aged from inciting events, such as hypotension complicating volume depletion, major surgery or adverse drug reactions. In the acute situation the patient may experience rapid decline in function, obtundation and oligemia. A proportion of patients with oligemia become dysfunctional, and this initiates medical contact. Patients also develop symptoms of associated problems which are discussed elsewhere in this chapter, such as hyperkalemia, hyponatremia or acidosis.

The symptoms of chronic renal failure are often more subtle with gradual decline in function. The patient may become dyspneic due to associated anemia. Pruritus, a common problem anyway in this population, may also occur and prove difficult to manage.

Objective

Renal failure, or insufficiency, is usually a 'laboratory diagnosis', from the findings of raised plasma urea (BUN) and creatinine. Physical findings are non-specific – there may be pallor (anemia) or a discoloration of the skin (uremia). Severe uremia, a rare situation, is marked by a uremic odor or by petechial hemorrhages in the skin. Abdominal examination may reveal enlarged or abnormal kidneys. The bladder size should be checked carefully – obstructive uropathy is an important problem to diagnose.

Assessment

The history of onset together with physical findings should indicate the acute or chronic nature of the problem. Blood levels of urea, creatinine and other electrolytes will be obtained. Urinalysis and urine culture may help define etiology. Patients with chronic renal failure may benefit from ultrasound and plain radiograph. If obstructive uropathy is indicated, other imaging techniques may be indicated. With the frail elderly other diagnostic techniques such as biopsy are rarely indicated.

Plan

Treatment is aimed at reversing any precipitating condition that is identified – replacing fluid loss and correction of volume depletion. Management of acidosis and electrolyte abnormalities are discussed elsewhere in this chapter. Dietary control of protein, to 40 gms and control of electrolyte and fluid intake are important. Most patients are managed conservatively.

Dialysis is rarely indicated in these patients because of associated disease burden. Hemodialysis is usually contraindicated. Some patients with limited disease burdens will benefit from peritoneal dialysis – the indications being the same as in the healthy elderly and other age groups.

Suggested reading

Lye, M. D. (1985). The milieu interieur and aging. In: Brocklehurst, J. C. (ed.) *Textbook of Geriatric Medicine and Gerontology*. Churchill Livingstone, Ch. 11, pp. 201–29.

Timaras, M. L. (1988). The kidney, the lower urinary tract and body fluids. In: Timeras, P. S. (ed.) *Physiological Basis of Geriatrics*. MacMillan, London.

21

Abnormalities of acid-base metabolism

Acid base disturbances

Acid-base status is determined by both the metabolism of hydrogen ions (kidney) and of carbon dioxide (lungs). The primary disturbances involve changes in the pCO_2 (respiratory) or bicarbonate (metabolic). These disturbances initially give rise to acidemia (decreased pH) or alkalemia (increased pH) but are then compensated through a variety of mechanisms and the pH is returned towards normal (about 7.4). Except in chronic respiratory alkalosis and minor degrees of respiratory acidosis, compensation is never complete and overcompensation never occurs.

Acid-base disturbances are usually suspected from the clinical setting and/or by results of electrolyte estimations. Hyperkalemia occurs in acidosis (as potassium moves out of cells in exchange for hydrogen ions) and hypokalemia is a feature of alkalosis (as potassium moves into cells). Reductions in plasma chloride concentration occur in metabolic alkalosis and in compensated respiratory acidosis. Estimation of the plasma bicarbonate concentration (sometimes called total CO_2) provides considerable information about possible acid base disturbances. A reduced plasma bicarbonate concentration suggests a metabolic acidosis or compensated respiratory alkalosis and an elevation suggests a metabolic alkalosis or compensated respiratory acidosis. Calculation of the anion gap is also very useful in acid-base disturbances and this may be done by subtracting the sum of the chloride and bicarbonate concentrations from the sodium concentration (normally 12 ± 4 mmol/l). A high anion gap suggests metabolic acidosis even in the presence of a normal bicarbonate concentration.

In most circumstances, suspicion of an acid-base disorder requires the taking of an arterial blood sample for measurement of pCO_2, pH and bicarbonate concentration. It should be remembered that the pH scale is logarithmic and small fluctuations in pH may reflect marked changes in hydrogen ion concentration and some laboratories also report the actual hydrogen ion concentration. The bicarbonate concentration obtained from blood gas analysers is calculated from pH and pCO_2 using the Henderson-Hasselbach equation and, unlike the plasma bicarbonate (total CO_2) obtained from 'electrolyte' measuring instruments, represents the real bicarbonate ion concentration. Two other values are often given with 'blood gas' reports, the standard bicarbonate and the base excess. The standard bicarbonate is a calculated value and represents the bicarbonate concentration with the respiratory component removed. The base excess, like the standard bicarbonate, is a measure of the metabolic component of an acid-base disorder. Negative values outside the normal range indicate acidosis and positive values, alkalosis.

Age changes in acid-base mechanisms

Hydrogen ion and bicarbonates are formed from carbon dioxide and water within the cells of the tubules. Hydrogen ions are excreted into the tubular lumen in exchange for sodium which is transferred to the blood together with the bicarbonate. This process may be attenuated in old age because of decreased production of aldosterone.

The hydration of CO_2 into hydrogen and bicarbonate ions is controlled by the CO_2. CO_2 excretion in the lungs is controlled by respiratory rate and area of lung available. Aging is associated with a diminished ventilatory response to hypercapnia and implies an impairment therefore in the rapid adjustments to alteration in acid base balance. Phosphate intake tends to be reduced in old age which would limit the amount available in the phosphate buffer system. The capacity to increase ammonia production is reduced in old age probably secondary to reduction in number of nephrons. The available evidence therefore suggests that aging is associated with a reduced ability to respond to disturbances in acid base balance.

Metabolic alkalosis

Metabolic alkalosis is probably the commonest acid-base disturbance encountered in geriatric practice and is defined as an elevation in bicarbonate concentration. When it arises as a primary disorder the compensatory change is hypoventilation and retention of carbon dioxide. The hypoventilation also induces hypoxia which stimulates ventilation and thus limits the elevation in pCO_2. In simple, compensated metabolic alkalosis the pCO_2 does not rise much above 55 mm Hg and higher values suggest the presence of a respiratory acidosis.

Metabolic alkalosis arises from either loss of hydrogen ions from the extracelluar fluid or from an accumulation of bicarbonate. Losses of hydrogen ions may originate from the stomach (vomiting, nasogastric suction), in the urine (usually in the setting of diuretic therapy in edema states but may also be seen in severe potassium deficiency, renal artery stenosis, carbenoxolone therapy and other conditions giving rise to hyperaldosteronism such as ectopic secretion of adrenocorticotrophic hormone by tumours). Diuretic therapy deserves special mention since it can give rise to alkalosis through a variety of mechanisms; volume depletion, chloride depletion, secondary aldosteronism and potassium depletion.

Bicarbonate excess is an unusual cause of alkalosis and arises from the ingestion of alkalis or substances metabolized to bicarbonate such as lactate and citrate.

Symptoms and signs attributable to the metabolic alkalosis are rarely severe and the major features are likely to relate to the underlying disorder. Vomiting and/or nasogastric suction should be obvious. A drug history is important, relating particularly to diuretics, ingestion of alkalis and organic acid salts (citrate, lactate and acetate) and carbenoxolone. Signs of fluid depletion should be sought. Features of the alkalosis relate to enhancement of calcium binding to proteins; lethargy, twitching and positive Chvostek and Trousseau signs (Chapter 22).

The majority of cases are associated with fluid volume depletion and respond to treatment with saline infusion. The urine chloride concentration is less than 20 mmol/l (and often less than 10 mmol/l). This may not be so after taking a dose of diuretic and urine chloride should be repeated later. Patients without fluid volume depletion are almost invariably potassium depleted and the urine chloride concentration will be greater than 20 mmol/l. Treatment should be aimed at correcting the underlying cause. Fluid deficits and potassium depletion should be corrected. It is very rarely necessary to give intravenous acids.

Respiratory alkalosis

This disorder arises from hyperventilation and is either centrally driven (in hypoxemia, hepatic encephalopathy, gram negative septicemia and CNS dysfunction such as stroke) or is driven by activation of receptors within the lungs (as in pulmonary embolism, congestive cardiac failure, asthma and pneumonia). The fall in hydrogen ion concentration is buffered by non-bicarbonate buffer systems in blood and the plasma bicarbonate concentration rarely falls below 18 mmol/l. If the disorder persists there is a further fall in bicarbonate concentration to between 12 and 15 mmol/l but rarely less. This is due to renal retention of hydrogen ions and a decrease in bicarbonate reabsorption in the proximal convoluted tubule. As the concentration of bicarbonate falls, that of chloride rises.

Clearly, features of likely underlying conditions should be sought (see above). Since respiratory alkalosis may be completely compensated, it may be confused with mixed respiratory alkalosis and metabolic acidosis. The clinical setting is important when faced with this dilemma (see later). Unlike the situation with metabolic alkalosis, features of the alkalosis are often prominent findings. Neuromuscular features may be severe and hypophosphatemia marked. Serious cardiac dysrhythmias may occur.

Treatment is aimed at the underlying condition but if the features of alkalosis are severe, it might be considered reasonable to administer a carbonic anhydrase inhibitor, ammonium chloride or even parenteral hydrochloric acid.

Metabolic acidosis

Metabolic acidosis is characterized by a decrease in the plasma bicarbonate concentration. In the primary disorder this fall in bicarbonate concentration gives rise to acidemia which in turn stimulates ventilation and lowers the pCO_2 as the compensatory response. Metabolic acidosis is frequently associated with other acid-base disturbances and a pH value below 6.9 suggests a co-existing respiratory acidosis. A near normal pH suggests a co-existing respiratory alkalosis.

Metabolic acidosis may be due to an increase in hydrogen ion production, to diminished hydrogen ion excretion and to excessive bicarbonate losses. Acid production is increased in ketotic states (uncontrolled diabetes mellitus, starvation and ethanol intoxication), following certain toxins (e.g. ethylene glycol, methanol and salicylates), following treatment with ammonium chloride and in lactic acidosis. Lactic acidosis is most often seen with overt hypoxia (so-called type A) as might arise in circulatory shock, respiratory failure, cardiac failure and severe anaemia. It may also arise without overt hypoxia (so-called type B) in uncontrolled diabetes mellitus, liver failure, after ethanol and methanol ingestion and after treatment with biguanides – principally phenformin which is no longer available in the UK. Acid excretion may be diminished in renal failure and in renal tubular acidosis types 1 and 4. Bicarbonate losses may be increased in severe or persistent diarrhea, type 2 renal tubular acidosis and with diversion of urine into the gut (ureterosigmoidostomy, vesico-colic fistula and ileal conduit).

Type 1 renal tubular acidosis is characterized by hyperchloremic metabolic acidosis with an alkaline urine. The defect in urinary acidification seems to be located in the distal nephron. Sodium losses in the urine may be profound and be associated with extra-cellular fluid volume concentration and secondary hyperaldosteronism with hypokalemia. In old age it is an acquired disorder associated with chronic urinary obstruction and certain autoimmune disorders including Sjögren's syndrome, systemic lupus erythematosus and primary biliary cirrhosis. It may also be associated with lithium therapy and with nephrocalcinosis.

Type 2 renal tubular acidosis is characterized by defective bicarbonate absorption in the proximal nephron and is very rare in geriatric practice.

Type 4 renal tubular acidosis is a disorder largely confined to adults and arises in association with hypoaldosteronism (common in old age), usually together with some impairment of glomerular filtration. It is most commonly associated with diabetes mellitus with renal involvement, with chronic renal failure of interstitial origin (e.g. in chronic pyelonephritis) and with chronic urinary overflow obstruction. There is also a strong link with chronic treatment with non-steroidal anti-inflammatory drugs (which can cause hyporeninemic hypoaldosteronism. A similar picture may also be seen with potassium sparing diuretics (spironolactone, triamterene and amiloride). The disordered hydrogen ion excretion is attributable to inadequate production of ammonia. The urinary pH is low and there is usually hyperkalemia.

The most useful investigations are the anion gap, the plasma chloride and the plasma potassium concentration. A high anion gap metabolic acidosis occurs in renal failure, ketoacidosis, lactic acidosis and after methanol, ethylene glycol, paraldehyde and salicylate poisoning.

When the plasma chloride is raised, further classification can be made on the basis of the plasma potassium concentration. Hyperkalemia is associated with hypoaldosteronism as may be seen with non-steroidal anti-inflammatory drugs and type 4 renal tubular acidosis. Hypokalemia suggests gastrointestinal losses, urinary diversion procedures, renal tubular acidosis types 1 and 2 and treatment with carbonic anhydrase inhibitors.

Consideration of the clinical setting, following the diagnostic steps just outlined, should allow a reasonably secure diagnosis to be made. The mainstay of treatment is to correct the underlying disorder, if possible. Hyperkalemia may be life threatening and should be managed as described. The decision whether to give alkalis depends on the degree of acidemia. They are almost always needed if the pH falls below 7.2. Remember that diabetic patients can usually generate their own bicarbonate once fluid and insulin treatment have commenced. Intravenous sodium bicarbonate may be given to raise the plasma bicarbonate concentration to about 15 mmol/l. The amount needed in mmol is the difference between plasma bicarbonate concentration and 15 multiplied by half of the body weight in kilograms. Care should be taken to avoid sodium overload, hypokalemia and hypocalcemia. Oral treatment with Shohls solution (citric acid plus sodium citrate) may be used. One ml contains the equivalent of 1 mmol sodium bicarbonate. Potassium citrate can be substituted for the sodium salt if there is hypokalemia. Oral sodium bicarbonate may also be given. Oral alkali treatment is usually needed in types 1 and 2 renal tubular acidosis. Type 4 renal tubular acidosis may respond to mineralocorticoids such as fludrocortisone and may also improve with frusemide treatment. Both drugs decrease hyperkalemia and enhance ammonia production.

Respiratory acidosis

Respiratory acidosis is defined by an elevation in the pCO_2 in the blood. Acutely, the bicarbonate concentration is proportional to the pCO_2 and rarely exceeds 30 mmol/l. Eventually the kidneys increase hydrogen ion excretion and bicarbonate production. There is a further rise in plasma bicarbonate concentration, but rarely above 45 mmol/l. In this situation the expected bicarbonate (in mmol/l) is given by the equation: $0.36 \times pCO_2 + 10$. As the plasma bicarbonate increases, the plasma chloride falls in association with the decrease in renal ammonia excretion.

Causes may be conveniently classified into central (with respiratory depression) and peripheral causes interfering with the mechanics of ventilation. The most important 'central' causes are head injury, major vascular lesions, intracranial neoplasms and overdose of medications suppressing consciousness/ventilation. The commonest 'peripheral' causes in geriatric practice are chest wall disease (e.g. severe scoliosis) and severe pulmonary infections (often with cardiac failure). Less common causes include neuromuscular problems (e.g. myasthenic crisis, Guillain–Barré syndrome), severe asthma, the adult respiratory distress syndrome and the sleep apnea syndromes.

Clinical findings vary from patient to patient. In general, chronic disorders are better tolerated and are associated with fewer symptoms. Symptoms of hypercapnia are attributable to cerebral arterial vasodilatation which increases blood flow and eventually increases intracranial pressure. Findings include headache, drowsiness, stupor and coma. Hyperkalemia occurs but is rarely significant (though it may be useful to help distinguish respiratory acidosis from metabolic alkalosis).

Blood gas findings may suggest co-existing disorders. If the pH is almost normal one should suspect a metabolic alkalosis (e.g. diuretic treatment or vomiting), though respiratory acidosis with pCO_2 below 60 mm Hg may be fully compensated.

Treatment is directed towards the underlying cause where possible. Carbon dioxide retention is most effectively treated by assisted ventilation and should be considered in acute respiratory acidosis. Parenteral bicarbonate treatment has little role to play but may be used if the pH is very low and there is no immediate access to a ventilator. Chronic carbon dioxide retention is usually well tolerated and the acidemia is rarely severe. These patients are often very difficult to wean from ventilators and other means should be sought where possible.

Mixed acid-base disorders

Respiratory and metabolic acidosis

This is suggested by a very low pH, low bicarbonate (metabolic acidosis), high pCO_2 and high anion gap. It most commonly occurs with severe pulmonary edema, severe chronic airflow obstruction, drug overdose and with cardiopulmonary arrest. These are all conditions giving rise to respiratory acidosis and the metabolic component is due to poor perfusion causing excessive lactate production.

Respiratory and metabolic alkalosis

This combination is suggested by a high pH, low pCO_2 and a normal or high bicarbonate. It is most likely to arise in the setting of pneumonia with vomiting, diuretic treatment in liver failure and in patients on ventilators with nasogastric suction.

Respiratory acidosis and metabolic alkalosis

This mixed disorder is most often seen in patients with chronic airflow limitation who are also taking diuretics. The clue to a mixed disorder is that compensatory responses for primary disorders are greater than expected. The pH is usually near normal. The pCO_2 is higher than expected as compensation for metabolic alkalosis (i.e. >60 mm Hg) and bicarbonate is higher than would be expected as compensation for respiratory acidosis (i.e. >45 mmol/l).

Respiratory alkalosis and metabolic acidosis

The pH is usually (but not always!) near normal. The pCO_2 and bicarbonate are both decreased. The bicarbonate is rarely below 18 mmol/l as compensation for respiratory alkalosis. This mixed disorder is most often seen with pulmonary embolism and in shock states, particularly septic shock.

Metabolic acidosis and alkalosis

This disorder should be suspected if the pCO_2 and bicarbonate are inappropriate for the clinical situation. The bicarbonate may be near normal in diabetic ketoacidosis or renal failure, especially with a high anion gap. This mixed disorder is most often seen in patients with a long-standing metabolic acidosis (e.g. renal failure) who develop vomiting, or in those with a long-standing metabolic alkalosis (e.g. long-term diuretic therapy associated with the development of diabetic ketoacidosis).

Suggested reading

Adlcr, S., Lindeman, R. D., Yiengst, M. J., Beard, E. and Shock, N. W. (1968). Effect of acute loading on urinary acid excretion by the aging human kidney. *J. Lab. Clin. Med.*, **72**: 278–89.

Rubin, S., Tack, M. and Cherniack, N. S. (1982). Effect of aging on the respiratory responses to CO_2 and inspiratory resistance loads. *J. Geront.*, **37**: 306–12.

22

Abnormalities of serum calcium

The serum ionized calcium in a healthy individual is maintained constant within a narrow range throughout the different times of the day and different dietary conditions. This constancy is mainly the result of a complex interaction between parathyroid hormone (PTH), 1,25 dihydroxycalciferol and calcitonin. Other variables which influence calcium regulation are glucocorticoids, thyroid hormone, prostaglandins, interleukins and growth-stimulating factors.

PTH increases serum calcium by: increasing bone resorption; increasing distal tubule resorption of calcium; stimulation of 1,25 dihydroxycalciferol production; and decreasing renal tubular resorption of phosphate. The synthesis of vitamin D is complex but basically 7-dehydrocholesterol is converted in the skin to vitamin D by ultraviolet light, which is then hydroxylated in the liver to 25 hydroxycalciferol. Finally this is converted to the active hormone, 1,25 dihyroxycalciferol, in the kidney. This final step is stimulated by low serum calcium levels mediated through PTH. At physiological levels the major effect of 1,25 dihydroxycalciferol is to increase intestinal absorption of calcium. Calcitonin is secreted in response to hypercalcemia and acts to reduces serum calcium levels by decreasing bone resorption. It has a relatively minor role to play in the maintenance of serum calcium levels.

1. Aging and calcium regulation

With aging there appears to be an increase in the level of PTH necessary to maintain a normal serum calcium. This may be compensatory to a reduction in PTH mediated 1,25 dihydroxycalciferol production secondary to a smaller renal mass.

Serum levels of 1,25 dihydroxycalciferol are normal with aging but there is evidence of a blunting of responsiveness to PTH or a low serum calcium. Serum 25 hydroxycalciferol levels are commonly lower in the elderly probably secondary to dietary factors and reduced sun exposure.

2. Hypocalcemia

Definition and Pathophysiology

Normal serum calcium concentrations range between 8.8 and 10.4 mg/dL (2.2 to 2.6 mM). Approximately 45 per cent is bound to serum proteins, 5 per cent is complexed with anions and 50 per cent is ionized. It is the ionized fraction which affects cellular function and is normally maintained between 4.8 to 5.42 mg/dL (1.2 to 1.3 mM). The proportion of ionized to total calcium is affected by not only the amount of protein- and anion-binding to ionized calcium but also by the pH of the blood. Acidosis decreases protein-binding and alkalosis increases it. Changes in pH therefore modify the symptoms of hypocalcemia thus tetany is more likely at an alkaline pH. Changes in K and Mg concentration also alter the response to calcium. Hypocalcemia can be defined as a serum calcium of less than 8.8 mg/dL (2.2 mM) or ionized calcium less than 4.4 mg/dL (1.1 mM).

The finding of a low serum calcium is common in the frail elderly but most are an artifact of a low serum albumin. The commonest causes of hypocalcemia in the elderly are abnormalities of vitamin D (osteomalacia or renal rickets) and parathyroid hormone (PTH) status. The commonest causes of a deficiency in PTH are: surgical; drugs such as calcitonin, diphosphonates and cytotoxic agents; and acute pancreatitis. Less common causes are idiopathic, severe magnesium deficiency and hyperphosphatemia. Rarely a PTH resistance state exists, pseudohypoparathyroidism.

Subjective

Symptoms depend not only on the level of blood calcium but also on the rate at which it develops and the time for which it persists.

A rapid onset of hypocalcemia is associated with neuromuscular excitability which may lead to painful spasms of the small muscles of the hands and feet. So-called 'tetany equivalents' are more common and comprise peripheral and peri-oral paresthesia and muscle cramps. Fits are uncommon in adults. Movement disorders such as Parkinsonism, chorea and athetosis may be seen. Psychiatric changes include irritability, depression and even frank psychosis.

Within a week or two some adaption occurs, but the above symptoms may re-emerge under stress (e.g. acute infection). More gradual onset of hypocalcemia is associated with ectodermal changes such as cataracts, skin rashes and brittle nails which are peculiarly sensitive to candida infections. Headaches are common and if associated with papilloedema, the syndrome is known as pseudotumour cerebri. Calcification of the basal ganglia may further confuse the picture.

Objective

The major objective finding is a low calcium level after correcting for serum albumin. Trousseau's sign of painful carpal spasms produced by occlusion of blood supply to the arm may be present.

Another classical sign is Chvostek's sign which is demonstrated by percussing the facial nerve in front of the ear and is regarded as positive if the mouth twitches. These signs may be positive in normal people, in those with hypomagnesemia and those with alkalosis. They may occasionally be negative in patients with severe hypocalcemia.

A prolonged Q–T interval on the ECG and slow wave activity on the EEG.

Assessment

The information required for assessment is usually available from the initial screen. In the presence of hypocalcemia it is recommended that the serum phosphate, serum albumin, alkaline phosphate and serum magnesium be measured and that renal function be assessed.

Plan

Diagnosis

The clinical setting may be of very great importance in the interpretation of hypocalcemia. If it is found in the setting of thyroid or parathyroid surgery, many diagnostic steps can be passed over. Cytotoxic therapy and rhabdomyolysis are usually obvious.

If no clue is apparent from the clinical setting, a logical approach should be applied. The first step is to ensure that the hypocalcemia is not due to magnesium deficiency (since it may be cured by adminstration of magnesium salts). Older patients seem particularly susceptible, usually in the setting of diuretic therapy, diarrhea or alcohol abuse. Although this is rare, it is a condition that requires different treatment and it is important to exclude.

If there is no magnesium deficiency, renal function should be examined. As the glomerular filtration rate (GFR) falls the plasma phosphate will tend to rise and calcium fall. This stimulates PTH secretion which restores the calcium level to normal. As the GFR falls to around 40 ml/min there is some impairment of 21-hydroxylation of vitamin D in the kidney. The calcium level therefore falls which further stimulates the parathyroid glands. One would therefore expect to find a raised urea and creatinine associated with raised phosphate and evidence of chronic renal failure.

In the absence of renal failure, a raised plasma phosphate may help to elucidate the problem. Again, the result is often already to hand. Phosphate administration via the oral, rectal or intravenous routes are the most likely causes, though it may occur in patients on cytotoxic chemotherapy or who have rhabomylysis.

If the patient has a normal serum alkaline phosphatase level, the possible diagnoses include primary hypoparathyroidism (confirmed by measuring PTH levels), pancreatitis (confirmed by the clinical setting and serum amylase estimation), chelating agent administration (usually obvious) or raised calcitonin levels (either exogenous or endogenous).

A raised alkaline phosphatase is suggestive of osteomalacia from whatever cause and will usually be associated with a low phosphate. A check for anticonvulsant therapy is easy. The history may suggest malabsorption. A bone scan is useful at this stage. The diagnosis of osteomalacia may be confirmed by bone biopsy or a trial of therapy. If a cause has not yet been determined it is likely that dietary deficiency of vitamin D is responsible.

Further tests are indicated depending on the findings and include measuring serum PTH levels, vitamin D metabolites or performing bone biopsy.

Treatment

If the situation is urgent (tetany, distressing involuntary movements) give 40 ml of 10 per cent calcium gluconate in 500 ml of fluid over 4 to 6 hours. Convulsions or laryngospasm warrant direct injection of 10 ml of 10 per cent calcium gluconate over 10 minutes (20 minutes in hypokalemic patients or those on digoxin because of the risk of ventricular fibrillation). No amount of calcium will help hypomagnesemic patients and this must be corrected by intramuscular magnesium.

In less urgent situations, therapy is aimed at the underlying cause (chelating agents, calcitonin and phosphates should be stopped). Renal osteodystrophy is treated with aluminum hydroxide gels to bind gut phosphate. Vitamin D is usually required. The dose is tailored to the patient's needs and changes should not be made at less than 6-weekly intervals. Patients stabilized on a particular dose may be destabilized by thiazide administration. Regular follow-up of stable patients (at least 6-monthly) are needed to detect toxicity. It is essential to watch for deteriorating renal function. If vitamin D is withdrawn, follow up should continue for at least one year before deciding it is no longer needed.

If phosphate is being given, it should be stopped. When hyper-phosphatemia is associated with chemotherapy it is treated symptomatically. It is due to tumour lysis and is self-limiting. Any chelating agents should be stopped. Hypoparathyroidism is treated with vitamin D by titrating the dose. The treatment of malabsorption is discussed elsewhere. The need for anticonvulsants must be reassessed. Since they are usually needed, vitamin D therapy will be given at the same time. Dietary deficiency of vitamin D can usually be successfully treated with calcium and vitamin D tablets BPC (two per day) and the situation checked in three months. Other causes of hypocalcemia will usually demand referral for a specialist opinion.

3. Hypercalcemia

This is said to be present when the serum calcium (after correction for the serum albumin level) exceeds the upper limit of normal (10.4 mg/dL or 2.6 mM). Hypercalcemia may be an unsuspected abnormality detected on routine biochemical screening or it may be suspected because of symptoms. The causes of hypercalcemia in the elderly are summarized in Table 22.1. The two commonest causes of hypercalcemia are hyperparathyroidism and malignant disease, and these are found with comparable frequencies. Vitamin D toxicosis and thyrotoxicosis are uncommon and other causes are rare. False hypercalcemia can arise from hemoconcentration and rarely in some cases of myeloma where the abnormal immunoglobulin binds calcium strongly.

Table 22.1 Causes of hypercalcemia in the elderly

Increased bone resorption
primary hyperparathyroidism
tertiary hyperparathyroidism
metastatic malignancy
humoral hypercalcemia of malignancy
immobilization
hyperthyroidism
Increased intestinal absorption
vitamin D toxicity
sarcoidosis
milk-alkali syndrome
Other's
Addison's disease
recovery phase of acute renal failure

Subjective

Below about 2.8 mmol/L, hypercalcemia is frequently asymptomatic, though renal stones may develop and may be passed in the urine. Above this level, the frequency of symptoms increases. These include vague aches and pains in the bones, abdominal pain and constipation. Polyuria, ocular discomfort and muscle weakness are not rare. Mental changes are often overlooked. Above a level of 3.25 mmol/L, renal function may progressively deteriorate with the patient presenting in renal failure. Patients with primary or tertiary hyperparathyroidism with florid bone disease may present with pathological fractures through brown tumours.

The severity and rate of onset of the hypercalcemia often gives a clue to the etiology. Mild, prolonged elevations of calcium are usually due to hyperparathyroidism and less commonly hyperthyroidism and sarcoidosis. In contrast severe and rapid elevation of calcium is usually due to malignancy or one of the other causes when dehydration is superadded to the picture.

Objective

A raised calcium level following an uncuffed venepuncture is the main finding. Physical signs are frequently absent. Corneal calcification may be apparent, although slit lamp examination is usually required to demonstrate it. Muscle weakness may be observed in severe hypercalcemia. Brown tumours may be palpable in patients with primary or tertiary hyperparathyroidism, although this is rare.

The ECG may show shortening of the Q–T interval.

Assessment

The information to make a diagnosis will normally be available from a thorough history and examination together with a blood count, ESR and biochemical profile. In some cases, the diagnostic process must give way to urgent therapeutic intervention (to be described later). Some investigations are obligatory in cases of hypercalcemia while others are suggested by the results of these. Additional investigations including serum PTH, serum magnesium or bone scan may be indicated depending upon the findings

Plan

Diagnosis

The steps to follow are straightforward. Vitamin D ingestion may be immediately obvious or only diagnosed by assaying the level of 25-OH D3. Patients with sarcoidosis (tuberculosis and berylliosis) are hypersensitive to vitamin D. Hypercalcemia in renal failure may occur in the setting of alkali ingestion (milk-alkali syndrome), vitamin D administration or as a pre-terminal event.

Lithium therapy will be obvious. Hypercalcemia in association with adrenal failure is usually associated with characteristic electrolyte abnormalities and signs of volume depletion.

Familial hypocalciuric hypercalcemia (FHH) may be very difficult to distinguish from primary hyperparathyroidism and may present late in life. It is a benign disorder which is not associated with progressive renal impairment. A useful feature to aid diagnosis is that hypermagnesemia and hypomagnesuria also occur.

It is believed that immobility (especially in patients with Paget's disease of bone) can lead to the development of hypercalcemia which responds to mobilization. Other rare causes include the administration of drugs such as gonadal steroids and tamoxifen and vitamin A toxicity. Vitamin A stimulates osteoclasts which cause resorption of bone. Clinical features include painful hyperostoses (especially in the shafts of long bones), tendon calcification, skin peeling, angular stomatitis, peripheral neuropathy, alopecia and localized areas of skin pigmentation.

Malignant disease may be obvious or very difficult to diagnose. Only very general guidelines can be given here. It may give rise to hypercalcemia in several different ways. Bony metastases can cause local resorption of bone, probably via locally released chemical substances. Prostaglandins (especially E2) have recently been implicated and it might be anticipated that prostaglandin synthetase inhibitors (e.g. indomethacin) will be of value here. Myeloma (and occasionally prostatic carcinoma and lymphoma) secretes osteoclast activating factor (OAF) which stimulates osteoclasts to mobilize calcium. This is usually associated with a normal serum calcium. Calcitonin is a specific inhibitor of this mediator and is the drug of choice to control hypercalcemia in myeloma. Ectopic secretion of PTH-like peptides (usually by squamous carcinomas) is a well-documented cause of hypercalcemia.

Treatment

Serum calcium levels below 3 mmol/L often require no intravenous therapy. Above this, intravenous hydration with sodium chloride will be needed in most cases. Frusemide has been used in doses up to 120 mg 3 hourly, but this requires very strict fluid and electrolyte balance studies. Fluid regimens may not be appropriate in patients with renal or cardiac failure, in which case, there are two other major lines of attack. One is to reduce calcium absorption and the other is to inhibit osteolysis. The former can be achieved with oral phosphates and glucocorticoids. Most cases of severe hypercalcemia are due to osteolysis. Mobilisation from bone can be inhibited (calcitonin, mithramycin); calcium can be chelated (diphosphonates, inorganic phosphate) and calcium can be removed by dialysis. Calcitonin would be preferred over mithramycin in patients with myeloma or lymphoma, but its results are unpredictable in other situations.

If phosphates are given, 50 mmol of neutral sodium phosphate buffer are infused over 6–8 hours. This causes an immediate fall in the plasma calcium and this continues for several hours. This treatment should not be given more frequently than once in 24 hours. Complications include metastatic calcification, hypocalcemia, hypotension and acute renal failure.

Oral treatment is used in mild hypercalcemia and comprises hydration and oral phosphate administration. Phosphate may cause metastatic calcification, nausea, diarrhea and fluid retention. Oral diphosphonates are a useful alternative.

Primary hyperparathyroidism is traditionally treated by surgery. However, the natural history of asymptomatic hyperparathyroidism is unknown. Some workers are beginning to adopt a conservative approach to these patients, especially the elderly.

Suggested reading

Adams, P. H. (1982). Conservative management of primary hyperparathyroidism. *J. Royal Col. Phys. Lond.*, **16**: 184–90.

Becker, K. L. (1978). Hypercalcaemic emergencies – how to proceed. *Drug Therapy (Hosp.)*, May, pp. 12–13.

Fisken, R. A., Heath, D. A., Somers, S. (1981). Hypercalcemia in hospital patients. *Lancet*, **1**: 202–207.

Hodkinson, H. M. and McPherson, C. K. (1973). Alkaline phosphatase in a geriatric inpatient population. *Age and Ageing*, **3**: 76.

Kallis, J. A. (ed.) (1982). Hypercalcemia. Aetiology and medical management. *Metab. Bone Dis. and Rel. Res.*, **2**(3), pp. 00–00

23

Abnormal liver function test

Liver function tests and aging

The liver appears to decrease in size with advancing age. Hepatic drug metabolism alters only slightly with age (hepatic oxidative microsomal pathways), the half life being prolonged for many drugs, but this does not appear to be of great clinical significance. The liver function tests that are routinely performed are not good indicators of liver function. The tests are relatively crude and indicate damage to the liver which does not correlate with function. In some situations liver enzyme elevation may indicate extensive damage to hepatocytes but liver function with regard to drug metabolism may continue unaffected. The normal range for bilirubin (<26 umol/l) does not change with advancing age.

Aspartate aminotransferase, AST (glutamic oxaloacetate transaminase) and alanine aminotransferase, ALT (glutamic pyruvic transaminase) are found in liver as well as skeletal and cardiac muscle. It is said that ALT is more specific to the liver, but in practice although two tests are usually performed one would suffice. The range for transaminases is the same in old age as in younger age groups, there being no difference in the standard assay or after stimulation with pyridoxal 5-phosphate.

There is no evidence that the normal range for alkaline phosphatase changes with advancing age. Surveys of the elderly, have revealed that a proportion have elevated values above the upper limit of normal. However investigation of such patients usually reveals underlying problems.

Gamma glutamyl transpeptidase (Gamma GT) is of liver origin, and there is no change in normal range with advancing age. It is one of the more sensitive tests of liver dysfunction. The enzyme is increased with the administration of certain drugs. This enzyme is used in many places to determine if elevated alkaline phosphatase is of liver origin. This test has replaced the need to do alkaline phosphatase isoenzymes or ribonucleotidase.

Serum albumin is produced in the liver. The normal range in the healthy elderly is the same as in younger age groups. Albumin may be reduced by a number of different conditions including malnutrition, nephrotic syndrome, protein losing enteropathy, infection and chronic liver disease. It is of limited value as a liver function test, although it will be reduced in the presence of cirrhosis or chronic hepatitis. It is of some value in younger age groups in determining the chronicity of hepatitis.

There are other tests of liver function, for example bromsulphthalein retention test, but none of real value in geriatric practice. None of these would be indicated without clear clinical pointers from the examination and history.

Jaundice

Jaundice is defined as an elevation of Bilirubin above the normal range. An elevated bilirubin, 'jaundice', should be approached in the same way as in younger age groups, the appropriate diagnostic tests being dictated by the pattern of elevation of the other liver function tests.

Values of serum bilirubin above the normal range are usually detectable as clinical jaundice. It should be remembered that in some elderly patients with aged sclerae that take on a yellow tinge, this becomes more difficult. Thus values that would be detectable clinically in younger people may go unnoticed in the elderly. In the same way jaundice is sometimes suspected and biochemical tests reveal that this is not the case.

The etiology, diagnosis and treatment of jaundice or disturbed liver function is the same in the elderly as in other age groups, with the proviso that associated disease burden may modify approach.

As the data base is gathered it is important to be aware of the different types of jaundice and their relative frequency in old age (Table 23.1). Jaundice can be classified as:

1. Unconjugated Hyperbilirubinemia, which would include hemolytic causes
2. Hepatocellular – essentially hepatitis, cirrhosis and metastatic cancer
3. Cholestatic – which includes intrahepatic cholestasis and obstructive jaundice.

Table 23.1 Types of jaundice

Early problem definition of jaundice	Groupings for diagnosis	Highest level problem solution
Unconjugated	Hereditary enzyme deficiency,	Gilbert's
	Hemolytic	Drugs
Hepatic	Acute hepatitis	Viral (Hepatitis B)
		Drugs
		Alcohol
	Chronic liver disease	Alcohol
		Idiopathic (Cryptogenic)
		Genetic (iron)
	Malignancy	Primary
		Metastatic
Cholestatic	Intrahepatic chronic liver disease	Drugs
		Primary biliary cirrhosis
	Obstructive	Stones
		Cancer (type and site)

From studies that have been done unconjugated hyperbilirubinemia is uncommon comprising 2 to 5 per cent of patients with jaundice over the age of 65. The other two groups are approximately equally divided in most of the series. The most frequent single cause is difficult to define but it would appear that malignancy with associated obstruction is slightly more common than gall stones.

Subjective

If the patient has been aware of jaundice then the duration needs to be determined. In considering the possible causes it is important to make a detailed and accurate inquiry from the patient or care provider about drugs, including non-prescription items, about alcohol intake and of course about previous surgery and blood transfusion. Alcoholic liver disease may be difficult to recognize in the elderly patient, because of denial, the inability to give a history or in some because of a documented intake that appears to be small. Alcohol related problems are of increasing concern amongst elderly patients and is one that is more frequently recognized in our practices. It would appear that alcoholic liver disease presents in a similar way to younger age groups and with similar associated problems.

Associated symptoms like pruritus and pain should be looked for. Pruritus is a common problem with geriatric patients and may be unrelated. Pain is not a good discriminator between stones and malignancy, and may be absent when stones are present and may be quite significant with malignant obstruction. However the finding of typical biliary colic would point to biliary calculi.

Objective

As noted above jaundice may be apparent on examination. General examination may reveal some of the stigmata of chronic liver disease, or other signs of liver failure like hepatic encephalopathy or fluid retention. Abdominal examination is mandatory and may reveal the presence of an enlarged liver, ascites or the presence of a mass within the liver or elsewhere, due to an enlarged gall bladder or pancreatic carcinoma for example. There may be signs of pruritus with extensive scratch marks.

Assessment

The approach to diagnosis, and the treatment of jaundice will be influenced by the likely etiology (Table 23.1 and Fig. 23.1). This in turn will be determined by the nature of the abnormal liver function tests and will therefore be dealt with as the different patterns are discussed.

High Transaminases

Any type of liver injury will cause elevation of the transaminases but the degree of elevation may indicate the nature of the liver problem. For example very high values of a thousand or more are said only to occur as a result of viral hepatitis. Other

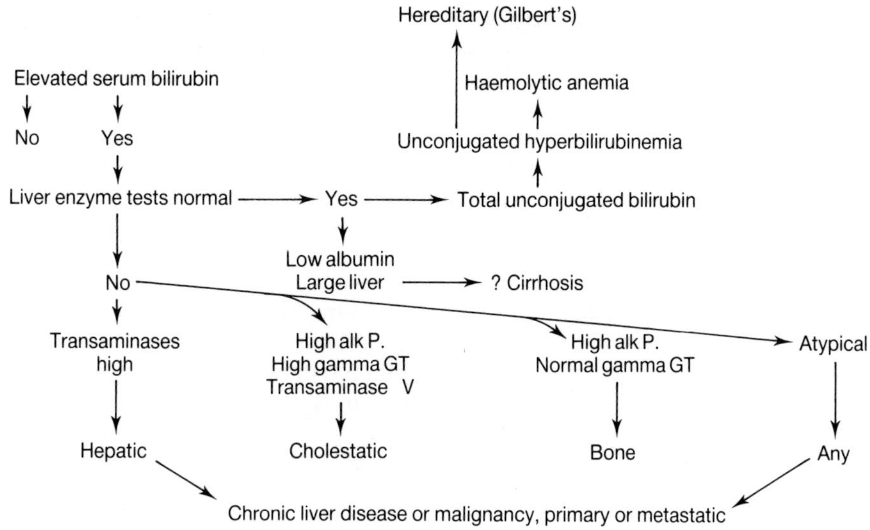

Fig. 23.1 Diagnostic approach – jaundice.

types of hepatitis, secondary to drugs for example, will cause significant but lower elevations. Values two or three times the normal upper limit are found in patients with predominantly obstructive problems. It should be remembered that these are simply guidelines and exceptions do occur.

If there is marked elevation of the serum transaminases then the problem is likely hepatocellular, and the most important etiological factors in this age group are alcohol, drugs and viruses. Chronic liver disease such as cirrhosis and chronic hepatitis can also elevate the liver enzymes. These possibilities will need to be confirmed by the use of appropriate tests such as serum for hepatitis B antigen, liver and spleen scan or liver biopsy (Table 23.2). When serum lactate dehydrogenase is also markedly elevated then metastatic cancer in the liver is a strong possibility, and this will need to be confirmed by appropriate testing which would include liver scanning (ultrasound, isotope or computerized tomography) and liver biopsy. Performance of such tests is dictated by the need to know the diagnosis, and whether management will be affected. When the clinical situation is such that the patient is obviously very ill then further definitive testing may well not be indicated.

Table 23.2 Atypical pattern of enzyme elevation

1. Serological investigations
   - viral hepatitis screen
   - iron, IBC, ferritin
   - alpha fetoprotein
   - antibodies
2. Scan
   - ultrasound or radioisotope
3. Further investigations
   - liver biopsy
   - visualization (CAT, ERCP, etc.)
   - bone scan
   - bone marrow

Serological tests are easy to perform and carry no increased risk. Liver biopsy should be done if this will help in the management of the patient. The normal routine of ensuring the absence of any bleeding tendency and that prothrombin time is normal, is done first. Needle biopsy carries no increased risk in the elderly population. A test that is likely to yield a definitive answer is preferred to a battery of less invasive tests that will never yield definitive results. Of course all tests are only worthwhile if the management of the patient is helped, and should never be done if the result will not affect decision making. For example in the question of metastatic cancer, when this looks a likely diagnosis yet the patient's condition is such that chemotherapy or surgery are not to be considered, further invasive testing should not be contemplated. On the other hand invasive tests are indicated if likely to help and the therapeutic possibilities remain open.

High Alkaline Phosphatase and Gamma GT (cholestasis)

A serum alkaline phosphatase value above the

upper limit of normal should be investigated. Modest elevation can be found in the presence of disease elsewhere, for example pneumonia. When the value is found to be elevated the first question is the site of origin of the alkaline phosphatase – bone or liver. Determination of the isoenzymes will reveal which is the case. The gamma GT if also elevated would support the conclusion that the elevated alkaline phosphatase is from the liver. An elevated alkaline phosphatase with normal gamma GT points to the possibility of bone disease.

Both alkaline phosphatase and gamma GT may be elevated nonspecifically and modestly in the presence of a variety of liver problems. It is therefore important to look carefully at the other liver function tests. It should also be remembered that patients may have abnormal liver function tests with only modest elevation of the gamma GT and very high alkaline phosphatase. In this situation one may be dealing with coexistent disease, for example the presence of hepatitis and associated Paget's Disease of bone.

The finding of a high alkaline phosphatase and gamma GT with only modest elevation of the other enzymes indicates that cholestasis is present. The purpose of further investigation is to determine the nature of the problem and specifically whether there is an intrahepatic cause or whether there is a mechanical obstruction (Fig. 23.2 and Fig. 23.3). The course of investigation depends upon the nature of the presentation. If the finding is a result of routine blood testing, with no significant history then the approach might be to arrange for further serological testing. For example by looking for autoantibodies – specifically antimitochondrial antibody – in this way primary biliary cirrhosis (PBC) or cryptogenic cirrhosis may be uncovered. Antimitochondrial antibody would appear to be specific for PBC and an extremely useful test. Routine screening will detect an unexpected number of elderly patients with asymptomatic PBC. If the patient has presented with non specific decline or the presence of jaundice then antibody screening tests will be performed but the next investigation should be ultrasonography looking closely at the diameter of the bile duct.

Patients who are shown to have mechanical obstruction may also have the site and nature of the obstruction revealed by ultrasonography. The investigation is usually successful and elderly patients do not present any major problem. It is important to recognize that this is so and that a significant number of elderly patients with biochemical evidence of cholestasis with dilated bile

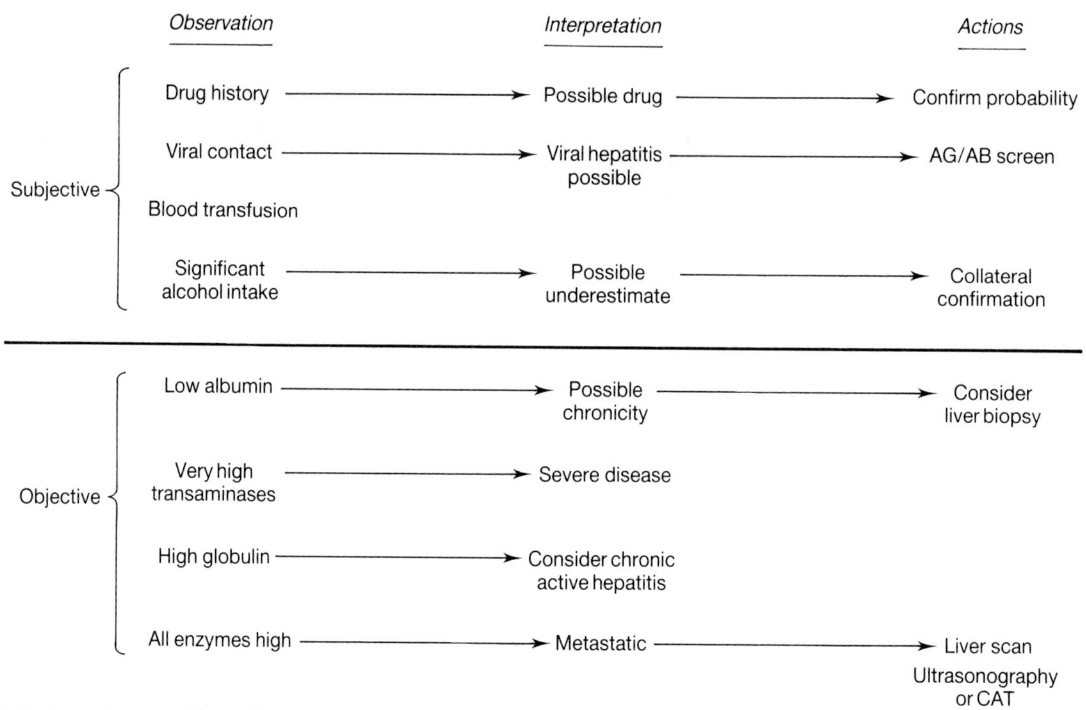

Fig. 23.2 Investigation of hepatic group.

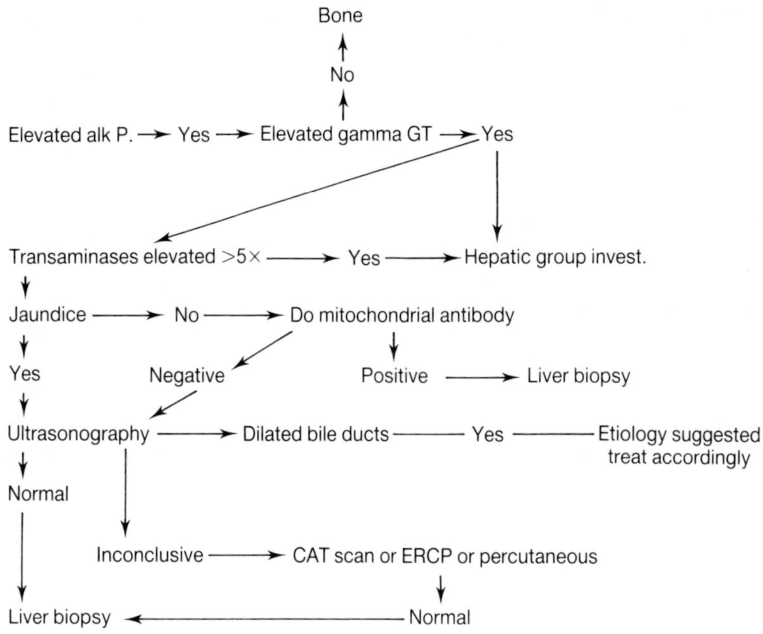

Fig. 23.3 Investigation of cholestatic group.

ducts have a surgically correctable cause. Ultrasound may not be definitive and in that case further investigation will be necessary. The nature of further testing depends upon the expertise and the resources that are available locally – for example endoscopic retrograde cholangiopancreatography, percutaneous transhepatic cholangiography or computerized axial tomography. All of these tests are valuable, although the latter is non-invasive and to be preferred for that reason. Again there appear to be no special risks or problems with the elderly patient.

High Alkaline Phosphatase

When the alkaline phosphatase is elevated and the rest of the liver function tests are normal then the likely origin is bone. There may well be clinical pointers that would support this hypothesis. For example, bone pain in the case of Paget's disease, or muscle stiffness with osteomalacia. In the case of osteoporosis there will only be an elevated alkaline phosphatase when there is a complication like fracture. The degree of elevation points to the likely cause – very high levels, >1000 U/L, for example being characteristic of Paget's disease. Confirmation of bone disease is obtained by performing appropriate skeletal radiographs, bone scanning and if necessary bone biopsy. Additional biochemical data is sought such as the serum calcium level, acid phosphatase level, urinary hydroxy proline excretion and serum PTH level, to clarify the likely nature of the underlying bone problem.

There is a real difference in the incidence of osteomalacia between the Old and the New World. High alkaline phosphatase of boney origin is not uncommon in the UK but is much less common in the elderly patient in Canada.

Treatment

Therapy will be dictated by the diagnosis. There is no reason to modify approach in the elderly except because of associated disease burden.

When drug sensitivity is suspected then the drug should be stopped immediately. Test administration of the drug should only rarely be considered necessary.

If viral hepatitis is confirmed then appropriate precautions need to be followed and the patient is treated conservatively and followed. There is no evidence that viral hepatitis is an important problem with the institutionalized elderly.

When gall stones are found obstructing the common bile duct or producing any other complications, appropriate treatment is indicated. Endoscopic removal may be possible and is useful for some elderly patients. The lithotripter is also likely to play an important role in those elderly unfit for surgery although at the present time this is only considered for those with 3 or fewer stones within the gall bladder.

Patients with metastatic cancer rarely need other than palliative therapy. At the present time, for most types of metastatic cancer surgery, radiotherapy and chemotherapy have nothing to offer. Palliative techniques for relief of jaundice may be possible with endoscopy, for example the placing of prosthetic tubes within bile ducts for drainage of bile. Such technology has the potential to be of great benefit to the elderly patient when major abdominal surgery can be avoided.

Suggested reading

Coles, J. A., Beynon, G. P. J. and Lees, W. R. (1982). The use of ultrasound in geriatric medicine. *Age and Ageing*, **11**, 145–52.

Eastwood, H. D. (1971). Causes of jaundice in the elderly: a survey of diagnosis and investigations. *Gerontol. Clin.*, **13**: 69–81.

Hodkinson, H. M. and McPherson, C. K. (1973) Alkaline – Phosphatase in a geriatric inpatient population. *Age and Ageing*, **3**, 76.

Huete-Armijo, A. and Exton Smith A. N. (1962). Causes and diagnosis of jaundice in the elderly. *Br. Med. J.*, **283**, 521–3.

James, O., MacKlon, A. F., Watson, A. J. (1981). Primary biliary cirrhosis – a revised clinical spectrum. *Lancet* **i**: 1275–7.

Munoz, L. E., Thomas, H. C., Scheuer, P. J., Doniach, D. and Sherlock, S. (1981). Is mitochondrial antibody diagnostic of primary biliary cirrhosis? *Gut*, **22**: 136–40.

Naso, F., Thompson, C. M. (1967). Hyperbilirubinemia in the patient past 50. *Geriatrics*, **22**, 206–12.

O'Brien, G. F. and Tan, C. V. (1970). Jaundice in the geriatric patient. *Geriatrics*, **25**, 114–27.

O'Malley, K., Stevenson, I. H., Ward, C. A., Wood, A. S. and Crooks, J. (1977) Determinants of anticoagulant control in patients receiving warfarin. *Brit. J. Clin. Pharmacol.*, **4**: 309–14.

Shepherd, A. M. M., Wilson, N. and Stevenson, I. H. (1977). Age as a determinant of sensitivity. *Brit. J. Clin. Pharmacol.* **4**: 309–20.

Succari, M., Ponteziere, C., Meneguzzer, E., Desmoulins, D., Amoros le-fay, A., Mioque, M. and Boy, P. (1987). Aminotransferases in elderly people: influence of pyridoxal 5-phosphate addition on the determination of aminotransferases in healthy elderly subjects. *Age and Ageing*, **16**, 94–100.

Woodhouse, K. W., Mutch, E., Williams, F. M., Rawlins, M. D. and James, O. F. W. (1984). The effect of age on pathways of drug metabolism in human liver. *Age and Ageing*, **13**: 328–34.

Woodhouse, K. W., James, O. F. W. (1985). Alcoholic liver disease in the elderly; presentation and outcome. *Age and Aging*, **14**, 113–18.

24

Abnormal blood glucose

The blood glucose level should be determined as part of the assessment of geriatric patients. The normal range of blood glucose varies throughout the day depending upon the timing of previous meals and the length of time fasting. Thus measurement of a random blood sugar without knowledge of previous food intake is of little help – unless grossly abnormal.

Fasting venous blood glucose levels should be below 7 mmol/litre. Values above this are considered abnormal, hyperglycemia. The level should not be below 3.5 mmol/litre, and if it is this is referred to as hypoglycemia. Hyper- and hypo-glycemia are not infrequent findings in geriatric practice and both require further assessment and further treatment.

The patient with sustained hyperglycemia has diabetes mellitus. This is usually divided into two types:

1. Type 1 insulin dependent diabetes mellitus which is mainly a disease of younger age groups and is characterized by an abrupt onset with ketoacidosis and insulin dependence.
2. Type 2 non-insulin dependent diabetes. This is more likely to have an insidious onset in older individuals, the patients are not dependent upon insulin, although they may benefit from it and do not develop ketoacidosis.

Hyperglycemia

Mild glucose intolerance occurs with increasing frequency with advancing age and this has been well recognized since its first description in the 1920s. The fasting blood glucose rises by approximately 0.14 mmol/litre per decade after the age of 50. Two fasting blood glucose values of greater than 8.5 mmol/litre or a random blood glucose of greater than 12 mmol/litre represent criteria for the diagnosis of diabetes mellitus.

Much of the glucose intolerance that occurs with advancing age is related to the increase of adipose tissue. There are no consistent changes in the pancreatic islets nor in insulin secretion. However serum insulin levels tend to rise with age which is interpreted as being due to more insulin resistance, less insulin degradation and decreased removal. Thus the slight rise in insulin levels that occurs is predominantly post-receptor and multifactorial.

Diabetes mellitus is diagnosed more frequently with advancing age and has a prevalence of about 6.9 per cent in men and 8.9 per cent in women over the age of 65 in the United States. It represents one of the major chronic disorders that affect the elderly population and the diagnosis is often delayed due to its insidious onset. The complications of diabetes are common and result in morbidity and frequent hospitalization.

It is commonly stated that those individuals with marginal hyperglycemia are not at any increased risk of diabetic complications. However, it is thought that glycosylation of proteins occurs in association with the hyperglycemia of aging. Indeed, protein glycosylation is thought to play a role in the pathogenesis of microvascular disease and therefore plays a central role in aging effects. There is an increased risk of cardiovascular disease in those individuals with the glucose intolerance of aging. It should also be noted that there is an increase in glycosylated hemoglobin levels in elderly subjects with normal glucose levels and normal glucose tolerance.

Subjective

Hyperglycemia produces an osmotic diuresis. This results in polyuria and thirst secondary to the dehydration, which are two of the classical symptoms of diabetes mellitus. Polyuria may, however, be difficult to distinguish from the nocturia that is so common in the elderly. Thirst may also be difficult to detect as it may pass unnoticed by some aged individuals. There are other non-specific symptoms such as weight loss, lethargy and fatigue which are frequently seen but many other conditions can cause these as well.

Unfortunately, diabetes in the elderly is more likely to present with symptoms of one or more of the many complications that may occur. For example, genital candidiasis, visual problems, neuritic pain, vascular complications or foot problems.

The pathophysiological changes that occur as a result of the sustained hyperglycemia may lead to profound dehydration and hypotension. The patient may decline in function resulting in a typical geriatric presentation with confusion, falling, loss of mobility and incontinence of urine. The assessment of such patients will be discussed but such changes necessitate a very detailed investigation looking for the features of a hyperosmolar non-ketotic state.

Objective

Objective findings on examination are often limited particularly in the case of new diabetics. Patients may be dehydrated and in the case of impending coma. This may be marked, with hypotension. Rarely, elderly patients will have the signs of ketoacidosis with typical fetor. More often the tongue will be coated and dry – sometimes the tongue has a very thick 'black fur'.

The patient may have signs of some of the complications of diabetes. For example diabetic retinopathy is found in about 20 per cent of diabetics over the age of 55 and the prevalence increases with advancing age. Other manifestations such as infections or neuropathies may be found. Autonomic neuropathies in the form of postural hypotension are quite common.

The most important objective feature that alerts the physician is the blood glucose which may have been done because of the initial non-specific decline and the requirement for a full geriatric assessment.

Assessment

There is likely to be additional information that will help in the full assessment of the patient. Apart from the blood glucose, electrolytes, blood urea nitrogen and creatinine should be available to determine the state of hydration and renal function.

Plans

Diagnosis

Diabetes is diagnosed by the finding of an elevated blood glucose – fasting or post-prandial, and the levels have been mentioned. When this is found in association with the typical symptoms no other diagnostic tests are necessary. Sometimes there are no symptoms and the glucose elevation is modest, in rare instances a glucose tolerance test will need to be done.

Treatment

The prognosis of maturity onset diabetes is not good and less than half of the patients will be alive 10 years after diagnosis. Mortality increases with advancing age, but not beyond the age of 75.

Patients presenting with hyperglycemia can frequently be controlled by diet alone. Those patients that are obese need to reduce their total calorie intake. The majority of elderly patients with diabetes are not overweight and the introduction of a calorie restricted diet in this type of patient, particularly over the age of 70, is not a good idea. High fibre diets can be of value in smoothing out the glycemic response to meals, but should be introduced with care in the immobile patients. Meals should be well balanced and nutritious. For many elderly subjects simple sugars should be excluded from the diet and the patient introduced to a simple exercise program. This will result in adequate control.

As long as the patient remains asymptomatic then additional treatment will not be necessary. But if the glucose remains above 14 mmol/litre despite adherence to a diet additional methods of treatment need to be instituted. The speed with which such treatment is begun depends upon the severity of illness of the patient. Many patients can be followed with a diet for several weeks before additional therapy is commenced. Others with a more acute presentation will need more immediate aggressive therapy.

Those patients with very high blood sugars and perhaps with an associated hyperosmolar state should commence on insulin. Insulin is also indicated if there is an associated acute condition such as infection. Soluble (Toronto) insulin is used for immediate control and regular administration (every 6 hours) on a sliding scale is preferred. It will soon become apparent as to how much insulin is required and the frequency can be reduced to twice daily or once daily as required. Depending upon the amount of insulin that is necessary to control the blood sugar it may be possible to stop insulin in many patients and revert to an oral hypoglycemic agent. Those patients requiring continued insulin usage should be reduced to a single injection in the morning if at all possible. This may need to be a combination of immediate and delayed action varieties. It is important that the patient is as active in hospital as they will be on their return home.

For those patients with inadequate control on dietary measures and in whom insulin does not appear to be necessary, good control can usually be obtained with oral hypoglycemic agents. There are a variety of agents to choose from. Sulphonylureas which stimulate the pancreas to produce more insulin can provide adequate control in most elderly diabetics. Chlorpropamide should not be used. It has an unacceptably long half life which gives a higher incidence of hypoglycemic episodes, and because of its effect on free water clearance hyponatremia is a common side-effect. Glyburide needs to be given only once daily and can be started in a dose of 2.5 mg before breakfast. Most patients are controlled on 5 to 10 mg per day with a maximum permissible of 20 mg daily. Tolbutamide needs to be given more frequently to reduce gastric intolerance. Glipizide is another agent that requires only once daily dosage and provides satisfactory control. Metformin, a biguanide, still has a limited role in the management of elderly diabetics despite the risk of lactic acidosis. It is our practice to reserve this agent for those patients not completely controlled by a single hypoglycemic agent especially if obesity is present. The addition of metformin 500 mg 3 times a day to those patients on the maximum dose of a sulphonylurea may improve control and avoid the requirement for insulin. The biguanides do not increase insulin production or release but are thought to enhance the effects of insulin on peripheral receptors.

Ketoacidosis is a rare condition in the geriatric population of frail elderly. When it does occur the treatment principles are the same as in other age groups. The patients will need close monitoring of blood glucose as well as the fluid status, electrolytes and acid/base/blood gas.

Hyperosmolar non-ketotic coma is a much more common presentation in the frail elderly. Many of these patients may not have a previous diagnosis of diabetes. Fluid is replaced with normal saline provided the serum sodium is below 150 mmol/litre. Half strength is used when there is hypernatremia. The fluid replacement needs to be monitored with a central line and insulin needs to be given frequently and closely monitored.

In addition to the management of the diabetes itself the physician will often need to treat the complications of diabetes. Most of the complications are related to vascular disease and are dealt with elsewhere. Infections require immediate and appropriate treatment. The risk of foot complications may be lessened and this is discussed under patient education.

Education

Education of the patient with regards to their illness represents a real challenge with the elderly population because of the associated cognitive decline in a significant proportion of the frail elderly. There is evidence that memory retrieval is more impaired in those patients with poorly controlled diabetes. In the event that the patient does have difficulty in learning then the major care providers will require to be educated.

Patients should receive education about the nature of their illness and about methods of treatment. In many centres there are diabetic clinics which provide such education. Video tapes and other aids can be used for the in-patient. Patients should understand the treatment that they require and be able to recognize side-effects such as hypoglycemia. Dietary counselling should be given by a dietician and this will need to be shared with the individual responsible for meal preparation.

Once the treatment regimen is established this must be explained to the patient, with oral agents the pharmacist can provide this counselling. If there is a memory problem then someone will need to be enlisted to ensure that the drugs are taken at the correct time and in the right amount. This is of the utmost importance and if there is any doubt the patient should be tried out on a self medication program in hospital and closely monitored.

If insulin is being used it needs to be determined

if the patient is capable of self-administration. If so the patient is taught how to do this and then practises under nursing supervision. If this is not possible then arrangements will need to be made for the patient returning home to have someone give the insulin injections. This can sometimes be a family member but more frequently a nurse will have to be brought in on a daily basis. Twice-daily injections are more problematical. Once this is achieved it needs to be determined if the patient can safely and accurately draw up the correct insulin dose. Because of failing vision this is impossible in many elderly patients. In this case a family member or a nurse can be brought in to draw up the insulin injections and put them in the refrigerator for use during the following week. These requirements will become apparent during the education of the patient. The education is of a very practical nature, and is not simply the transfer of theoretical information.

Patients need to be well-informed about proper hygiene and also of appropriate foot care. They should be advised to have regular chiropody visits for nail trimming. They will be able to avoid some of the common foot problems by the use of proper fitting foot wear.

Patients should be advised to avoid non-steroidal anti-inflammatory agents if at all possible because of the risk of side-effects particularly in the face of renal insufficiency. Patients should be advised to receive influenza vaccination each year to avoid unnecessary illness and complications.

Failing vision is a common problem in the elderly and even more common with diabetics and patients need regular ophthalmological examination. This should be stressed with initial diagnosis during the education sessions.

Monitoring

Diabetes needs to be monitored by regular blood glucose measurement. In the early stages of treatment the blood will need to be taken several times daily – fasting, and two hours post-prandial. In hospital, laboratory measurement rather than paper strips or bedside measurement, is preferred. As control is achieved the frequency of measurement can be reduced to once daily. Home glucose monitoring can be achieved using paper indicators or glucometer. The frequency of testing will vary between patients some requiring at least daily, others weekly and others rarely. Patients need to be monitored by their physician and blood glucose can be supplemented by measuring glycosylated hemoglobin levels every two or three months. It is just as desirable to maintain good metabolic control in the elderly as in younger patients. It should be appreciated though that frequent hypoglycemic reactions are potentially more dangerous and may present atypically in the elderly. Urine testing is of no value in monitoring these patients due to altered renal thresholds to glucose.

In addition to controlling the diabetes the patients should be seen regularly for foot care and for eye examination. Weight should be checked on each doctors visit and should be maintained at a steady level.

Hypoglycemia

Spontaneous hypoglycemia is a rare occurrence in elderly patients without diabetes and should be investigated in the same way as in patients of other ages. Occasionally patients *in extremis* with septicemia will develop hypoglycemia which is a bad prognostic sign and extremely difficult to manage.

Hypoglycemia in elderly diabetics is a relatively common clinical problem and is related to the use of hypoglycemic agents – insulin or oral agents. It has been considered by many to be more dangerous in the elderly in that the brain is more susceptible to damage because of coexisting cerebrovascular disease. It has been postulated that there is a normal early morning rise in blood sugar which disappears with aging, the so-called 'dawn' phenomenon. Some have postulated that the absence of this phenomenon makes the elderly diabetic more susceptible to hypoglycemia in the early hours, although others have not found this to be the case.

Subjective

The initial symptoms are well recognized by clinicians but are not so easily recognized by many elderly patients. This may be because the symptoms are less florid in the elderly, although this is not well documented and the pathophysiological mechanisms that would account for this are not easily identified. Early symptoms are related to catecholamine release and include shaking, sweating, palpitations, weakness and hunger. A variety of neurological symptoms may also occur including blurred vision, headache and behavioral changes. These may rapidly progress to drowsiness, confusion and coma. Occasionally there are convulsions and focal neurological signs.

In some patients the hypoglycemia is not so marked and the major change is increasing confusion and cognitive impairment. The most important aspect of the history is the previous diagnosis of diabetes and the type of treatment that the patient is receiving. The treatment that the patient is receiving, dosage and route of administration, needs to be determined; as well as knowledge of the diet and the timing of the last meal in relation to last dose of insulin or other agent.

Objective

The findings on examination vary, depending upon the degree of hypoglycemia. The patient may be confused and agitated and indistinguishable from other causes of delirium. The patient may be in coma with focal neurological signs. In many elderly patients with hypoglycemia there are no unique features which point to the etiology. In fact the most important information will be the history of diabetes, for which the patient is receiving treatment and the blood glucose level.

Assessment

In the patient with recent cognitive decline without the manifestations of acute hypoglycemia, the diagnosis should be suspected if the glucose is below 5 mmol/litre together with the appropriate history. In an individual who has had persistently raised glucose levels, a sudden fall to 'normal ranges' may be associated with 'hypoglcemic symptoms'.

Blood glucose needs to be determined in any patient presenting acutely with a change in conscious state, a history of diabetes and the use of insulin or oral hypoglycemics.

Plans

Diagnosis

The diagnosis is made by the finding of a blood glucose below 3.5 mmol/litre. No other tests are necessary.

Management

The early symptoms of hypoglycemia can be reversed by the use of oral carbohydrates. Once the patient is uncooperative or unconscious then glucose needs to be administered intravenously.

If the hypoglycemia has occurred at home and the patient is alone then occasionally spontaneous recovery will occur. If not then the physician is usually faced with not only treating the hypoglycemia but also the complications that have resulted – for example pneumonia, hypothermia or brain damage. Individuals who have had hypoglygemia reversed are more vulnerable for several hours to neurological sequelae of further episodes. Careful monitoring of the individual should take place for 12–24 hours, especially if long-acting hypoglycemic agents are implicated.

Once the acute problem is controlled then the cause of the problem needs to be determined and a decision made as to whether the ongoing management of the patient and their diabetes needs to be changed. Insulin or oral hypoglycemic agent may need to be reduced or changed. With regards to the oral agents it is most commonly seen in association with chlorpropamide which has a prolonged half life. For this reason this agent is best avoided in the elderly. Those patients with some degree of cognitive impairment may well take too many pills too frequently. The meals need to be looked at and adjusted if necessary. If the patient is confused and having problems with management then alternative methods of monitoring the diabetes needs to be looked at.

Suggested reading

Arnetz, B. B., Kallner, A., Theorell, T. (1982). The influence of aging on hemoglobin A1c. *J. Gerontol.*, **37**: 648–50.

Cerami, A. (1985). Glucose as a mediator of aging. *J. Amer. Ger. Soc.*, **33**: 626–634.

Fink, R. I., Kolterman, O. G., Olefsky, J. M. (1984). The physiological significance of the glucose intolerance of aging. *J. Gerontol.*, **39**: 273–8.

Grobin, W. (1970). Diabetes in the aged: under-diagnosis and over-treatment. *Can. Med. Assoc. J.*, **103**: 915–23.

Jarrett, R. J., McCartney, P., Keen, H. (1982). The Bedford Survey: ten year mortality rates in newly diagnosed diabetics, borderline diabetics and normoglycemic controls and risk indices for coronary heart disease in borderline diabetics. *Diabetologia*, **22**: 79–84.

Matz, R. (1986). Diabetes mellitus in the elderly. *Hosp. Pract. (Off.)*, **21**: (Suppl. 3): 195–218.

Morley, J. E., Mooradian, A. D., Rosenthal, M. J., Kaiser, F. E. (1987) Diabetes Mellitus in elderly patients. Is it different? *Amer. J. Med.*, **83**: 533–44.

Perlmuter, L. C., Hakami, M. K., Hodgson-Harrington, C. et al. (1984). Decreased cognitive functioning in aging non-insulin dependent diabetic patients. *Am. J. Med.*, **77**: 1043–48.

Podgor, M. J., Leske, M. C., Ederer, F. (1983). Incidence estimates for lens changes, macular changes, open angle glaucoma and diabetic retinopathy. *Amer. J. Epidemiol.*, **118**: 206–12.

25

Abnormal thyroid function tests

Establishing firm criteria for the diagnosis of thyroid disease in the elderly presents special problems. There are many similarities between the aging process and some of the usually accepted external manifestations of thyroid disease. As in many other diseases some of the classical symptoms and signs are absent or modified. Thus ophthalmic signs are often absent in hyperthyroidism and the picture may be more that of apathy and fatigue, quite different from that seen in younger populations. A number of diseases and drugs commonly used in the elderly are known to modify thyroid function tests. Normal ranges for some of the commonly used thyroid function tests appear to be altered with age.

Regardless of the above mentioned problems, in many cases a clear therapeutic approach is indicated. It is usually estimated that the prevalence of thyroid disease in over 65 year olds is 0.5–1.5 per cent hypothyroidism, and 0.5–3.0 per cent hyperthyroidism. A further 0.5–4.0 per cent have Sub-clinical Hypothyroidism with a raised TSH but normal T4 levels, approximately half of whom have a history of previous thyroid surgery or radioactive iodine therapy.

1. Aging and the Thyroid

There is probably no major change in thyroid size with age in the absence of nodules. However, it does appear that the prevalence of nodules, particularly microscopically, increase with age. In non-goitrous areas 27 per cent of elderly subjects are found to have nodules at post-mortem.

Serum T4 levels show little change throughout life in healthy individuals. Some investigators have reported lower mean levels in older patients but still well within the normal quoted ranges. Anomalous high results may be seen in the hospitalized elderly in relation to drugs and disease. In some cases this may be due to a lowered peripheral conversion rate to T3 in ill old people.

Decreases in serum T3 levels with age have been noted of the order of 10–50 per cent. This appears to occur earlier in men. In many cases the fall in serum T3 relates to non-thyroid illness rather than age itself.

In the Baltimore Longitudinal Study of Aging; serum TSH levels were 38 per cent higher in the elderly. In another study 5.9 per cent of the older subjects had levels above 10 and 20 per cent above 7. In half of those with results above 10, a lowered serum T4 was also found. In a community survey of the elderly 5.0 per cent had TSH levels above 10 with normal serum T4. Half of these had previous histories of thyroid surgery, radioactive iodine treatment or were on T4 replacement therapy. In a third of the rest the serum T4 was found to be fall to sub-normal levels within 12 months, suggesting they were detected in the transition phase of developing frank hypothyroidism. The remainder however, after a two year review had either normalized their TSH or continued with a raised TSH but normal serum T4.

Thyroid antibodies are found more commonly with increasing age, for example antibodies to thyroglobulin were found in 2 per cent in women aged 25 years and 20 per cent of those age 75 years or older. Many of these individuals have no evidence of thyroid disease. The presence of a thyroid antibodies in asymptomatic subjects with raised TSH makes it more likely for overt hypothyroidism to develop.

2. Hypothyroidism

Autoimmune thyroiditis is traditionally the commonest cause of hypothyroidism in the elderly with about 80 per cent having auto-antibodies in classical studies but other causes are increasingly seen. The common use of radioactive iodine as the preferred treatment of autoimmune hyperthyroidism in the elderly is producing an increasing pool of ablated thyroids. Surgery for goitre or malignancy may result in hypothyroidism in the short-term because of amount of tissue removed or in the long-term because of an autoimmune process. Overdosage with antithyroid drugs may rapidly produce hypothyroidism. Other drugs such as the sulphonylureas, PAS and lithium carbonate are mildly goitrogenic and have been reported as causing hypothyroidism.

Subjective

The insidious onset and the non-specific nature of its symptoms of lethargy, dry skin, weight gain, constipation, poor memory, depression and cold intolerance raises diagnostic problems since these are found in many other situations without thyroid disease. The symptom of cold intolerance does not indicate an increased likelihood of hypothyroidism in the elderly. The possibility of hypothyroidism has to be considered in many geriatric patients. A history of previous thyroid disease, surgery or radioactive iodine treatment is relevant.

Objective

Swelling of the face, with course and dry skin, yellow tint to the skin (due to carotene deposition) and loss of hair especially over the lateral third of eyebrow is characteristic but not diagnostic. These changes to some degree can be seen in normal aging.

The gruff voice if present can be characteristic but can also be misleading. Asher (1949) described it as a bad gramophone record, running down, of a drowsy and slightly intoxicated person with a bad cold. Deafness may be present due to a serous effusion of the middle ear, which may improve with thyroxine therapy, but deafness is very common in the elderly.

The inclusion of hypothyroidism as a cause of secondary dementia is common to many a differential diagnosis list but unfortunately its detection rarely alters the clinical course. In the Northwick Park study, there was no excess of mental impairment amongst hypothyroid patients and no patient with dementia improved on therapy. The functional mental disorders, of depression, paranoia and psychosis were however, more common than in controls and often responded to treatment.

Some of the weakness and lethargy may have an objective basis in myopathy or entrapment neuropathies. Muscle weakness may also occur because of low total exchangeable potassium.

Complaints of hand paraesthesiae especially at night should raise the possibility of a carpal tunnel syndrome. Arthralgia in the form of synovial thickening, joint swelling and pain may be seen as a direct result of thyroid hormone deficiency.

Ataxia may be present with other evidence of cerebellar dysfunction. This is usually reversed with thyroxine replacement therapy.

The slow relaxation phase of the ankle jerk in hypothyroidism is well described. It is, however, not specific and may be absent in the presence of overt hypothyroidism.

The cardiovascular signs of thyroid disease; slow pulse, quiet heart and heart failure, are non-specific and rarely of help in diagnosis. The presence of pleural and/or pericardial effusions in the absence of obvious hemodynamic cause should raise the suspicion of thyroid dysfunction. Ascites may also be seen. The ECG is commonly abnormal with low voltages and flattening or inversion of T waves.

A number of non-specific laboratory findings may be seen in hypothyroidism. Anemia is present in perhaps one-third of cases. Macrocytosis is also commonly present. Hypercholesteremia is often seen.

Assessment

The common occurrence of hypothyroidism, the insidious and often non-specific nature of its symptoms and signs has contributed to the common practice of routine thyroid function tests during geriatric assessment.

The thyroid – stimulating hormone (TSH) level is by far the most sensitive test for hypo- thyroidism. A level in excess of 10 with a subnormal serum T4 and or serum T3 is diagnostic. However, in the presence of a normal T4 or T3 the position is less clear. If the T3 is normal but the T4 suboptimal the patient's condition is T3 euthyroidism or compensated hypothyroidism.

The condition of mild elevation of TSH but normal T4 and T3 is commonly referred to as sub-clinical hypothyroidism. Individuals with sub-clinical hypothyroidism and thyroid autoantibodies are likely to develop overt hypo- thyroidism.

Plan

The value of treatment of overt hypothyroidism is readily apparent and many of the symptoms and signs respond to therapy. Many such patients have co-existing cardiac problems and may be extremely sensitive to small doses of L-thyroxine. Treatment should commence therefore at 0.025 mg in such cases and proceed with similar increments at 2 weekly intervals. The usual maintenance dose is 0.075–0.10 mg daily. Thyroid function tests should be repeated once these levels have been reached for more than 7 days. The aim should be a TSH and T4 within the normal range.

The efficacy of treating sub-clinical hypothyroidism is however, less clear. They require very small doses to suppress TSH secretion. A study of treatment in younger patients failed to show clinically significant benefits. We suggest treatment with L-thyroxine not be commenced but the individuals be kept under review. Thyroid autoantibodies should be tested for, as their presence alters prognosis. In their presence TFTs should be checked 3-monthly for 12 months and then 6-monthly for 12 months followed by annually. In their absence TFTs should be checked at three months and then annually. Following this regimen cases requiring therapy will be readily detected and excess repetition of tests minimized.

3. Hyperthyroidism

The main causes of hyperthyroidism in the elderly are Graves' disease, toxic multinodular disease, Plumner's disease, thyroiditis and iodine induced hyperthyroidism. Classical Graves' disease seems to be relatively uncommon with increasing age. The clinical presentation differs with a much reduced incidence of proptosis, ophthalmoplegia and pretibial myxoedma. Most cases of hyperthyroidism in the elderly occur in the presence of multinodular glands. The solitary adenoma of Plumner's disease usually presents with 'toxicity' signs rather than the 'neck mass' of the younger patient.

Subjective

Once again the symptoms are less helpful than one associates with a younger group of patients. The nervousness of the hyper-metabolic state is less of a feature, often the patient is apathetic. An increased appetite is less common; in fact seen in only one-third of elderly patients. Loss of weight suggestive of malignancy and cardiac failure are common presenting pictures. The presenting picture of apathy and cardiac failure is seen in nearly a third of cases and referred to as 'apathetic thyrotoxicosis'.

Patients may present with confusion or other psychiatric problems. Such patients will usually have no specific symptoms that point to thyrotoxicosis and will be detected because of the routine investigations ordered as a result of the geriatric presentation.

A family history of thyroid disease and other autoimmune diseases such as pernicious anemia, is often seen.

Objective

As indicated the thyroid gland is often nodular rather than having the features of smooth enlargement of younger patients. Exophthalmos is seen in less than 10 per cent and retraction of the upper eyelid in only 25 per cent. Tremor is present but is not useful because of its common presence from a variety of causes in the elderly.

Cardiac findings are common. A modest tachycardia is often seen. The commonest rhythm disturbance is atrial fibrillation and seen in half of patients. Edema of the legs is seen in 50 per cent of the patients but reflects cardiac failure in only half. The cardiac failure is often relatively refractory to therapy a situation which improves with treatment of the thyroid disease.

The weight loss of hyperthyroidism is in part due to muscle wasting. Myopathic changes are present in the limb girdle muscles in as many as 90 per cent of thyrotoxic elderly patients. About half will complain of weakness and may have difficulties with rising from a chair or climbing stairs.

Osteoporosis is seen more commonly in hyperthyroidism and fractures may be a presenting feature. Occasionally hypercalcemia occurs which may give rise to symptoms of depression, thirst and polyuria.

Assessment

A number of difficulties arise in the interpretation of laboratory tests. In patients with systemic illness T3 and T4 levels may be abnormal in the absence of thyroid disease. Some of these abnormalities are accounted for by impaired peripheral conversion of T4 to T3. It is usually suggested that in such cases T3 levels are more reliable than T4, in establishing or confirming the diagnosis of hyperthyroidism. Some 22–43 per cent of ill patients with an elevated serum T4 and a normal T3 are eventually found to be hyperthyroid.

The serum T4 level, which is elevated in 90 per cent of patients and the free T4 index, which is elevated even more frequently, provide highly sensitive and useful tests for the diagnosis of hyperthyroidism. The free T4 has the advantage of not being influenced appreciably by changes in serum protein levels.

Thyroid-stimulating hormone levels are low or undetectable in thyrotoxicosis. In the case of the TRH test the ability of the pituitary gland to respond to stimulation is suppressed. A normal response excludes hyperthyroidism.

Radioactive isotope uptake studies are no longer necessary for diagnosis of hyperthyroidism but are still of use in assessment of patients with a nodular goiter. A scintiscan enables the function of a nodule to be determined, whether it is 'hot' or 'cold' and whether the rest of the gland is suppressed or functioning. When there is a solitary nodule, needle aspiration biopsy with cytological examination, is indicated. No other special diagnostic tests are indicated in most patients with thyroid disease.

Plans

Hyperthyroidism as in the young can be treated with drugs, surgery or radioactive iodine. The current preferred treatment tends to be radioactive iodine although this carries a long-term risk of developing hypothyroidism requiring L-thyroxine therapy. Antithyroid drugs such as propyl thiouracil are effective but since a smaller proportion of the elderly suffer from Graves' disease fewer go into spontaneous remission so treatment might need to be life-long. Surgery is usually only considered where nodules are cosmetically distressing or producing a compression syndrome.

Suggested reading

Barzel, U. S. (1988). Endocrinology and Aging. In: Reichel, W. (ed.) *Clinical aspects of Aging*. William and Wilkins, ch. 30, pp. 374–77.

Bharkri, H. L., Fisher, R., Khadri, A. and MacMahon, D. G. (1990). Longitudinal study of thyroid function in acutely ill elderly patients using a sensitive TSH assay – defer testing until recovery. *Gerontol.*, **36**: 140–44.

Hodkinson, H. M. and Irvine, R. E. (1985). The endocrine system – thyroid disease in the elderly. In: Brocklehurst, J. C. (ed.) *Textbook of Geriatrics and Gerontology*. Churchill and Livingstone, Edinburgh. Ch. 34, pp. 686–714.

Rosenthal, M., Hunt, W. C., Philip, G. and Goodwin, J. S. (1987). Thyroid failure in the Elderly. *JAMA*, **258**: 209–13.

26

Chest infection

1. Definitions

There are several questions that are important in the management of patients with chest infection:-

1. Is an infection present?
2. Where is the infection?
3. What is the most likely organism?
4. Is there underlying or associated disease?

The first question seems obvious but is an important step in that it recognizes the possibility of a chest infection being present. As will be described in more detail later the elderly commonly present with a chest infection in a non-specific and atypical manner. It is unfortunately common for these presentations to be taken at their face value and the diagnostic search for a chest infection not even entertained.

The second question on localization of infection is an important one and leads in to the definitions that will be used here. Infections of the respiratory tract are best divided broadly into two groups: lower respiratory tract infections (LRTI) and upper respiratory tract infections (URTI). LRTI can be further subdivided into pneumonia and bronchitis, an inflammation of the bronchi. The latter can be further subdivided into acute bronchitis, and chronic bronchitis with exacerbation.

The most important problems in geriatric practice are pneumonia and exacerbation of chronic bronchitis and will be dealt with in the problem oriented format. Only those patients with chronic bronchitis can develop exacerbations of the problem. Chronic bronchitis is defined as a chronic recurrent productive cough present on most days for a minimum of three months in two successive years. Such patients are most likely to develop exacerbations during the winter months. During these exacerbations a variety of microbial flora may be isolated including various viruses, mycoplasma, streptococcus pneumoniae and Hemophilus influenzae. Such exacerbations are frequently self-managed by the patient with antibiotics, such as amoxycillin, tetracycline, a cephalosporin or cotrimoxazole.

Patients with serious exacerbations or with pneumonia complicating chronic lung disease will be considered along with other pneumonias, however the importance of complicating diseases like emphysema will become apparent.

2. Lower respiratory tract infection

Predisposing factors

Aging, whether primary or secondary to environmental factors, produces changes in the respiratory tract which predispose the individual to infection. Such changes need to be looked at in two ways:

1. Primary changes in the defence mechanism
2. Secondary factors which increase the exposure to pathogenic organisms or modify host response effectiveness.

Primary Age Changes in Defence

Mucus provides a natural barrier to invading organisms. The organisms need to be cleared from the respiratory tract and this is done by ciliary action and the cough reflex. Organisms that manage to get through the filtration system in the upper airway, and are not trapped and cleared by the mucociliary defence may reach the alveoli. Here there are important cellular defence mechanisms, namely the alveolar macrophages and the tissue histiocytes. There is no good evidence that these mechanisms deteriorate with age.

With advancing age there is, however, loss of lung elasticity. With loss of elastic recoil there is increased susceptibility to collapse, there is also an increase in anatomical and physiological dead space. The cough reflex becomes depressed with advancing age. These changes undoubtedly contribute to the increased incidence of LRTI with advancing age.

Secondary Changes in Defence

Elderly individuals who become disabled often find themselves in settings where there are many other elderly people, – for example day care centres. Or indeed there may be living in environments with many other dependent elderly, in nursing homes or long-term care hospitals. In these situations there is an increased likelihood of exposure to a variety of organisms. For example an increased risk of exposure to tuberculosis has been clearly documented. With advancing age there is an increasing risk of admission to hospital and it is well-recognized that the elderly are more prone to nosocomial infection.

Associated disease burden is an important factor in susceptibility to chest infection, as well as perhaps the most important factor in morbidity and mortality. Pulmonary problems like chronic bronchitis, emphysema or neoplasm clearly predispose to infection. Cardiac failure may result from chest infection, but pulmonary edema will also predispose to infection. Other problems may make aspiration or impaired clearance more likely and include stroke, Parkinson's disease or dementia and the administration of medications, sedatives or tranquilizers.

Precipitating factors

It can be seen that there are many factors that predispose the elderly to chest infections, for example exposure to a general anesthetic, abdominal surgery, loss of consciousness or excessive sedation In this predisposed group a sudden change, or dramatic increase in one of these factors may precipitate an infection.

The etiological agents that are of most importance are:

1. Streptococcus pneumoniae
2. Gram negative rods, in the hospital setting Klebsiella aerogenes.
3. Legionella pneumophila
4. Staphylococcus aureus
5. Hemophilus influenzae for exacerbations of chronic lung disease.
6. Viruses

Obviously exposure to these organisms in sufficient quantity is the actual precipitant. The chest infection or pneumonia is determined by the dose of inoculum as well as the susceptibility of the host. Certain organisms are more likely in different situations and this knowledge is useful in deciding the most appropriate treatment.

Subjective

The typical symptoms of pneumonia are found in all age groups, even in the elderly although they may need to be looked for more closely. Typical symptoms would include abrupt onset of cough, pleuritic chest pain, fever, chills and breathlessness. Chills are significantly less frequent in those patients over 65 with pneumonia. Published reports have not revealed a significant difference in the frequency of the symptoms of fever, cough or chest pain between those under 65 compared with those over 65.

Clinical experience leads us to believe that the geriatric presentation occurs more frequently with advancing age. It is likely that the other more non-specific features of falls, immobility, confusion and incontinence mask the more typical symptoms or signs. In this situation the chest infection has a more insidious onset with evidence of functional impairment. This has been confirmed in one study looking for the atypical or geriatric presentation and it was found in a long-term care setting that looking for functional decline and the development of one of the giants of geriatrics resulted in a doubling in the detection rate for chest infection and a reduction in mortality rate. An important conclusion from the various studies that have been done is that the typical symptoms (and signs) of pneumonia are usually present, even in the very old, but they need to be searched for.

Objective

Fever is usually present in patients with pneumonia. There is published evidence that with advancing age an increasing number of patients fail to develop fever in the presence of infection. However, in our study of patients in a long term care setting fever was detected at some time in all patients with pneumonia – although it is apparent that one needs to look more closely, and perhaps more frequently.

It is claimed that an increased respiratory rate is one of the best signs that infection is localized to the respiratory tract. The upper limit of normal being 25 per minute. There is no doubt that this is a useful sign in those with a non-specific presentation, but a note of caution needs to be introduced. Some patients with a raised respiratory rate and fever turn out to have infections elsewhere and false positives do occur.

The typical signs of pneumonia are found in elderly patients which allow the localization of the infection to the lungs. In the examination the physician may find features of consolidation at the lobar level. Adventitious sounds, rhonchi and rales, are found in equal frequency in the elderly as the young.

In advanced cases there may be respiratory failure and up to 25 per cent of patients may require ventilator assistance.

Assessment

Patients will have been identified as suffering from an infection or more precisely a chest infection. The nature of the findings on examination may indicate more and suggest a lobar pneumonia. It is important to determine where the likely infection was acquired since this will make certain etiological agents more likely.

It is also important to identify any disabilities that the patient has which might be predisposing factors.

Plan

Diagnosis

There are obvious clinical pointers from the history and physical examination that point to the diagnosis of chest infection and more specifically pneumonia. These features may be sufficient in certain settings, depending upon the patient, to make a presumptive diagnosis and to begin treatment.

The most important diagnostic aid is a chest radiograph, which is the hallmark for diagnosing pneumonia. It must be remembered that if this is done early in the course of the disease then the possibility exists that there will be no abnormality on the chest X-ray. It is not unusual to make a clinical diagnosis and to have to wait for the radiographic changes to develop.

Other tests are aimed at determining the nature of the etiological agent. Again the setting in which the patient is seen determines the extent of the investigations. Where there is access to a microbiological laboratory sputum should be collected for immediate stain and for culture. It needs to be recognized that the yield is low. In the first instance specimens are difficult to collect and perhaps only a third of patients will have successful collection of a specimen. Up to a half of the patients may have already received antibiotics by the time they are seen in hospital. In this case sputum culture is unlikely to be of any benefit.

Blood cultures are easier to perform in the hospital setting, but produce a positive yield of only about 5 per cent–10 per cent. A positive result, however, is often of immense value in terms of directing the therapy.

Patients with features of chronic lung disease, those with involvement of more than one lobe and those who are obviously critically ill need further investigation in the form of arterial blood gas measurement. Further sampling will depend upon the results and the clinical course of the patient.

At the present time there is no evidence that more invasive diagnostic approaches to establish etiology are routinely needed. This has to be qualified, and individuals who prove resistant to initial therapies may need such tests as transtracheal aspiration, needle biopsy or aspiration.

Other tests may be indicated depending upon the general problems of the patient.

Treatment

The approach to management is twofold. First of all, therapy directed at the pneumonia itself and secondly, supportive therapy. The circumstances of the patient, the site that the pneumonia was acquired are important in the choices with regard to treatment. The reason for the separation is that the antibiotic choice for initial therapy is different.

All patients require a similar diagnostic approach and work up. Similar attention needs to be given to the general measures with regard to maintaining comfort, maintaining hydration, ensuring adequate oxygenation and dealing with the accompanying problems that are so common in the geriatric population such as confusion, incontinence and immobility. It is important to recognize that pneumonia is often accompanied by other acute medical problems that require medical management, and perhaps the most important of these is cardiac failure. Pneumonia may precipitate cardiac failure which needs to be recognized and treated. Patients with cerebrovascular disease, may well have a deterioration in their functional state and an increase of their neurological deficit during the course of their pneumonia which may be interpreted as a fresh stroke.

The most frequent etiological agent for pneumonia in any setting is streptococcus pneumoniae. This needs to be recognized when the choice of antibiotics is being made. Patients with exacerbations of underlying chronic lung disease frequently have Hemophilus influenzae identified as the causative agent. Gram negative organisms play an increasingly important role with advancing age, and in the institutionalized elderly. The most frequent single gram negative organism being Klebsiella pneumoniae. Staphylococcus can be found in any setting, particularly in post-influenzal infections. Mycoplasma is not a consideration in this age group. Legionella appears to be of increasing importance in the more debilitated elderly in either the hospital or community setting. Legionella has yet to be implicated in the nursing home setting.

The following suggestions are made for initial treatment choices:

1. Community acquired pneumonia – amoxi-cillin or cefaclor for those treated at home. If the patient is sick enough to require hospitalization then additional laboratory data might be available to direct therapy but failing that amoxicillin is a reasonable choice, or alternatively cefamandole intravenously.
2. Nursing home acquired pneumonia – Again depending upon the severity, either cefamandole or amoxicillin plus an aminoglycoside. Such patients do not require expensive drugs like the third generation cephalosporins. In certain patients potent oral agents or intramuscular preparations that can be given only once a day are attractive.
3. Hospital acquired pneumonia – these patients should receive intravenous erythromycin plus cefamandole if an empirical choice is being made. The erythromycin is usually given in the dose of 500 mg every 6 hours, but if the patient is very ill and Legionella is seriously suspected the dose will need to be increased to 1 gm every 6 hours.

Patients who are quite ill, particularly with associated conditions, and those elderly who cannot get the support at home or within the nursing home will be admitted to hospital. In this situation further diagnostic help will be available in a significant percentage. A sputum smear that is considered to be diagnostic will have more than 25 polymorphonuclear leukocytes and less than 10 epithelial cells per low power (×100) field. In elderly patients with a routine laboratory one might expect that approximately one-third of patients will yield diagnostic smears. This means that the rest will require empirical choices, at least until results of blood or sputum cultures are returned. Choices can be made according to the results of the smear (Table 26.1). With the return of positive cultures or alternatively diagnostic titres such as for legionella, therapy might need to be changed.

Hydration should be maintained. Oral intake is usually adequate but elderly patients with associated problems like confusion may rapidly become dehydrated and will therefore require intravenous replacement. Mortality in elderly patients with pneumonia is for the most part from the effects of associated disease states. Patients should be watched for the development of cardiac failure and treated if necessary.

Patients with underlying chronic lung disease will need to have this treated at the same time. Approximately one-quarter of the patients admitted with pneumonia require ventilator support. The usual indication for such support comes from the arterial blood gas measurements, which would be $pO_2 < 50$ or $pCO_2 > 50$. The indications for performing blood gas measurements are not precise, and it is recommended that judgement needs to made with regard to the severity of illness, the degree of dyspnea the presence of chronic obstructive lung disease, etc.

Table 26.1 Antibiotic choices

Gram positive diplococci (strep. pneumoniae)	Penicillin I.V. unless allergic (erythromycin)
Gram positive clusters (staph. aureus)	Cephalothin or oxacillin I.V.
Small gram negative bacilli (hemophilus influenzae)	Ampicillin I.V. cefamandole
Large gram negative bacilli (klebsiella, etc.)	Cefazolin aminoglycoside

Patient education

The most important aspect of patient education is with regard to prevention of chest infection. Early death from pneumococcal infection, the most frequent etiological agent in pneumonia of the elderly, has not been affected by the advent of antibiotics. Pneumococcal vaccination has been shown to reduce this early mortality and it is therefore recommended for all elderly patients over the age of 65 living at home. Studies have not revealed whether it is beneficial in the institutional setting. It would seem that vaccination of nursing home subjects leads to elimination of infection from the serotypes present in the vaccine but the overall prevalence remains the same as the other serotypes increase in frequency. Pneumococcal vaccination appears to confer adequate protective titres in elderly subjects, although the antibody titres take longer to rise, fail to reach such a high peak as younger subjects and decline sooner. Nonetheless, the protection appears adequate. At the present time it is recommended that patients need booster vaccination after 5 years but more work needs to be done in this area.

It is recommended that all elderly individuals over the age of 65 be vaccinated against influenza on an annual basis. This should be done in the fall of the year when the appropriate antigenic strains have been predicted for the coming flu season. Present vaccines have few side-effects and confer significant benefit. Influenza epidemics continue to result in significant mortality amongst the elderly, particularly the frail elderly. The cause of death being usually from post-influenza pneumonia. Vaccination produces adequate protection in the elderly population even though the titres may be lower and the rate of seroconversion is lower amongst the frail elderly that reside in nursing homes. Despite the reduced seroconversion rate, vaccination is recommended for the elderly within nursing homes as morbidity and mortality is reduced. If a decision is made to vaccinate, then every effort should be made to ensure that the majority of residents are indeed vaccinated. Eighty per cent of residents need to receive the vaccine to ensure that there is adequate 'herd immunity'. Rates less than this will allow the development of significant outbreaks of influenza within the institution. Another important consideration is that the health care workers and care providers are vaccinated.

3. Upper respiratory tract infections

The common cold, coryza, occurs less frequently than in younger populations probably because of less frequent association with children of school age. Other upper respiratory problems such as otitis media are significantly less frequent.

There is nothing unique about these problems in the elderly except that care needs to be taken in using preparations for symptomatic relief. The side-effects from some preparation may be severe in elderly patients resulting in loss of balance, falling and confusional states. Upper respiratory infections like influenza are associated with significant increases in mortality. The death that occurs is due to the development of secondary bacterial infections, specifically pneumonia. Prevention of the primary influenzal infection by vaccination has been discussed in the previous section. In the face of an impending outbreak within a closed community like a nursing home, when herd immunity or adequate vaccination has not been achieved, amantidine in a dosage of 200 mg daily will protect the rest of the residents from developing influenza.

Suggested reading

Bentley, D. W. (1981). Pneumococcal vaccine in the institutionalised elderly: review of past and recent studies. *Rev. Infect. Dis.* 3 (supplement): S61–70.

Bentley, D. W. (1984). Immunisation in *Immunology and Infection in the Elderly.* ed. Roy, A. Fox, Churchill Livingstone, London.

Marrie, T. J., Haldane, E. V., Faulkner, R. S., Durant, H. and Kwan, C. (1985) Community acquired pneumonia. Is it different in the elderly? *J. Amer. Ger. Soc.*, **33**: 671–680.

Marrie, T. J., Durant, H. and Kwan, C. (1986) Nursing home acquired pneumonia. *J. Amer. Ger. Soc.*, **34**: 697–702.

Puxty, J. A. H. and Andrews, K. (1986). The role of chest radiography in the evaluation of the geriatric giants. *Age and Aging*, **15**: 174–6.

Valenti, W. M., Trudell, R. G. and Bentley, D. W. (1978) Factors predisposing to oropharyngeal colonization with gram negative rods in the aged.

27

Urinary tract infection

Bacteriuria means the presence of bacteria in the urine. The term significant bacteriuria is used to describe the presence of bacteria in numbers that exceeds that usually considered to be due to contamination from the anterior urethra (>100,000 bacteria/ml). When significant bacteriuria is accompanied by symptoms and signs it is referred to as urinary tract infection (UTI). UTI may be restricted to the lower urinary tract – the bladder, or may involve both upper as well as lower urinary tract.

Bacteriuria is an extremely common problem in old age, being significantly more common in the female than the male. In fact approximately 24 per cent of women and 8 per cent of men over the age of 65 have infection at any one time. Infection is more common with increasing disability or increasing disease burden.

Urinary tract infection can be a serious problem with significant morbidity and mortality. Symptomatic urinary tract infections need to be treated. Despite treatment there is a significant rate of recurrence. There is no doubt that in young individuals recurrent urinary tract infection can be a serious problem with the potential for renal scarring and chronic renal disease. Recurrent infection in the older patient does not carry the same prognosis and patients have been followed prospectively and show no evidence of progression of renal disease. In this chapter we will consider for the most part symptomatic urinary tract infection, and include in that category the geriatric presentation.

1. Predisposing factors

It has already been noted that with advancing age there is an increasing prevalence of urinary tract infection. The sick elderly with multiple chronic diseases and increasing disability also have an increasing incidence of urinary tract infection. It is important to understand the factors that contribute to this.

Predisposing factors can be considered under two main headings: normative age changes and changes secondary to disease.

Normative Age Changes;

The normal urethra provides a barrier to ascending infection, being less efficient in the female. With the development of atrophic vaginitis the bacterial flora changes and the risk of contamination with pathogenic bacteria increases. Changes occur within the epithelial cells and the rate of adherence of certain bacteria increases. Mucus production decrease with aging but it is not clear as to whether this contributes to the predisposition to infection. Waning of the immune response has been widely reported and investigated, however studies that have been done on the secretory immune response do not reveal any deterioration. It seems unlikely that waning immunity contributes to the increasing incidence of urinary tract infection in old age.

Changes secondary to disease

Changes within the urinary tract that promote stagnation or reduction of flow of urine will predispose to infection (Table 27.1). One of the normal defence mechanisms is the flow of urine so that potentially adherent bacteria will be washed away. Any condition causing reduced flow of urine and stasis will predispose to bacteriuria. In the female, genital prolapse may cause obstruction to flow.

Table 27.1 Factors linked to the etiology of urinary tract infections

Predisposing	Precipitants
Dehydration	Instrumentation
• Reduced flow	
Obstruction	Foreign body
Incontinence of feces	Environmental exposure
Aging	• epithelial changes
• mucus reduction	
• waning immunity	

Urethral stricture may occur in either sex. Prostatic hypertrophy in the male is a major predisposing change. Flow may be reduced by an obstructing tumour or other masses within the pelvis, the most common of these being fecal impaction. Reduced flow may have a neurogenic cause, a large atonic bladder having a significant residual volume of urine. Reduced fluid intake also results in limited urine flow and undoubtedly predisposes to infection.

Conditions that increase the contamination of the perineal area predispose to infection. This is increased further if the normal defence is impaired. Thus fecal incontinence and poor hygiene will increase contamination and will increase the likelihood of infection.

The presence of chronic disease outside the urinary tract predisposes to infection. Diabetes Mellitus is associated with an increased incidence of urinary tract infection.

2. Precipitating factors

In certain instances UTI arises by the haematogenous spread of organisms – for example, with mycobacterium tuberculosis, salmonellosis or schistosomiasis. It is accepted however, that the usual route of infection for all other UTI is ascending, via the urethra. Thus anything that carries infection into the bladder from the perineum may precipitate infection – for example catheterization or other forms of instrumentation. Other foreign bodies may promote colonization, for example calculi or tumours. When patients are admitted to hospital they are exposed to a variety of pathogenic organisms, urinary tract infection is the second most frequent type of nosocomial infection.

Some of the factors that have been discussed as predisposing to infection may also precipitate. For example the sudden development of obstruction or rapid dehydration (Table 27.1).

Subjective

Many of the elderly present in a similar manner to other groups with UTI. They may suffer constitutional symptoms found in the presence of any type of infection – for example feeling tired or a loss of appetite. Such symptoms may be mild in the presence of a localized infection and become more marked with increasing severity. Systemic features may therefore dominate the clinical picture when there is bacteremia or septicemia.

The typical symptoms of UTI include dysuria, increased frequency of micturition and urgency. Pain may be localized to the suprapubic region or in the case of pyelonephritis to the flanks. A significant number of frail elderly will however, present less typically. Their local symptoms of a UTI are less obvious and features of malaise, fatigue, confusion, falls, immobility and incontinence dominate. It is not unusual to find increasing impairment of those functions that are already impaired – a confused patient becoming more confused. For this reason urine is always collected for culture and sensitivity in those patients with a geriatric presentation.

Bacteriuria becomes increasingly common with advancing age so that the older and more debilitated the patient the more likely is that patient to have bacteriuria. In an ill patient who has presented 'geriatrically' with decline in function, the clinician needs to proceed with caution before attributing the functional decline to asymptomatic bacteriuria. If treatment of the urinary tract infection results in improvement of function then the UTI can be assumed to have been causative. If there is no change in function then another explanation for decline in function must be sought and any recurrence should be ignored and accepted as asymptomatic bacteriuria.

Objective

Patients with UTI are usually febrile, whatever their age or degree of impairment of function. Examination may reveal tenderness in the abdomen in the suprapubic region, or in the flanks. In the male the external genitalia should be carefully examined since epididymo-orchitis is a relatively common complication and is frequently missed. Apart from the enlargement and tenderness there may not be any systemic manifestations of infection.

Urinalysis may reveal the presence of pus cells and counts above 20 leucocytes per high power field have been considered to be indicative of bacteriuria. This is not an accurate way to make a diagnosis and this finding or the detection of bacteria on microscopy indicates the need for culture.

The most important objective evidence for UTI is the finding of significant bacteriuria. Specimens can usually be collected by the mid-stream voiding technique. Failing that, catheter specimens or those obtained by needle aspiration may be necessary. Finding of >100,000 gram negative bacteria per ml indicates significant infection and is unlikely to be due to contamination. Lower counts of gram positive organisms may be significant.

Plan

Diagnosis

An approach to the assessment, diagnosis and treatment is suggested in Fig. 27.1. The diagnosis is reached by the finding of significant numbers of bacteria in the urine specimen. False negative or positive results may occur and one should take precautions to avoid this. For example specimens are best collected first thing in the morning and excessive disinfection is to be avoided. Fresh specimens should be used. Most infections are due to a single species, the most common being Escherichia coli which accounts for up to 80 per cent. When the patient has an indwelling catheter then multiple species is the rule. The results of culture will also give some idea as to susceptibility to antibiotics.

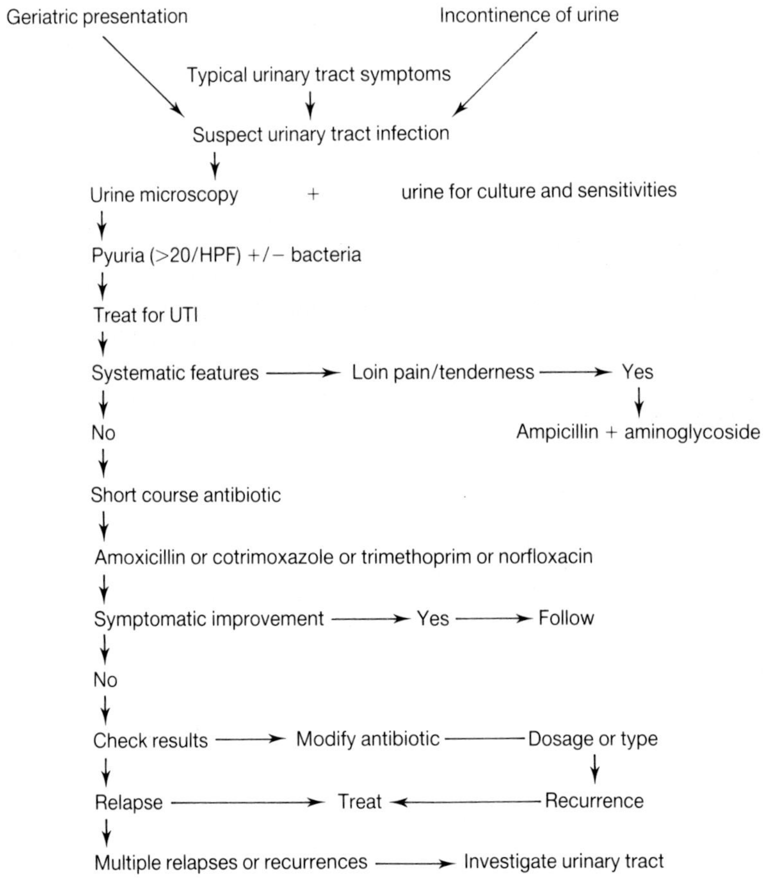

Fig. 27.1 Urinary tract infection.

The clinical response of the patient should be followed as the best guide to efficacy. This may be difficult with the non-specific presentation but repeat specimens will tell if the organisms are eradicated.

It is not necessary to localize infection to upper or lower urinary tract. The use of tests such as antibody coated bacteria do not result in any therapeutic improvement.

When there is significant pyuria but no growth on culture then early specimens should be collected and cultures for acid fast bacilli obtained. If the pyuria persists then suprapubic needle aspiration will determine if the pus cells originate in the bladder or from the organs distal to this. This is of particular importance in diagnosing prostatism for example.

Patients with recurrent infection may need to be investigated by visualizing the urinary tract directly (cystoscopy), by ultrasonography or radiographically (pyelography with contrast media).

Treatment

Symptomatic UTI should be treated. Patients with recent functional decline and specifically those with incontinence of urine need to be treated as symptomatic UTI. There has been a great deal of discussion about the need to treat asymptomatic bacteriuria. The consensus is that this is a benign situation that does not need to be altered by antibiotic administration. For this reason routine cultures of urine are not recommended for asymptomatic elderly individuals even within an institutional setting. Treatment may well have an adverse effect by encouraging the development of organisms which are resistant to common antibiotics.

Successful culture of urine will also reveal the sensitivities of the organisms and antibiotic therapy can therefore be directed. In practice antibiotics may be prescribed before laboratory reports are available. Escherichia coli account for approximately 80 per cent of infections outside of hospital, and the usual initial choice would be ampicillin or cotrimoxazole. However, there is an increasing incidence of serious side-effects with the use of cotrimoxazole in the elderly. This has led to the use of trimethoprim alone or to alternatives like the newer quinolones, norfloxacin or ciprofloxacin. We recommend that the fluorinated quinolones should be reserved for difficult resistant strains particularly pseudomonas. Ciprofloxacin is particularly useful when parenchymal disease is present or the prostate is involved.

In the majority of patients a short course of antibiotic only is required – from 3 to 5 days. A single dose of amoxicillin (3 gm) is effective in 90 per cent of patients. If the patient appears to have a complicated UTI with pyelonephritis or septicemia then antibiotics will need to be given for 10 days and parenteral antibiotics are likely to be required. When symptoms and signs persist for 48 hours, the choice of antibiotic or dose need review.

Relapse suggests that there is kidney parenchymal involvement, local anatomical problems or that treatment has been inadequate. Urine cultures should be repeated and treatment decisions reviewed.

The frail elderly with persisting functional impairment and/or incontinence of urine despite adequate treatment, will often redevelop bacteriuria once treatment is stopped. This should not be looked upon as recurrence but rather as asymptomatic bacteriuria. Treatment should not be repeated.

Those who have eradication of their symptoms for at least 2 weeks with return when the infection returns, need to be treated again. If recurrence or relapse is frequent then patients might need long-term antibiotic or antiseptic therapy. Such patients should be looked at to determine if there are factors contributing to the reinfection – for example the presence of a foreign body or any of the factors that predispose to infection. If any exist these should be modified – for example ensuring, adequate hydration, eliminating fecal incontinence or constipation, relieving obstruction or removing a foreign body.

It is important to attend to other aspects of therapy and to ensure adequate relief of pain, to control incontinence and to promote adequate urine flow.

Patients with indwelling catheters or external collection devices have a very high incidence of infections. The most important aspect of treatment is prevention. The collecting devices and the catheters are handled taking strict hygiene precautions with closed drainage systems. The external genitalia are kept clean. Silastic catheters are recommended and changed when required due to blockage or encrustation, with bag changes at least weekly. Antibiotics or antiseptics should not be administered on a long-term basis. Such patients will almost always have a number of bacteria growing in their urine. The urine should not be cultured routinely.

If the patient with an indwelling catheter

develops septicemia cultures should be taken from the urine and the blood. For most patients a reasonable empirical choice in this situation would be ampicillin and an aminoglycoside or a cephalosporin like cefamandole. Such patients should have their urinary flow maintained by adequate hydration – intravenous if necessary.

Patient education

When possible patients should be educated with regard to matters of hygiene of the perineal area. Incontinence of urine can be managed successfully using external containment systems that is adult diapers. These appear to carry a lower risk of infection as compared to indwelling catheters and external collection devices (condom catheter).

3. Other genitourinary infections

Male

Acute prostatism is not a common problem in geriatric practice. The most common organism being *E. coli*. Patients are usually ill and toxic and complain of dysuria, perineal heaviness and pain on defecation. Chronic prostatism may be asymptomatic or may present with pain in the perineum or rectum. Diagnosis is made by bacterial culture. Treatment is with antibiotics unless there is abscess formation.

Acute epididymo-orchitis is not an uncommon problem. Patients may complain of a dull ache in the groin and then develop pain and swelling of the testis. The scrotal wall is often edematous and shiny red. These patients are often afebrile. Treatment is with appropriate broad spectrum antibiotics, analgesia and scrotal support.

Female

Fungal and bacterial infections of the vulva or groin (intertrigo) are common. Treatment consists of the use of antifungal agents or antibiotics and appropriate hygienic care.

Vaginal infections with discharge are not infrequent in elderly females. Thick creamy discharges with whitish plaques on inspection are indicative of candida infections. Therapy is with antifungal agents. Greenish discharges indicate bacterial infections, which are related to the increased susceptibility of the atrophic vagina. A variety of organisms may be found, usually gram negative rods. The infection may spread to give endometrial infection with pyometra and occasionally pelvic and systemic infections. Such infections can cause non-specific declines and geriatric presentations. Treatment should be twofold – using estrogens and antibiotics.

Suggested reading

Brocklehurst, J. C., Dillane, J. B., Griffiths, L. and Fry, J. (1968). The Prevalence and symptomatology of urinary tract infections in an aged population. *Gerontol. Clin.*, **10**: 242–53.

Dontas, A. S., Kasviki-Charvati, P., Papanayioutou, P. C., Marketos, S. G. (1981). Bacteruria and survival in old age. *New Eng. J. Med.*, 304; 939–43.

Freedman, L. R. (1975). Natural history of urinary tract infection in adults. *Kidney Internat.* [Suppl] Suppl. 4; S96–100.

Horan, M. A., Puxty, J. A. and Fox, R. A. (1983). Gynecological sepsis as a cause of covert infection in old age. *J. Amer. Ger. Soc.*, **31**: 213–15.

Nicolle, L. E., Mayhew, J. and Bryan, L. (1987). Prospective randomized comparison of therapy and no therapy for asymptomatic bacteruria in institutionalized elderly women. *Amer. J. Med.* **83**: 27–33.

Nicolle, L. E., Bjornson, J., Harding, G. K. M. and MacDonell, J. A. (1983). Bacteruria in elderly institutionalized men. *N. Engl. J. Med.*, **309**: 1420–25.

Nicolle, L. E., McIntyre, M., Zacharias, H., MacDonell, J. A. (1984). Twelve month surveillance of infections in institutionalised elderly men. *J. Amer. Ger. Soc.*, **32**: 513–19.

Rubin, R. H., Rang, S. T., Jones, S. R. et al. (1980). Single dose amoxycillin therapy for urinary tract infection. Multicentre trial using antibody coated bacteria localisation technique. *J. Amer. Med. Assoc.*, **244**: 561–4.

Sourander, L. B. (1966). Urinary tract infections in the aged. An epidemiological study. *Ann. Int. Med. Fenniae*, **55**: Suppl. 45;1–55.

28

Geriatric psychiatry

1. Depression

Depressive symptoms within the aged community are very common, the prevalence in surveys ranging from 5-15 per cent. They are equally distributed between the two sexes. Major depressive episodes are however, much less common and of the order of 1-3 per cent.

The suicide rate in the elderly peaks for men between the ages of 80 and 90 years, and for women at 50 to 65 years. The highest risk group for suicide are single, socially isolated, physically disabled white males. Psychotically depressed patients are also at high risk.

Predisposing Factors

The aged may be predisposed to depressive mood disorders in a variety of ways:

1. There may be a life-time history of mood disorders.
2. Normal aging and retirement may be mistakingly perceived as a time of loss of function, role and self-esteem.
3. An increasing proportion of the population with aging suffer from multiple chronic health problems creating disabilities and handicaps which create dependency with resultant loss of self-esteem.
4. Sensory deprivations may interfere with long-established activities and hobbies.
5. A number of medications such as antihypertensives may contribute to a depressive mood state.
6. Conditions such as Cerebrovascular disease, Parkinson's Disease and Alzheimer's disease are often associated with a higher incidence of depression.

Precipitating Factors

A number of medical conditions may cause depression (Table 28.1.). It is important therefore to consider the possibility of a depression as one of the presenting features of these conditions.

A number of diseases which result in chronic impairment, disability and/or pain may precipitate a depressive disorder. Nearly 50 per cent of stroke patients develop clinically important depression. There are three critical periods: immediately post-stroke, at discharge from acute care, and on cessation of active treatment. It is usually stated that the left hemisphere or left frontal strokes are most commonly associated with post-stroke depression (although this is controversial). It is thought to correlate with loss of brain catecholamines. This type of depression usually occurs within six months of the stroke but can occur years after.

A number of psychiatric conditions may have depression as a feature including: bipolar affective disorders; schizophrenia; borderline personality; and grief reaction.

Table 28.1 Medical conditions associated with depression

Metabolic
thyroid disease, hypercalcemia, Cushing's, Addison's, hypoglycemia, hypokalemia
Nutritional deficiencies
iron, B_{12}, folate
CNS disease
Parkinson's, MS, SDAT, mass lesions, head trauma
Miscellaneous
viral infections, malignancy, pernicious anemia, sleep apnea

Some drugs which cause depressive symptoms are alcohol, amantadine, antipsychotics, cimetidine, clonidine, cytotoxics, digitalis, guanethidine, immunosuppressives, methyldopa, propranolol, sedatives, steroids, reserpine.

Subjective and Objective Features of Depression

The clinical picture can include many of the classical features of major depression (Table 28.2) or minor depression, but not uncommonly in the elderly more atypical features are seen (anxiety, insomnia, hypersomnia, phobia, somatization, pseudodementia). The picture may be dominated by vegetative symptoms (weight loss, early morning wakening, etc.). Symptoms of fatigue, thoughts of death, changes in weight and changes in sleep pattern are common in the elderly, often representing the presence of organic disease. The elderly often therefore present a challenge in the diagnosis of depression. Some of the features one might look for at the bedside are summarized in Table 28.1

A great deal of prominence is given to the presentation of depression as a disturbance of cognition (Pseudodementia). It should be appreciated that estimates of 20 per cent prevalence are based on observations made in institutionalized populations of two decades ago and are unlikely to be true of more modern practices. In many cases the picture of depression is readily distinguishable from that of dementia by features of datable onset, excessive memory complaints and inconsistency of mental state assessments. It has been observed that some cases of 'pseudodementia' are not as benign as was previously thought. As many as 50 per cent of such cases diagnosed in memory disorder clinics on follow-up subsequently present with a true dementia. It is possible that in those cases mild, early cognitive changes have been exacerbated by a mood disturbance, and so present early with apparently reversal with anti-depressive therapy. With time, however, the pathological process advances and a later representation occurs with irreversible dementia. Minor depression is a more chronic form of depression, and the symptoms are similar to major depression but are milder. Patients are

Table 28.2 The features of a major depression according to DSM IIIR criteria

A. At least five of the following symptoms occurring nearly every day during a 2-week period, representing a change from previous functioning (one of the symptoms must be criterion 1 or 2):
   1. depressed mood most of the day
   2. markedly diminished interest or pleasure in all, or almost all activities most of the day
   3. significant weight loss, weight gain, decrease or increase in appetite
   4. insomnia or hypersomnia
   5. psychomotor agitation or retardation
   6. fatigue or loss of energy
   7. feelings of worthlessness or excessive or inappropriate guilt, which may be delusional
   8. diminished ability to think or to concentrate or indecisiveness
   9. recurrent thoughts of dying or suicide

B. Exclusion of other causes of symptoms:
   1. organic factors
   2. normal reaction to the death of a loved one

Note: must distinguish between primary depression, and depression secondary to other medical and psychiatric disorders and drugs

At the bedside, major depression can be seen as:

Behaviour	Retardation/agitation, anxiety, negativism, anorexia symptoms are worse in the morning
Mood	Worried, perplexed
Thought	Poor concentration, hypochondriasis, 'I don't know',
Delusion	Poverty, catastrophe, guilt, suicide
Other	Somatization ⟶ pain, itch, burning
Depression	Previous depression &/or family history of

Fig. 28.1 Features of depression.

usually worried about health problems but have no delusions or vegetative symptoms. There can be a history of poor adjustments to major life losses and neurotic tendencies. Symptoms are present intermittently for at least two years.

Assessment

Evidence of organic disease should be sought in any suspected case of depression. Laboratory investigation should include CBC, ESR, urea and electrolytes, liver function tests, thyroid function tests and screening for syphilis. Attempts have been made to develop more specific tests for depression such as the dexamethasone suppression tests but their sensitivity and specificity are too low to be of value in routine clinical practice.

Plan

Supportive therapy is *always* indicated. Guidelines indicating a discrete depressive illness to be treated with antidepressants include:

1. a discrete change from baseline emotional state
2. affective symptoms are of recent onset
3. symptoms are sustained and do not react to changes in the environment
4. symptoms are out of proportion to an identifiable precipitant
5. the patient is anhedonic and has lost interest in usual activities

The above recommendations come from studies of young patients and have not been well validated in the elderly. Usually more aggressive therapy is considered if the depressive symptoms have been present for greater than 6 weeks and are causing symptoms or signs resulting in a disruption of normal life. Usually antidepressants are tried first, the choice being based on the individuals presenting features (agitation versus retardation), and co-existing diseases states (heart disease, renal or hepatic dysfunction, presence of dementia etc.) A summary of the major antidepressants is included in Fig. 28.2

Tertiary amines:
Imipramine, Amitriptylline, Doxepin
- more likely to cause postural hypotension
- prominent anticholinergic and sedative effects
- Doxepin may have less orthostatic effect
- anticholinergic side effects include:
  Central – delirium, cognitive impairment
  Peripheral – tachycardia, urinary retention, blurred vision, dry mouth

Secondary amines:
Desipramine, Nortriptyline, Trimipramine
- tend to have less anticholinergic effect and less sedative effect

Heterocyclic (second generation) compounds:
- Trazodone (Desyrel)--selective seretonin uptake blocker sedating but little anticholinergic or orthostatic effect
- Maprotiline (Ludiomil)–little anticholinergic effect and does not produce orthostatic hypotension

Generic	Trade	Daily dose	AC effect	SED. effect	POST hypot.
Amitriptylline	Elavil	25–100	+++	+++	+++
Doxepin	Sinequan	25–150	+++	+++	+++
Imipramine	Tofranil	25–100	+++	++	+++
Desipramine	Norpramine	25–100	+	+	+++
Nortriptyline	Aventil	25–100	++	++	++
Maprotiline	Ludiomil	25–150	++	+++	+
Trazodone	Desyrel	50–150	+	++	+

AC = anticholinergic; SED = sedative; POST hypot. = postural (orthostatic) hypotension.

Fig. 28.2 Antidepressive agents.

Depressed patients with psychotic features require both an antidepressant and an antipsychotic agent. Such a combination at therapeutic doses will be effective in 70 per cent of cases which compares favorably to only 30–40 per cent of either agent alone.

Monoamine oxidase inhibitors are often used as second-line agents after a trial of tricyclic or polycyclic agent. The major potential problem with their use is possible interactions with a number of food products and other drugs. With careful attention to precautions they can be extremely useful agents (Fig. 28.3).

Electroconvulsive therapy (ECT) is probably the single most effective therapy for depression alone or with psychotic features. It has been shown to be safe and effective in the elderly providing it is used appropriately. Its use should be considered in non-responsive cases to medications, perceived high risk of suicide, presence of dehydration/malnutrition, evidence of poor compliance or tolerance to medications. To minimize memory impairment, ECT is administered to the non-dominant hemisphere whenever possible. The only absolute contraindication is the presence of increased intracranial pressure.

2. Paranoid Disorders in Late Life

Persecutory ideations are seen in 2–4.5 per cent of the elderly community. In studies of the elderly with psychiatric disorders 10–17 per cent will suffer from delusions of a paranoid nature. Cooper noted the higher prevalence of deafness in patients with paranoid psychosis. Patients with early dementia may develop delusions and hallucinations at any stage of the illness. Characteristically they may occur early on, and be the first sign of deterioration. Acute onset may be a feature of delirium precipitated by another problem such as infection or change in medications. Patients with dementia who develop paranoid ideation may have a personality that has always been suspicious. It is also true that many of these patients have sensory impairment – poor vision or hearing – and misinterpret things. It becomes problematical to determine if such patients have intermittent delirium, as they decline cognitively they often get mixed up with their medications and confusion increases; drug handling worsens and the patient enters a deteriorating spiral. This scenario is much more frequent in practice and easier to handle than the patient with true paraphrenia or schizophrenia.

The two main paranoid psychotic disorders in the elderly are paraphrenia and schizophrenia. Paraphrenia usually refers to those individuals who are cognitively intact but have well-circumscribed paranoid delusions. Their personalities are often well preserved and generally they are moderately well compensated to their delusions. Often the delusions take an auditory nature. They have to be distinguished from the more common paranoid delusion seen as part of a delirium response to acute illness. Such patients require treatment with antipsychotic agents only if there is interference with their normal life.

Many physicians are reluctant to make the diagnosis of Schizophrenia at an age greater than 40 to 50 years. The onset of paranoid symptoms in this age group most often results in a diagnosis of Organic Mental disorder. Nevertheless, most stud-

Must adhere to a diet free of Tyramine, avoid some medications including 'over the counter' medications
No anticholinergic effect and less sedating than tricyclics
Most frequent side effects are hypotension and insomnia
Most frequent serious side effect is hypertensive crisis caused by ingestion of tyramine or drugs, i.e. meperidine, sympathomimetics, amphetamines
Generally well tolerated in the elderly

MAO inhibitors	Trade	Daily dose	AC effect	SED. effect	POST hypot.
Phenelzine	Nardil	15–45	–	+	+++
Tranylcypramine	Parnac	5–20	–	+	+++

Fig. 28.3 Monoamine oxidase (MAO) inhibitors use precautions.

ies of geriatric psychiatric in-patients with a diagnosis of schizophrenia, reveal about 5 per cent with an onset of symptoms after age 45, and a smaller proportion with onset of symptoms after age 60.

The symptoms of late onset Schizophrenia may not be different from the younger patients. First rank symptoms including auditory hallucinations and thought withdrawal, are not infrequently described in paraphrenics. Auditory hallucinations are usually discussed by the patient in the third person. They lack the religious or mystical quality of the hallucinations frequently observed in younger patients. In one retrospective study of 658 elderly patients with a clinical diagnosis of Schizophrenia, however, only 25 per cent showed a clinical course clearly compatible with Schizophrenia. A further 18.7 per cent showed substantial affective symptomatology, and 40.6 per cent showed signs of organic mental disease.

Some classic symptoms are milder in the elderly with late onset including: affect incongruity, thought blocking, verbal incoherence, grimacing and manneristic movements.

The personal history of these patients may include:

1. suspicious, aggressive personalities
2. history of involvement in cults, sects
3. increased incidence of hearing difficulties
4. often have few friends, surviving relatives

Schizophrenics with onset early in life tend to improve, or at least plateau, with advancing age. The reason for this is unclear. The treatment of the elderly schizophrenic involves the use of neuroleptics. The physician should be aware of the increased incidence of side effects in the elderly:

1. tardive dyskinesia
2. extrapyramidal signs
3. orthostatic hypotension
4. sedation
5. cardiac toxicity
6. anticholinergic effect

Suggested reading

Blazer, G. (1986). Suicide in late life, review and commentary. *JAGS*, **4**: 519–525.

Craig, T. J. and Bregman, Z. (1988). Late onset schizophrenialike illness. *JAGS*, **36** (2), February: 104–107.

Goff, D. C. (1986). Treatment resistant depression in the elderly. *JAGS*, **34**: 63–70.

House, A. (1987). Depression after stroke. *Brit. Med. J.*, **294**: 76–8.

Jenike, J. A. (1988). Assessment and treatment of affective illness in the elderly. *J. Ger. Psych. Neurol.*, **1**: 89–107.

Karlinsky, H. (1984). The clinical use of electroconvulsive therapy in old age. *JAGS*, **32**: 183–6.

Mielke, D. H. Multiple monitored electroconvulsive therapy. *JAGS*, **32**: 180–2.

Peabody, C. A. (1986). Antidepressants and the elderly. *JAGS*, **34**: 869–74.

Post, F. (1980). Paranoid, schizophrenialike, and schizophrenic states in the aged. In: Birren, J. E. and Sloane, R. B. *Handbook of Mental Health and Aging*. PrenticeHall, Englewood Cliffs, NJ. Ch. xx, pp. 591–616.

Robinson, R. G. (1986). Poststroke mood disorders. *Hosp. Prac.*, April.

29

Bioethics

Introduction

Bioethics is important to all physicians in all areas of medical practice, and much has been written. In the practice of geriatric medicine bioethics is extremely important because the physician is grappling with difficult decisions every day. Often these decisions are whether to start or to stop treatments which might be considered life saving. The physician often has to deal with the patient who is no longer capable of making decisions for themselves or who may not be able to express themselves. The geriatrician should be aware of the principles of bioethics and for his/her practice to be ethical will be putting these principles into practice every day.

In a book of this sort it is not appropriate to simply reiterate all the teachings of medical ethics, but we have attempted to define the important problem areas. Although the result is quite comprehensive it is neither exhaustive nor complete. There are areas that we have not touched upon, but we hope that by application of the principles that we have espoused the fresh problems can be approached in a logical and ethical manner to the satisfaction of all concerned. We will deal with the principles that should govern the practice of geriatric medicine, and then move on to discuss three problem areas – placing limits on treatment, dealing with the incompetent patient and finally special issues with regard to research.

1. Principles

Patient autonomy

All people experience losses as they age, and for many elderly people it is loss of function which leads to loss of independence. With loss of independence the individual becomes dependent upon others for various types of care. As significant others take over the care, they often take over the decision-making which removes the patient's autonomy. Within some societies it has become almost acceptable to deny elderly individuals the right to speak for themselves, with others (family or 'society') making decisions for them. This has resulted in the elderly being less vocal within their society and perhaps accepting of their position so that their expectations are reduced. It is easy to see why in this environment it becomes easy for the individual's wishes to be overlooked and for physicians and other health care professionals to make decisions for their elderly patients.

An important principle in geriatric practice is that the patient's wishes are paramount. It is now generally accepted that patients have the right to self determination and that should they choose to refuse life saving treatment that this should be honored by physicians as it is honored within the courts. There are of course some important exceptions;-

1. Protection of a third party. When treatment is necessary to prevent the spread of infection then individual autonomy can be overridden for the benefit of the state.
2. Administration of justice In certain instances prisoners have been treated against their will so that justice can be administered an example would be force feeding.
3. Suicide: Until recently suicide was a criminal offence, and there remain instances when physicians and others have made appeal to the courts when treatment would be life saving and relatively free of burden. In most instances despite the states interest in preserving life and despite possible appearance of self-homicide, individual autonomy usually wins.

Some might argue that refusal of treatment might compromise the integrity of the medical profession, but such a challenge has not been used successfully to override individual autonomy. This principle of autonomy should be uppermost in the mind of the physicians working with their elderly patient. To enable older, dependent patients to make up their minds they should be aware of all the potential benefits and burdens of proposed treatments. This means that the physician has to be knowledgeable in this area and recognize potential for recovery. A positive caring attitude makes a great deal of difference and patients soon recognize the interest and dedication of their physicians and other members of the team. Patients may well make different decisions when they are being cared for properly than when they are being neglected. If a health care team shows little interest and offers no hope for improvement, a patient may well become resigned to no treatment and continuing deterioration. On the other hand, a patient who is surrounded by health professionals who enjoy working with the elderly, who recognize their patient's disabilities and help set goals and objectives for the patient to achieve and who encourage independence, is likely to do better and develop a more positive attitude.

The important principle here is that autonomy is recognized, so that patients can make up their mind under optimal conditions. It is also important to recognize that when a patient wishes to place certain limits on his/her treatment this does not prevent continuing optimal therapy up to that point. It is also recognized that during times of stress and illness some patients wish to relinquish their autonomy in so far as they hand over medical decision-making to their physician. The patient will usually want to be kept fully informed, will wish to give consent, but will rely upon the medical expertise of the physician, asking them to act in their (the patient's) best interest. Respecting a patient's autonomy will include being prepared to respect their wishes in this regard and for the physician to accept this responsibility. The physician must be continually aware of the patient's feelings and hopefully will help patients to take back the responsibility for decision making as soon as they are able.

Treatment should be medically appropriate

In patients who have a number of interacting problems due to disease or aging, treatment decisions are often difficult. It is well recognized that treatment of one problem may exacerbate another. It becomes difficult to determine when treatment is no longer beneficial and that deterioration is inevitable. For these reasons, such elderly patients need to be looked after by individuals experienced with this type of patient and their problems. It is often the case that such patients are looked after by physicians who do not know them well, and whose experience rests with younger patients with simpler problems. Inappropriate decisions can therefore be made which add unnecessary burdens to the patient and may simply prolong the dying process.

If physicians are capable of making decisions which do not benefit the patient it is easy to see how patients and family members can also make requests of physicians for care and treatment that are inappropriate. For example, in a patient with advanced obstructive lung disease and a previous cerebrovascular event it is known that in the event of cardiac arrest resuscitation is almost always ineffective. In all studies that have been done which have shown that age is no barrier to successful resuscitation, it has been shown that disease burden is a barrier, and that resuscitation is not successful for the type of patient described above. If this is so then it is not an appropriate medical option. A physician has the responsibility not to offer inappropriate types of treatment and should not be asking patients or their family whether they want something done that is known to be useless.

This argument can be taken further, in that when patients are dying from an illness such as cancer or even dementia it needs to be recognized that death will take place. Physicians need to recognize that when death is expected it is not identified as a cardiac arrest. Technology is often being applied or considered inappropriately. Cardiac resuscitation is successful for sudden unexpected death during the course of myocardial infarction and recovery from it, it is not a procedure that should be extended to every episode of death. Yet this is the situation that has occurred in most places and many hospitals have a policy that cardiac resuscitation will always be instituted unless ordered otherwise. Fortunately, when some patients are asked, they understand the stupidity of the question and elect for no code. Many others do not, but it is the physicians responsibility to inform patients and families of appropriate treatment.

The situation becomes more complex when we start dealing with other forms of technological intervention. In some societies certain decisions have been made for economic reasons – for example that none over the age of 65 will be dialysed if they have renal failure. In other places no such ruling applies and age is not considered a barrier. Does a very old patient with multiple problems including cardiac failure and renal failure have the right to ask for dialysis when it is known that it is not going to be successful? Or does a family member have that right if the patient is incompetent?

Physicians have the responsibility to identify the treatment options that are appropriate and point out the benefits and burdens to the patient or appointed decision maker. The physician should not give options that are medically inappropriate. By paying more attention to this area there will be significant savings in terms of suffering as well as cost.

Ageism and disease burden

If a society decides to place limits on treatment options for the very old, for example by limiting access to patients of 75 or older to an intensive care unit, then when a 78 year old has respiratory failure for the first time that person's death on a geriatric ward would be unfortunate. Death might have been preventable by appropriate treatment of the pneumonia and short-term intubation and ventilator support. But society had made a rule therefore the result is unfortunate but not unfair. There have been many examples of decisions such as the one mentioned above, where the older patient has suffered misfortune because of restrictions placed on treatment options. With better understanding of aging and more people working with the elderly patient it has become clear that many decisions have been made with insufficient information or because of mistaken assumptions. Inappropriate attitudes have been revealed and ageism fostered.

An important principle or value that ought to govern health care of the elderly is that management decisions will not be made on the basis of age. Patients will not be denied access to certain types of treatment or to certain facilities simply because they have achieved a certain age. Rather, treatment decisions will be based upon medical problems that the patient has and the associated disease burden and functional impairment. For example, it might be appropriate not to admit a 75 year old patient to an intensive care unit for intubation and ventilator support if that is what the patient wishes or if the pulmonary disease is end stage and there are associated significant problems in other systems. It would not be appropriate to refuse admission simply because that person was 75 years old, remembering that such a decision is reached if such a patient is automatically admitted to a geriatric unit isolated from a hospital which has such facilities!

Economic issues

Many of us would like to practice medicine in an environment where one does not have to think about the cost. Such a situation does not exist and physicians have an obligation to consider the cost of the treatment that they request, and to behave responsibly with regard to expenditure in keeping with what is accepted as normal practice within society. If government places an upper limit on expenditure then care has to be rationed. Physicians will have to practice within limits set, but must continue to practice humane and ethical medicine. When decisions are needed physicians have to do the best with what they have, a situation which is imposed by the society of which the physician is a member. This does not mean that physicians do not have the right to demand and fight for change. If one considers the development of the speciality of geriatric medicine one realizes that this is exactly what the practitioners of this speciality have had to do, and are continuing to do.

The principle is that elderly individuals have as much right to appropriate treatment as younger members of our society, and should not be rejected or treated with benign neglect. It is our contention that if elderly patients are treated appropriately – neither being neglected (rejected) nor being subjected to unwarranted investigation or treatment – then money would be saved. Without question there would be relief of much suffering. There is now ample evidence in the literature that geriatric programs like assessment (evaluation and management) units, reactivation (rehabilitation or restorative care) units, day hospitals and consultation services have a significant and positive impact on health care of the elderly. This means that in times of fiscal restraint when new programs are not being developed there needs to be reallocation of resources. An important aspect of geriatric practice is to ensure that this is realized and that new programs continue to develop. Such programs do cost money, and it is unfortunate that they tend to lose out during allocation when competing against the more glamorous high technology programs. Physicians need to be involved in this area for the foreseeable future.

2. Placing limits on therapy

Introduction

Deciding upon what treatment is medically appropriate is the role of the physician. It is what the physicians have been trained for and for what they are paid. This has already been discussed. With advancing age the probability of the patient having more than a single problem increases dramatically. Each patient may have several diseases that require simultaneous treatment and investigation as well as attention to functional impairment that has occurred as a result of the aging process or specific pathology. Each day in the practice of geriatric medicine one is faced with options – to treat or not to treat. Usually the choice is difficult because the predicted outcomes are not clear cut. Often it is clear that there should be limits placed upon therapy because of the unacceptable burdens that will be imposed. The concept of the 'limit' applies to technological intervention or aggressive therapy. Perhaps a better way of defining it is 'as an alternative treatment protocol'. Decisions are made for example that treatment will not include admission to an intensive care unit. Many consider this a limit with the mistaken belief that such treatment is always beneficial and the best. We argue that this is not always the case and that such treatment has the potential to be harmful to certain patients and would merely add undesirable and unnecessary burdens or prolong the dying process. The 'alternative or appropriate treatment protocol' is to recognise that other forms of treatment which are equally demanding, but require less technology, is more appropriate. For example instituting palliative care, or perhaps continuing active geriatric care but accepting that if sudden deterioration occurs then death will be accepted as an inevitable and nonreversible outcome. Appropriate treatment is the preferred term because many consider placing limits means no treatment. Such practice would be unacceptable morally and ethically and would reflect, perhaps, ageism. How are such problems defined and how are decisions such as these made?

The decision–maker

The patient

The patient has the right to decide which treatment options they would wish to pursue, given that they are in a position to exercise judgement and that they are fully informed. When a decision is being sought the physician seeking the decision should be fully informed and knowledgeable. Elderly patients have as much right to expertise as any other patient. The point being that elderly patients with complex interacting problems have the right to have physicians with training in geriatric medicine looking after them. Care for such patients should not be relegated to physicians with no specific training and lack of experience.

The physician has the responsibility to determine that the patient is equipped with the facts, as far as they are understood and that their mental competence is not clouded by cognitive impairment or mental illness. The physician must guard against assuming that because a patient disagrees with their decision and has different priorities, that their competence is suspect. The physician should not try to persuade the patient to change his or her mind unless it is clear that a different decision would be life saving with no significant added burden. Ethical practice implies respect for a patient's autonomy. In geriatric practice it is common to see patients who have experienced that their autonomy is ignored or not respected.

Patients should be involved in decision-making about their care from the beginning of the physician patient interaction. Even in those patients who have lost their ability to reason there is a great deal of scope for meaningful involvement in their care. A patient may not be able to balance a cheque book but may have clear ideas about what makes them happy and where they want to live. They may not be able to give consent, but should be able to assent. Apart from the ethical considerations it is much better to have an involved and willing patient for any diagnostic or therapeutic intervention.

It is not always possible to accede to a patient's wishes – for example a male patient of 78 is admitted because of continuing deterioration and the development of fecal incontinence. He has long-standing hypertension, controlled cardiac failure, peripheral vascular disease, cerebrovascular disease with a previous stroke, degenerative osteoarthritis and chronic lung disease. He is dependent in most activities of daily living and requires a wheel chair for mobilizing. He is found to be in renal failure with end-stage renal disease. In discussing the problem with the patient he says that he wants everything done including a kidney transplant. Requests like this need to be handled by sensitive discussion and the patient needs to be made aware that such treatment is not a medical option, and although the patient may want this it is not a choice that is available. There is no ethical dilemma here, not providing that particular treatment is not compromising the patient's autonomy. The standard of practice that is required is that the patient is kept aware of his condition and the treatment options that are possible.

The physician

The physician is responsible to make medically appropriate decisions, incorporating the various principles that have already been discussed. Patients, or their families, contract with the physician to provide medical care. The physician is expected to make decisions, in conjunction with the wishes of a fully informed patient. There are many instances in geriatric practice when the alternatives in choice are not clear cut, for example when the choice between treatment or no treatment is not always life or death, but rather the degree or type of burden. In this situation the physician may advise but the decision is with the patient.

In the personal contract between physician and patient there may well be an unwritten understanding. The patient wanting full autonomy when comparatively well and able to cope with decision-making; but wishing to hand over the burden of decision-making to the professional when ill and dependent. In the past there has been an assumption that this is often the case and that this is paternalism. It is important to recognize that patient's have the right to hand over this aspect of their care when they wish to do so and it is the responsibility of the physician to accept this.

In decision-making it is important for the patient to be aware of all options and the relevant information. In our present-day obsession with truth telling one must ask the question as to whether the physician has to reveal everything. The answer of course, is no. Only that information that is relevant to decision-making needs to be shared. Furthermore, truth needs to be shared at the appropriate time. Information is like a drug, timing and amount are important. Everything should not be unloaded on a patient as soon as known, and in geriatric practice when assimilation of new data takes longer there needs to be time for this to take place.

Is it ethical to withhold the truth? The answer must be no. The information should be revealed to the best of the ability of the physician, and always when requested. There is no place for withholding important information to protect the well being of the patient. Some would argue that 'white lies' are permissible and that this represents benevolent obfuscation. There is no moral justification for this. However it is not necessary to reveal information that is not requested neither is it justified to reveal uncertainties unless there is a treatment choice which the physician cannot make.

The family

Those individuals who are unable to make decisions for themselves, who are incompetent because of cognitive or communicative impairment, should have a significant other as proxy decision-maker. There are some elderly who have thought of this eventuality and have drawn up living wills with designated decision-makers or who have appointed someone with enduring power of attorney. Others have legally appointed guardians. For many others there are a number of family members who prefer to act by consensus. The proxy decision-maker is treated in the same way as the patient, is fully informed and shares in the decision-making process with the physician. The proxy decision-maker takes over and exercises the patient's autonomy. It has been suggested that the main role of the family is to provide information to reveal the patient's wishes and to act in accordance with those wishes. This is so and is the moral obligation of the proxy. The same restrictions with regard to useless treatment and nonviable options pertains to the proxy decision-makers as it does to patients.

In this setting the physician needs to be aware of the potential for abuse, when the needs of the family are served rather than the patient. It is the responsibility of the physician and other members of the health care team to ensure that all decisions are made in the best interests of the patient.

In order to support appropriate decision-making, communication needs to be encouraged with regular meetings. When there are multiple family members dissent can be kept to a minimum by good communication. When conflict remains, a decision needs to be made that does not add unnecessary burdens to the patient, consensus may not be reached but the assent of all members may be achieved. When the problem is continuing dissent between family members and physician then arbitration must be sought. This can often be achieved by means of an ethics consultation or referral to a bioethics committee. In rare instances courts will need to be approached for legal decision-making.

Appropriate (limited) treatment protocols

When treatment is given to a patient it is hoped that it will be beneficial and this outcome can usually be detected. Similarly in many instances it can soon be detected that treatment is futile. Between these two black and white extremes there is a grey area or ambiguous zone. In elderly patients with multiple problems it is often very difficult to determine when treatment is futile or when the burden is too great. Whilst being difficult it is also of increasing importance that physicians can recognize the point at which it is appropriate to switch from aggressive to palliative therapy. This timing is likely to be influenced by the personal wishes of the patient or family. Because it is a switch in therapy one should think of appropriate treatment protocols, rather than limitation of treatment. However it is the use of highly technical medicine, such as is found within an intensive care unit, that is seen as needing to be limited – hence the term.

It has been discussed that treatment that is useless should not be used. When further treatment is considered futile and that it will only prolong the process of dying or alter the mode of death, then there is no reason, moral or otherwise, to continue therapy. The difficulty arises when doctors who know nothing about the premorbid state of the patient, and know nothing about the wishes of the patient are called upon to treat in emergency or acute situations. A nursing home resident deteriorates and is sent to the emergency room of the acute hospital. Resuscitation measures are instituted and cannot be stopped – the patient is 'caught by the machines' and endless resources are poured into the 'black hole of natural death'. This is the problem. One solution has been to identify treatment options for patients in long term care settings, where many of the patients have a significant disease burden.

Patients may be classified into four basic categories:

- Class A The patient may be fully independent or partially dependent but has no medical problems that can be considered terminal.
- Class B The patient is dependent in activities of daily living, at home or within an institution. The dependency resulting from chronic disease, psychiatric, medical or a combination of both. None of the problems can be considered to be terminal.
- Class C The patient is extremely dependent with a combination of major medical problems, which will not lead to death in the immediate future but may well limit life-span.
- Class D The patient is terminally ill from one or more major medical problems and death is considered to be both inevitable and imminent.

This classification was developed to help in decision-making with patients residing within institutions on a long-term basis. The boundaries are not clear cut. For example, a patient with advanced Alzheimer's disease might be considered to be terminally ill and therefore Class D. However time of death is difficult to predict and many would not consider death to be imminent, thus putting the patient in Class C because of extreme dependency. The classification helps in decision-making and provides guidelines. The wishes of the patient should be determined first of all, and if the patient is incompetent the proxy decision-maker will need to be consulted. Thus some patients whatever their level of dependency or degree of 'illness' will decide that they would not want heroic measures whatever the circumstance. The guidelines for treatment choices would be as follows:

- Class A In the event that acute illness develops or a sudden emergency like cardio-respiratory arrest there will be maximum therapeutic efforts. Such patients are candidates for intensive care units. Age is no barrier.
- Class B Maximum therapeutic efforts may be instituted and these patients should be transferred to an acute care hospital. Treatment will stop short of emergency resuscitation or transfer to an intensive care unit either because it is the patient's wishes or because of the nature of the chronic diseases that provide medical contraindications.
- Class C The treatment choice here is likely to be palliative with therapeutic efforts being designed for comfort rather than cure. Such patients may well require the facilities of an acute care hospital but are not candidates for an intensive care unit, for emergency resuscitation or other types of aggressive therapy. In order to alleviate suffering diagnosis and appropriate treatment is indicated in certain circumstances. In this category it is possible to make statements on certain

treatment options – for example artificial feeding by nasogastric tube or by gastrostomy, dialysis, antibiotic use, blood transfusion.

Class D Treatment is palliative and is aimed at comfort, not cure and not prolongation of life. Further investigation and invasive monitoring are not indicated and would be considered unacceptable.

It can be seen that this approach has the potential to prevent unnecessary transfer to hospital from nursing home and to limit unnecessary aggressive therapy. It is *not* designed to restrict admission to hospital of those that need it. It means that more physician involvement is required within the institutional setting to determine approaches before the event. It means that the records of such decisions need to be available to the physicians that look after these patients – for example, within the emergency room. It should also be remembered that these are guidelines and as such can be flexible. The physicians that are involved with the patient in making decisions should be knowledgeable in this area. There is a risk that the old patient with chronic disease is put in a lower category than is justified because the potential for improvement with expert treatment is not identified. This makes it essential that all physicians who will be dealing with elderly patients should receive training in geriatric medicine. Theory is important, but physicians need to gain experience within geriatric units to understand the potential for recovery that elderly patients may have.

Cardiac resuscitation

In most hospitals there is a policy that unexpected 'collapse' is recognized as an emergency and that the cardiac arrest team is summoned. The emergency team that arrives is trained to identify the nature of the problem leading to collapse and to institute emergency resuscitation measures. An important cause of sudden collapse is cardiac arrest, and prompt medical intervention may reverse a rhythm problem and save a patient. It has been shown that age is no barrier, and the results within coronary care units are as good for the old as the young (Table 29.1). Associated disease is a barrier and patients with cerebrovascular disease or chronic lung disease fare much worse and are unlikely to get out of hospital. In the setting of an intensive care unit where the patient is being closely monitored the chances of successful resuscitation from an arrest are considerably higher than if the same thing occurs at home, in a nursing home or at a distant site in a hospital.

Table 29.1 Outcome of cardiac arrest

No discernible effect	Definite effect
Age	Disease burden: worse with CVA, COPD, etc. Location: better in ICU in hospital Team: better with more experience Delay after event: worse with longer time

Emergency resuscitation is a technique that has been developed to deal with sudden unexpected death when this is due to a cardiac problem – specifically a sudden rhythm problem. Such a technique should be utilized when appropriate and not offered when inappropriate. In other words it should be recognized that patients die in hospital, and that for many conditions the inevitable outcome is death. When death occurs in this setting it should not be considered as a cardiac arrest. Many hospitals have a no resuscitation policy, which allows a physician to write an order that there will not be a code call in the event of death or collapse. The patient may request this, or the health care team might suggest because of the nature of the patient's problems. The patient who is dying is allowed to die if sudden collapse occurs.

It seems that common sense has left the medical and nursing professions if we offer such a technique to those where death is inevitable and imminent. It is inappropriate and illogical. When treatment is being discussed with a patient, or proxy decision maker, if death is acknowledged as inevitable and imminent, the physician should make it clear that arrest calls with the potential for further high technology medicine and intensive care units will not be offered – it is not offered as an option for the patient or significant others to make a decision about.

For patients who are residing at home this is not an issue. For those within nursing homes it may be. If there is a trained arrest team and there is proximity to an acute care hospital then emergency resuscitation might be instituted. In one such institute with approximately 150 patients such a team has been in existence for several years. In this same institution there has been a no resuscitation protocol for about 4 years. During this time a decision has been reached on every patient, and in approximately half the patients a no code order is written. There is a significant death rate, but a code is called only rarely. A successful cardiac resuscitation has not occurred and one must therefore ask if such an emergency procedure should be made available.

Patients need to be made aware of the fact that on admission to hospital if there is sudden collapse then emergency resuscitation will be commenced. Thus all patients should be prompted to consider if they would like limits to be placed on their treatment. This is best done at the time of admission rather than when there are changes. Discussion of emergency resuscitation in a very ill patient is not helpful to the mental well being of the patient. The alternative treatment protocols that have already been discussed are appropriate for all patients, and this has been recognized in some areas so that the living will is legal. The living will outlines the wishes of the patient which is binding on the physician. In this context the question of emergency cardiac resuscitation should also be considered.

The decision not to offer this is a medical one. Such a decision should not compromise medical treatment in other ways. There is a tendency to interpret 'no code' as being palliative therapy only. 'No code' means that in the event of cardiopulmonary arrest, cardiopulmonary resuscitation measures will not be instituted. It might be appropriate to respond to other emergencies such as a sudden bleed or aspiration of food. Because of this difficulty perhaps the style of ordering should be changed. When patients are dying it is identified, and in these circumstances there is no emergency. In other circumstances where the issue is that intensive care and high technology medicine is contraindicated, and death is not imminent or expected then a code is called but the team only responds to the immediately remediable such as a blocked airway. External cardiac massage will not be instituted.

At the present time it is ethically acceptable to write orders for no resuscitation. Hospitals should be encouraged to have such a protocol in place.

Stopping treatment

Physicians and other health professionals have great difficulty in stopping treatment, once started. Because of this some physicians decide not to start treatment in the first place. This is unfortunate since it may prevent a patient from having treatment that would not only be life prolonging but also life saving.

For example, an old person sustains a major cerebrovascular accident which results in a reduction in the level of consciousness and impairment of swallowing. Nutrition and hydration become significant management problems. Medical nutrition should be commenced and continued until the prognosis is clear. If the patient gets no recovery of swallowing and the impaired consciousness does not improve or gets worse then medical nutrition can be stopped. The procedure that is used in such situations should be of a temporary nature because of this possibility of stopping, it is much more difficult to reverse a permanent feeding gastrostomy for example.

Stopping treatment has been the subject of wide discussion by ethicists and it is generally agreed that the decision to stop is ethically no different to the decision not to treat in the first place. The same considerations of benefits and burdens apply, the only difference is that prognosis has become clearer. Since the prognosis is clearer then one might conclude that to decide not to treat in the first instance on the grounds that one would have difficulty in stopping is in fact unethical.

The same reasoning holds whatever the treatment. Thus patients always have the right to change their mind and assert their autonomy. With time, conditions change and prognosis often becomes clearer. This may well change the decision. Although in practice physicians feel uncomfortable with this it should be seen to be not only ethical but also of most potential benefit to the patients.

Medical nutrition

Important aspects of medical nutrition have been covered in the Chapter 16. The question of stopping such treatment has been discussed in the previous segment. Medical nutrition remains one of the difficult and controversial areas of medical care today.

There is debate as to whether medical nutrition represents ordinary or extraordinary means of support. We would recommend that for ethical decision-making medical nutrition represents extraordinary support, it is beyond routine nursing care. As such the decision to use any extraordinary means of treatment should only occur after due ethical consideration.

The important factors are the benefits to the patient in terms of cure of their problem, prolongation of life, relief of suffering and ability to return to their former state of well-being. On the other hand one has to consider the burdens – those imposed by the treatment itself as well those imposed by the prolonging of life. In most instances there is enough time to consider the different options before treatment is commenced, but if not treatment can be commenced to be discontinued, if necessary, as the prognosis becomes clearer.

In the case of the patient who is terminally ill, where death is inevitable and imminent, medical nutrition is usually not indicated. Palliative care units have shown quite clearly that there are alternatives to medical nutrition, such as good mouth hygiene, if the intent is to relieve suffering. In some situations it is clear that the patient is terminally ill but the imminence of death is in question. One court decision concluded that imminence was in fact within one year. It is very difficult to make sound prognostic judgements of this type. When feeding is simply prolonging life which can be considered biological or non-cognitive, and there is no evidence of suffering by not feeding then it is ethically acceptable not to feed or to stop feeding. When the patient is actively resisting feeding by pulling out a tube or spitting out food, as in the patient with advanced dementia, then feeding is providing an unnecessary burden and should not be started or may be discontinued.

There are no clear guidelines which help in decision making of this type. Any decision should be ethical, which means that the wishes of the patient (or proxy decision-maker) are taken into account and that no treatment which can be considered either useless or imposing unnecessary burdens is instituted. When there is doubt about comfort of the patient, where failing to provide nutrition or hydration is thought to be producing suffering then there should be no question that this should be relieved. Physician's and nurses, like any person, may have very different perceptions as to what is the correct treatment and what is minimal accepted standard. Thus individuals with the same training and cultural background might conclude that going without food is inhuman and imposes unnecessary suffering even for the patient in a persistent non-cognitive (vegetative) state, and others would see this as perfectly acceptable and that prolonging life for no reason is inhuman. Such arguments are difficult to reconcile and it would appear that providing medical nutrition or withholding it are equally acceptable ethical decisions. It needs to stressed that when decisions of this sort are made that the physicians determines the benefits and the burdens, and that these are discussed openly with patient or proxy decision maker.

The incompetent patient

For ethical decision making the autonomy of the patient has been stressed. In deciding upon investigations and treatment, particularly when the outcome in terms of benefits and burdens is not clear, the patient has the final word. In order to make a decision the patient has to be adequately informed. And for consent to be informed the patient must understand the information that is being transmitted.

The physician has a double responsibility. First to ensure that he/she him/herself is well informed. This will be achieved by experience and by learning, acquired from didactic instruction and self-direction. The physician also has to be able to communicate this knowledge to the patient. Secondly, the physician has to determine that the patient can receive this information, interpret it and communicate the decision. The ethical physician ensures that knowledge and practice is up to date. In geriatric practice the physician needs to be able to assess the patient to determine that communication is open, that the patient can comprehend and interpret this material and then act upon it. In other words determine that the patient is competent.

To be competent means to be well qualified, capable, fit, sufficient or legally qualified *(Webster's Dictionary)*. In the context that we are discussing here we are talking of being capable of making decisions about care. Competence implies comprehension. To comprehend one must receive. Thus the patient who cannot receive information is rendered incompetent by the inability to understand. The totally deaf person can be communicated with by writing, but when there is blindness as well there is no way to communicate. The aphasic patient may understand one-or two-step commands with gesturing but is unlikely to understand abstract concepts. Furthermore, such a patient is unlikely to be able to express their wishes and probably not be able to read.

In geriatric practice incompetence in decision making usually stems from a failure to comprehend, secondary to cognitive impairment. The geriatric physician is also called upon to make decisions with regard to ability to live alone, the amount of help that is required for a safe and comfortable existence, the ability to operate a motor vehicle and the ability to manage financial affairs.

To define competence in decision-making the physician relies upon information gathered from the patient, the family and care providers. The patient will need to be examined, preferably over a period of time and on several occasions. Apart from a formal test of mental status, the patient's understanding is judged using relatively simple methods of seeking interpretations of stories, proverbs, sayings, and so on.

At the present time, although many jurisdictions define a legal age for a child to be considered competent in decision-making, it is now widely accepted that competence does not come at a particular time but instead there is increasing competence or increasing ability to participate in decision-making – ultimately resulting in full competence. The same is true of elderly patients with cognitive impairment. A patient may be unable to manage their own financial affairs, it may be unsafe to leave the patient in the home alone, but he/she may be able to maintain an ability to understand certain aspects of care and treatment and therefore have a major input into any decision. When there is cognitive impairment the physician will usually need to bring a proxy decision-maker into the process. For all but those with advanced dementia it is possible to sit down with patient and family member and obtain consent in that setting. Such an approach demonstrates a continuing respect for the individual and maintains the focus on the patient as the key decision-maker.

When a patient is considered to be incompetent, and there is no close family and no designated proxy decision-maker then the physician needs legal appointment of such a decision-maker. The patient needs to be made a ward of Court. This can be done rapidly and frequently the Chief Executive Officer of a Hospital will be given that role, particularly for emergency decision making. It is obvious that prior declaration of intent is invaluable in such situations. Patients can have living wills which contain clear statements as to their wishes as well as a designated decision-maker. Conflicts may be avoided when patients have already been considered with regard to appropriate treatment protocols.

Physicians and decision-makers must weigh all things carefully and ensure that the patient is treated within the basic norms of what is considered just and fair. Recognition of incompetence means that physician and proxy decision-maker need to be aware that the patient may be burdened by failing to understand what is happening and thus suffer psychic as well as physical pain. For example, moving a very confused patient to another hospital for a special investigation such as a CAT scan may be very distressing. The result often not contributing to management. Thus the burden of investigation and treatment is different for the cognitively impaired when they do not understand what is happening. For this reason decisions may well be different, and the switch from aggressive to palliative therapy may occur sooner than in the cognitively intact patient.

Other areas of competence

The ethical practitioner of geriatric medicine recognizes obligations to society as well as the patient. Because of impaired cognition patients may be a danger to others as well as themselves.

For example the confused patient living in an apartment block may represent a fire hazard, particularly if a smoker. In such situations the physician needs to identify the danger and ensure that living arrangements are such that these dangers are reduced to an acceptable level.

The cognitively or neurologically impaired elder represents a danger to others as well as himself when operating a motor vehicle. When such a potential problem is identified the physician has an obligation to reduce the danger. In most places this would mean writing to the authority that handles driving licences suggesting that a medical report is furnished and that further testing be done if considered appropriate. The physician should inform the patient and the family that this is being done. In many instances families will have recognized that this is a problem and will have already stopped that patient from driving. At other times this is not so and it might be that the cognitively intact spouse cannot drive and therefore has a vested interest in their partner continuing to drive. In such instances the intact spouse needs to be counselled with regard to alternative arrangements. At times this is hard on the impaired patient who experiences even more restrictions in an ever shrinking world. The physician is usually protected by law against any legal action for informing in this way and in many jurisdictions it is compulsory to inform. It should be realized that the patient has the opportunity to furnish a full medical report and the opportunity to be tested. It is better to be done in this way rather than waiting for an accident to occur and precipitate action.

If in the course of investigation it may become clear that a patient is no longer competent to manage their own financial affairs and it also needs to be recognized that such individuals are prone to abuse and financial exploitation. Family members need to be informed that power of attorney is no longer valid when a patient is declared incompetent unless it is enduring power of attorney which is legal in many areas. If this is not the case one of the family should apply for appointment as legal guardian by the courts. If there is no family the patient needs to be protected by application for the Public Trustee to ensure that financial matters are taken care of. For such patients there may be a persisting problem of who will act in terms of medical decision making, since public trustees are often not willing to take this on. There are some innovative approaches to this, such as recruiting and training 'volunteer' guardians – individuals who are strangers to the patient but who are prepared to become involved and act as proxy decision-maker.

3. Research

There is much to be learned about aging and the diseases of the aged. There is a need to improve health care of the elderly and to introduce more innovative methods of management. To achieve these things there is a requirement for research. It could be argued that those involved in this field of medicine have a moral obligation to be actively involved in research in some way – either directly or indirectly. On the other hand there is a need to ensure that patients are not exploited. Patients who find themselves captive within certain environments, such as a long-term care institution with academic affiliations, may be over-involved in research. Such patients represent a 'captive group' who are approached time and time again for participation. We have to ensure that this is not the case and that patients do not feel coerced into participating for fear that their care will be adversely influenced by nonparticipation. The issue of research using incompetent patients is also difficult. It would seem that 'society' has accepted the view that research into conditions like Alzheimer's disease is desirable. That the next of kin who would be making decisions with regard to treatment has the right to give consent for participation in research studies. Most would agree that there are unwritten guidelines with regard the research, and that the burdens to the patient will be minimal. Consent to invasive research that will produce suffering and no clear benefit to the individual will need to be looked at very carefully. The questions that are being asked need to be considered, together with the likely yield in new information. In other words, for the research to be ethical it needs to be scientifically valid.

Suggested reading

Besdine R. W. 1983 'The decision to withhold treatment from nursing home residents' *J. Amer. Ger. Soc.* **31**: 602–606

Dresser R. 1985 When patients resist feeding. *J. Amer. Ger. Soc.* **33**: 790–794.

Elford R. John ed. 1987. *Medical Ethics and Elderly People* Churchill Livingstone, (Edingburgh)

High D. M. 1987 Planning for decisional incapacity. J. Amer. Ger. Soc. **35**: 814–20

Jahnigen D. W. and Schrier R. W. 1986 *Ethical Issues in the Care of the Elderly* Vol 2, No. 3, *Clinics in Geriatric Medicine.* W. B. Saunders Philadelphia.

Thomasma D. C. 1984 Freedom and dependency in the very old. *J. Amer. Ger. Soc.* **32**: 906–14

30

Long-term care

It was from within institutional long-term care that the specialty of geriatric medicine developed. From its early beginnings with such pioneers as Dr Marjorie Warren, geriatric medicine has progressed into rehabilitation, acute care and prevention. Geriatric medicine still has an important role to play within institutional long-term care, but emotional attachment to the historical roots has prevented many from rational consideration of exactly what that role should be.

With deterioration and increasing functional impairment comes an increased likelihood of medical contact. As patients become disabled due to a combination of chronic problems, and dependent upon others for activities of daily living, there is an increased need for ongoing medical care. Thus long-term care is a term that can be used for the ongoing care of the frail or dependent elderly – either within the patient's home or within an institution of some sort.

1. Principles

There are several important principles that can be put forward to help in the management of patients in long-term care (Table 30.1). Perhaps the most important principle, is that the aim of 'medical' treatment and social supports is to allow the patient to live as independently as possible, or to function at as high a level as possible. The patient's level of care should be commensurate with the real need that is established by expert assessment. Expert assessment will also identify those patients who have a disability gap, who consistently function at a level lower than they are capable of. With recognition and identification of the problem the patient can be treated by the team including the psychologist in an attempt to narrow the gap. If this is not possible the expert team identifies the gap and makes appropriate recommendations with regards to future care.

Table 30.1 Principles of long-term care

1. The patient's level of care should be commensurate with the real need of the patient established by expert assessment.
2. Patients have the right to expert geriatric assessment by those trained to do so, namely geriatric specialists.
3. The physicians, primary care and consultant, must be trained in working with groups or teams of health care workers.
4. Primary care by those physicians trained in primary care – whatever the setting.

Many of these patients are complex and require expert assessment at various stages during 'long-term' care. Patients have the right to expect the most expert medical help available which is from specialists in geriatric medicine and geriatric psychiatry. An important principle would be to ensure that this kind of support is available to primary care physicians to help them in their management. Such consultants have the advantage of knowing the environment as well as the patient on a long-term basis. This does not preclude the intervention of other specialists as necessary, but it is suggested that multiple physician involvement can lead to over investigation, inappropriate treatments and iatrogenic problems.

A third principle is that the physician of record must know how to function within the setting of a health care team. This is essential for good care within an institution and is of increasing importance within the community. There is a real difference here between different societies. Family practitioners in the United Kingdom, routinely act in this way in the community, but in North America most still function as individual practitioners. The role within the team will be analysed more fully in the next section.

One problem that has arisen with the development of the specialty of geriatric medicine has been the controversy over who should look after the institutionalised elderly. This has arisen because of the system within the United Kingdom where virtually all hospital care is provided by specialist physicians and junior doctors in training. Traditionally geriatricians have controlled large blocks of hospital beds for long-term care. This has given rise to much emotion when this topic has been debated.

The fourth principle that we would put forward at this point is that the primary care of elderly patients should be carried out by those physicians who are trained to do it. In other words for most countries this would be the family physician or general practitioner. This would be true if the patient is either at home or within an institution. In some countries, such as the United States primary care is performed by those with specialist training in internal medicine as well as family practitioners. Most internal medicine training programs do not have a large component of geriatric medicine and do not cover some of the important areas such as family dynamics, team leadership, rehabilitation and psychiatry of old age. In any event primary care physicians should do the primary care, and should receive appropriate training for this. In some countries, for example the United Kingdom and United States, such training and knowledge can be recognized by examination. This is important since there are an inadequate number of specialist in the field of geriatrics and geriatric psychiatry and freeing them from the necessity of primary care allows them to do the consulting and advisory work for which they are trained.

2. Assessment

The primary care physician may well respond to an individual patients needs without recourse to other physician's or other health professionals. As dependency increases the need for other professional involvement increases and an important part of the training of primary care physicians is to learn how to work with the other health professionals and with consultants. The primary care physician needs to decide when it is necessary to call in additional help and when a more complete assessment should be carried out. Assessment is the technology of geriatric medicine and has been discussed at some length in Chapter 1.

The whole question of what constitutes a geriatric patient has been discussed in the first chapter of this book. The geriatric status scale was presented. It would be unusual for any patient with completely normal function to be housed within a long-term care institution – although it does occur. Assessment is indicated for any patient who deteriorates from independent function to impaired function. Any patient who deteriorates non-specifically so that their level of care of increases (in other words their level of care needs reclassification) needs to be looked at very carefully and should be fully assessed to determine if they can be treated and helped to return to their former level of function.

Those patients who are completely dependent and at the highest levels of care tend to be complex with several interacting medical problems (often physical and mental). Such patients often require time to be able to sort out the different problems to determine if there is treatment which can improve the patient's quality of life and to relieve suffering. This is the area of expertise possessed by the geriatric specialists and these patients need geriatric assessment. It should be pointed out that such assessment does not imply transfer to another unit since this can be done with the other health care professionals who are on site in long-term care. This aspect will be discussed further.

3. Team role

In long-term care the assessment team includes the physician with specialist training in geriatric medicine, the primary care physician, the nurses and other health professionals that are allocated. In many ways the team is no different to that which is found in acute geriatric assessment, but in practical terms such luxury is usually not available. The nucleus or core team in long-term care may be quite small and consist of nursing and medicine, the other members being called upon when required. The other health professionals need to be available – including social work, physiotherapy and occupational therapy. In this setting recreation plays a much more important role and together with pastoral care can be considered core members.

The team has several important roles. Assessment has already been completed to determine that the patient requires this level of care. Further assessment is necessary by those individuals who are providing the ongoing care. The thrust of the assessments being to develop a program of care to assist the patient (now a resident) to continue to function at as high a level as possible – with as high a quality of life as possible. The team will meet early on to share knowledge and information and then come up with the care plan. The care plan needs to be shared with the patient and it is often useful in this setting to include the patient and family in the initial conference to make sure that objectives are mutually agreeable.

Most residents need to be reviewed frequently during the first several months to ensure that there are no untoward effects of institutionalization and that all is well. Following this all residents should be reviewed by the physician, in detail, at least every six months. This is usually enough if all is going well, although one of the outcomes of these regular reviews is that it is recognized that a full geriatric assessment is in order – at this time other health professionals such as physiotherapy, occupational therapy and nursing will be asked to review and to meet in the setting of the team conference.

Change in function will necessitate 'crisis' assessment which is discussed in the next section.

Another important role of the team in long-term care is to work with the patient and immediate family or surrogate decision maker to make decisions about future level of care. The health care team, the patient and the family need to be aware of the current medical condition which might influence the extent of treatment in the future. In other words if the patient is considered to be in the terminal stage of an illness then this needs to be acknowledged so that inappropriate treatment of new problems will not occur. Patients with multiple problems for whom technological intervention would not be indicated will be identified. Most important of all the wishes of the patient and if appropriate the family will be identified so that the dying process will not be prolonged by unwished for intervention. This approach is referred to as the development of 'Limited treatment protocols' the term that we prefer is 'Appropriate treatment protocols' and this is discussed in the chapter on Bioethics (Chapter 29).

4. Crisis management

From time to time crises occur with decline in function or development of one of the common geriatric problems and when such decline occurs, or when there is the development of fresh problems with potential interaction, full geriatric assessment is indicated. Consultant support by specialist geriatricians is indicated and patients may require periods of more active intervention. This may occur at the site of residence, home or institution, but if the facilities are not available it may be necessary to transfer to an acute unit. Obviously the need for this would depend upon the functional level of the patient and the potential for improvement.

There are long-term care hospitals where full health care teams are involved and in this situation regular assessment occurs and crisis management can usually be handled on site. In many situations there is only a limited amount of nursing care that is available. In many nursing homes the ratio of nurses or personal care workers, to resident is quite low. When the level of function declines to total dependency as a result of illness, there is not enough nursing care to continue to look after the patient in this setting. It is unfortunate that this is so and that the usual result is transfer to an acute care facility. It is necessary for the care providers and the patient to be fully aware of the most appropriate options available. When continuing care within the institution is the most appropriate option, then steps should be taken to ensure that more nursing and medical care can be brought to that site. In many facilities this is handled by having areas for 'concentrated care'. Undoubtedly this approach is cost effective as well as being more appropriate in terms of quality of life. It is not an excuse to restrict appropriate entry into hospital nor to accept an inferior quality of care.

Other types of crises occur, for example with behavioral problems. These may be dealt with by various members of the team, including the physicians. Psychologists have a particularly important role to play here.

5. Education and development

Geriatric medicine grew from a base within long-term care and there is a long history of involvement. The geriatrician has an important role to play in the education of those involved in this type of care. Particularly with the family practitioners. This can be done during their early training or later. On the job training can also occur within the setting of team conferences when both family physician and geriatrician are present. Consultation is another effective way of providing education.

In many areas there is a great deal to be done in terms of development of better services within long-term care - institutional and community. Geriatricians have an important advisory role in this area. Some areas of need would include the development of policies on alternative treatment protocols, the place for cardiac resuscitation and development of units for higher acuity (concentrated) care.

6. The future

It would seem that in some countries, such as Canada, the greatest emphasis until very recently has been on institutional long-term care. This country has 8-9 per cent of the population over the age of 65 within various institutions. In most Provinces in Canada there is tremendous pressure on these institutional beds with long waiting periods for entry – whether these are hospital or homes for special care. There has always been social assessment, but very limited emphasis on expert medical assessment. One concludes from this that one could never build enough long-term care 'beds' to meet the perceived need. The way of the future is to make sure that all patients are receiving the level of care that is commensurate with their expertly assessed needs and that there are comprehensive geriatric services to provide this assessment, treatment, rehabilitation and respite care. Additional emphasis is needed in developing appropriate programs in home care to maintain a greater percentage of the disabled elderly at home.

In North America and other countries the future will see a great increase in comprehensive geriatric services and services for home support. There is likely to be a slowing down of building institutions, but an improvement in the type of care that occurs within them. Such changes are already occurring - but slowly. The geriatric specialists need to be involved in these changes, in promoting and advising.

In the United Kingdom there has been a commitment to community care at the expense of institutional care. There is a low percentage (3.8 per cent) of patients within long-term care institutions. However there is a considerable amount of stress as a result of this. In the future there will need to be more emphasis on the needs of care providers and relieving strain. It is likely that institutional care will increase slightly.

The population of the very old will continue to increase dramatically over the next few years and if present trends continue the number of frail elderly will also climb. With these increases will come an increased demand for long-term care, institutional and at home. It is difficult to predict the exact number of long-term care institutional beds that are required, and what is the optimal or minimal number (at the present time we suspect that this is close to 6 per cent of the over 65 year olds). As geriatric services improve and as assessment and rehabilitation improve it is hoped that the number will decrease. Also the role of prevention has to be taken into account. Programs designed to maintain mobility, to ensure better nutrition, to reduce iatrogenic drug problems and immunization to prevent infection will all have an impact.

Within the setting of long-term care there will also be an increasing need for other roles, for example the physician and health care team trained for palliative care. Geriatric medicine will continue to have an important role in long-term care since there will continue to be those patients who are severely disabled and for whom there is no anticipated improvement. But the role in prevention, acute care and assessment, and rehabilitation or restorative care will overshadow this. As these roles become more consuming there will be a major contribution to long-term care in that the number requiring it will be kept to a minimum.

Suggested reading

Applebaum, G. E., King, J. E. and Finucane, T. E. (1990). The outcome of CPR initiated in Nursing Homes. *J. Amer. Ger. Soc.* **38**: 197–200.

Berman P., Hogan D. B., Fox, R.A. (1987) The atypical presentation of infection in old age. *Age and Ageing* **16**: 201–207.

Cohen M. A., Tell, E. J., Wallack S. S. (1988) The risk factors of Nursing Home entry among residents of six continuing care retirement communities. *J. Gerontol. Soc. Sci,* **43**: S15–S21.

MacAdam, M., Capitman, J., Yee, D., Prottas, J., Leutz, W. and Westwater, D. (1989) Case management for frail elders. *Gerontologist*, **29**: 737–44.

Mott P. D., Barker, W. H., (1988). Hospital and medical care use by Nursing Home patients: the effect of patient care plans. *J. Amer. Ger. Soc.*, **36**: 47–53.

Schneider E. L., Ory, M. and Aung, M. L., (1987). Teaching nursing homes revisited *J. Amer. Med. Assoc.*, **257**: 2771–5.

Shaughnessy P. W. and Kramer A. M. (1990). The increased needs of patients in nursing homes and patients receiving home health care. New Engl. J. Med. **322**: 21–27.

31

Drug prescribing and iatrogenic disease in the elderly

In this chapter we are concerned with the main aspects of drugs as they relate to the elderly. This will include a discussion of the epidemiology of drug prescribing and consumption and a section on iatrogenic disease.

1. Drug Prescribing

The elderly present particular problems to the physician in terms of therapy. The capacity to metabolise drugs and the response to them may be modified.

In view of the multiplicity of problems often seen in an elderly patient, it is to be expected that prescribing habits will be affected. Polypharmacy is unfortunately often the rule, rather than the exception. In Britain, although those over 65 years of age comprise 15 per cent of the population, they in fact account for 30 per cent of the national drug expenditure.

In a recent survey of the elderly in the community, we found 83 per cent of those over 75 years of age were taking regularly prescribed drugs. There was an average of 2.7 different drugs per person but 6 per cent were taking 6 or more different drugs. The commonest prescribed were diuretics (32 per cent) hypnotics and sedatives (17 per cent), non-steroidal anti-inflammatory agents (15 per cent) and analgesics (11 per cent). Comprehension problems concerning the indications for the drugs, and on the times they should be taken were present in 12 and 16 per cent respectively. Particularly worrying was the fact that once the number of drugs rose to three or more, comprehension problems increased sharply (Table 31.1). Similar observations have been noted by others. Labelling was felt to be unclear in 8 per cent of all subjects, but this rose to 17 per cent of those with poor understanding of their medication.

One particular problem seen is the habit of 'repeat prescriptions', often without the patient being seen by their physician.

Drug compliance is thought to be a particular problem in the elderly. It has been suggested that among the elderly living alone, failure to comply with a therapeutic regimen may be as high as 80 per cent. Sometimes, there is deliberate non-compliance, but more often it is for other reasons such as poor instructions, unclear labelling, multiple agents and unpalatable preparations. Instructions should be as clear and simple as possible. It is important to use containers that the patient can open which bear a clear label that the patient understands.

We have found that the hospital pharmacist can be very helpful in this situation. It has become our practice to try to prescribe drugs which need

Table 31.1 Problems with comprehension and number of drugs taken

Number of drugs	% Comprehension problem	% Labelling unclear
1	1.4	0
2	5.4	8.1
3	16.4	10.6
4	26.2	14.3
5	19.8	15.4
6	27.3	19.2
6+	30.0	20.0

only be given on a once or twice daily basis. If multiple drugs must be given, the pharmacist can often prepare a powder, capsule or syrup containing all the drugs. Some drugs can only be given by infrequent doses because of a special formulation such as enteric coating. It is obviously important not to interfere with such a preparation.

2. Pharmacokinetics in the elderly

Pharmacokinetics refers to the study of drug absorption, distribution and clearance of drugs. The effects of aging on a variety of anatomical structures, physiological functions and homeostatic mechanisms are likely to modify pharmacokinetics.

A number of age related changes have been described which may influence distribution, including reduction in lean body mass and total body water, and an increase in body fat. An increase in body fat and a reduction of total body water means that a lipid soluble drug will pass into fat in a greater proportion, with a prolongation of plasma half life. This seems to occur with diazepam where the half life is prolonged but the clearance is unaltered. The actual plasma levels fall. For polar drugs, the volume of distribution will fall but the levels rise for a given dose.

Falls in levels of serum albumin have been described with advancing age but only in the presence of disease or immobility. The synthesis and degradation of albumin appears to decrease with age. Although the number of albumin binding sites may be reduced in some elderly patients, this does not usually achieve therapeutic effects in the case of single drugs. Problems are more likely to arise when several drugs are used, which are competing for fewer binding sites. The free drug concentrations of phenylbutazone, salicylate and sulphadiazine have been noted to be greater in elderly patients on multiple-drug therapy.

The binding of drugs to red blood cells is decreased with advancing age. Pethidine and chlormethiazole display reduced binding to red blood cells in elderly compared to young subjects.

Hepatic blood flow decreases with age which increases the bioavailability of drugs, such as propranolol, with a high first pass metabolism. The decline in blood flow does not seem to affect the metabolism of drugs with small hepatic extraction ratios. Changes in hepatic oxidative enzymes systems with age have been noted and may have some relevance in the metabolism of some drugs.

The glomerular filtration rate tends to decline with age. This is of importance in the elimination of polar drugs and metabolites. Examples include aminoglycosides, tetracyclines, penicillins, digoxin, cimetidine, chlorpropamide and atenolol. It is necessary to make a dose adjustment to prevent dangerous accumulation of the drug.

It is important to appreciate that creatinine not only reflects the glomerular filtration rate but also the lean body mass. The lean body mass falls with age and so a deterioration in renal function may not be associated with an elevation in serum creatinine.

Some drugs are actively excreted in the tubules (organic acids), but this may be blocked by probenecid. It appears that the effect of tubular blocking drugs is very dependent on renal function, since probenecid has very little effect on the half life of penicillin (which is already prolonged) in the elderly.

In order to clear bladder infections it is thought that the concentration of an antibiotic must exceed the minimal inhibitory concentration (MIC) for the organism. As glomerular filtration falls with age, the plasma levels and half life increase, but urine concentration is lowered and infection may not be cleared.

3. Iatrogenic Disease

This may be defined as 'disease or disability caused or compounded by a doctor's attitude or action'. This definition is deliberately wide, so as to avoid excluding those not induced by drugs. The non-drug related iatrogenic conditions may be more important in determining morbidity and mortality but are seldom stressed.

Non-drug related iatrogenic conditions

Ageism

This is an attitude of mind which 'switches one off' to the problems of old age. A typical example would be the comment 'what do you expect at your age, dear?'. Not only is this comment negative, but it is patronizing and the underlying attitude is likely to be effectively communicated to the patient. The patient and relatives themself may foster this attitude, which contributes to late reporting of treatable conditions.

Inadequate Assessment

This follows on naturally from ageism and is responsible for the 'pseudo-silent' presentation of disease in old age. The presentation of pneumonia as an acute confusional state with incontinence and social crisis is inappropriately labelled as dementia and/or a social problem. Appropriate investigation and therapy is inadvertently withheld, and instead responses of sedation and confinement commenced, which hinder recovery and may result in permanent decompensation.

Adverse reactions to drugs may not be recognized for what they are and may be treated with another drug rather than by the withdrawal of the first.

Sick-role Induction

This is another problem which arises from the doctor's and paramedical staff attitudes – for example 'Hospitals are for 'sick' patients who should be in bed'. In many hospitals it is considered to be more convenient for examination and investigation that patients stay in night clothes. More attention is given to the 'ill, frail, dependent patient' thereby reinforcing the sick-role. If patients lose their independence for long enough, it may be very difficult to retrieve the situation. It is for this reason that most geriatric units get patients up as soon as possible and encourage dressing in normal clothes, and set great store by training in the 'activities of daily living ' (ADL). If at all possible, patients should participate in any decisions made concerning their own care, and should not be talked *about* or *at*, but *with*.

Regimentation

Hospitals often appear to be run more for the convenience of staff than the patient. The timing of ward rounds and drug rounds are usually such, that patients have to be woken at an early hour and are then expected to sit quietly, whilst everything is prepared. Lights out coincide with nursing rotas, rather than the patients preferences and long established habits. It is more convenient for the patient to use a bed-pan at night, despite the totally artificial nature of it. In such a setting it is surprising that many patients do manage to maintain their personality and independence, although by doing so they risk being labelled 'awkward and troublesome' and being sedated.

Physical environment

Wards are often not designed with the physically and mentally frail elderly patient in mind. Toilets are often hidden in small areas some distance from the beds and lack clear sign-posting. Illumination may be poor. The space available may restrict the use of aids.

Aids

Usually this is understood to imply objects that are intended to improve mobility (canes, tripods, frames, wheelchairs). It should however, be extended to include the use of furniture or any instrument which optimizes independence. The provision of a chair of the correct height, depth and firmness which is used perhaps 12 hours a day may be more important than a 15 minute session with a physiotherapist and a zimmer-frame (walker). An unsuitable chair may undo all of the therapists efforts.

It is essential to ensure that the aid is appropriate in nature, size and state of repair. No aid should be prescribed without proper assessment. Most wheelchairs have inflatable tires, and if these are not at sufficient pressure, the brakes do not work. There are many other aids designed for specific problems such as callipers, back braces, long-handled shoe horns, etc., which in certain circumstances may dramatically improve independence, if used appropriately. These are usually prescribed by the occupational therapist, an integral member of the geriatric team.

Drug related iatrogenic disease

It is widely believed that the elderly are especially prone to drug side-effects. Much of the available information derives from drug surveillance programmes. These are systematic (usually hospital based) inquiries aimed at the detection of adverse reactions. Such a programme comes from Boston in the United States and demonstrates a definite relationship between adverse reactions and age for Chlordiazepoxide, Diazepam, Flurazepam, Nitrazepam, Heparin, Lignocaine and Propanolol. No definite relationship was established for over 90 other commonly used agents.

The collaborative study of the British Geriatrics Society, yielded data on 677 men and 1321 women. Fifteen per cent of patients suffered adverse reactions, and these contributed to hospital admission in 10 per cent of cases. It is believed that the underlying disease(s) modifies the response to drugs and this study emphasised the high frequency of multiple disease. Over 75 per cent of patients in the study had one to three diagnoses and the rest had four or more.

The increased occurrence of adverse reactions to drugs seen with advancing age, is probably due in part to the greater number of drugs being taken. The changes in drug binding sites, with increasing age, mean that individuals taking multiple drugs are more at risk of undesirable changes in the amounts of active free drug available. Alterations in hepatic metabolism and renal excretion are likely to increase drug half life and thereby result in accumulation. Errors in drug taking and problems with compliance are more likely as discussed above.

Recommendations for prescribing to the elderly

The prescription of aids or drugs are not uncommon antecedents of disability. Clearly, a precise diagnosis with effective definition of a therapeutic objective is paramount. Sometimes a mode of treatment is used which entails known risks and these must be specifically sought. Problems often cannot be predicted, but it is essential to be conversant with the manufacturer's data sheet before embarking on any drug therapy, and the indications for particular drugs. Other non-therapeutic factors, such as environment and staff attitudes, may be just as important in determining final outcome.

The principles of prescribing to the elderly are summarized in Table 31.2. The patient must be fully assessed and the problem(s) identified. Careful consideration is needed as to whether a treatment should be given, and if it is, a specific goal should be defined. After defining the goal, the best regimen should be chosen to achieve this. In the case of drugs allowance for the patient's age, sex, build, renal and hepatic function must be made. The reasons for the treatment and its method of use must be carefully explained. Any labelling must be appropriate and legible to the patient. Special prepacked formulations or calender packs may be of value in some instances. The containers must be manipulable by the patient.

Table 31.2 Principles of drug prescribing in the elderly

1. Review indications for drug treatment.
2. Consider factors modifying choice:
   - untreated condition risk versus drug risk
   - formulation and palatability
   - avoid complex regimens
3. Alter dosage according to age, sex, body build, renal and hepatic function.
4. Other points:
   - patient education
   - suitable container
   - meal relationship
   - consider compliance problems

Having commenced treatment it is incumbent upon the doctor to reevaluate the patient. If the therapeutic goal has not been achieved, it must either be redefined or another treatment regimen used. If therapy is continued a decision must be made as to its duration, in order to avoid its continuation in perpetuity.

Suggested reading

Bliss, M. R. 1980 Prescribing for the elderly. *Br. Med. J.* **283**: 203–206.

Caird F. I., Evans J. G. (1981). *Advanced Geriatric Medicine*, Vol. 1, Pitman Medical, London.

Chan, J. Kendall M. J., Mitchard, M. and Wells W. D. E. (1975). The effect of aging on plasma pethidine concentration. *Br. J. of Clin. Pharmacol.* **2**: 297–302.

Cluff, L. E., Thornton, C. F. and Seidl, L. G. (1964) Studies on the epidemiology of drug reactions. I. Methods of surveillance. *JAMA*, **188**: 976–983.

Dall, J. L. C. (1970). Maintenance digoxin in elderly patients. *Br. Med. J.* **2**: 705–706.

D'Arcy, P. F., Griffin J. P. (1981). Iatrogenic Diseases. 2nd Ed, Update, Oxford University Press, London.

Dass, B. C., Maddock, S. G. and Whittingham G. C. (1977). Special problems of medication in a survey of 114 elderly people at home, in welfare homes and hospital. *Mod. Geriat.* **7**: 22–25.

Dass, B. C., Williams, B. D. H. and Williams, A. (1981). Labelling medicine: a new system evaluated. *Geriatric Med*, September, 82–85.

Dennis, P. J. (1979). Monitoring of psychotrope prescribing in general practice. *Br. Med. J.* **2**: 1115–16.

Friedman, M. (1982). Iatrogenic Disease. *Postgraduate Medicine* **71**: 123–129.

Greenblatt, D. J., Sellers E. M. and Shader, R. I. (1981). Drug disposition in old age. *New Eng. J. of Med.* **306**: 1081–88.

Grymonpre, R. E., Mitenko, P.A., Sitar, D. S., Aoki, F. Y. and Montgomery, P. R. (1988). Drug Associated Hospital Admissions in Older Patients. *J. Amer. Ger. Soc.* **36**: 1092–98.

Judge, T. G. and Caird, F. E. (1978). *Drug treatment of the elderly patient.* Pitman Medical, London.

L'Estrange–Orme M. (1981). Major drug interactions. *Hospital Update*, October, pp. 1013–24.

Lindenbaum, J., Rund, D. G., Butler, V. P., Tse–Eng D., Raha J. R. (1981) Inactivation of digoxin by the gut flora: reversal by antibiotic therapy. *New Eng. J. of Med.* **305**: 789–94.

McDevitt, D. G. *et al.* (1976). Plasma binding and the affinity of propranolol for a beta receptor in man. *Clin Pharamacol. Ther.*, **20**: 152–7

Nations, R. L., Triggs, E. J. and Selig, M. (1977). Lignocaine kinetics in cardiac patients and aged subjects. *Br. J. Clin. Pharmacol.* **4**: 439–48.

Nolan, L., O'Malley, K. (1988). Prescribing for the Elderly. Part I: Sensitivity of the Elderly to Adverse Drug Reactions. *J. Amer. Ger. Soc.* **36**: 142–49.

Richey, D. P. (1975). Effects of human ageing on drug absorption and metabolism. In: Goldman, R. and Rockstein, M. (eds) *the Physiology and Pathology of Human Ageing*. Academic Press, London, pp. 59–99.

Squires, R. F. and Brasetrup, C. (1977). Benzodiazepine receptors in rat brain. *Nature*, **266**: 732–4.

Wallace, S., Whiting, B. and Runcie, J. (1976). Factors affecting drug binding of elderly patients. *Br. J. of Clin. Pharmacol.* **3**: 277.

Williamson, J. (1979). Adverse reactions to prescribed drugs in the elderly. In: Crooks, J. and Stevenson, I. H. (eds) *Drugs and the Elderly.* Macmillan, London, pp. 239–46.

Wood, A. J. J., Vestal, R. E., Wilkinson, G. R., Branch, R. A. and Shand, D. G. 1979 Effect of ageing and cigarette smoking on antipyrine and indocyanate green elimination. *Clin. Pharmacol. Ther.*, **26**: 16–20.

32

Rehabilitation of the elderly

We used to think of rehabilitation as the management of disability by physical methods. The concept has now broadened and rehabilitation includes not only techniques to improve physical function but also ways of restoring psychological health and enabling the disabled to enjoy social activities. By rehabilitating elderly people we are trying to help them to achieve their optimal level of ability and well-being. As most disabled old people are living at home, successful rehabilitation also involves educating and supporting the family and other carers (Andrews, 1987).

Before beginning to treat the patient we must have a detailed medical assessment. Having established the medical diagnoses and formulated a problem list, we should then make a full assessment of the patient's previous abilities. Only by knowing the types of person they are, their experiences and expectations, can we begin to help them to reach their full potential.

It is important to plan ultimate goals with the patient and family. Much of rehabilitation involves problem solving. We should identify specific aims (e.g. enabling the patient to stand unsupported; to walk safely without assistance; to dress; to manage the toilet; to be able to prepare a meal or enjoy a hobby). If these aims cannot be achieved we must ask why and see if we find other ways of enabling a patient to do the required task – a different therapeutic technique perhaps; the provision of aids; alterations to the environment; personal help.

In this short chapter we will not attempt to be encyclopedic but will limit our considerations to some important components of rehabilitation and focus on those common problems that tend to be omitted in standard textbooks.

1. Basic considerations

If we are to rehabilitate our elderly patients successfully we need:

1. timing of treatment
2. the team
3. techniques

Timing of treatment

There must be time to listen. There is a danger that because we are so busy, we might only make time for what we consider to be the essentials. The problem of the individual patient we are seeing at home, in clinic or on the ward should be the most important thing in the world to us at that moment. We must listen – and show that we are listening. We should make ourselves accessible to the family: ensure that the ward staff tell relatives that the consultant is available to hear of their anxieties and discuss diagnoses, treatment and future management and support. Many geriatricians set aside time for appointments with relatives, for example the first hour or so of each day or a special family conference. This is prime time well spent: the family will be heartened by the doctors' interest, recognize them as allies, and trust them to be available to help long after the patient has left hospital. They will furnish a more complete picture of the patient – his personality, background, fears, wishes for the future. This information is of inestimable value in guiding our approach to the disabled elderly person and helps us to set appropriate therapeutic goals. It is also vital when plans are being made for discharge and ongoing care.

When does rehabilitation begin.

A traditional view has been that rehabilitation starts when the doctor has completed the medical treatment. Indeed, rehabilitation has sometimes been considered as something which therapists do when doctors have become therapeutically bankrupt or have lost interest. The demarcation between 'medicine' and 'rehabilitation' is arbitrary and is not in the patient's best interests. Waiting to see how a stroke patient gets on in the first few weeks before involvement of the rehabilitation team is bad practice. It may result in complications, which could have been prevented, and low morale. In stroke, rehabilitation should begin on day one – ensuring that the limbs are frequently put through a range of motion; involving the speech therapist or occupational therapist in the assessment and treatment of swallowing disorders and the physiotherapist in positioning the patient correctly.

Rehabilitation of Parkinsonian patients should not be deferred until the patient has developed side-effects with medication. Indeed, it may be possible to postpone the introduction of anti-Parkinsonian drugs or keep the dosage at minimum levels for longer periods if the patient is taught techniques of turning and standing and is provided with a chair of appropriate height, a raised toilet seat, grab rails and bath aids. Rehabilitation should therefore start as soon as possible. Delay helps no-one.

Frequency and intensity of therapy.

We have few clinical trials to help us determine the optimum treatment periods for different disabling conditions. The amount of therapy received by a stroke patient or an old lady recovering from a hip operation varies from hospital to hospital and country to country. Dysphasic stroke patients in Britain may by lucky to get one or two speech therapy sessions per week. In parts of the United States this level of treatment is considered to be merely token: higher staffing levels allow several sessions per day (Wertz 1987). It may be that more frequent contact with therapists results in a greater degree of recovery and a more rapid improvement, but this is unproven. In very elderly disabled patients, fatigue may be a limiting factor.

It is a mistake to consider rehabilitation as something done to the patient by a therapist. Most therapy will be done by the patient, helped and encouraged by the family and nursing staff. At case conferences, therapists should advise on what the patient should be encouraged to do – and prevented from doing. Many physiotherapists will not want a hemiplegic stroke patient to attempt to walk before his balance has returned and he has good hip and knee control. Attempting to 'walk' a stroke patient between two nurses too early may result in an unacceptable gait pattern.

When to stop?

If we continue rehabilitation efforts for many months, therapists may become dispirited because of the patient's diminishing rate of progress. They will not be able to give adequate time to other disabled old people who might benefit more from their skills. We should therefore set limits: otherwise staff morale will decline and rationed resources not used most efficiently and effectively. On the other hand, when a disabled person is discharged from active treatment he may feel very disappointed and rejected. He may not maintain his progress but lapse into inactivity and despair. What are we to do? We must discuss the purpose of rehabilitation and the likely end-points with patient and family.

Some conditions are self-limiting in their extent after the initial insult (e.g. hip fracture, amputation of a leg). In these instances the end-points are usually obvious: the patient's aim will be to walk independently and return to as full a life as possible. Barring complications and further medical problems, they should maintain progress once these goals have been reached.

Another group is those with progressive disorders (such as Parkinsonism and motor neurone disease) where despite favorable responses to therapy the underlying condition will likely continue to worsen. In these instances long-term regular review will be necessary, the frequency depending on the rate of progression of the disabling disease. As the patient's condition declines, new ways should be found to help him cope with reduced levels of ability.

A third group are those who make an incomplete recovery either because of the primary deficit (e.g. many stroke patients) or because of other chronic conditions which adversely alter the prognosis (chronic pulmonary disease, severe arthritis, cancer). In these instances we provide the patient and family with the best estimate possible of the prognosis for recovery. It is then necessary for them to give some guidance in what are reasonable end-points to strive for. In some instances this may require review over a number of months with establishment of new end-points if necessary. Some will wish to see the consultant every few months, as well as being followed regularly by the family practitioner: this is entirely reasonable.

We know very little about the longer term care of the disabled elderly, particularly those who are in the community. The problems that affect them should be of particular concern to us and stimulate us to do research into such neglected problems as falls, post-stroke epilepsy, constipation, depression, the cold hemiplegic arm. Some will find clinic attendance wearisome and prefer support at home. In those who are seriously incapacitated, long-term day hospital is useful – not only to maintain function but to give the carer a much-needed regular break.

In short, the duration of therapy should be tailored to the needs of the individual. We should study the best ways of providing continuing rehabilitation to those with residual disability. We will not go far wrong if we tell the patient and family the range of options available and ask them what they want.

The Team

Rehabilitation of the elderly person who has complex disability can be a very difficult undertaking which requires the skills of a number of people who work closely together. There are several features of a successful rehabilitation team:

1. involvement of patient and family
2. team coordinator
3. involvement of nurses in rehabilitation (enablement)
4. focusing on goals
5. concern with the well-being of the team

The patient and family are the key people. Their views should be sought; they should be involved and informed at all times. As discussed earlier, they must have a clear understanding of the goals and methods being used within the rehabilitation process. The family are important motivators of the patient and by following desirable practices can supplement the treatment process.

The team usually needs a coordinator. This is usually the doctor. The traditional medical stereotype of the omniscient consultant who makes ex-cathedra statements with an exaggerated sense of importance is not in keeping with the true spirit of an interdisciplinary team. The team coordinator should be aware of the skills – and limitations – of all members of the team. This includes him or herself: it does no harm to admit to ignorance or to mistakes, or to have one's suggestions rejected by other team members who may have better ideas. The successful team coordinator should ensure that each member of the team is involved in discussion and should welcome everyone's observations and opinions. These aspects of team function are also discussed in other chapters.

The role of the nurses in rehabilitation is central. They provide round-the-clock care and continue much of the work initiated by therapists. It is therefore vital that nurses understand the principles and techniques of physiotherapy, occupational therapy, speech therapy as well as the social and psychological dimensions of disability. Their input at case conferences is of particular importance: without their observations and suggestions the other team members will gain only a limited perspective of the patient.

The team discussions should focus on ultimate goals (ideally, to help this person return to their own home); specific aims (e.g. helping the stroke patient improve balance and weight-bearing through the affected leg before beginning to walk); and barriers to progress. Barriers may be overcome by medical intervention, different rehabilitation techniques or by providing aids and appliances or services. It is important to be specific: what have we achieved this week? What do we hope that the patient will be doing this time next week? Why has he not progressed as quickly as we would have liked? Is there anything else we can do to make this patient feel better? Has anyone any other suggestions?

The well-being of the team must be a major concern of the team leader (Coordinator). Rehabilitation of old people with multiple problems can be demanding and exhausting. There should be a balance of patients on the unit: those who are going to progress quickly; slower-stream patients, and those who are unlikely to make much more recovery but who may deteriorate if they are not given regular rehabilitation. Positive achievements should be praised; frustrations expressed; laughter encouraged. Limits should be set: the team leader should say when little further functional recovery can be expected. Research should be encouraged – the most arduous rehabilitation problems can be converted into a source of fascination once we begin to ask fundamental questions about them and try to find the answers by designing research projects.

Techniques

Details of specialized techniques can be found in textbooks dealing with specific disorders. Here we will list some of the basic principles in rehabilitation.

Accurate assessment and recognition of all problems

We will not know what to do unless we are certain of what we are dealing with. It is easy to overlook Parkinsonism in a poorly mobile old person who has no tremor; we may not identify subtle signs of cerebrovascular disease; we must not forget common problems in the elderly such as depression, thyroid disorders, osteoarthritis and osteomalacia which may prevent an old person responding well to rehabilitation.

Prevention of complications

An important element of rehabilitation is the avoidance of problems that are going to make the patient worse - aspiration of fluids in the acute stroke patient who cannot swallow liquids properly; pressure sores; constipation; pain and oedema in the leg as a result of deep venous thrombosis; the painful hemiplegic shoulder.

Physical agents

Ice can be helpful in stimulating the swallowing reflex in neurological dysphagia; heat may relieve muscle and joint pain for a short time, thus allowing the patient to perform movements; faradism may be helpful in treating lower motorneurone disorders; sensory feedback training (biofeedback) may prove to be valuable in restoring neuro-muscular control.

Physical techniques

Each member of the inter-disciplinary team will have techniques that may be useful in specific disorders. Some of these involve general encouragement and can be done with individuals or groups by partially trained volunteers (e.g. stimulation of speech in selected dysphasic stroke patients). More specialized techniques require the skills of highly trained therapists – breaking down hypertonicity in stroke; restoring balance to unsteady old people who fall; treating dysphagia, dysarthria and dysphasia.

Compensating for disability

Many patients will not recover completely. They will benefit from learning new ways of performing activities of daily living from occupational therapists. The use of aids, appliances and adaptations can be of enormous value in overcoming disability (Mulley, 1988).

Rating Scales

Unless we measure what we are doing, we will not know whether our rehabilitation efforts are effective. It is curious that doctors will carefully measure the blood pressure and pulse and document cardiac enzymes and peak flow rates but make little attempt to measure disability. Hospital case notes often include *qualitative* impressions ('seems to be improving', 'no progress'). We should also record *quantitative or objective* measurements of activity. Measurement in rehabilitation is not easy and those aspects of recovery which are easiest to quantify reliably may not be relevant to the patient (Tallis 1987). However, by using rating scales we can not only plot a patient's progress but also identify areas where improvement is not being made. We can then determine whether alternative strategies may help.

Simple 2- or 3-point scales have the advantage of close inter- and intra-observer agreement. Examples are yes/no answers; noting whether a person has no movement/some movement/full movement in a limb; no use/some use/full use in a hand. The disadvantage of these scales is that they only provide a coarse assessment. They do not tell us about subtle improvements that may be important to both patient and therapist.

More detailed scales can be used for specific physical problems (e.g. the Motricity index for motor power (Demeurisse, et al., 1980); the Frenchay Dysarthria assessment (Enderby, 1982)) for measures of general health (the Nottingham Health Profile (Ebrahim, 1986)) and of ability to perform everyday activities (the Barthel Scale (Snaith, et al., 1971)). Some of these are discussed in Chapter 1 in the section on assessment.

Morale and motivation

In our attempts to make rehabilitation more scientifically respectable by careful definitions and measurement, we may have tended to de-emphasize more nebulous concepts such as morale and motivation. Yet successful rehabilitation depends on these: a severely disabled person who is strongly motivated may achieve more independence than a less disabled person who is less determined. Declining morale is one factor in the decline in function often seen after discharge from day hospital (Andrews and Stewart, 1979).

2. Assessment

Assessment is discussed in Chapter 1 and will be reviewed here with particular reference to rehabilitation. Each member of the interdisciplinary team needs to assess the patient. Although the emphasis of these assessments will differ according to the specialty of the rehabilitation worker, they should all include details of patient's previous abilities; an evaluation of current problems; a statement of treatment aims and objectives, and measurement of progress.

Three areas which might be of help to the geriatrician are the plotting of the patient's previous capabilities by documenting disability 'milestones'; determining what problems the patient has during a normal day; and ascertaining the patient's truc needs.

Previous abilities and current disabilities

We might expect different attitudes to disability in the person who retired in their late 50s because of ill health compared with someone who continued to do two or three part-time jobs until their early 80s. The individual who has taken pride in working with hands or muscle will be more distressed by diminishing physical prowess than a former office worker; those who have made a living by using words and ideas will be especially handicapped by language impairment or the shortened attention span that may occur after a stroke. The patient who proudly recalls winning prizes for sporting achievements will find it hard to adjust to serious disability, especially if the condition causing a reduction in activity came on abruptly.

Disability Milestones

Pediatricians use developmental milestones to monitor the progress of children. In order to understand our elderly patients better, determine how they are affected by disability and to successfully plan their rehabilitation, it is helpful to plot the course of their disability. Much rehabilitation effort is concerned with improving motor performance; we should therefore pay particular attention to how the patient's physical activities have declined.

Plotting the time course of disability can be done by asking the patient: when did you last walk to the shops or post office without help? When did you last go to the end of the road or walk to the garden gate? How long have you been housebound? When were you last able to go up and down stairs unaided? How long have you been confined to this room? Failure to document these milestones may cause the rehabilitation team to aim unrealistically high; this will result in ultimate disappointment.

Typical day

Successful rehabilitation involves attention to detail - paying particular attention to those small, undramatic aspects of patient care (Dunkle and Schmidley, 1987). To identify those aspects of self-care which cause problems it is a good idea to ask the patient and family about a day in their lives (Table 32.1).

Some of these questions may be incorporated into such assessment instruments as Barthel's (see

Table 32.1 Checklist for identifying problems with everyday activities

What time do you wake up?
Do you have difficulty getting out of bed?
Do you need assistance with washing, grooming, dressing?
Are you able to bathe or have a shower?
Can you get on and off the toilet unaided?
Do you need help with wiping your bottom or other aspects of personal hygiene?
Can you descend the stairs safely? Do you need help? Have you fallen on the stairs?
What problems do you have with preparing food, eating, drinking?
Can you reach to retrieve dropped objects? Do you clean the house and do the washing?
Do you go outside? If not, what prevents this? How could you be helped to go out more easily and more often?
How do you spend your time during the day?
Do you need help going upstairs and getting into bed?
Are there any sexual difficulties?
Do you sleep well? Can you roll over in bed?
Do you need help with toileting during the night?

Chapter 1) and using them will help in this area. Bathing is difficult for a third of healthy people aged 75 or more living at home (Clark, et al., 1984); it is a problem for anyone with physical disability. If a disabled person cannot bathe he feels uncomfortable and is at risk of skin problems. Helping disabled old people to bathe regularly can improve morale: this can be achieved by the provision of appropriate bath aids, though many people will also need personal help. Over two-thirds of women over 85 years of age are unable to get to and from the toilet without aids or assistance. The provision of mobility and toilet aids can do much to help.

Another common problem is tedium. The immobile, housebound disabled elderly person will spend long hours in front of a television set. In order to shake off the 'basket-weaver' tag, occupational therapists have tended to move away from 'diversional' therapy. This is regrettable: many old people would love to rekindle previous skills or learn new creative activities. We should pay more attention to improving patients' abilities to perform leisure activities. In the setting of rehabilitation there is an important role for recreation therapists (recreologists), art therapists and music therapists for example.

Ascertaining the patient's true need

The disabled elderly usually have many problems: indeed, if the problem list is short, the clinician has probably taken an inadequate history. There is a danger that by concentrating on aspects that health professionals consider important, we may overlook those things which really trouble the patient. Unless we identify the worries that cause patients most concern, we will fail to provide comprehensive care. One tip is to say to the patient 'If I could wave a magic wand, what is the one thing that you would like me to improve more than anything else?' This can produce interesting answers: the amputee may unrealistically yearn for a new leg; the stroke victim whose flaccid arm has been immobile for six months may wish for full recovery of manipulative function. Patients may harbour other inappropriate ideas about recovery. Alternatively, their main concerns may be social or financial – the wish to see a daughter who lives miles away; distress that the garden is now overgrown; the worry about returning to a burgled flat; concern about not receiving their pension while in hospital. There may be other anxieties – perhaps their reading spectacles are at home, their dentures are loose, their feet painful. Our patients will not reach their fullest capabilities if they are troubled by these considerations. We should therefore consider these problems as priority.

3. Some rehabilitation problems

Variable Performance

Rehabilitation staff may become impatient with the patient and exasperated with themselves when an older person does something on one occasion but not on another. On certain occasions the patient functions below the level that they are known to be capable of – a disability gap. The change in performance can alter with time, place or person:

Time

A patient may find movement difficult in the early morning (especially if he is arthritic or Parkinsonian). Mobility may improve as the day progresses. If there is some cognitive impairment, 'sun-downing' may occur – an increase in confusion in the late afternoon, making cooperation with nursing and rehabilitation staff more difficult. It is important that rehabilitation is done at the time of day when the patient is able to give of his best. This time will vary from patient to patient.

Many patients have 'good' and 'bad' days. This day-to-day variability is a universal experience but marked swings in ability are particularly noticeable in patients with cerebrovascular disease. The mechanism is unclear. The rehabilitation team should recognize that this variability is related to the underlying disease. They should not accuse the patient of being 'lazy', of 'not trying'. Indeed, these judgmental comments should stimulate the geriatrician to review the patient in some detail. Although some old people are lazy and others do not wish to improve, many do want to achieve independence. The patient who has been labelled 'difficult' or 'poorly motivated' may be depressed, deaf, dysphasic or dyspraxic; he may be constipated, in pain or have heart failure. The 'difficult' rehabilitation patient presents to us a diagnostic challenge. We will have great difficulty restoring him to well-being and optimum function until the reasons for his apparent behavioral difficulties have been identified.

Place

The patient may be independent in all aspects of daily living when he leaves hospital. Once he is home, he may quickly revert to immobility, incontinence and independence. The general practitioner and community nurse may understandably believe that the hospital team has not done its job properly and that the discharge has been premature. The patient may then be returned to hospital where he spontaneously reverts to independent activity – sometimes within hours. This marked contrast (disability gap) between behaviour in a therapeutic setting and that at home has been called the 'Jekyll and Hyde syndrome'. Its psychopathology is poorly understood. An awareness that this is a recognized condition may cause some relief to perplexed relatives and may prevent mistrust between hospital and community health professionals. It is important to identify the disability gap and to discuss with the patient and the family in the setting of a conference. This may improve things and reduce the gap, but if not realistic plans for coping need to be formulated with appropriate planning for the worst scenario.

Person

The patient who depends on two nurses to be transferred from chair to commode may walk with minimal support from a physiotherapist. When the geriatrician asks her to walk during his ward round, she may smile sweetly, stand confidently and walk safely without any assistance. This also occurs on home visits: the patient who has been bedfast or chairbound and causing great physical stress to the relatives will produce a virtuoso performance for the visiting doctor. This variability (disability gap) according to perceived status of the observer is a curious yet common phenomenon. Unless they are told that it is a recognized entity, rehabilitation staff will feel that their assessments have been imprecise (they only rarely assume that the physician has supernatural powers) and family carers will feel dispirited. The difference may be reduced by good team communication and by having the therapists work with the nursing staff and relatives so that everyone, including the patient, knows that everyone knows what level of function is possible.

Failure

'This patient is a rehabilitation failure.' This sad admission is often mistaken. True, there are rehabilitation disasters – patients who received no therapy for several weeks because the doctors wanted 'to wait and see how things went'; stroke patients with painful shoulders because of incorrect handling of the paralysed arm; old ladies with hip fracture who are constipated, dehydrated and have painful sores on heel and sacrum. But the patient whose recovery has been minimal and remains dependent on others for self care should not be dubbed a 'failure' – some old people with complex disability are unable to make much progress because of the nature of their illnesses. The geriatrician should be sure to explain to the team that minimal improvement in these circumstances is not a reflection of their lack of skills or dedication. Rather, the fact that the patient is obviously free from pain and distress, is able to do something for himself (even if it is only drinking through a straw or being able to enjoy an outing in a wheelchair to a park or pub) and has come to terms with his disabilities are successes which should be applauded.

Meeting the many needs of disabled old people can be very demanding and the nurses, doctors, rehabilitation staff and social workers need support and recognition for their hard work. Explaining that the 'rehabilitation failure' could not possibly have received any better care helps to heal the healers.

4. Carers

Those who work exclusively in hospital can be forgiven for failing to realize that most disabled old people are at home and that the burden of their care falls on their relatives. Hospital workers may also mistakenly believe that many relatives opt out of their responsibilities and are content to leave the care of their disabled and disadvantaged elders to the state (Lowther and Williamson, 1966). True, there are relatives who refuse to care, sometimes for selfish reasons. However, many relatives who appear to care no longer have reached breaking point. This is because their plight has not been appreciated and they have received no recognition, support and relief; or, sadly, that support has been promised but failed to materialize. These carers – the majority of whom are women – have struggled on under enormous strain until they can no longer cope (Anderson, 1987).

Most carers go on providing care week in, week out for years. These front line workers are probably the most undervalued group in our community. They have very high expectations of themselves and though they are often old and frail, continue to work long hours without time off in order that the disabled patient can remain at home.

Although we have known about the problems of informal carers for many years, it is only recently that supporting the carer has been recognized as a vital part of rehabilitation. We must therefore be familiar with the many physical, psychological and social difficulties experienced by carers (Table 32.2); what their unmet needs are (Table 32.3) and how to help them (Table 32.4). Care for the carer should be the concern of everyone in the rehabilitation team. We should ensure that we are approachable, open and helpful. Physicians, geriatricians and family doctors, have a particularly important role. They know who does what in providing help and support for the disabled person and his family and can coordinate community support; make representations on the patient's behalf to housing departments; try to accelerate the provision of aids and appliances. Above all, they can provide a life-line for the carer who may be struggling to keep afloat. Simply knowing that there is someone who is interested, informed, involved and able to provide appropriate help is enormously reassuring. The 'production line' approach to hospital medicine is not appropriate

Table 32.2 Carers' problems

Physical
- back pain
- ischemic chest pain
- breathlessness
- herniae
- weakness
- aging
- fatigue

Psychological
- emotional strain
- anxiety
- tiredness
- depression
- loneliness
- resentment – patient
  – other relatives
  – the system
- conflicting loyalties
- loss of control of their lives
- dependence on tranquilizers, alcohol

Social
- financial problems
- no free time
- no holidays

Spiritual
- loss of purpose
- lack of meaning in their role

General
- ignorance – who to ask?
  – what to ask for?
  – am I doing it correctly?

Table 32.3 What do carers want?

1. Help – immediate in a crisis (fall; illness in patient or carer)
   – regular
   – sustained
2. Honesty
   No false promises: do not promise services, support unless you are certain that they can be provided
   Openness: be open about the likely outcome of the disabling illness
3. Recognition
   Carers are often unrecognized by professionals, who are not always aware of the heroic support provided by this large hard-working group
4. To talk to someone
   To express feelings of rage, frustration, guilt, violence, ambivalence
5. To relax
   To switch off, have fun, have something to look forward to

Table 32.4 Care for the carers: a check-list

1. *Identifying problems*
   Have you pinpointed difficulties which are causing stress and may result in carer breakdown? For example:
   - disturbed sleep
   - disturbing behavior
   - incontinence (especially fecal soiling)
2. *Education*
   - informal discussion with doctors, nurses, therapists, social workers
   - information meetings
   - publications
   - agencies (Parkinson's society; Arthritis and Rheumatism Council; Stroke Association
3. *Emotional support*
   - counselling
   - pastoral care
   - carer groups
   - regular visitors – professionals
     – volunteers (Age Concern; church
     – groups)
4. *Practical help*
   - services
   - aids and appliances
   - money – are the family receiving their full entitlement of grants and allowances?
5. *Relief*
   - an hour or two – sitters; volunteers who arrange outings
   - a day or two – day hospital; day centre
   - a week or two – holiday admission to appropriate facility (hospital, nursing home, residential home, family placement scheme)
   - regular intermittent relief care

to providing imaginative long-term care to the disabled, at home or in a long-term care institution.

Disabled patients with functional impairment due to stroke, arthritis or chronic chest disease for example, should be followed regularly. Support from the geriatrician can be offered by review once or twice a year or, if coming to the clinic is difficult, by the general practitioner (family physician) contacting the geriatrician at any time that problems arise. One of the worst aspects of being disabled and caring for disabled people at home is that no-one seems to care. The number of people calling to the house dwindles with time. The family become isolated, anxious and despondent. There is little point putting considerable effort into the early stages of rehabilitation if later the patient is simply going to sit at home becoming more immobile and depressed. Therefore before discharging a person from hospital, clinic or day hospital, detailed discussions should take place with the family who should be told about the range of help and services available. If they do not wish to avail themselves of support at this stage, they should be told that this will in no way bar them from receiving help if and when they change their minds.

5. Conclusion

Rehabilitation is difficult and demanding. It requires time, teamwork and a lot of energy. The geriatrician needs to be enthusiastic, available and interested. By paying attention to numerous small details he can encourage others to appreciate the satisfaction of providing comprehensive, imaginative care to the patient and family, and ensure that those for whom he is responsible receive the highest possible standard of care and support.

References

Anderson, R. (1987). The unremitting burden on carers. *Brit. Med. J.*, **294**: 73–4.

Andrews, K. (1987). *Rehabilitation of the Older Adult*. Edward Arnold, London.

Andrews, K. and Stewart, J. (1979). Stroke recovery: he can but does he? *Rheumatology and Rehabilitation*, **18**: 43–8.

Clark, M., Clark, S., Odell, A. and Jagger, C. (1984). The elderly at home: health and social status. *Health Trends*, **16**: 3–7.

Demeurisse, G., Demol, O. and Robaye, E. (1980). Motor evaluation in vascular hemiplegia. *European Neurology*, **19**: 382–9.

Dunkle, R. E. and Schmidley, J. W. (1987). Stroke in the elderly. New issues in diagnosis, treatment and rehabilitation. Springer, New York.

Ebrahim, S., Nouri, F. and Barer, D. (1986). Use of Nottingham Health Profile with patients after a stroke. *J. Epidemiol. and Com. Health*, **40**: 166–9.

Enderby, P. (1982). Franchay Dysarthria Assessment. College Hill Press, San Diego.

Goldberg, D. (1972). The detection of psychiatric illness by questionnaire: Maudsley Monograph, No. 21. Oxford University Press, London.

Lowther, C. P. and Williamson, J. W. (1966). Old people and their relatives *Lancet*, **ii**: 1459–60.

Mahoney, F. I. and Barthel, D. W. (1965). Functional evaluation: the Barthel Index. *Maryland State Med. J.*, **14**: 61–5.

Mulley, G. P. (1989). *Everyday Aids and Appliances.* British Medical Journal, London.

Snaith, R. P. Ahmed, S. N., Mehta, S., Hamilton, M. (1971). Assessment of the severity of primary depressive illness: Wakefield self-assessment depression inventory. *Psychological Medicine*, **1**: 143–9.

Tallis, R. (1987). Measurement in rehabilitation: an introduction. *Clinical Rehabilitation*, **1**: 1–3.

Wertz, R. T. (1987). The efficacy of language therapy for aphasia. In: Dunkle, R. E. and Schmidley, J. W. (eds). *Stroke in the Elderly: New Issues in Diagnosis, Treatment and Rehabilitation.* Springer, New York.

33

The elderly surgical patient

This chapter aims to be more than simply a check list of questions to ask an elderly patient the night before an operation. While medical assessment prior to surgery is discussed, we also look at four broad problem areas encountered in surgery in the elderly within which the reader will be able to construct smaller problem lists relevant to their patients. Because of the need for brevity, the references in the text have been kept to a minimum and some of the statements may appear over-dogmatic. For a more detailed discussion the interested reader is referred to Seymour (1986), Seymour and Vaz (1987) and Seymour et al. (1992).

1. General principles in the elderly surgical patient

(a) Age itself should be no bar to surgery and elderly patients, once committed to operation are, as Reiss (1980) contends, just as entitled to high technology intervention as patients in a younger age group. Indeed, arguably, the elderly are the very patients most often in need of this intervention because of accompanying, often complex, medical problems.
(b) Increasing economic constraints on western medical systems are creating debate about health care priorities. There is now a growing trend to quantify these priorities through methods derived from economics, one example being the Quality Adjusted Life Year (QALY) system. As Harris (1987) points out, the elderly are at risk of doing poorly in such analyses.
(c) Post-operative mortality rates and complications tend to be higher in elderly patients than in younger patients with comparable surgical problems. The major reason for this difference, however, is age-associated disease rather than physiological changes due to aging. Careful preoperative medical assessment is therefore of key importance in elderly surgical patients and should lead to a reduction in surgical risk.
(d) Over the last 20 years, developments in anaesthesia and surgical technique have been dramatic. As the Confidential Enquiry into Peri-operative Deaths (CEPOD, 1987) has shown, anaesthesia on its own is a very uncommon cause of post-operative mortality, the main causes being underlying disease combined with surgical and medical complications.
(e) Non-elective admission, advanced age and high rates of post-operative problems are related to one another in a complex fashion. Thus, non-elective admission and age over 75 are both associated with a two to four times increase in post-operative mortality, but these two factors are also positively correlated with one another.

It has been tentatively estimated that about a third of non-elective surgical admissions in the elderly might be preventable (Seymour and Pringle, 1983). It is also suspected, although not proven, that a negative attitude on behalf of elderly patients, their relatives and their medical attendants may be an important reason for late referral for necessary surgery. Not all emergencies are foreseeable in advance, however. When emergency surgery is inevitable, the principle should be that the older the patient is, the more experienced the surgeon and anaesthetist should be (CEPOD, 1987). The CEPOD Report also makes an important distinction between true surgical emergencies, where no delay is possible before sending the patients to the operating room, and urgent surgery where a few hours delay is acceptable and potentially beneficial so that urgent medical therapy can be instituted.

2. The path to elective surgery

It will be apparent from the above remarks that the medical, surgical and anesthetic decisions to be made in the non-elective surgical patient are quite different from those to be made in the elective case. In the former situation, the room for maneuver may be considerably limited and it is in the elective patient that the interested physician can make the major contribution. For this reason the path by which an elderly patient with an elective surgical problem achieves, or fails to achieve, an operation is dealt with here. Discussion centres around those elderly patients who are not terminally ill and who are able to give informed consent. The dying or the demented patient presents special ethical dilemmas which deserve more attention than we are able to give in this chapter.

There are four major problem areas that will be discussed.

Perceiving the need for surgery

The Patient

The medical systems in Britain and North America primarily depend on the patient (or a close relative of the patient) bringing an elective surgical problem to medical attention. One barrier to consultation is the feeling that surgery in old age is not worthwhile because the patient feels they are about to die any-way. An inspection of Tables of Life Expectancy will soon dispel this argument because a healthy women of 65 can expect to live over 17 years in the West, and even at 80 the expectation of life is around 8 years.

Another misconception of many elderly patients is that mortality rates after surgery are high. It must be remembered that some elderly patients (and perhaps their relatives and even their doc-tors) formed their opinions about the risks of sur-gery three or more decades ago. With modern tech-niques the mortality rates of elective surgery are low even into extreme old age and morbidity rates are acceptable. Some recently published figures are shown in Table 33.1. Individual elderly patients however, might find statistics less convincing than

Table 33.1 Post-operative mortality rates in the elderly surgical patient

Reference	1	2	3	4
Type of surgery	colonic	all types	abdominal	general
Lowest age	70	70	70	65
Number	163	1000	1000	288
Mortality rates %				
Elective	7.5	4.0	9.7	2.8
Non-elective	23.3	20.4	19.7	12.7
Excluding cancer	–	4.8	10.9	3.8
Total	10.4	5.8	13.6	5.2

References:
1. Greenburg et al. 1981
2. Stephen 1986
3. Reiss et al. 1987
4. Seymour and Vaz 1988

personal contact with an elderly patient who has received successful surgery. There may be a case for family practitioners and hospitals keeping a 'panel' of such patients on hand to help in counselling (in much the same way as mastectomy counsellors operate in some areas).

Another barrier to self-referral may be the fail-ure to realize that a surgically important problem is present. It is well recognized by geriatricians that rectal bleeding may be dismissed as due to haemorrhoids or even as 'normal' in old age, and a change in bowel habit may not be seen as indicative of bowel pathology. Atypical presentations of the 'acute abdomen' (Clinch et al., 1984; Telfer et al., 1988) complicate the picture and the patient may not present to a doctor until a surgical emergency has arisen.

The barriers discussed above are all amenable to education provided the doctors themselves have the necessary information. An age-related component to surgical education of medical students should play an important role here.

The Doctor

Four important factors have been identified in the decision to proceed to surgery – quality of life pre- and post-operatively, capability of giving informed consent, attitude of the surgeon and economic considerations (Reiss, 1980). In addition, forces moving surgeons and physicians toward and away from surgery have been recognized (Reiss, 1980). In the first instance, however, a surgical problem has to be brought to light. A surgical problem such as a lump in the breast, a mass in the abdomen, an inguinal hernia or a change in bowel habit may be detected by a doctor while examining a patient for another purpose. A 'surgical' explanation for an apparently 'medical' problem must also be kept in mind. One of the most tragic situations in general surgery occurs when a patient who has been known to have an iron deficiency anemia for a year or more, subsequently turns out to have a large bowel malignancy which has passed beyond the stage of surgical therapy. Iron deficiency anemia in old age should be assumed to be due to blood loss until proved otherwise, and the possibility of a bowel tumour should be constantly borne in mind.

A few formal analyses have been carried out to compare the effects of surgical and non-surgical therapy. For example, Neuhauser (1977) looked at inguinal hernias in elderly patients. He examined the expected outcome of elective surgery compared with the outcome of a 'wait and see' policy. Under this second policy, the hernia received surgery only if it strangulated. With the 'wait and see' policy any operations that were necessary had a higher mortality but some patients did not require surgery at all. In the case of inguinal hernia the conclusion was that, from a mortality point of view, there was nothing to choose between elective surgery and a 'wait and see' policy. The decision, therefore, hinged on the quality of life of the patient and in particular their attitude to surgery or conservative management. In the case of femoral hernias the strangulation rate was much higher and the mortality analysis favored early surgery in all cases.

Early case detection of surgical problems in the elderly may be worthwhile, but very little information is available. Case-finding could be carried out at any patient-doctor consultation. Problem lists compiled on every elderly patient should include formal consideration as to whether a surgical problem exists. With respect to specific case-finding programmes there is already a wide discussion in the literature on the strengths and weaknesses of screening for colorectal cancer by looking for fecal occult blood (Winiwer and Miller, 1987). The case for screening for more benign surgical conditions in the elderly has been less well addressed, although possible areas would include questions about changes in bowel habit, bleeding from any site, symptoms of prostatism or early detection of hernias. Further studies with community questionnaires or primary care screening programmes to assess current surgical need would be helpful.

Practical Points for the Referring Doctor

1. *What is the range of expertise in local surgeons?*
   This may tip the balance for or against referral, for instance in the case of moderate osteoarthritis of the hip.
2. *What are the attitudes towards the elderly of local surgeons?*
   A technically excellent surgeon with a negative attitude to the elderly may not be the best person to refer an elderly patient to.
3. *What are the patient's alternatives and how accurate is the information supplied to the patient?*

In order to decide between surgical and non-surgical therapy, the patient able to give informed consent needs accurate and correct information about likely risks and benefits. If the referring doctor does not have all the relevant information then it is important to give patients the benefit of the doubt and refer them to someone who has. It would appear vital in the case of a patient refusing an operation to ensure that this refusal is also an informed one.

A special circumstance may arise when surgery has been recommended for a condition which may be malignant. While again it is the patient's right to refuse surgery for a carcinoma, even if this is the only prospect of cure, we would argue that the diagnosis must be made explicit to the patient under such circumstances. It seems to us unjustifiable ethically to use euphemisms such as 'an ulcer in the bowel' when a patient is refusing surgery for a known or suspected large bowel carcinoma.

The barriers to surgery in the elderly

Medical Barriers

The decision as to whether the patient is medically fit for surgery is one to be made in hospital by a team which includes the surgeon and anesthetist responsible. However, it is very helpful if medical problems are identified well in advance, particularly as the rate of incidental medical disease in elderly surgical patients is likely to be high. In a recent study of general surgical patients aged 65 years and over in Cardiff, only one patient in five had no medical problems of any kind. While some of the medical problems were minor, 29 per cent of patients had evidence of significant respiratory disease, 14 per cent had a history of past congestive cardiac failure, 9 per cent had symptoms of angina,

5 per cent had had strokes in the past and 9 per cent had an abnormal preoperative score on a mental status questionnaire. Such problems by no mcans precludc surgery, but it is highly desirable for them to be recognized in advance. It is very distressing to elderly patients when an operation needs to be cancelled at the last moment because of the late detection of a medical problem.

Some medical findings are obviously of more importance than others, although the relative risks of individual findings are rarely given in standard textbooks of surgery. This is particularly true for the elderly. The available data has been summarized by Seymour (1986) Seymour et al. (1992) and more briefly by Seymour and Vaz (1987). Many of the essential facts are listed in Tables 33.2 and 33.3, which can also be used as a check list when assisting respiratory and cardiac risk in the preoperative patient.

Table 33.2 Preoperative risk factors and post-operative respiratory complications in the elderly

Preoperative risk factor	Relative risk of postoperative respiratory complication
Age over 75	approximately 1.5x
Male sex	1.3–4x
Smoking	1.5–7x
> 120% ideal weight	2x
Emergency surgery	1.5–2.5x
Dyspnea on minimal exercise (NYHA grade 3 or 4)*	2x
ASA class 3 or 4*	2–5x
Incision near diaphragm	2x
Past respiratory history or recent symptoms	2x
Acute respiratory disease	2–3x
Peak flow < 250 litres/min	1.5–2x
FEV, FVC < 70%	approximately 2–3x

Note: * See Seymour, 1986, pp. 49, 94, and Seymour and Pringle, 1983
Note: Based on Seymour, 1986, pp. 43–61

Functional Status

Three functional scales are shown in Table 33.4. The American Society of Anethetists (ASA) score and the NYHA score are mainly used in hospitals by anesthetists and cardiologists respectively. In elderly patients we have found the ASA score to be closely correlated with post-operative mortality (Seymour and Vaz, 1987), but the correlation between a poor NYHA score and an adverse post-operative outcome has been less clear-cut. The reason for the poor performance of the NYHA score in elderly people may be that the older patient with heart disease deliberately limits his or her activity so that the symptom of dyspnea is not experienced. Seymour and Pringle (1983) suggested that the mobility score was better guide to post-operative outcome than the NYHA score as it looked at what the patient actually could do rather that the symptoms complained of. In a recent study

Table 33.3 Preoperative risk factors and post-operative cardiovascular complications in the elderly*

		Postoperative CVS complications – increase in relative risk		
		Myocardial infarction	Cardiac death	All CVS complications
Age over 70		2–4X	2–12X	2–3X
Emergency admission			4X, in cardiac surgery	2X
Myocardial infarction within 3 months**		5–8X	5–8X	
Myocardial infarction 3–6 months before**		2–4X	2–4X	
Stable angina controlled heart failure			1·5–2X	2–3X
Acute heart failure	?	2X	10–15X	
Dyspnea on moderate exercise		2–4X	2–4X	2–4X
Sex, obesity, smoking diabetes, systolic BP		No proven correlation with adverse CVS outcomes in the elderly		

Notes: * See Seymour, 1986, pp. 89–106 for references
** Relative to patients with infarctions more than six months old

Table 33.4 Scales which have been used in physical assessment*

1. American Society of Anesthetists' (ASA) Grading of Physical Status:	
CLASS I	A normally healthy patient
CLASS II	A patient with mild systemic disease
CLASS III	A patient with severe systemic disease which is not incapacitating
CLASS IV	A patient with an incapacitating systemic disease that is a constant threat to life
CLASS V	A moribund patient who is not expected to survive for 24 hours with or without operation
2. New York Heart Association (NYHA) Scale	
CLASS I	Heart disease but no limitation of activity
CLASS II	Some limitation on heavy exertion, but patient could climb one flight of stairs or walk three blocks without shortness of breath
CLASS III	Some limitation on ordinary activity with difficulty walking three blocks or climbing one flight of stairs
CLASS IV	Shortness of breath at rest
3. Mobility Score	
Grade 1	Above average activity, e.g. underoing regular
Grade 2	Fully active, doing own shopping, cooking, housework or more
Grade 3	Out of the house three or more times a week (by own efforts) but needing some help with shopping, cooking or housework
Grade 4	Out of the house twice a week or less
Grade 5	Housebound
Grade 6	Chairfast

Note: * For reference see Seymour, 1986, pp. 49, 94, and Seymour and Pringle, 1983

of general surgical patients in Cardiff, patients who were unable to leave the house had four times the mortality of patients with more favorable mobility scores. When a patient has been referred for a consideration of surgical operation, particularly an orthopedic procedure, then a description of their normal level of activity and other major barriers to rehabilitation (such as poor eyesight) are useful pieces of information.

Patients' Fears about Surgery

So far we have talked about objective risks of surgery, but it must be realized that some patients who are referred for elective surgery in their 80s have been superbly fit all their lives and have probably not seen the inside of an out-patient department let alone an operating room. Such patients need to be reassured and given a brief description of what they can expect. Patients may also have irrational fears based on the surgical mishaps (real or imaginary) of near relatives or friends. It is as well to enquire about these and confront them rather than let them become magnified in the patient's imagination. The fear of cancer is often unspoken and many a patient has been concerned that their hernia was a malignant tumour. The patient may also have very strong views on whether they want an operation done under general or local anaesthetic. While the final decision on this must take into account the technical considerations and the opinion of the anesthetist, if the patient has strong preferences, these are best mentioned in the original referral letter.

Getting the patient ready for surgery

The timing of preoperative assessment

There is much to be said for a complete assessment of the patient two or three weeks before admission so that any necessary medical problems can be identified and, if possible, treated. In special high risk situations, such as in patients with chronic respiratory problems, then a brief admission to an appropriate respiratory unit or perhaps a geriatric service may need to be arranged to 'fine tune' the patient.

The role of routine preoperative screening

While there is a general feeling that in the younger patient routine pre-operative electrocardiography, chest radiology and multiphasic biochemical screening are not cost-effective, our conclusion to date is that a routine ECG, chest X-ray, full blood count, urea and electrolytes, blood sugar and possibly calcium and liver function tests are indicated in older patients (Seymour, 1986). Further information may change these recommendations. In the patient with no history of abnormal bleeding, routine screening for coagulation disorders appears not to be indicated (Seymour, 1986).

Prophylaxis against thromboembolism

This is a decision that needs to be made by the hospital team, but age is one of the recognized factors increasing the risk of post-operative deep venous thrombosis and pulmonary embolism. In general surgery, subcutaneous heparin is probably sufficient prophylaxis, but in orthopedic surgery and extensive pelvic surgery, extra precautions may need to be taken (Seymour et al., 1992).

Prophylaxis against infection

An antibiotic given intravenously shortly before operation appears to be able to reduce the risk of sepsis in higher-risk groups of patients. Again this is a decision that needs to be made primarily by the surgical team, but a summary of recent recommendations is given by Kaiser (1986).

The continuation of medication through the operative period

Most elderly patients are on one or more medications and it may be difficult to decide on whether these medications should be continued over the operative period. The decision obviously depends on the agent and the clinical circumstances. In the case of drugs such as beta-blockers and digoxin, however, the usual advice is to continue them through the operative period unless they are causing toxicity, as the risks of sudden withdrawal are high. However, the practice of giving 'prophylactic' digoxin in elderly patients who were not previously receiving the drug, has now largely been abandoned (Seymour, 1986). The question of the treatment of moderate hypertension over the anesthetic period is a complex one. Prys–Roberts (1979) has pointed out that hypertensive patients tend to have swings of blood pressure during anaesthesia whether or not they are on anti-hypertensive therapy. He therefore advocates that moderate degrees of hypertension (e.g. a diastolic of less than 110 mm Hg) noted for the first time in a patient prior to surgery should probably be tolerated and treated at leisure post-operatively. When the patient is already established on anti-hypertensives the risk of withdrawal must be balanced against side-effects such as hypotension during anesthesia.

Nutritional therapy in the elderly

A decade ago a number of publications appeared suggesting that general surgical patients of all ages had a significant incidence of malnutrition. It now appears that many of these studies used inappropriate methods of measurement, and widespread nutritional supplementation has not found a place in routine surgical therapy. The interpretation of low serum albumin in surgical patients has also caused confusion. While protein malnutrition certainly causes serum albumin to fall, low serum albumins are often encountered in elderly patients with acute or chronic illness and under conditions of physiological stress. A study in Cardiff (Seymour et al., 1988) has shown that patients with a preoperative serum albumin below 35 G/L are at an increased risk of post-operative mortality and a wide range of post-operative complications. However, the reason for this increased risk is not necessarily malnutrition, as many of the patients had low albumins as the result of illness. The beneficial effects of brief periods of nutritional supplementation in surgical patients, even those who are unequivocally malnourished, are still disputed by many. A good account of the present position in general surgery is given by Hill (1988). The patient with a fractured neck of femur however, may have special nutritional needs (Bastow, et al., 1983)

The efficacy of surgery

Curiously, this is an area we know remarkably little about. Long-term morbidity and mortality statistics are few and the main study on long-term survival after surgery (Anderson and Ostberg, 1972a, b) was completed many years ago when surgical and anesthetic techniques were less advanced.

'Quality of life' as seen earlier, is quoted as an important ingredient in the decision to operate. At the present time with regard to outcome of surgery in the elderly 'surgical success' is largely a subjective judgment. We badly need objective data on which to base decisions, and follow up studies of 'quality of life' indices in the weeks and months post-operatively will be an important contribution to the field of surgery in the elderly.

3. Conclusion

The path to an elective surgical operation in an elderly patient presents many medical, surgical, technical and ethical challenges. Age on its own should not be used to deny anyone potentially useful surgery. However, safe surgical passage requires more than good intentions. We undoubtedly need accurate and up-to-date information about the risks and benefits of surgical treatments in the elderly, but all of these will be to no avail if the patient is not identified and referred in the first instance. A recognition of the barriers which currently prevent elderly patients with surgical problems reaching surgical help is the first step to overcoming them. After the operation is over, we need to pay more attention to the short and long-term outcome, measuring the latter both in terms of quantity and quality of life.

References

Andersen, B. and Ostberg, J. (1972a). Survival rates in syrgery of the aged. Assessment of long-term prognosis according to coexisting disease. *Geront. Clin.* **14**: 354–60.

Andersen, B. and Ostberg, J. (1972b). Long-term prognosis in geriatric surgery: 2-17 year follow-up of 7922 patients. *J. Am. Ger. Soc.*, **20**: 255–8.

Bastow, M. D., Rawlings, J., Allison, S.P. (1983). Benefits of supplementary tube feeding after fractured neck of femur: a randomized controlled trial. *Brit. Med. J.*, **287**: 1589–92.

Clinch, D., Banerjee, A. K. and Ostick, G. (1984). Absence of pain in elderly patients with peptic ulcer. *Age and Ageing*, **13**: 120–3.

CEPOD (1987). The Report of a Confidential Enquiry into Peri-operative Deaths. Buck, N., Devlin, H. B. and Lunn, J. N. (eds). Nuffield Provincial Hospital Trust, London.

Greenburg, A. G., Saik, R. P., Coyle, J. J. and Peskin, G. W. (1981). Mortality and gastrointestinal surgery in the elderly. Elective versus emergency procedures. *Arch. Surg.*, **116**: 788–91.

Harris, J. (1987). QALYfying the value of life. *J. Med. Ethics*, **13**: 117–23.

Hill, G. L. (1988). Surgical nutrition: time for some clinical common sense. *Br. J. Surg.*, **75**: 729–30.

Kaiser, A. B. (1986). Antimicrobial prophylaxis in surgery. *New Engl. J. Med.*, **315**: 1129–38.

Neuhauser, D. (1977). Elective inguinal herniorrhaphy versus truss in the elderly. In: Bunker J. P., Barnes, B. A., Mosteller, F. (eds). *Costs, Risk and Benefits of Surgery*. Oxford University Press, New York, 223–39.

Prys-Roberts, C. (1979). Hypertension and anesthesia – fifty years on. *Anesthesiology*, **50**: 281–4.

Reiss, R. (1980). Moral and ethical issues in geriatric surgery. *J. Med. Ethics*, **6**: 71–77.

Reiss, R., Deutsch, A. A. and Nudelman, I. (1987). Abdominal surgery in elderly patients: statistical analysis of clinical factors prognostic of mortality in 1000 cases. *Mount Sinai J. Med.*, **54**: 135–40.

Seymour, D. G. (1986). *Medical Assessment of the Elderly Surgical Patient*. Croom Helm, London.

Seymour, D. G. (1988). Medical aspects of surgery. In: Stanton, E. L. (ed.) *Bailliere's clinical obstetrics and gynaecology*, **2**: 269–287.

Seymour, D. G., Rees, G. A. D. and Crosby, D. L. (1992). Introduction and general principles. In Crosby, D. L., Rees, G. A. D. and Seymour, D. G. *The Ageing Surgical Patient: Anaesthetic Operative and Medical Management*, Wiley, Chichester. 1–90.

Seymour, D. G. and Pringle, R. (1983). Post-operative complications in the elderly surgical patient. *Gerontol.*, **29**: 262–70.

Seymour, D. G. and Vaz, F. G. (1988). Aspects of surgery in the elderly: pre-operative medical assessment. *Br. J. Hosp. Med.*, **37**: 102–12.

Stephen, C. R. (1986). Risk factors and outcome in elderly patients: an epidemiologic study. In: Stephen, C. R. and Assaf, R. A. E. (eds). *Geriatric Anaesthesia: Principles and Practice.* Butterworths, Boston, pp. 345–62.

Telfer, S., Fenyo, G., Holt, P. R., de Dombal, F. T. (1988). Acute abdominal pain in patients over 50 years of age. *Scand. J. Gastroenterol*, **23**: (suppl. 144), 47–50.

Winawer, S. J. and Miller, D. (1987). Screening for colorectal cancer. *Bull. World Health Org.*, **65**: 105–11.

34

Medical education and geriatrics – an overview of critical problems in undergraduate, graduate, and continuing medical education

During his tenure as British Prime Minister, Lloyd George had to contend with the First World War, an economic crisis, and rebellion in Ireland among other difficulties. When asked how he retained his equilibrium, Lloyd George replied, 'Well, I find that a change of nuisances is as good as a vacation'.

Medical educators interested in gerontology and geriatrics often feel like Lloyd George. In response to the demographic imperative there is a consensus that physicians today and in the future will require better training on how to deal with elderly patients. The 1978 Institute of Medicine report on 'Aging and Medical Education' made a number of recommendations which would have led to increasing undergraduate and graduate education in geriatrics. To this date the North American medical establishment has been slow in responding to these recommendations. In this Chapter I wish to review some of the key problems in the domains of undergraduate, graduate and continuing medical education which appear to be hampering the development of geriatric medicine.

1. Undergraduate Medical Education

During the 1970s and 1980s the undergraduate medical curriculum has changed mainly in response to pressure groups, each championing their own particular interest (Rosinski, 1983). Additions have been made to the curriculum with the development of new or expanded courses often with no accompanying subtraction. Areas which have been added in at least some medical schools include medical ethics, human sexuality, medical economics, nutrition, substance abuse, and palliative care. There has been a tendency in some quarters to view the impulse for greater offerings in gerontology/geriatrics as, in essence, the same as for any other – the particular interest of a pressure group. It is my perspective that the necessity to respond in this area is at least quantitatively different.

There is general agreement that physicians practicing clinical medicine, except for some specialized areas such as pediatrics and obstetrics, will spend a large proportion of their time dealing with elderly patients. The elderly as a group present with complex, compounding problems which necessitate the acquisition of specific attitudes, skills, and knowledge. As most graduates of medical schools will be dealing with elderly patients and will require a basic level of competency to deal effectively with them, it is hard to dispute the incorporation of gerontology/geriatrics within the required undergraduate curriculum. Generally accepted educational objectives in geriatrics have been developed and an example of such a list is shown in Table 34.1 (Robbins, 1982).

What is the current status with regards to undergraduate medical education? In the United Kingdom, 28 out of the 30 clinical medical schools (93 per cent) provide formal teaching in geriatric medicine (Stout, 1985). At most schools (83 per

Table 34.1 Undergraduate medical education objectives

1. To be able to take an accurate medical history from an elderly patient which would include a functional history such as a patient's ability to perform daily activities and a psychosocial history, including factors such as motivation, morale, family and social interaction, household composition, and productivity.
2. To conduct and record a complete physical examination of an elderly patient with specific attention to normal physical signs of aging, functional assessment including mental status testing, and activities of daily living.
3 To distinguish 'normal' from pathological aging.
4. To demonstrate clinical decision-making skills, taking into account the altered clinical presentation of disease, multiple illness complexes, patient's lifestyle, cost-effectiveness factors, and prognosis.
5. To apply ones' knowledge to clinical pharmacology in the treatment of elderly patients.
6. To apply ones knowledge of rehabilitative medicine in managing elderly patients.
7. To identify available community resources in planning the care of an elderly patient.
8. To co-ordinate and provide for a continuum of care.
9. To provide personalized and empathetic care to patients and their families.
10. To co-ordinate assessment and management as part of an interdisciplinary health care team (Robbins, 1982).

cent) all medical students receive some teaching in geriatric medicine but clinical rotations are provided to only a proportion. In the United States the situation appears to be less sanguine. Most US medical schools have clinical geriatric offerings but the courses tend to be elective – i.e., not required (Vivell et al., 1987). Only 2 per cent to 3 per cent of American medical students participate in these experiences. Obviously there is limited exposure to the concepts of geriatric medicine within American medical schools. The reasons are complex and include factors such as lack of qualified faculty, competition from other offerings for available curricular time, conflict among the key clinical departments (Internal Medicine, Family Medicine, Psychiatry) as to who has responsibility, and lack of recognition of the necessity of geriatrics within the upper echelons of some medical schools. Another key issue appears to be the organizational framework in which geriatrics must evolve. Medical schools in some respects can be viewed as feudal kingdoms with basic science and clinical departments representing the various warring principalities. Curricular development is at least partially a political process with negotiation and conflict between the various key players. Unless geriatrics has an academic 'home' with both the interest and power required to effect change it is unlikely to be very effective in obtaining greater curricular time. This is particularly important because of the over-crowded state of the undergraduate curriculum. Whether this 'home' is a separate department, a subdivision of an established department, or a course committee with real power, will obviously depend on local circumstances.

After setting basic general objectives and obtaining curricular time other critical questions would include determining who should teach and how (or where) should the teaching be done. It is my bias that there is a requirement for full-time academic physicians in geriatrics who would be responsible for at least a proportion of the geriatric teaching. Obviously their prime responsibility should be to teach those areas which cannot be taught by other members of the faculty. In the main this would relate to the clinical practice of geriatrics such as the assessment and management of falling, immobility, confusion, incontinence of urine and bowel dysfunction in the elderly. Gerontology (which relates to the scientific study of aging) could be taught by these individuals but would probably be more appropriately handled by basic science faculty. If anything the teaching of gerontology appears to be less developed than the teaching of geriatric medicine – in the UK only 25 per cent of the clinical medical schools offer formal teaching in gerontology which compares to 93 per cent which provide formal teaching in geriatric medicine. For the development of appropriate clinical skills and attitudes, it is essential that part of the training occurs in a clinical setting. To paraphrase Osler, to study geriatrics without seeing patients is never to have studied geriatrics at all. Determination of which settings is a crucial issue and requires careful attention. In addition to acute in-patient units there is a need to expose students to domiciliary care, ambulatory facilities and long-term care institutions.

Once an undergraduate medical education program is established it is obviously necessary to evaluate it. The evaluation should be congruent with the objectives developed for the program. While factual knowledge is important it is essential not to neglect areas such as clinical skills and attitudes, although they are more difficult to assess. Evaluation data obtained should be used to modify and improve the program.

In summary, the necessity to develop undergraduate educational offerings in gerontology/geriatrics is obvious and irrefutable. In order to act as agents for change it is necessary to situate the geriatric faculty within an appropriate structure so that they can function effectively within the organizational universe of the medical school. As in any educational program it is important to delineate educational objectives which in this circumstance may be critical clinical competencies felt necessary for all graduates. Following this there should be careful consideration of the methods of teaching with emphasis on developing the specific settings to be utilized. In addition to student evaluation, there should be rigorous evaluation of the educational program itself with the data obtained being used for course improvement. Times of curricular renewal are particular windows of opportunity to expand geriatric offerings which should not be missed.

2. Graduate Education

It is very hard to separate this area from the entire question of the role of geriatric medicine within the health care system. How will practitioners in geriatric medicine function? Are they to be nearly inaccessible consultants limited to academic centers, being heavily involved in teaching and research, or will geriatricians become primary care physicians dealing with elderly patients? The answer to this question will be critical in designing the type of graduate training necessary for practitioners in geriatric medicine.

One of the hallmarks of twentieth-century medicine has been the increased specialization of practice. Since 1977 in Canada geriatric medicine has been accepted as a medical specialty while recently in the United States the American Board of Family Practice and the American Board of Internal Medicine have announced an examination in geriatric medicine which will lead to the awarding of a Certificate of Added Qualifications in Geriatric Medicine. These developments are encouraging for a number of reasons. Hopefully the examination process will lead to an ensured level of basic competency on the part of practitioners. The examination adds credibility to the field of geriatrics. Finally, if individuals are labelled as having special competency in geriatrics, then there may be some changes in financial compensation favoring these individuals. While this will aid in the recruitment of individuals into geriatrics, it may leave other physicians feeling excluded from this area of practice.

In North America it is not clear exactly how specialists in geriatrics will practice in the future. Questions of territoriality with other specialties have to be addressed – exactly which patients should specialists in geriatrics be dealing with? At this stage in its development an interesting question is whether the training programs will drive the style of practice or if the style of practice will eventually drive the structure of the training programs. Currently the training programs have a major influence on the shaping of geriatric practice – people tend to do what they have been trained to do particularly if they have that option. Optimally the training programs should be designed to meet the health care needs of the population but this is no easy exercise. In Table 34.2 is given a list of competencies required for the practice of geriatric medicine as a consultant, derived by seeking the opinion of Canadian specialists in geriatrics (Fox et al., 1989.)

By September of 1987 11 of the 16 Canadian universities had accredited training programs in geriatric medicine. In 1980, the United States had 25 programs with a total of 67 residency positions. By 1986 this had grown to 66 programs with 204.5 positions. In spite of this rapid growth the number of available trained geriatricians to fill faculty positions, even aside from providing clinical care, falls far short of the need.

In Canada it is felt that most of the primary care and general consulting work in geriatrics will be the responsibilities of family physicians and general internists respectively. As such it is critical that these individuals have appropriate grounding in the basics of geriatric medicine. Individuals in Departments or Divisions of Geriatric Medicine often feel that a rotation through geriatrics should be mandatory for all these trainees. This is not the current situation in many training centres and it is unlikely that this will change quickly. The reasons are multiple and relate to the lack of qualified faculty, competition with other services for a limited number of residents, and debate with regards to the necessity of a mandatory rotation in geriatrics. The development of stronger divisions or departments of Geriatrics would aid by providing a larger cadre of faculty and increasing the prestige of geriatrics which should improve the chances of competing favorably with other services for residents.

In conclusion, geriatric medicine is accepted as a bona fide specialty in North America but because

Table 34.2 Competencies required for the practice of geriatric medicine as a consultant physician

Knowledge:

1. To demonstrate competence in general internal medicine, which is required for effective diagnosis and therapy of disease in elderly patients referred for consultation. This includes knowledge of pharmacologic alterations associated with aging and the special problems of polypharmacy, overmedication and iatrogenic disease.
2. To demonstrate an awareness and knowledge of sensory losses resulting from aging and disease, as well as familarity with current modes of treatment.
3. To demonstrate particular expertise in areas of clinical neurology and assessment of musculoskeletal problems as they relate to the elderly.
4. To demonstrate awareness and competence in dealing with psychiatric problems – in particular, acute confusional states, the dementing illnesses, depression and the paranoid states.
5. To have a mastery of the principles of rehabilitative medicine as it relates to frail elderly patients with co-existent acute and chronic illnesses.
6. To have an awareness and a comprehension of social issues as they relate to the care of individual patients.
7. To demonstrate appropriate knowledge of basic gerontology, including areas such as the biology of aging and the relevant social sciences.
8. To have knowledge of the epidemiologic issues of aging, diseases of the aged, health care delivery, health promotion and disease prevention.

Attitudes:

1. To manifest the appropriate attitudes required for managing ill, elderly patients and their families. The practitioner needs to be compassionate, patient and sensitive to negative stereotyping of elderly patients (ageism) and be able to educate others about such stereotyping.
2. To practice a comprehensive (holistic) type of medicine, the various factors that come into play in the appropriate management of elderly patients being kep in mind. This individualization of care underscores the emphasis given to ensuring as much patient autonomy as possible in decision-making.
3. To demonstrate appropriate attitudes toward other members of the health care team, to recognize their unique contributions as health care professionals and to foster an interdisciplinary team approach. To demonstrate appropriate attitudes to all care providers in various settings, including nursing homes and other long-term care institutions.

Skills:

1. To perform or interpret a comprehensive geriatric assessment (including assessment of physical health, mental health, functional status, socioeconomic status and environmental factors) and to evaluate the following clinical problems: confusion or memory failure, falling or postural instability, reduced mobility, incontinence of urine, bowel dysfunction (constipation or fecal incontinence) and difficulties in activities of daily living.
2. To deal effectively with patients with several interacting problems that may be related to specific diseases, aging or various combinations. To perform preoperative assessments in such patients and provide support in post-operative management.
3. To develop a critical approach to the interpretation of scientific information and foster research involvement to improve understanding of aging as well as diseases of the aged and to apply these skills to clinical practice.
4. To demonstrate an awareness of the dangers of inappropriate use of technology in the management of elderly patients and to demonstrate a balance between excessive intervention and a nihilistic approach. This would require knowledge of the precepts of medical ethics.
5. To deal with interpersonal relationships and family dynamics.
6. To demonstrate a knowledge of group dynamics and the ability to work effectively in the setting of health care teams.
7. To have an understanding of and be able to participate in health care planning and policy-making as it relates to the management of elderly patients.
8. To know when to use the various resources that may be called into play to meet the needs of elderly patients, including health services, social programs, informal help from families and various support groups (e.g. the Alzheimer Society of Canada).
9. To demonstrate competence as a physician working with patients in long-term care institutions and to provide consultant support to primary care physicians and other health care professionals in this setting.

of its newness it is still establishing its territory with regards to both academic and clinical activities. Training programs in geriatrics are expanding rapidly but at the present time still appear to be insufficient to produce the required number of qualified physicians. At this juncture the training programs will probably have a critical role in defining exactly how geriatrics will be practised in the future. While mandatory geriatric rotations for trainees in family medicine and general internal medicine are an ultimate goal, currently it would be both logistically impossible and politically unrealistic to expect in many training centres.

3. Continuing Medical Education

One of the commonly stated goals of medical schools is to produce life-long learners. As part of this process continuing medical education has become, to use an American expression, a growth industry with increasing opportunities available to the practitioner.

Continuing medical education can be defined as 'processes aimed at improving health care outcomes through learning, either by individual efforts or as part of activities, products, and services provided by continuing education provider units' (Green, et al., 1984). Up to the present continuing medical education has emphasized the traditional 'classroom' approach with the transmission of knowledge and, occasionally, the demonstration of technical skills.

In certain critical ways adult learners (which is what practicing physicians are) differ from the student learners that academic physicians have most of their contact with (Kriscols, 1978). Adult learners tend to be more self directed. To the learning encounter they bring a rich resource of their own past experiences. They usually demand that the knowledge learned be directly applicable to problems they encounter in their work. As such their orientation to learning tends to be problem centered. The teacher generally must be both collaborative and informal, trying to foster mutual respect. Ideally the learner should be part of the planning process for the educational experience. This would include diagnosing the problem areas and formulating educational objectives.

Over the last ten years there appears to have been increased continuing educational offerings dealing with geriatrics – at least in the United States. For the 30-month period beginning 1 January, 1975 there were 36 courses dealing with geriatrics. For the 24-month period beginning 1 January, 1984 there were 85 (Vivell, 1987). In spite of this it has been estimated that over the 2 year period beginning 1 January, 1984 only 8000 of the 450,000 practicing physicians in the United States (1.8 per cent) participated in a continuing medical education offering dealing at least partially with geriatrics.

A particular problem geriatrics has in recruiting individuals to continuing education offerings is that most practitioners have had no experience with formal geriatric teaching. (You don't miss it if you don't know what it is.) Even when physicians do attend these courses one must wonder if they are the most appropriate venue for transmission of what is felt to be important in geriatrics. Improved care of the elderly probably depends at least as much on reordering values and attitudes as on the transfer of knowledge and technical skills. One must also question the whole concept of traditional passive courses in view of what is known about adult learners. There are multiple ways that physicians continue their learning after medical school and I suspect that it would be fruitful for individuals interested in geriatric education to consider options other than the classroom technique.

Theoretically it would be more appropriate to promote self-directed learning among physicians. Some areas to consider would include contract learning (here the learning plan is devised after negotiation between the physician and the educational specialist), information brokering (linking physicians with consultants and community resources), collegial networking (discussion groups), and special interest groups. A potentially fruitful approach would be a 'mini'-residency in geriatrics of preferably one to six months duration followed by ongoing contact, possibly by enrolling the 'student' physician in a special interest group dealing with geriatrics.

To summarize, it is time to consider the various ways of facilitating continuing medical education in geriatrics. The traditional lecture approach will probably lead to a minimal impact on a minimal number with little resultant improvement in health care as it relates to the elderly.

4. Conclusion

One could become discouraged by the complexity of the problems facing medical educators with an interest in this field until one realizes the distance already covered. Initially our goals will have to be somewhat limited. Changes will not be revolutionary but rather evolutionary. This limitation in goals is reflected by a story told about Konrad Adenauer. While he was still Chancellor of the Federal Republic of Germany he developed an upper respiratory tract infection near his 90th birthday. His personal physician was unable to do much to alleviate his symptoms and had to put up with a great deal of verbal abuse. Finally he told the Chancellor that 'I'm not a magician, I can't make you young again.' Adenauer responded, 'I haven't asked you to, all I want to do is to go on getting older.'

Recommended reading

Fox, R. A., Clarfield, A. M. and Hogan, D. B. (1989). Competencies required for the practice of geriatric medicine as a consultant physician. *Can. Med. Assoc. J.*, **141**: 1045–47.

Green, J. S., Grossworld, S. J., Suter, E. and Waltball, D. B. (1984). *Continuing Education for Health Professions*. Jossey-Bass, San Francisco.

Institute of Medicine (1978). Aging and Medical Education. Washington, DC, National Academy of Sciences.

Kriscoles, M. *The Adult Learner – A neglected Species*. Gulf Publishing, Houston.

Robbins, A. S., Fink, A., Kosecoff, J., et al. (1982). Studies in Geriatric Education. *J. Am. Ger. Soc.*, **30**: 281–8.

Rosinski, E. F. (1983). Curricular trends In: *Handbook of Health Professions Education*. Jossey-Bass, San Francisco, pp. 164–194.

Stout, R. W. (1985). Teaching gerontology and geriatric medicine. *Age & Aging (suppl.)*.

Vivell, S., Solomon, D. H. and Beck, J. C. (1987). Medical education responds to the 20th century's success story. *J. Am. Ger. Soc.*, **35**: 1107–15.

35

Geriatrics internationally

The Diseases of the aged are worthy of the most careful study . . . Let us not dismiss (their) ailments with the facile diagnosis: You are old.

Ignatius Nascher (1914)

There is much to recommend geriatrics as a specialty comparable to pediatrics. The creation of such a specialty would stimulate those with a leaning to this type of work and raise the standard of the work done.

Marjory Warren (1946)

1. Introduction

The raison d'entre of geriatric medicine, succinctly captured in the words of Ignatius Nascher, the American physician who coined the term 'geriatrics', is rejection of the passive acceptance of disease and disability as inevitable consequences of aging. In its stead, geriatric medicine advocates careful assessment, treatment and continuing care for health problems of older people, with a goal of maintaining or restoring maximal independent function. This point of view was first fully articulated in Britain in the 1940s and 1950s, epitomized by the pioneering work of Marjory Warren. The essence of Dr Warren's work was to bring thorough medical assessment and multidisciplinary rehabilitation to large numbers of institutionalized elderly persons and in turn to recommend such approaches for older patients in the acute hospital and in the community. While the concept of geriatrics as a distinct branch of medicine has been debated in many countries, the fact that the field has attracted widespread adherents was clearly evidenced at a first ever symposium on 'Geriatric Medicine Worldwide' convened in Eastbourne, England in 1987. The symposium included professors and other identified leaders in geriatrics from countries throughout the developed and developing world (Brocklehurst, 1987).

The 'geriatric imperative' underlying this movement comprises the forces of demography, chronic disease and disability which characterize populations which are aged and aging throughout the world (Fig. 35.1) (Davies, 1985 and Grundy, 1983).

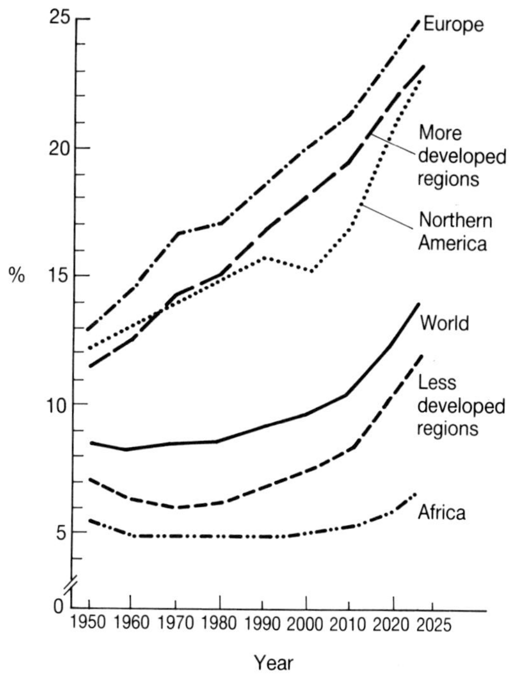

Fig. 35.1 Percentage of population 60 years and over in different parts of the world. (UN data and predictions, 1950–2025). (from Davies, M. (1985). Epidemiology and the challenge of aging. *International Journal of Epidemiology* **14**: 9–19.

A direct corollary is the challenge to individual countries to develop comprehensive health and health related services and appropriately trained professionals to meet the multi-faceted needs of their older citizens. In response to this universal challenge, the World Health Organization (WHO) in 1974 convened an expert committee to address the topic 'Planning and Organization of Geriatric Services' (WHO, 1974). This chapter begins with a summary of the WHO committee's principal recommendations. The extent to which these recommendations are being fulfilled is then examined using information gathered in a 1988 mail survey of selected participants in the 1987 Geriatric Medicine Worldwide Symposium and supplemented by reports on geriatric developments from individual countries. Findings from the author's comparative study of the experience in two societies, Great Britain and the United States, are illustrative of contrasting national responses to the 'geriatric imperative' (Barker, 1987). The chapter concludes with discussion of emerging epidemiological and ethical challenges to be met by geriatric medicine internationally.

2. The world health organization report

The 1974 report of the WHO expert committee addresses, respectively, organization of services, medical training and education, and research.

With respect to services, the report states:

Each country should assess the unmet needs of the aged and explore the most suitable pattern of care that fits into its health care system, giving special attention to the basic aspects of such a system, with its major elements of medical and social prevention, multidisciplinary assessment, home and institutional curative treatment, rehabilitation, long-term care, and supportive social welfare.

Recommendations for Training and Education

Countries where geriatrics is not yet recognized as a medical specialty should be encouraged to establish, on an experimental basis, geriatrics as a special branch of medicine in order to ensure the availability of professional personnel for teaching, research, and consultation in the geriatric field.

All medical schools should introduce into their curricula the study of adult human development and aging in all its physiological, psychological, pathological, clinical, epidemiological, and sociological aspects. This should entail both lectures and the clinical presentation of geriatric patients.

Whenever it is appropriate, chairs of geriatric medicine should be created in all countries.

Research Recommendations

It is recommended that there should be studies on a number of specific health problems related to aging. Due consideration should be given to the creation of special centers of gerontology and adult human development to be entrusted with research, the training of personnel, and the dissemination of knowledge.

The WHO should promote in-depth comparative studies of the different systems of providing geriatric services and of facilities for training and education in geriatrics that already exist in various countries.

3. Survey of selected countries

The WHO recommendations are being fulfilled to a considerable degree, according to information gathered from countries responding to the author's 1988 mail questionnaire survey. Principal findings are tabulated by country in Table 35.1.

Professional medical societies identified with geriatrics and/or gerontology exist in all of the responding countries. Virtually all of these organizations have assumed the important role of promoting interest and learning in the field of geriatrics by sponsoring one or more professional meetings a year. The majority also sponsor professional journals dealing with health and health care of older people.

Official recognition of geriatrics as an independent medical specialty or sub-specialty in internal medicine has occurred in all but a few countries surveyed. In most instances this has occurred in the past decade, for example, Norway (1975), Canada (1980), Netherlands (1983), United States (1988). In all countries specialty qualification in geriatrics requires successful completion of prescribed postgraduate training and in approximately half, a certifying exam must also be taken. Guidelines for specialty training and certification in several countries have been published (Dalgaard, 1981; Cape and MacDonald, 1986; Barker, 1987, pp. 87–100). Training guidelines for qualifying in the specialty are quite similar among countries. These include 2 to 4 years of training in general medicine or family practice, followed by 2 to 3 years training in geriatric medicine or closely related specialties. With respect to the latter, several countries specifically recommend or require rotations in psychiatry, rehabilitation, neurology and rheumatology.

Geriatrics and/or gerontology are taught as a required part of curriculum in the majority of medical schools in a number of countries; however in several countries such teaching is reported in none or few schools. Professorial chairs in geriatrics have been established in medical schools in most countries, but again, as with required curriculum, this is the exception rather than the rule in a number of instances. Historically, in a number of countries the establishment of specialty status for geriatrics has preceded the formal incorporation of the subject into medical school curricula and establishment of academic departments. Therefore with recent relatively rapid increase in recognition of the specialty, increased attention in academic centers may be anticipated.

Research institutes or agencies dedicated to aging exist in about half the survey countries. Of note, the United States, while the most recent country to recognize the specialty and a country lagging significantly in medical school involvement in geriatrics, has shown perhaps the greatest commitment to research with establishment of the prestigious National Institute on Aging in 1974.

In the critical realm of development of innovative geriatric services, experiences have varied widely around the world. The survey focused particularly on the status of special geriatric units in general hospitals and geriatric day hospitals, two service innovations central to the successful geriatric movement in Great Britain. With rare exception, reports that these geriatric service modalities were commonly in place were restricted to British Commonwealth countries (Australia, Canada, New Zealand). This pattern reflects in part the fact that leaders in geriatric medicine in these societies have frequently trained and consulted closely with the acknowledged world leaders in clinical geriatrics in Great Britain. Of equal importance has been the enactment of public policies to support and encourage development of hospital-based geriatric units and day hospitals. Examples of evolution of such policies have been described for Great Britain (Barker, 1987, pp. 20–32), Israel (Halot and Margulec, 1985), and New Zealand (Campbell, 1987) among others.

Table 35.1 Status of selected aspects of geriatrics in various countries*

Country	Professional society Meetings	Professional society Journal	Medical specialty Recognized	Medical specialty Exam	Medical schools Required curriculum	Medical schools Professorial chairs	Research institute or agency	Health services Hospital units	Health services Day hospitals	Health services Gov't long-term care
Australia	Yes	Yes	Yes	No	Yes	Majority	No	Common	Common	Yes
Brazil	Yes	Yes	Yes	Yes	No	Few	Yes	No	Few	Yes
Canada	Yes	Yes	Yes	Yes	Majority	Majority	Yes	Common	Common	Yes
Denmark	Yes	Yes	Yes	No	No	Few	Yes	Common	Common	Yes
Finland	Yes	No	Yes	Yes	Majority	Majority	No	No	Few	Yes
France	Yes	Yes	No	NA	No	None	Yes	No	Few	Yes
Germany	Yes	Yes	No	NA	No	None	Yes	No	Few	No
Great Britain	Yes	Yes	Yes	No	Majority	Majority	Yes	Common	Common	Yes
Ireland	Yes	No	Yes	No	Majority	Few	No	No	Few	Yes
Israel	Yes	Yes	Yes	Yes	Majority	None	Yes	Common	Common	No
Italy	Yes	Yes	Yes	Yes	Majority	Majority	No	No	Few	No
Japan	Yes	Yes	No	N/A	No	Few	Yes	No	Few	Yes
Mexico	Yes	Yes	Yes	No	No	Few	No	No	No	No
Netherlands	Yes	Yes	Yes	No	Majority	Majority	No	No	Common	No
New Zealand	Yes	No	Yes	No	Majority	Majority	No	Common	Common	Yes
Norway	Yes	Yes	Yes	No	No	Majority	Yes	No	Few	Yes
Spain	Yes	Yes	Yes	Yes	No	None	No	Few	Few	No
Sweden	Yes	Yes	Yes	No	All	All	Yes	Common	Common	Yes
Switzerland	Yes	Yes	No	N/A	No	Few	No	No	Common	No
United States	Yes	Yes	Yes*	Yes	Few	Few	Yes	Few	Few	Yes

*Based upon survey responses in 1988

4. Great Britain and the United States – a comparison

In reflecting upon how and why the field of geriatrics has developed in different countries, it is instructive to examine the contrasting experiences of Great Britain and the United States. Both of these countries, along with many others, began the twentieth century with a legacy of separately organized and financed services for acute and chronic medical care. With the introduction of the National Health Service in Great Britain in 1948, acute and chronic care were united under one system. Organized geriatric services in turn evolved in concert with community-based medical and social services to provide older persons and their families and physicians a much valued comprehensive system of care. In the United States, in the absence of a comprehensive national health program, a market driven and fragmented set of acute and chronic care services has evolved for old and young alike. Medicare, the government administered health insurance program for older Americans enacted in 1965 accentuated the fragmentation by largely restricting its coverage to acute care hospital and physician services, leaving out most preventive, rehabilitative and long-term care services. Confronted by the inadequacies and high costs of fragmented services, the country is beginning to explore ways to adopt more appropriate approaches to caring for older persons such as found in Great Britain.

Great Britain

Elements of comprehensive geriatrics and related health and social services in Great Britain are listed in Table 35.2. These include an array of community services, the most important being the general practitioners with whom virtually all old persons (and young persons) are enrolled. GPs work closely with practice-attached community nurses and have ready access to home helps and other community support services for their patients. General hospitals serve the elderly population within defined catchment areas and commonly include dedicated geriatric units staffed by multidisciplinary teams representing geriatric medicine, nursing, social

Table 35.2 Some specific elements of comprehensive health services for the elderly in Great Britain

Community	*Institutional continuing care*
Enrollment in primary care practice • general practitioner • attached community nurses • home visiting by GPs and nurses Social service liaisons • home helps • meals-on-wheels • domiciliary occupational therapy	Geriatric assessment and rehabilitation prior to admission Medical surveillance: avoid frequent transfer to hospital Multidisciplinary maintenance of function Social and recreational services
General hospital	*Education*
Acute geriatric services • defined catchment population • geriatric medicine specialists • multidisciplinary teams • rehabilitation emphasis • home visiting • day hospital • respite admissions Liaison consultation with other hospital services • medicine • orthopedics • psychiatry	Academic departments of geriatric medicine Required curriculum in medical schools Formal post-graduate specialty training Post-graduate training for primary care practitioners

Source: Adapted from Barker, 1987

work, physical and occupational therapy. These units, most of which are independent hospital departments, or divisions within general medicine departments, generally receive referrals of older patients with multidimensional problems for whom they provide acute assessment and treatment, rehabilitation and restorative care and, as needed, long-term care. The day hospital, which has become a ubiquitous feature of geriatric services in Britain (Brocklehurst and Tucker, 1980) serves both for initial assessment and rehabilitation of referred patients, in lieu of hospital admission, and as a site for continuing rehabilitation following discharge from hospital. Liaison between geriatric units and other hospital specialties, particularly medicine, orthopedics and psychiatry, extends the skills and resources of geriatric medicine to older persons admitted to these services. Introduction of such liaison services has been shown to reduce lengths of stay and improve post-hospital disposition for older patients on general medicine and orthopedic services (Kennie et al. 1988). Institutional continuing care of patients with chronic disease and disability remains a responsibility of the geriatric unit, which assesses all patients referred for such care and oversees ongoing health maintenance and medical care for intercurrent illness.

The structural relationships of a hospital-based geriatric medicine unit are illustrated in Fig. 35.2. A recent monograph based on a series of surveys conducted throughout the country provides detailed descriptions of staffing and operation of contemporary British geriatric medicine units (Andrews and Brocklehurst, 1987). Organizational patterns for linking the key components of acute, rehabilitative and long-term care are flexible as demonstrated in Table 35.3 which summarizes findings from some 220 geriatric units surveyed.

The emergence and success of comprehensive geriatric services as part of the British National Health Service, reflects in large part the commitment of a cadre of medical leaders and their trainees, who now comprise the large and well respected body of consultants in geriatric medicine in Great Britain. This group, through its professional organization, the British Geriatrics Society (founded in the 1940s), has issued numerous advisory reports setting standards for education, training, organization and practice for the field of geriatrics within the National Health Service. The most recent of these, a model for peers in other countries to consult, is a 4-page memorandum on: 'Provision of Services by Departments of Geriatric Medicine', published in 1988 (British Geriatrics Society).

Table 35.3 Organizational patterns of major service components among 220 geriatric units in Great Britain

Pattern	Per cent
Combined acute and rehabilitation; separate long term care	38
Separate acute, rehabilitation, long term care	24
Combined acute, rehabilitation, long term care	21
Separate acute; combined rehabilitation and long term care	8
Rehabilitation and long term care only	2
Other	7

Source: Adapted from Andrews and Brocklehurst (1987)

United States

In the absence of an organizing principle such as the British National Health Service, a wide array of health care delivery and financing modalities have emerged to meet needs of older persons in the United States. Primary care is provided by internists and family practitioners as well as sub-

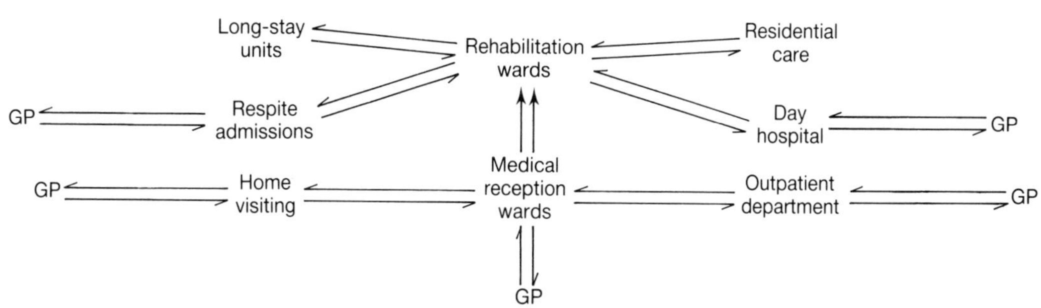

Fig. 35.2 Basic elements of a hospital-based geriatric medicine unit (Barker, 1987).

specialists, hospital clinics and emergency rooms. This care is financed by a variety of government and private health insurance mechanisms. Organized linkage with community nursing and social services is rare. Most such support services operate on a semi-autonomous referral basis and are limited to short term acute or subacute care. A variety of long-term care 'case management' experiments have explored approaches to maintaining frail elderly persons in the community, but such services have not been adopted as norms (Kane and Kane, 1987).

General hospital care for elderly Americans, financed by the Medicare program, is largely limited to short term acute medical and surgical care. As illustrated in Fig. 35.3, various models for incorporating special geriatrics assessment and rehabilitation services similar to those in Great Britain have been introduced as demonstrations in some American hospitals. Evaluative studies have documented the capacity of such services to reduce length of stay and cost, and improve patient outcome (Rubenstein et al., 1984; Barker et al., 1985). However, as 'demonstrations,' these modalities for dealing with multi-dimensional problems of hospitalized elderly persons have not been adopted as standard hospital services as has occurred in Great Britain and other countries. Such rehabilitation-oriented geriatric services are particularly vulnerable in the cost containment atmosphere current in the US in which prices for hospital care are set according to specific diagnoses (Diagnosis Related Groups – DRGs).

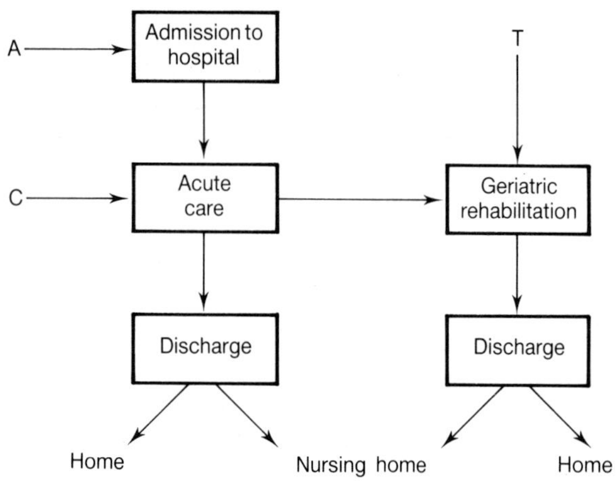

A = Admit to acute geriatric services.
C = Geriatric consultation on acute medical, surgical services.
T = Post-acute transfer to special geriatric rehabilitation unit.

Fig. 35.3 Potential intervention by special geriatric services in the course of acute hospital admission (Barker, 1987).

Nursing homes retain their traditional separate status from the mainstream of medical care, effectively excluded from coverage under Medicare and financed by either private savings or public welfare programs. Quality and continuity of medical care in nursing homes is highly variable and residents are frequently discharged to the costly acute hospital sector due to lack of onsite physician care (Barker, et al., 1987). An exception to this pattern, the 'teaching nursing home', a concept introduced in the 1980s, has resulted in affiliations between some nursing homes and academic medical centers with dramatic improvement in quality of medical care in some settings (Schneider, et al., 1987). The role of geriatric nurse practitioner in such demonstrations has been particularly impressive (Wieland, et al., 1986).

While various specific elements critical to successful geriatric services have been explored in the United States, as noted above, there is a clear lack of a system for integrating these elements into a continuum of care such as seen in Great Britain. Again there are exceptions. These include comprehensive geriatric health services provided in some parts of the country by the Veteran's Administration for its large aging cohorts of veterans of the First and Second World Wars (Wettle and Rowe, 1984) and the Social Health Maintenance Organization, a prepaid combination of acute and chronic care services available to Medicare beneficiaries in several demonstration sites (Leutz, et al., 1985).

The need for major national health policy reform to foster integrated acute and chronic care services has been addressed in a number of recent proposals from prominent sources, including the US Congress Special Committee on Aging, the Harvard University Medicare Reform Project, and the health policy subcommittees of the American College of Physicians and the American Geriatrics Society (Barker, 1987, ch. 10). In addition to organizational and financing aspects, all of these proposals address explicitly or implicitly, the evolving roles for physicians and other health professionals in providing a multidisciplinary continuum of health services for older persons.

5. Future concerns universally

As the practice of geriatric medicine and related health services, education and research evolve in countries around the world, several phenomena of global significance are emerging to challenge present and future leaders in the field. Among the most compelling of these are the epidemiological question of whether modern societies are experiencing 'compression of morbidity' late in life and the ethical question of whether the use of life-saving medical technology should be rationed late in life.

The compression of morbidity issue, first articulated by Fries in 1980 (Fries, 1980) asserts that the vigorous pursuit of healthful behaviors throughout adult life will (and has begun to) result in a fuller natural life span with less disabling chronic conditions in old age. This thesis has been challenged by epidemiologists and others who in the extreme assert the converse, that prolonged survival in modern society represents a 'failure of success', in which greater numbers of aging persons survive with physical and mental disabilities as a consequence of the use of life prolonging modern medical technology (Gruenberg, 1977). These two contrasting views of the present and future health status and by implication health service needs of modern aging societies clearly pose a challenging research agenda for geriatric medicine to be aware of and involved in. The best insight into this question will be provided by longitudinal studies such as one currently in progress involving consecutive cohorts of 70 year old persons in Goteborg, Sweden (Svanborg, 1983).

The rationing of life-sustaining medical technology in caring for frail elderly persons, while no doubt widely exercised on an informal or implicit basis by practitioners, administrators and policy-makers has begun to be addressed more explicitly. This concern is driven by confluence of the inexorable growth in costly technology on the one hand and a limit to the amount of resources which societies are willing or able to allocate to medical care on the other hand. In *Setting Limits*, a seminal book which explores these forces in depth, the American medical ethicist Daniel Callahan (1987) argues for the evolution of health policy which would restrict use of life saving medical technology on the basis of age. This view has been sharply questioned and rejected by critics who focus upon the arbitrary nature of such a policy. Others, cognizant that rationing of medical resources is inevitable and is in fact already widespread, take a broader view in which explicit limits on use of life-saving technology among the frail elderly is undertaken in the context of an overall policy that addresses what are appropriate levels and limits of health care for all segments of a society (Churchill, 1988). As participants in this pressing societal debate, geriatricians are particularly well situated and compelled to give close consideration to individual patients and their families with respect to their preferences for or against use of medical technology in life-threatening situations late in life. Such personal 'patient care planning' may in effect accomplish much of what is intended by those who are seeking a humane approach to rationing technology (Mott and Barker, 1988).

Suggested reading

Andrews, K. and Brocklehurst, J. (1987). *British Geriatric Medicine in the 1980s*. King Edward's Hospital Fund, London.

Barker, W. H. (1987). *Adding Life to Years. Organized Geriatric Services in Great Britain and Implications for the United States*. Johns Hopkins University Press, Baltimore.

Barker, W. H., Williams, T. F., Zimmer, J. G., VanBuren, C., Vincent, S. and Pickrel, S. G. (1985). Geriatric consultation teams in acute hospitals: Impact on back-up of elderly patients. *J. Amer. Ger. Soc.*, **33**: 422–28.

Barker, W. H., Zimmer, J. G., et al. (1987). Rates, predictors, causes and costs of hospitalization of nursing home residents. Proceedings of 1987 Public Health Conference on Records and Statistics: 'Data for an Aging Population'. DHHS Pub. No. (PHS) 88–1214. Washington, DC, pp. 171–6.

Brocklehurst, J. (1987). Personal communication. September.

British Geriatrics Society. (1988). Provision of Services by Departments of Geriatric Medicine. (Pamphlet).

Brocklehurst, J. C. and Tucker, J. S. (1980). *Progress in Geriatric Day Care*. King Edward's Hospital Fund, London.

Burley, L. E., Currie, C. T., Smith, R. G. and Williamson, J. (1979). Contribution from geriatric medicine within acute medical wards. *Brit. Med. J.*, **2**: 90–92.

Callahan, D. (1987). *Setting Limits. Medical Goals in an Aging Society*. Simon and Schuster, New York.

Campbell, J. A. (1987). Implications of policy

and management decision on access, quality and type of services for the elderly in New Zealand. *Int. J. Health Planning and Management.* **2**: 187–200.

Cape, R. T. and MacDonald, J. A. (1986). Integrated university training program in geriatric medicine accredited and evaluated by the Royal College of Physicians and Surgeons of Canada. *J. Amer. Ger. Soc.*, **34**: 787–8.

Churchill, L. R. (1988). Should we ration health care by age? *J. Amer. Ger. Soc.*, **36**: 614–17.

Dalgaard, P. Z. (1981). Care of the elderly in Denmark. Special aspects including geriatrics and long-term medicine. *Danish Med. Bull.*, **29**: 131–5.

Davies, M. A. (1985). Epidemiology and the challenge of aging. *Int. J. Epidemiol.*, **14**: 9–19.

Fries, J. F. (1980). Aging natural death and the compression of morbidity. *New Eng. J. Med.*, **303**: 130–35.

Gruenberg, E. M. (1977). The failures of success. *Milbank Memorial Fund Quarterly*, **55**: 3–24.

Grundy, E. (1983). Demography and old age. *J. Amer. Ger. Soc.*, **31**: 325–32.

Halot, B. and Margulec, I. (1987). Geriatrics-policy issues and models of care in Israel. *Israel J. Med. Sci.*, **21**: 203–04.

Kane, R. A. and Kane, R. L. (1987). Long-Term Care: Principles, Programs and Policies. Springer, New York.

Kennie, D. C., et al. (1988). Effectiveness of geriatric rehabilative care after fractures of the proximal femur; a randomized clinical trial. *Brit. Med. J.*, **297**: 1083–85.

Leutz, W. N., Greenberg, J. N., Abrahams, R., et al. (1985). *Changing Health Care for an Aging Society.* D.C. Health, Lexington, Mass.

Mott, P. D. and Barker, W. H. (1988). Hospital and medical care use by nursing home patients: the effect of patient care plans. *J. Amer. Ger. Soc.*, **36**: 47–53.

Nashcer, I. L. (1914). *Geriatrics: The Diseases of Old Age and Their Treatment.* Blakiston, Philadelphia.

Rubenstein, L. Z., Josephson, K. R., Wieland, G. D., et al. (1984). Effectiveness of a geriatric evaluation unit: a randomized clinical trial. *New Engl. J. Med.*, 311, 1664–70.

Schneider, E. L., Ory, M. and Aung, M. L. (1987). Teaching nursing homes revisited: survey of affiliations between American medical schools and long-term care facilities. *J. Amer. Med. Assoc.*, **257**: 2771–5.

Svanborg, A. (1983). The Gothenbug longitudinal study – health and well-being: a critical review of methods and interpretation of research data. In: Ageing. *Living conditions and quality of life.* International Seminar in Oslo, 18–19 October, 1982 sid. 56–63. Norsk Gerontologisk Institutt.

Warren, M. (1946). Care of the chronic aged sick. *Lancet* **1**: 841–43.

Wettle, T. and Rowe, J. W. (1984). *Older Veterans: Linking VA and Community Resources.* Harvard University Press, Cambridge, Mass.

WHO (1974). Planning and Organization of Geriatric Services. World Health Organization Technical Report Series No. 548. World Health Organization, Geneva.

Wieland, D., Rubenstein, L. Z., Ouslander, T. B. and Martin, S. E. (1986). Organizing an academic nursing home: Impacts on institutionalized elderly. *J. Amer. Med. Assoc.* **255**: 2622–7.

Guidelines for fellowship training programs in geriatric medicine. 1987 *J. Amer. Ger. Soc.*, **35**: 792–5.

Index